ULTIMATE GUIDE TO
HIIT
HIGH-INTENSITY INTERVAL TRAINING

GENERAL DISCLAIMER
The contents of this book are intended to provide useful information to the general public. All materials, including text and images, are for informational purposes only and are not a substitute for medical diagnosis, advice, or treatment for specific medical conditions. All readers should seek expert medical care and consult their own physicians before commencing any regimen for any general or specific health issues. The author and publishers do not recommend or endorse specific treatments, procedures, advice, or other information found in this book and specifically disclaim all responsibility for any and all liability, loss, or risk, personal or otherwise, which is incurred as a consequence, directly or indirectly, of the use or application of any of the material in this publication.

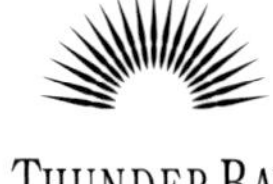

THUNDER BAY
P·R·E·S·S

Thunder Bay Press
An imprint of Printers Row Publishing Group
10350 Barnes Canyon Road, Suite 100, San Diego, CA 92121
www.thunderbaybooks.com • mail@thunderbaybooks.com

All notations of errors or omissions should be addressed to Thunder Bay Press, Editorial Department, at the above address. Author and illustration inquiries should be addressed to Moseley Road Inc., smoore@moseleyroad.com.

Thunder Bay Press
Publisher: Peter Norton
Associate Publisher: Ana Parker
Senior Development Editor: April Graham Farr
Editor: Stephanie Romero Gamboa
Senior Product Manager: Kathryn C. Dalby
Production Team: Jonathan Lopes, Rusty von Dyl

Produced by Moseley Road Inc., www.moseleyroad.com
President: Sean Moore
Art Director: Lisa Purcell
Production Director: Adam Moore
Editor: Finn Moore
Photography: Naila Ruechel. www.nailaruechel.com

Library of Congress Control Number: 2019943783
ISBN: 978-1-64517-044-0

Printed in China

23 22 21 20 19 1 2 3 4 5

ULTIMATE GUIDE TO HIIT

HIGH-INTENSITY INTERVAL TRAINING

WITH DETAILED INSTRUCTIONS AND ANATOMICAL ILLUSTRATIONS FOR 170 HIIT EXERCISES

Alex Geissbuhler

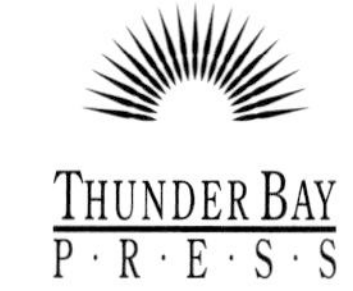

THUNDER BAY
P·R·E·S·S

San Diego, California

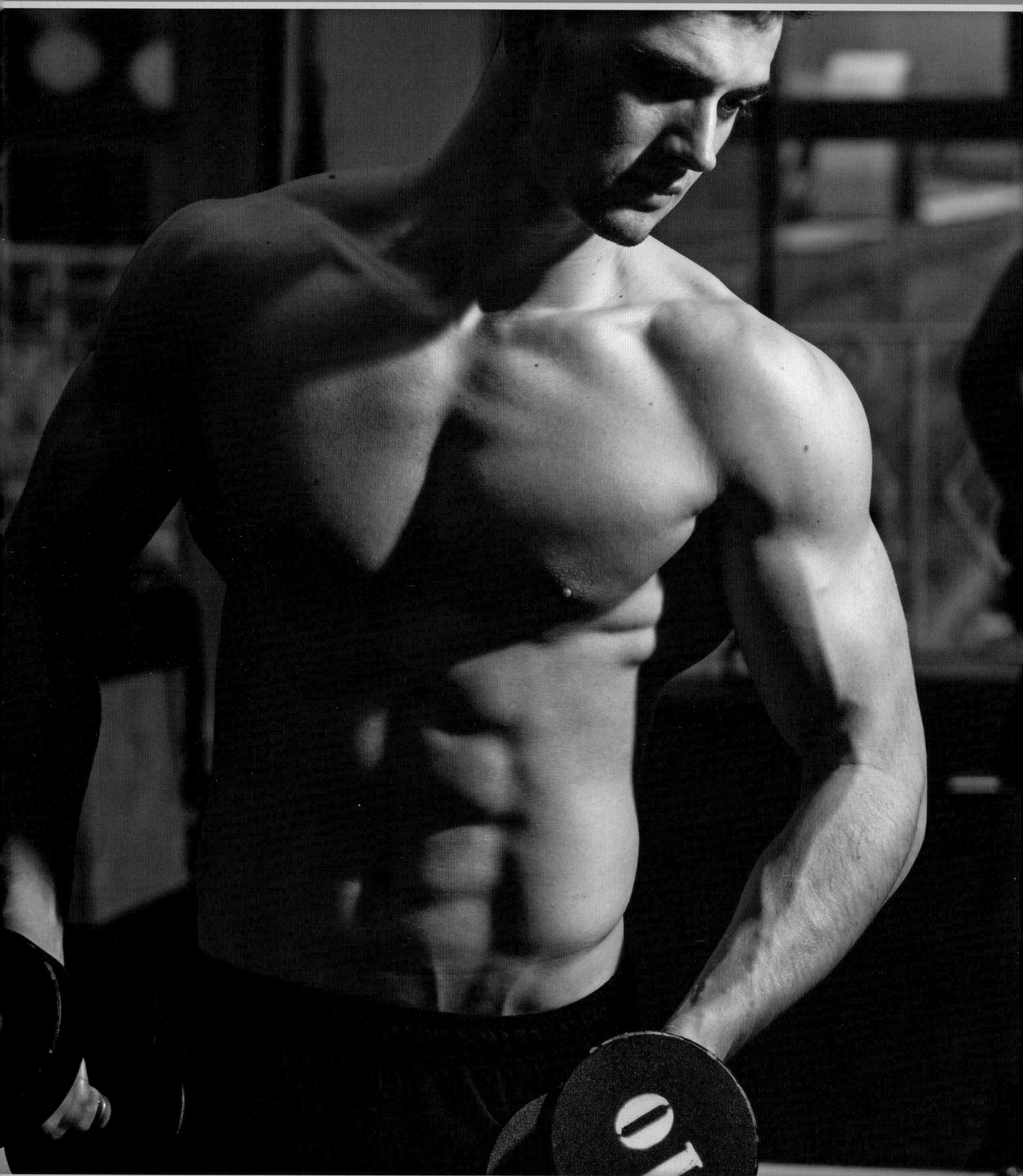
10

CONTENTS

What Is HIIT?

If someone were to tell you that there is a fitness program that can do incredible things for your health in half the time of most fitness regimens, you might respond with a disbelieving eye roll. But they would be right. According to numerous studies, high-intensity interval training (HIIT) does just that.

GET RESULTS FAST

HIIT efficiently builds muscle and ups your endurance levels. Not only do you burn more calories during a HIIT workout in half the time of most other fitness regimens, but the effect of all that intense exertion also kicks your body's metabolic cycle into hyperdrive. That means you burn more calories and more fat in the 24 hours after a HIIT workout than you do after a steady-pace workout.

HIIT defines an exercise program that alternates between intense bursts of maximum-effort activity interspersed with fixed periods of active or complete rest. This pattern of alternating between maximum-effort activity and rest is exactly what provides the numerous benefits that HIIT can bestow. The high-intensity exercise aspect involves an "all out" approach in which you push your body to maximal exertion levels, thus requiring a high demand of energy and calorie expenditure. Yet your body can sustain high-intensity activity for only a brief duration because all that activity depletes your energy stores. In other words, you get tired. What follows is a period of either active rest, which can consist of a relatively low-demand exercise, or complete rest.

The goal of the interval aspect of this type of program is to restore the energy required to perform more work through recovery intervals. The recovery interval replenishes you so that your body can give its all during the active phase. You will burn more calories, place your muscles under tension for longer, and perform a greater volume of work in a relatively short period of time.

HOW AND WHY IT WORKS

Exercise requires energy, otherwise known as adenosine triphosphate (ATP). The body will try to obtain this energy from whatever source it can obtain it from. There are three different energy-breakdown processes in which your body produces this ATP. The first two (the phosphocreatine cycle and the glycolytic cycle) are anaerobic, meaning that

---

Resources:

Foster C, Farland CV, Guidotti F, et al. "The Effects of High Intensity Interval Training vs Steady State Training on Aerobic and Anaerobic Capacity." *Journal of Sports Science & Medicine* 14, no. 4 (2015): 747–755.

Ouerghi N, Khammassi M, Boukorraa S, et al. "Effects of a High-Intensity Intermittent Training Program on Aerobic Capacity and Lipid Profile in Trained Subjects." *Open Access Journal of Sports Medicine* 5 (2014): 243–248.

Hussain SR, Macaluso AJ, Pearson S. "High-Intensity Interval Training Versus Moderate-Intensity Continuous Training in the Prevention/Management of Cardiovascular Disease." *Cardiology in Review* 24, no. 6 (2016): 273–281.

LaForgia J, Withers RT, Gore CJ. "Effects of Exercise Intensity and Duration on the Excess Post-Exercise Oxygen Consumption." *Journal of Sport Sciences* 24 no. 12 (2006): 1247–1264.

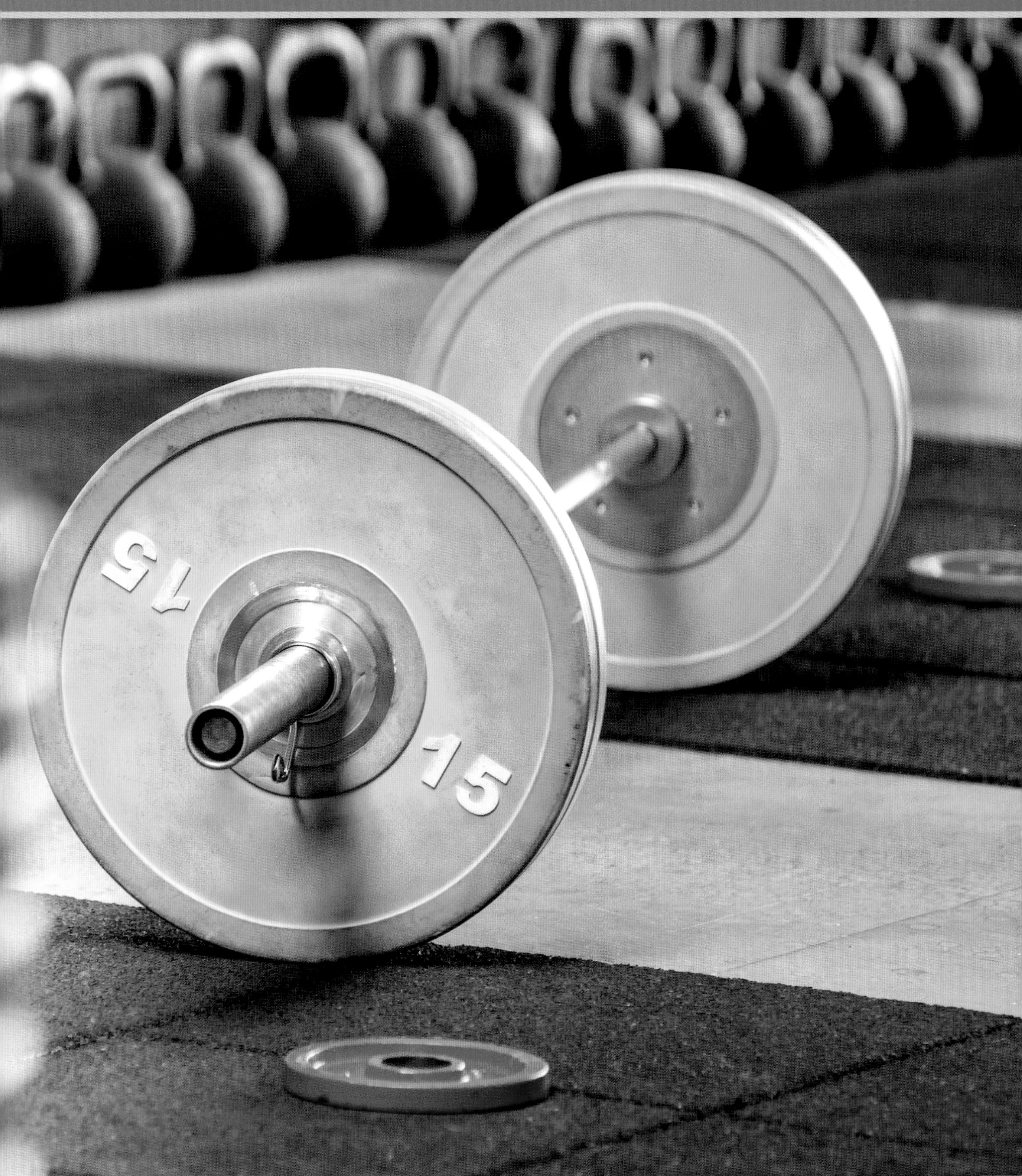
15
15

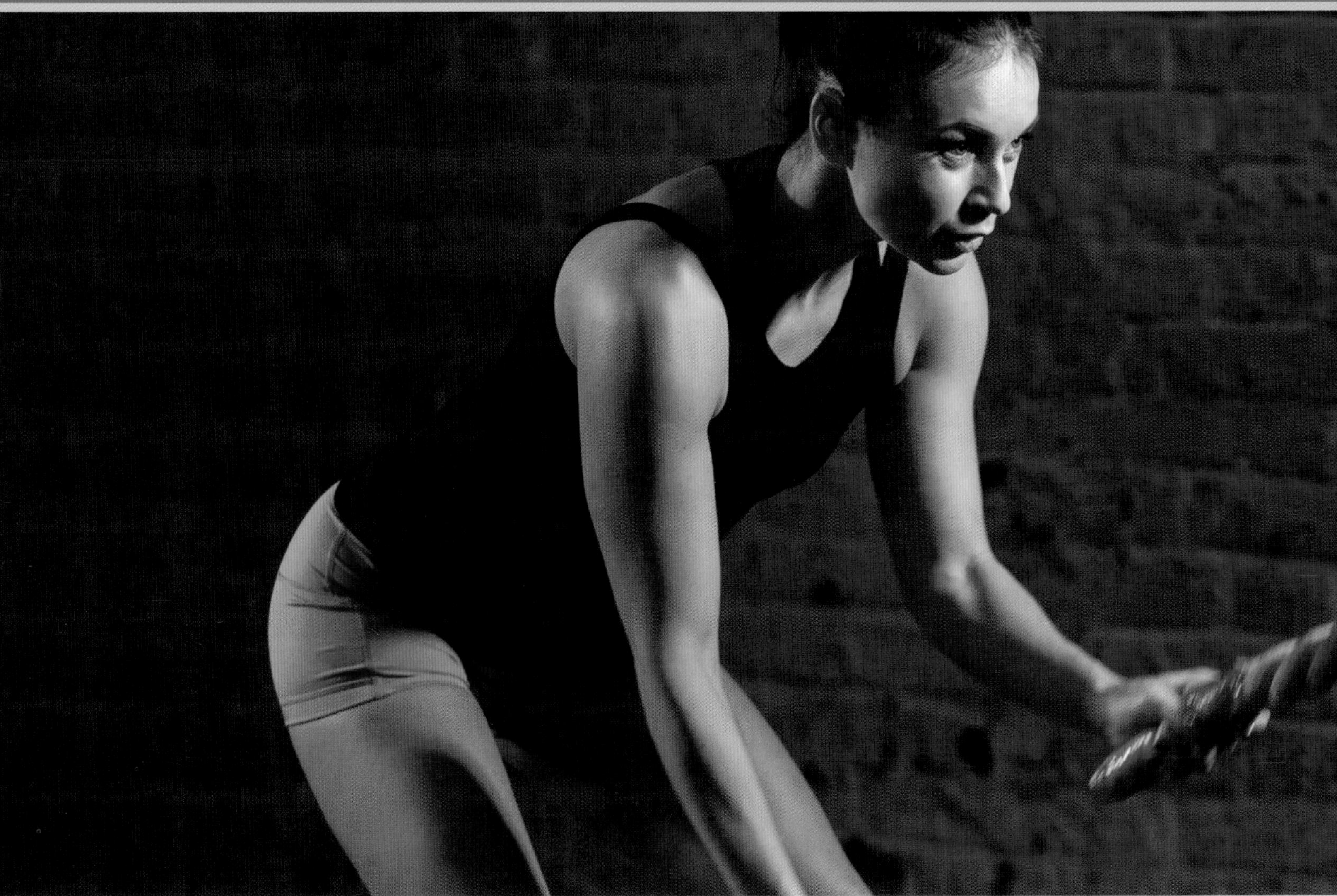

the process does not require oxygen for this energy production. It is these two energy systems that are typically used when one thinks of strength training.

Although effective in producing energy, these two systems do not last very long. Together, they last a period of about two minutes or so before the cycles have run their course and their energy is depleted. This is where the third process, the oxidative cycle—or the aerobic pathway—picks up. The aerobic system creates ATP through the breakdown of protein, carbohydrates, and fats. This is what we typically use when we think of steady-state, less-demanding, and longer-duration exercise, such as running. This aerobic cycle helps to replenish the first two energy systems. The aerobic system assists in clearing the lactate produced by the previous system and rebuilds the ATP that the anaerobic system can use again.

High-intensity workouts require a great energy demand from the anaerobic pathways and generate a greater post-exercise energy expenditure. This physiological effect is called excess post-exercise oxygen consumption (EPOC). Also known as oxygen debt, EPOC is the amount of oxygen needed to achieve homeostasis and restore your body to its resting

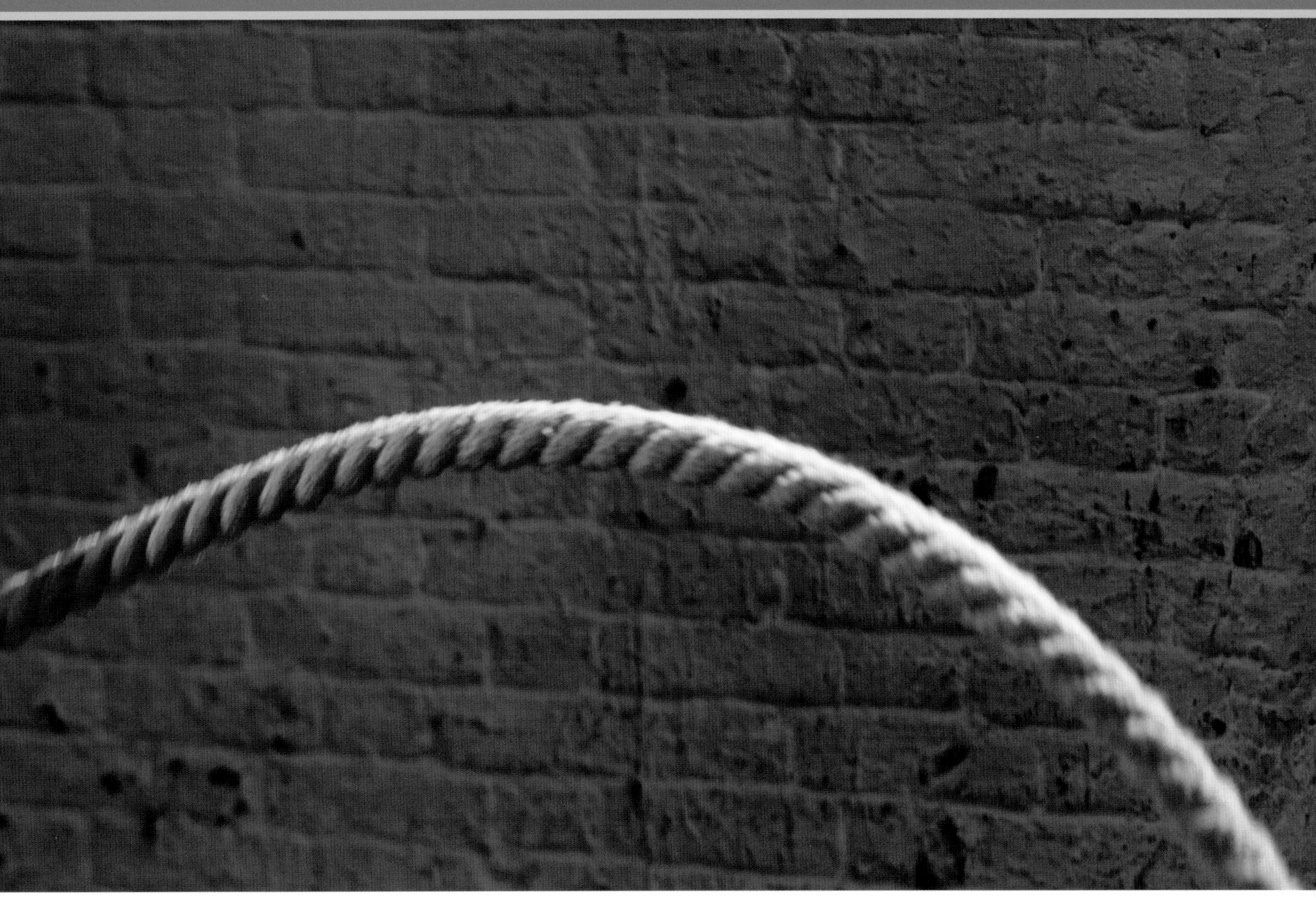

metabolic level. This demand continues to burn calories long after the stressor on your body has ceased. Studies have shown that HIIT programming is superior to steady-state exercise programs in producing workload in a shorter period of time and creating EPOC, and therefore burning more calories.

WHAT DOES ALL THIS MEAN?

This means that not only is it possible to build muscle and burn a tremendous amount of calories during your workout, but you will also reap benefits when you are done. After you have finished a HIIT workout, your body's metabolism is in a heightened state, and it will continue to burn even more calories for the 24-hour period afterward. This is why HIIT works.

The beauty of HIIT is that it requires the use of all of your energy-producing systems. Placing a high energy demand on your anaerobic system is great for conditioning and building muscular strength and cardiopulmonary health; the lower demand of the rest intervals requires your body to switch into the aerobic pathway, which is fantastic for endurance, burning calories from fat, and keeping your body active.

Who Is HIIT For?

HIIT is for anyone seeking a program that provides an effective and efficient way to decrease body fat, increase lean muscle mass, build strength, enhance endurance, and improve overall health.

The fast-growing popularity of this fitness regimen is well deserved. There are numerous benefits to adopting a HIIT program, including the following.

LOSE FAT

HIIT has been proven to be superior for weight loss when compared to steady-state aerobic exercise. The weight loss that comes from HIIT is not just your typical, overall weight reduction. This type of training substantially reduces subcutaneous body fat (the fat that sits under the skin) as opposed to visceral fat, which surrounds the organs. Although the traditional strategy of running on the treadmill for hours on end will technically burn calories from the infamous "fat-burning zone" for the duration of the workout, a HIIT program significantly increases the total caloric burn and fat breakdown.

BUILD MUSCLE

Time under tension is the basic methodology for all muscle building, whether it be pure strength, muscle hypertrophy, or muscular endurance. HIIT uses this methodology to its advantage, with muscular fatigue a certainty. There is also evidence to suggest that there is an increase in the body's human growth hormone production response during a HIIT workout, leading to a natural increase in muscle production.

INCREASE CARDIOVASCULAR ENDURANCE

Research indicates that beneficial adaptations for cardiovascular improvements are intensity dependent. In this way, a program of high-intensity exercise is more beneficial than traditional training. HIIT training has displayed evidence of greater improvements in VO_2 max (the way your body utilizes oxygen), endothelial function, blood pressure regulation, cardiac muscle contractility, and insulin signaling, among others, when compared with moderate-intensity exercise. These studies show indications for HIIT as not only a preventative strategy but also a tool for reversing the pathological processes of cardiac disease.

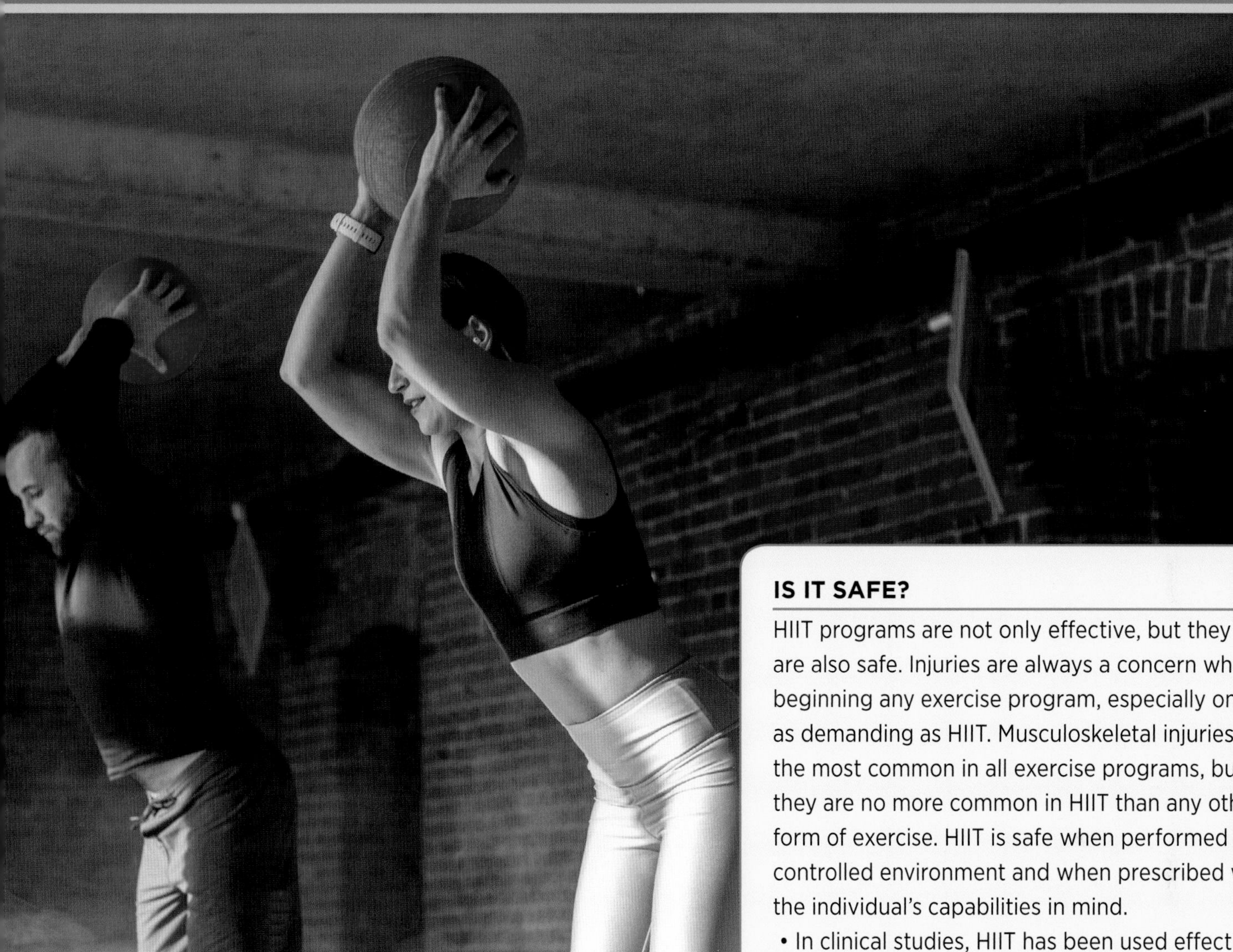

IS IT SAFE?

HIIT programs are not only effective, but they are also safe. Injuries are always a concern when beginning any exercise program, especially one as demanding as HIIT. Musculoskeletal injuries are the most common in all exercise programs, but they are no more common in HIIT than any other form of exercise. HIIT is safe when performed in a controlled environment and when prescribed with the individual's capabilities in mind.

- In clinical studies, HIIT has been used effectively in patients with diabetes, stable angina, heart failure and after myocardial infarction, post-cardiac stenting, and coronary artery grafting. Several studies have shown the benefits of HIIT training for those who are living with chronic coronary arterial disease, heart transplant, and decreased pulmonary function.
- Certain types of exercise are inadvisable for certain patient populations, and because HIIT is such a high-demanding program, some patients who are unfamiliar to exercise may require specific assessment or instruction in HIIT from a physiotherapist or exercise specialist.
- Consult your physician before starting any and all new exercise regimens, such as HIIT.

CONTROL HEALTH

There are numerous other health benefits of a HIIT program. Research has shown that maintaining a regular HIIT regimen can help manage certain conditions, such as diabetes, with evidence of increased insulin sensitivity and glucose regulation, and high blood pressure or heart disease, with research showing a decrease in LDL cholesterol. It might also boost your overall mood. It has even been found to improve emotional states with a release of "happy" hormones, such as endorphins.

How to Do It

Interval periodization is the most important aspect when designing a HIIT program. Understanding this concept will allow you to get the most from your efforts. It will give you the knowledge you'll need to create your own personalized routines geared to your specific goals.

HIIT is defined by work output, as well as work/rest interval duration. That is to say that this type of program is looking for a maximal effort for as long as one can sustain. Through this you will see the progressive benefits of muscular strength and endurance.

WORK AND REST

You can use a variety of work/rest in a HIIT program. A work/rest ratio is the duration of your exercise compared to the duration of your rest. For example, when you perform 60 seconds of work followed by 60 seconds of recovery, your HIIT ratio is 1:1. When you perform 15 seconds of work followed by 45 seconds of recovery, your HIIT ratio is 1:3. For those just starting out, a 1:4 ratio is best, with the rest interval being four times as long as the exercise interval (for example, you exercise at a high interval of 30 seconds, and then rest for 2 minutes). You can adjust the work/rest ratio as your physical fitness improves. For the more experienced exerciser, a 1:2 work/rest ratio produces favorable responses that enhance both aerobic and anaerobic energy system development. Remember work/rest ratios can be varied throughout a single workout and should be based on your fitness level.

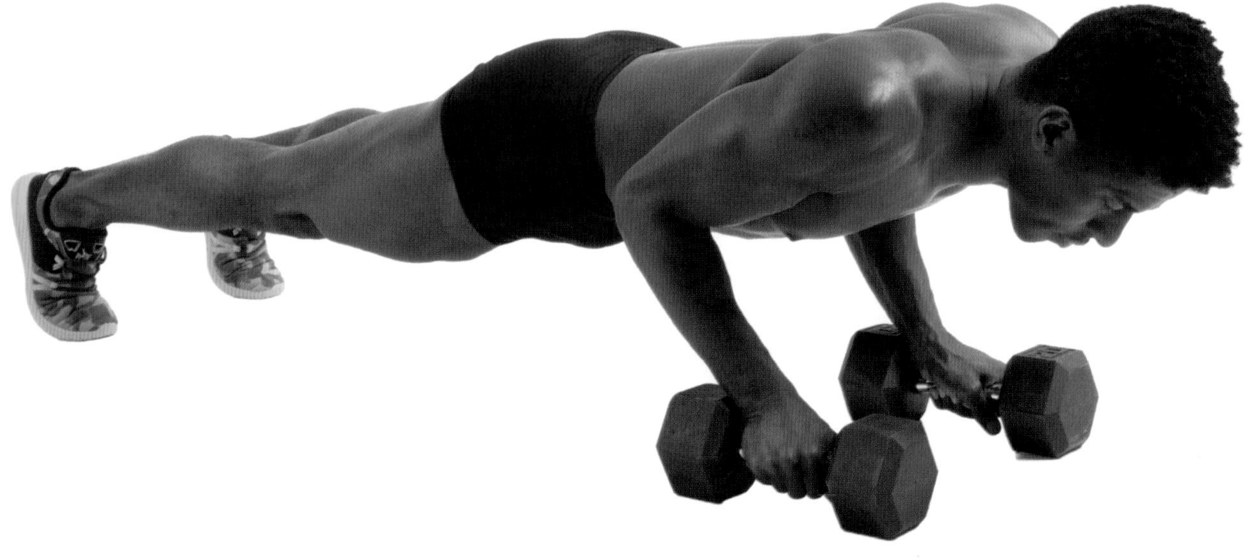

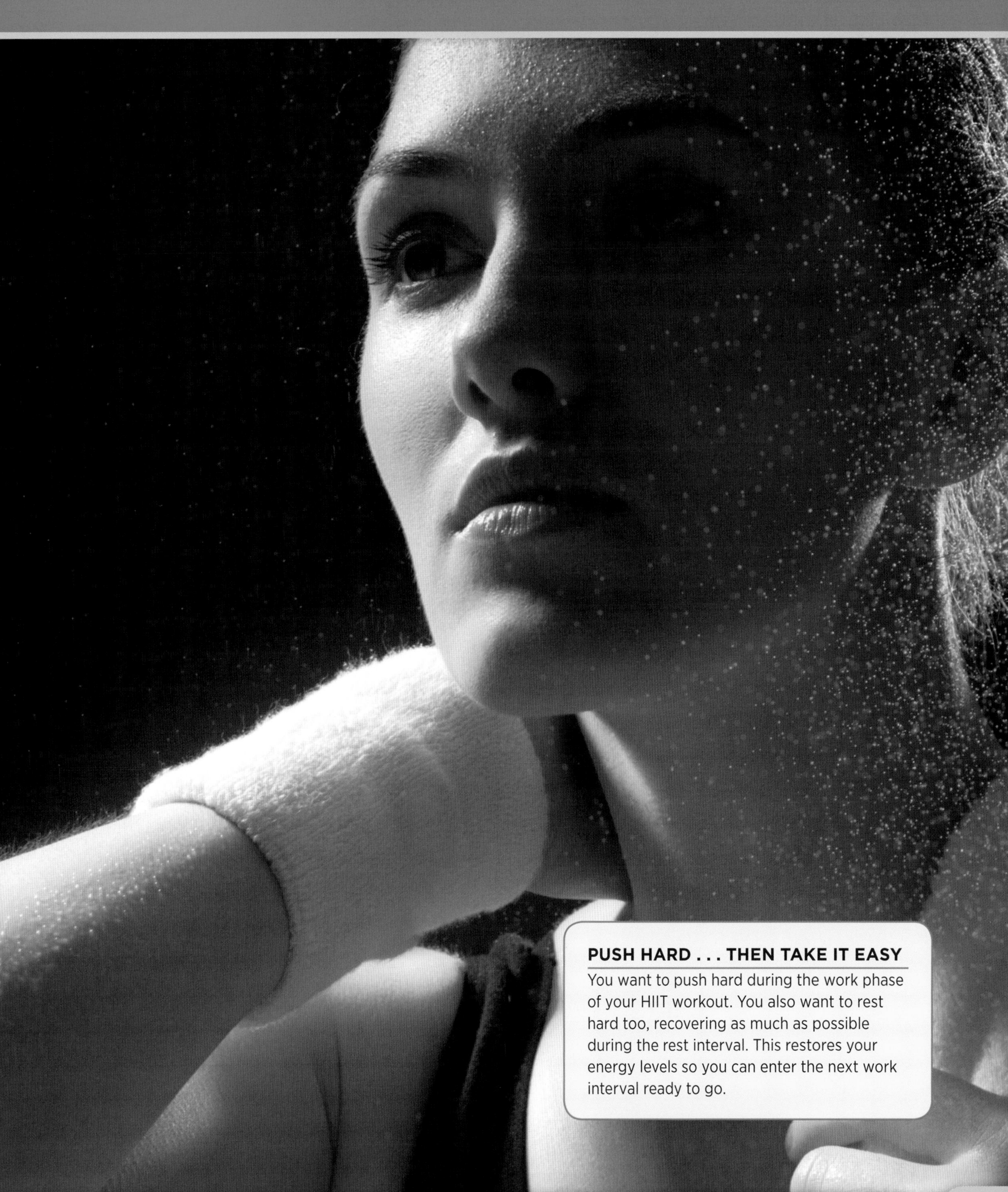

PUSH HARD . . . THEN TAKE IT EASY

You want to push hard during the work phase of your HIIT workout. You also want to rest hard too, recovering as much as possible during the rest interval. This restores your energy levels so you can enter the next work interval ready to go.

TAKING IT TO THE NEXT LEVEL

Progressions can be through equipment adjustment, exercise selections, or work/rest interval modifications. If you are a novice to an interval training program, a complete rest would be appropriate, allowing you adequate recovery before the next bout of exercise. If you become acclimated to a more intense HIIT routine, you can progress from complete rest intervals to active-rest intervals. In an active-rest interval you will perform exercises at a much lower intensity. In this way, your body can recover while still remaining active. At the end of this book, suggested routines with paired interval ratios are offered for the novice, intermediate, and experienced athlete.

HOW TO BUILD A HIIT ROUTINE

For HIIT routines, there are no specific number of repetitions or sets to accomplish. Instead, you'll use time as the foundation to build your program. Begin with the total amount of time you will give to a circuit. This can span any duration from 10 minutes to an hour.

Then, depending on your fitness level, separate that total time into the work/rest ratio that is appropriate for your fitness level. Take into consideration the complexity of the movements you are performing. For example, compound, complicated exercises may require more time to complete repetitions than relatively simple, quick movements. Resistance can also have an effect, with increased demand also requiring increased work time, as well as rest. You can adjust the resistance or complexity of movements, as well as the work interval, to craft a workout for a desired result. If your desired outcome is power, for example, a repetition range to strive for is 1 to 3 repetitions to be completed within one work interval. With this example, you would choose an appropriate weight that is challenging enough so that you can perform it only 1 to 3 times within the work interval. You can lower the weight if your goal is either hypertrophy or endurance.

On the opposite page are sample charts to help you understand how to create your own HIIT workouts. Chart A, at right, displays the appropriate repetition range for the desired fitness outcome. Chart B displays an example of a beginner routine for building muscle.

CHART A—FITNESS OBJECTIVES

OBJECTIVE	DEFINITION	REPETITION RANGE	PERCENTAGE OF MAXIMAL EFFORT
Power	Power is the ability to move weight with speed. This is using maximal strength with explosiveness.	1–3	85%–100%
Strength	Muscular strength is the ability of a muscle or muscle group to exert maximal force against resistance.	4–6	75%–85%
Hypertrophy	Muscle hypertrophy describes the process of muscle building, or the actual increase in size of skeletal muscle through a growth in the size of its component cells.	8–12	60%–75%
Endurance	Muscular endurance is the ability of a muscle to exert submaximal force against resistance for an extended period of time.	15+	< 60%

CHART B—HYPERTROPHY ROUTINE

FITNESS LEVEL: BEGINNER (5 exercises)	**WORK/REST INTERVAL (1:3)**	**TOTAL EXERCISE DURATION**	**SETS** (total rotations of circuit completed)	**REPS FOR GOAL: HYPERTROPHY**
Body-Weight Routine II 1. Squat 2. Triceps Push-Up 3. Arm Hauler 4. Bench Dip 5. Bent-Knee Sit-Up	20 seconds of work: 1 minute of rest	40 minutes	6	8–12 repetitions performed during work interval

What You'll Need

You can perform a HIIT workout just about anywhere, using just your own body weight. To get even more out of your hard work, adding a few fitness tools can amplify the benefits and add a bit of variety to your routine.

EQUIPMENT

When engaging in HIIT, you should avoid equipment such as the stationary, single-modality machines often found in commercial gyms, which are not an efficient use of your time when working through an interval program. In this book, you will find suggestions for exercises using equipment such as dumbbells, barbells, medicine balls, kettlebells, and more. These tools, which you can easily pick up and put down, add value without eating into your workout time. If you don't have access to any of this equipment, don't worry. There is a large section strictly for body-weight HIIT exercises to hit every major muscle group. Remember your most valuable piece of fitness equipment: your own body. Some of the most effective exercises in this book are done with nothing but you.

Dumbbell To add resistance to an exercise and increase its benefits, pick up a dumbbell. Start with very light weights, and then work your way up to heavier ones. You will see several varieties, including hexagonal and the iconic round shape. The hexagonal variety allows you to balance on them if an exercise calls for it. If you decide to invest in a set of dumbbells, check out adjustable models that allow you to easily vary the weight levels. If you don't have access to a pair of dumbbells, substitute unopened food cans or water bottles.

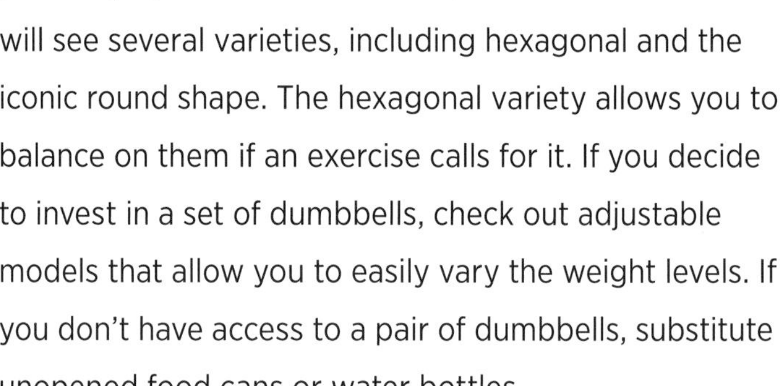

Kettlebell The kettlebell, a cast-iron or cast-steel ball with a handle at the top, is used to perform many types of exercises that combine cardiovascular, strength, and flexibility training.

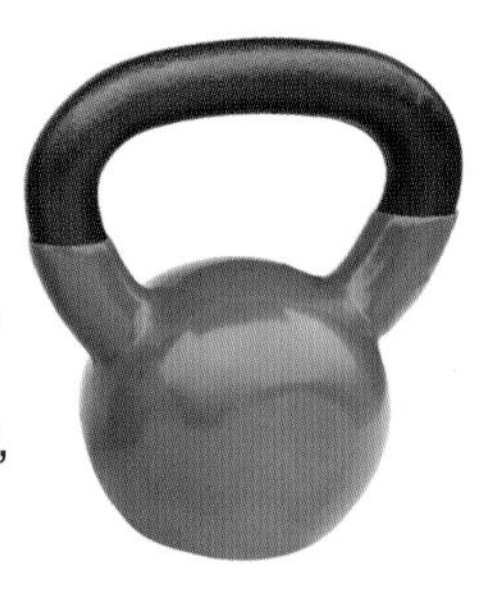

Barbell A barbell is a long bar, usually with weights attached at each end, used in weight training, bodybuilding, and powerlifting. If you are new to working with this kind of weight, practice exercises using just the bar. As you build strength, start adding the weight plates. The weight plates themselves are also handy tools for adding resistance to an exercise.

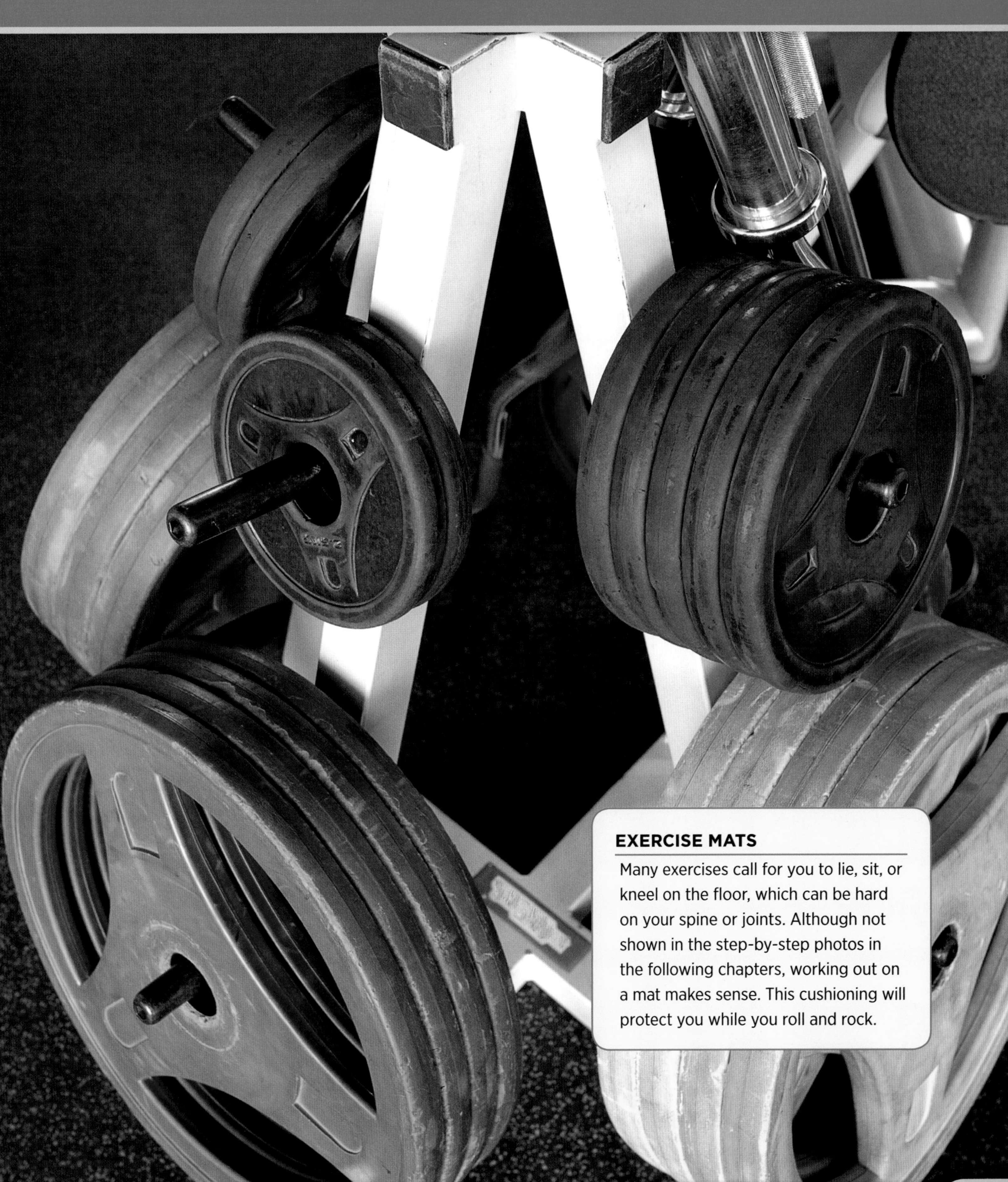

EXERCISE MATS

Many exercises call for you to lie, sit, or kneel on the floor, which can be hard on your spine or joints. Although not shown in the step-by-step photos in the following chapters, working out on a mat makes sense. This cushioning will protect you while you roll and rock.

Swiss ball Also known as an exercise ball, fitness ball, body ball, or balance ball, this heavy-duty inflatable ball comes in a variety of sizes. A Swiss ball really works your core, and because it is unstable, you must constantly adjust your balance while performing a movement, which helps you improve your overall sense of balance and your flexibility. To find the best size for your height and weight, sit on the ball. Your thighs should be parallel to or slightly above parallel to the floor.

Medicine balls Use these weighted balls to improve strength and neuromuscular coordination. Sizes vary from baseball to beach-ball size. You can use them for any exercise that calls for a hand weight.

Aerobics step This is a 4-inch to 12-inch raised platform used to step up, around, and down from the platform. Step exercises boost your heart rate and breathing, and strengthen your muscles. If you don't have one, use any stable raised surface, such as a box, a stair, or a low table.

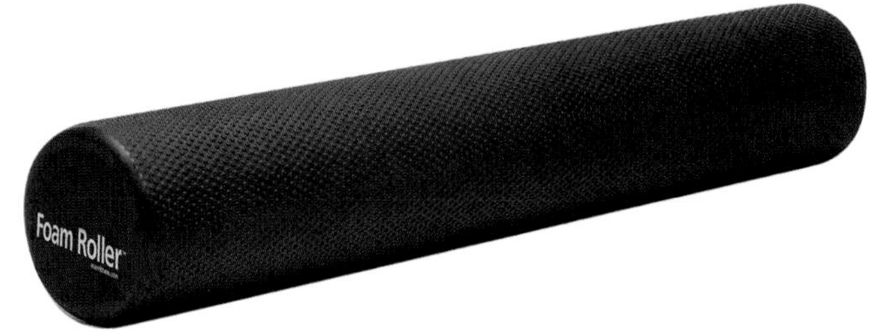

Foam roller Like a Swiss ball, the foam roller adds an element of instability to an exercise, which can help you hone your balance, improve your strength, and increase cardio endurance. To boost the challenge to the targeted muscles of a basic exercise, such as the push-up, perform it on the unstable surface of a roller. A foam roller, which is simply a dense foam cylinder (either smooth or knobbly), is relatively inexpensive and highly portable. If you do not have access to a foam roller, substitute a swimming noodle.

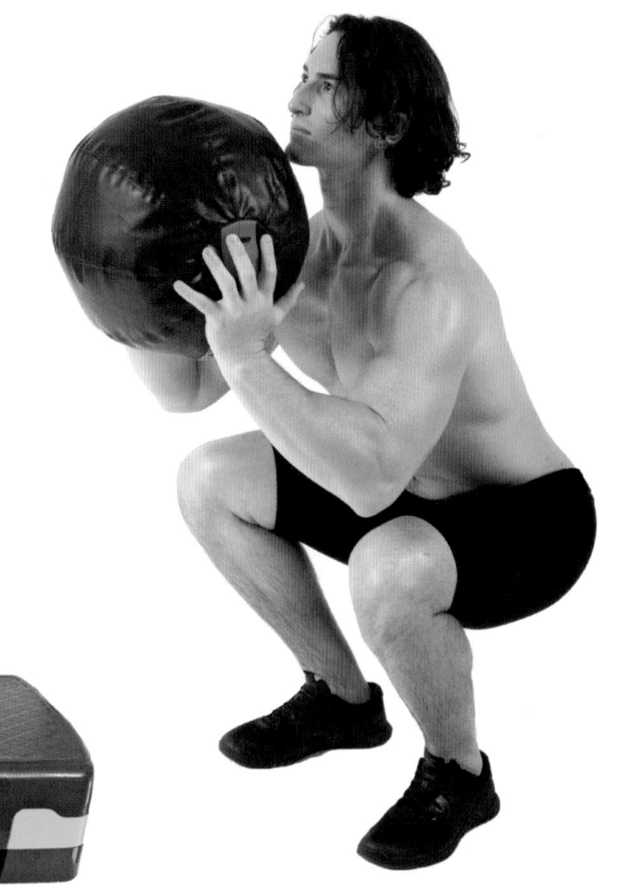

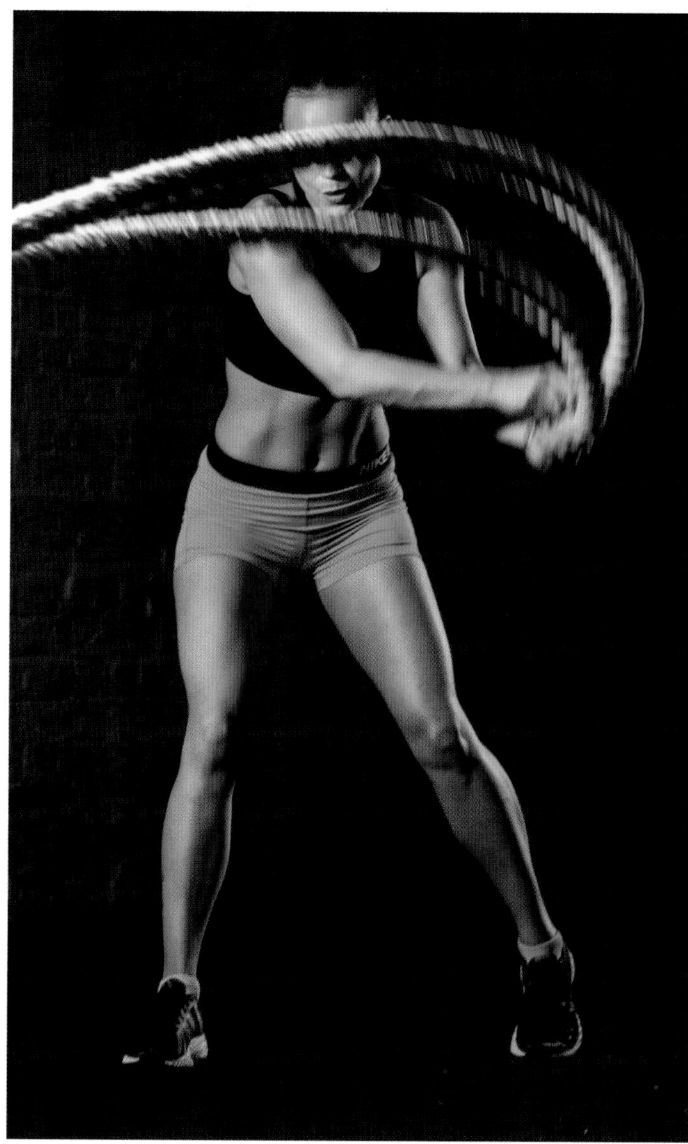

Battle ropes Standard equipment at military boot camps and on football training fields, battle ropes have hit the gym. Anchored to a wall or beam and used in pairs, they provide intense cardio workouts and help build total-body strength.

Pull-up bar Most gyms—and many urban playgrounds—feature a pull-up station. A pull-up bar is part of most multipurpose home gym machines. You can also

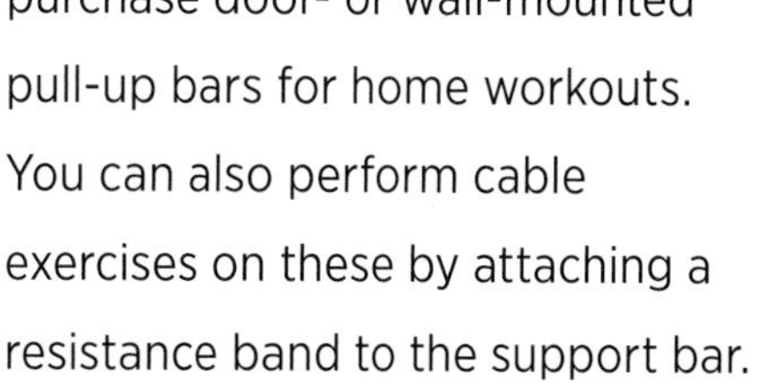

purchase door- or wall-mounted pull-up bars for home workouts. You can also perform cable exercises on these by attaching a resistance band to the support bar.

LOCATION

HIIT can be done virtually anywhere, with nearly any type

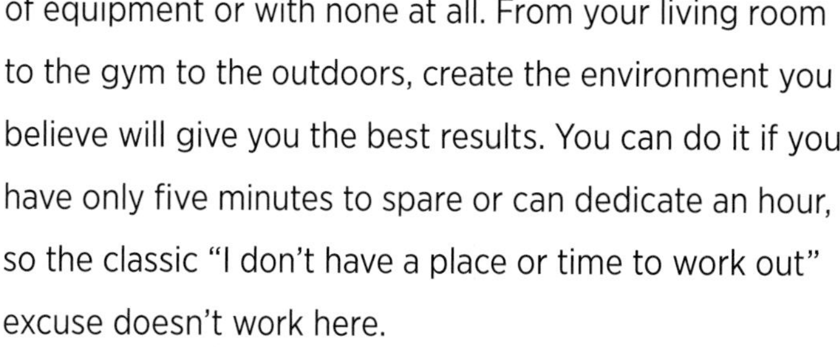

of equipment or with none at all. From your living room to the gym to the outdoors, create the environment you believe will give you the best results. You can do it if you have only five minutes to spare or can dedicate an hour, so the classic "I don't have a place or time to work out" excuse doesn't work here.

This book will provide you with the exercises and knowledge to safely start your HIIT journey, or, if you already have, to take it to the next level. There are endless combinations of exercises to build the right workout for you. You'll find some great, challenging workouts compiled for you at the end of this book, but don't be afraid to make up your own based on your capabilities and comfort level. You can make any HIIT workout as challenging as physically possible for you by pushing yourself during the interval—remember, you'll get a breather soon enough. Keep proper form with your exercises, push yourself, and, most of all, have fun!

How to Use This Book

Ultimate Guide to HIIT features step-by-step instructions to 170 exercises specially selected to fit into a high-intensity interval training regimen.

For each pose, you'll find a short overview of the position, photos with step-by-step instructions, tips on proper form, and anatomical illustrations that highlight the targeted muscles. A quick-read panel features key points. There may be pose variations shown in a Modification box.

CHAPTER BREAKDOWNS

Chapter One: Warm-Ups & Cooldowns Here you will find a selection of exercises that you can perform before or after your full HIIT routine.

Chapter Two: Body-Weight Exercises Featuring exercises that rely on your own body weight for resistance, you can take this chapter anywhere.

Chapter Three: Separable Free-Weight Exercises Get out your dumbbells and kettlebells for this chapter. This challenging group uses free weights for resistance.

Chapter Four: Exercise Equipment This chapter offers a selection of exercises that use a variety of fitness equipment. From gym classics, such as barbells and battle ropes, to at-home favorites, such as Swiss balls and aerobic steps, you will find effective tools to help you build a better body.

Chapter Five: Workout Routines Once you've familiarized yourself with the featured exercises, turn to this chapter to learn how to put them together in targeted HIIT routines.

KEY

EXERCISE SPREADS

1. **Category**
   Gives the overall body areas targeted: your back, arms, chest, core, legs, or total body.
2. **Exercise Info**
   Gives the name of the exercise and some key details you need to know about it.
3. **How to Do It**
   Step-by-step instructions detailing how to perform the exercise.
4. **Close-up**
   Highlights an important element of the exercise.
5. **Step-by-Step Photos**
   Images of the key steps to the exercise.
6. **Do It Right**
   Tips to help you perfect your form.
7. **Fact File**
   A quick list of key facts: the exercise's main targets, equipment needed to perform it, its principal benefits, and any cautions that may apply.
8. **Anatomical Illustration**
   Highlights the key working muscles. May also include an inset showing muscles not illustrated in the main image.
9. **Modification**
   Shows you how to do variations that may be easier, harder, or of similar difficulty.

WORKOUT SPREADS

1. **Routine Info**
   Gives the name of the routine and some key details you need to know about it.
2. **Exercise Info**
   Listed in the order you perform each exercise; shows the name, page number to find it, and how many repetitions to perform.
3. **Photo Icon**
   A quick view of exercise.
4. **Fact File**
   A quick list of key facts about the routine: its level of difficulty, its objective, the work/rest ratio, and how long it takes.

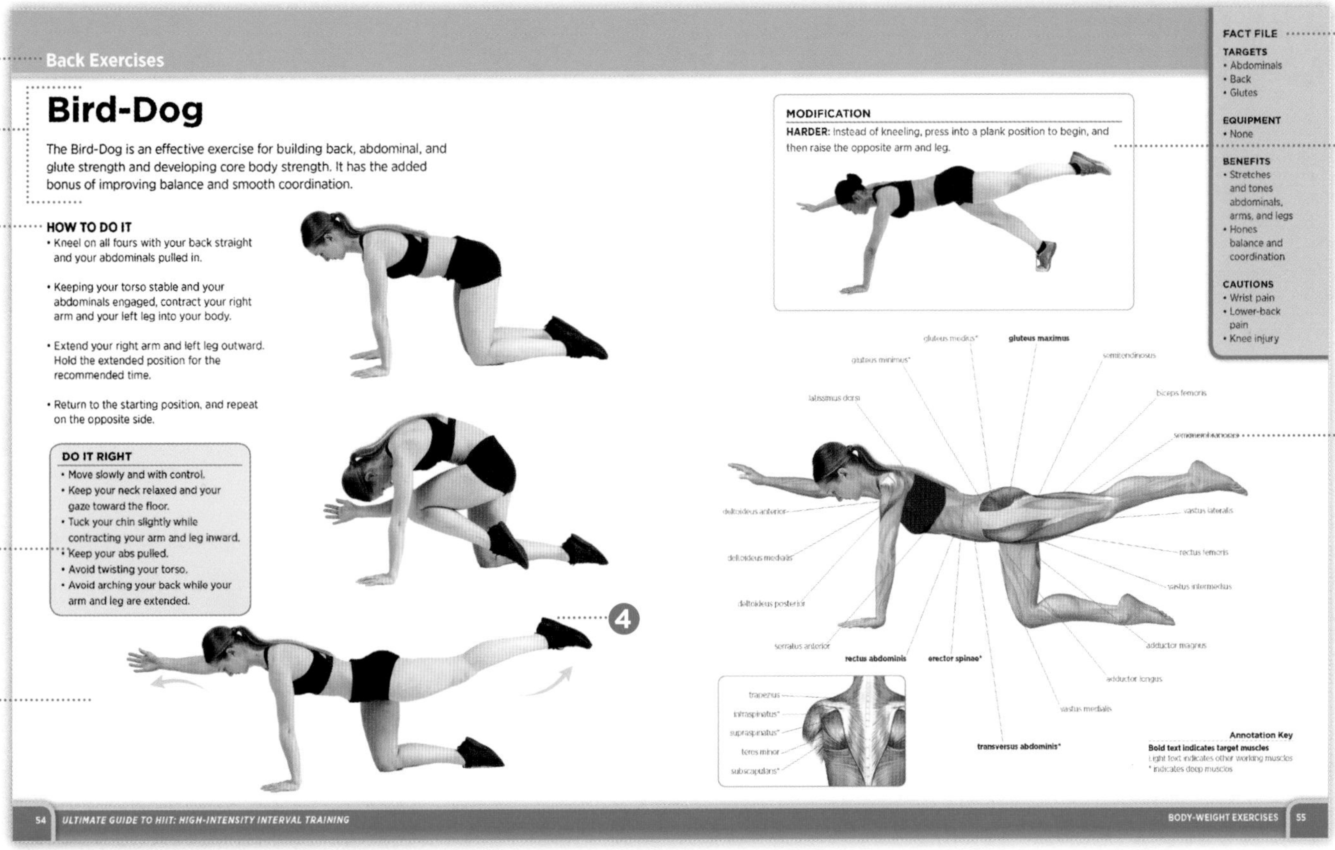

1 Back Exercises

2

Bird-Dog

The Bird-Dog is an effective exercise for building back, abdominal, and glute strength and developing core body strength. It has the added bonus of improving balance and smooth coordination.

3 **HOW TO DO IT**

- Kneel on all fours with your back straight and your abdominals pulled in.
- Keeping your torso stable and your abdominals engaged, contract your right arm and your left leg into your body.
- Extend your right arm and left leg outward. Hold the extended position for the recommended time.
- Return to the starting position, and repeat on the opposite side.

DO IT RIGHT

6
- Move slowly and with control.
- Keep your neck relaxed and your gaze toward the floor.
- Tuck your chin slightly while contracting your arm and leg inward.
- Keep your abs pulled.
- Avoid twisting your torso.
- Avoid arching your back while your arm and leg are extended.

4

5

MODIFICATION

9 **HARDER:** Instead of kneeling, press into a plank position to begin, and then raise the opposite arm and leg.

gluteus medius*
gluteus maximus
gluteus minimus*
semitendinosus
latissimus dorsi
biceps femoris
8 semimembranosus
deltoideus anterior
vastus lateralis
deltoideus medialis
rectus femoris
vastus intermedius
deltoideus posterior
adductor magnus
serratus anterior
rectus abdominis
erector spinae*
adductor longus
trapezius
infraspinatus*
supraspinatus*
teres minor
subscapularis*
vastus medialis
transversus abdominis*

Annotation Key
Bold text indicates target muscles
Light text indicates other working muscles
* indicates deep muscles

7 **FACT FILE**

TARGETS
- Abdominals
- Back
- Glutes

EQUIPMENT
- None

BENEFITS
- Stretches and tones abdominals, arms, and legs
- Hones balance and coordination

CAUTIONS
- Wrist pain
- Lower-back pain
- Knee injury

54 *ULTIMATE GUIDE TO HIIT: HIGH-INTENSITY INTERVAL TRAINING*

BODY-WEIGHT EXERCISES 55

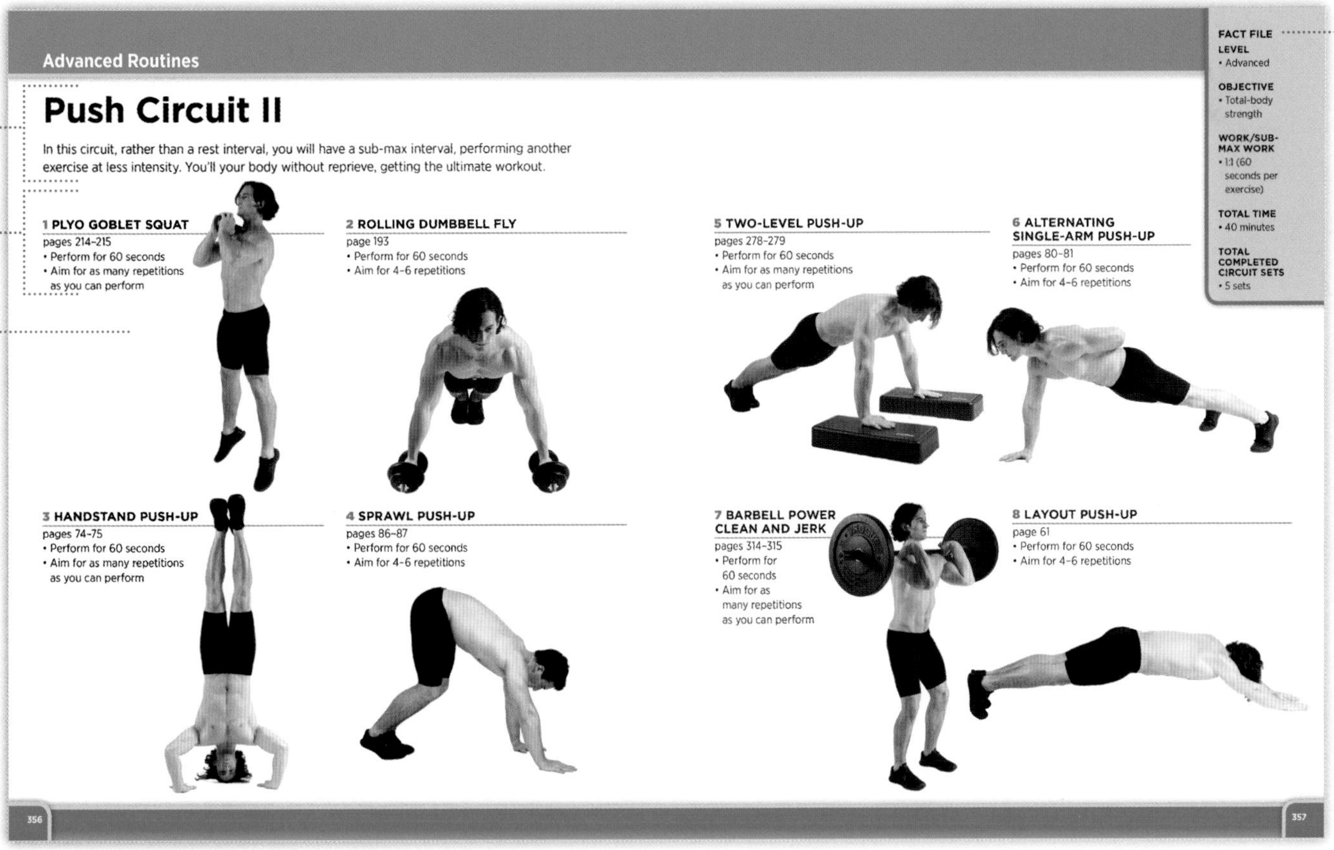

Advanced Routines

1

Push Circuit II

In this circuit, rather than a rest interval, you will have a sub-max interval, performing another exercise at less intensity. You'll your body without reprieve, getting the ultimate workout.

2 **1 PLYO GOBLET SQUAT**
pages 214–215
- Perform for 60 seconds
- Aim for as many repetitions as you can perform

3

2 ROLLING DUMBBELL FLY
page 193
- Perform for 60 seconds
- Aim for 4–6 repetitions

3 HANDSTAND PUSH-UP
pages 74–75
- Perform for 60 seconds
- Aim for as many repetitions as you can perform

4 SPRAWL PUSH-UP
pages 86–87
- Perform for 60 seconds
- Aim for 4–6 repetitions

5 TWO-LEVEL PUSH-UP
pages 278–279
- Perform for 60 seconds
- Aim for as many repetitions as you can perform

6 ALTERNATING SINGLE-ARM PUSH-UP
pages 80–81
- Perform for 60 seconds
- Aim for 4–6 repetitions

7 BARBELL POWER CLEAN AND JERK
pages 314–315
- Perform for 60 seconds
- Aim for as many repetitions as you can perform

8 LAYOUT PUSH-UP
page 61
- Perform for 60 seconds
- Aim for 4–6 repetitions

4 **FACT FILE**

LEVEL
- Advanced

OBJECTIVE
- Total-body strength

WORK/SUB-MAX WORK
- 1:1 (60 seconds per exercise)

TOTAL TIME
- 40 minutes

TOTAL COMPLETED CIRCUIT SETS
- 5 sets

356

357

Full-Body Anatomy

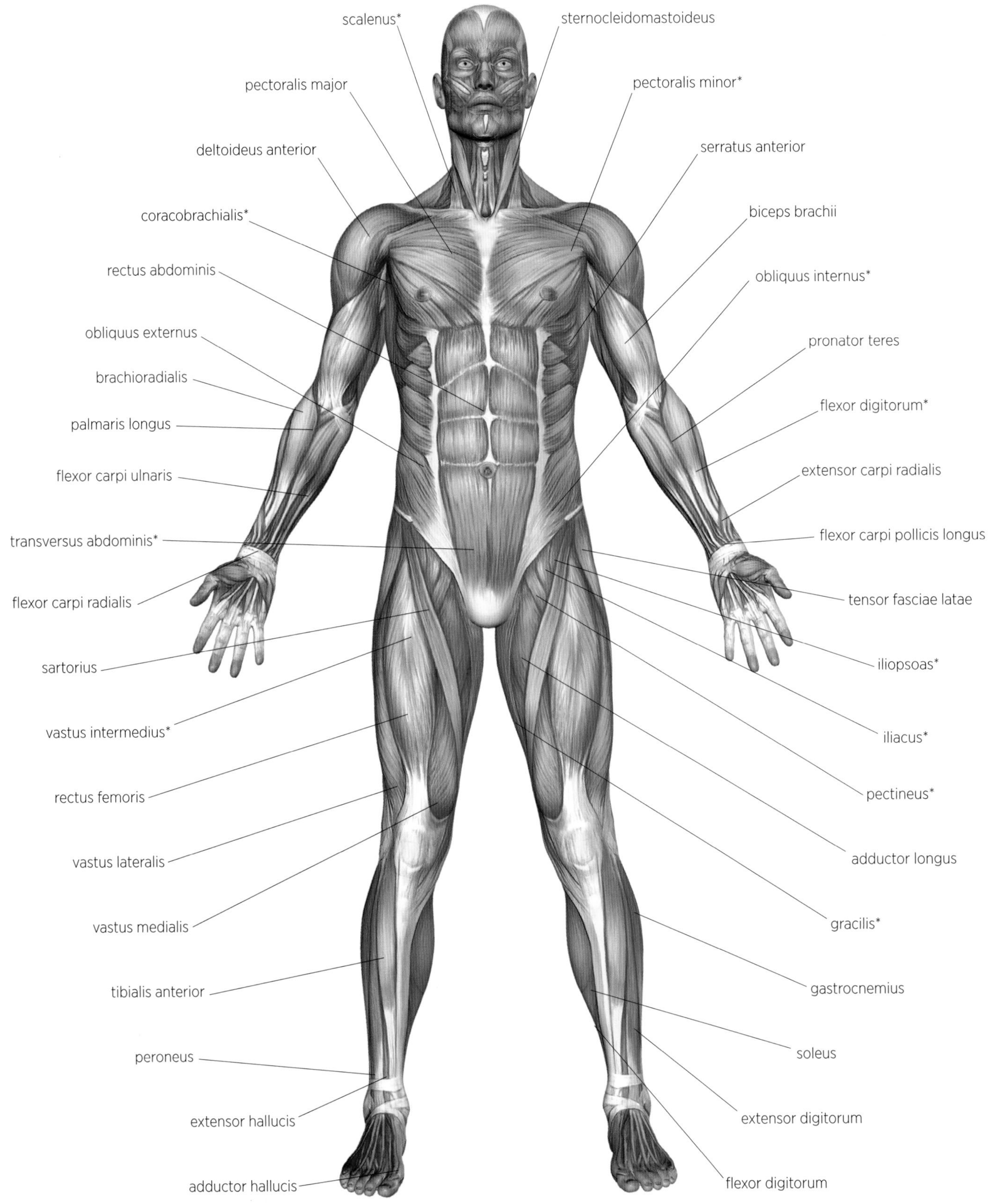

Annotation Key
* indicates deep muscles

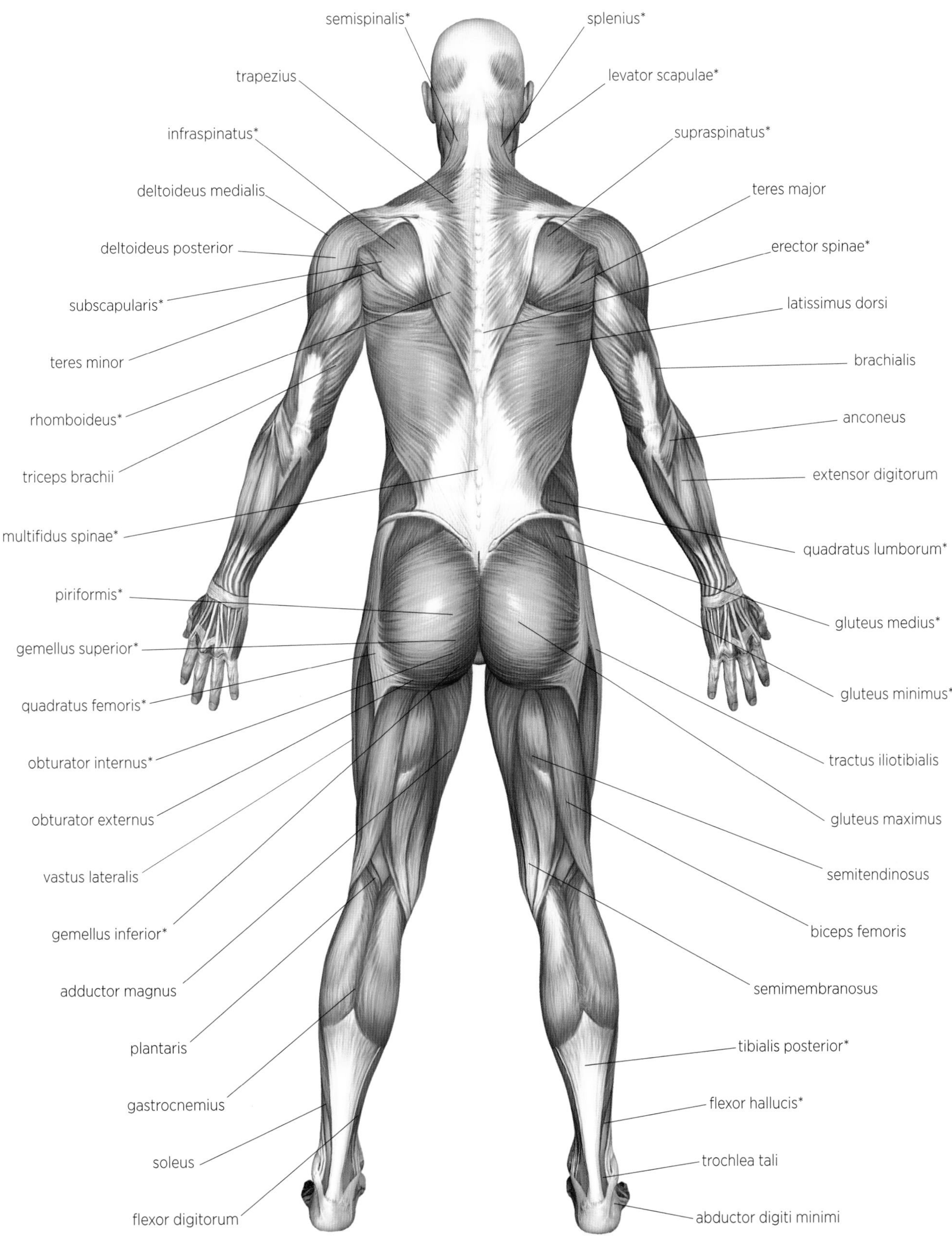

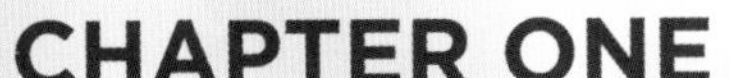

CHAPTER ONE

WARM-UPS & COOLDOWNS

Two crucial components to any exercise program are the warm-up and cooldown portions. It's absolutely necessary to prepare your muscles and other soft tissues, as well as your skeletal system, for rigorous exercise. Bringing your soft tissues through the ranges of motion that you will be using during your HIIT workout will get your muscles ready to engage within these ranges, reducing the risk of sprains and strains. All the included warm-ups are exercises in their own right, but they have been carefully selected because of their soft tissue warm-up potential, as well as the inherent flexibility each one imposes. A well-thought-out warm-up prepares you for anything you can throw at it. Don't be surprised if you sweat during the warm-up—that's the intention. Welcome to HIIT!

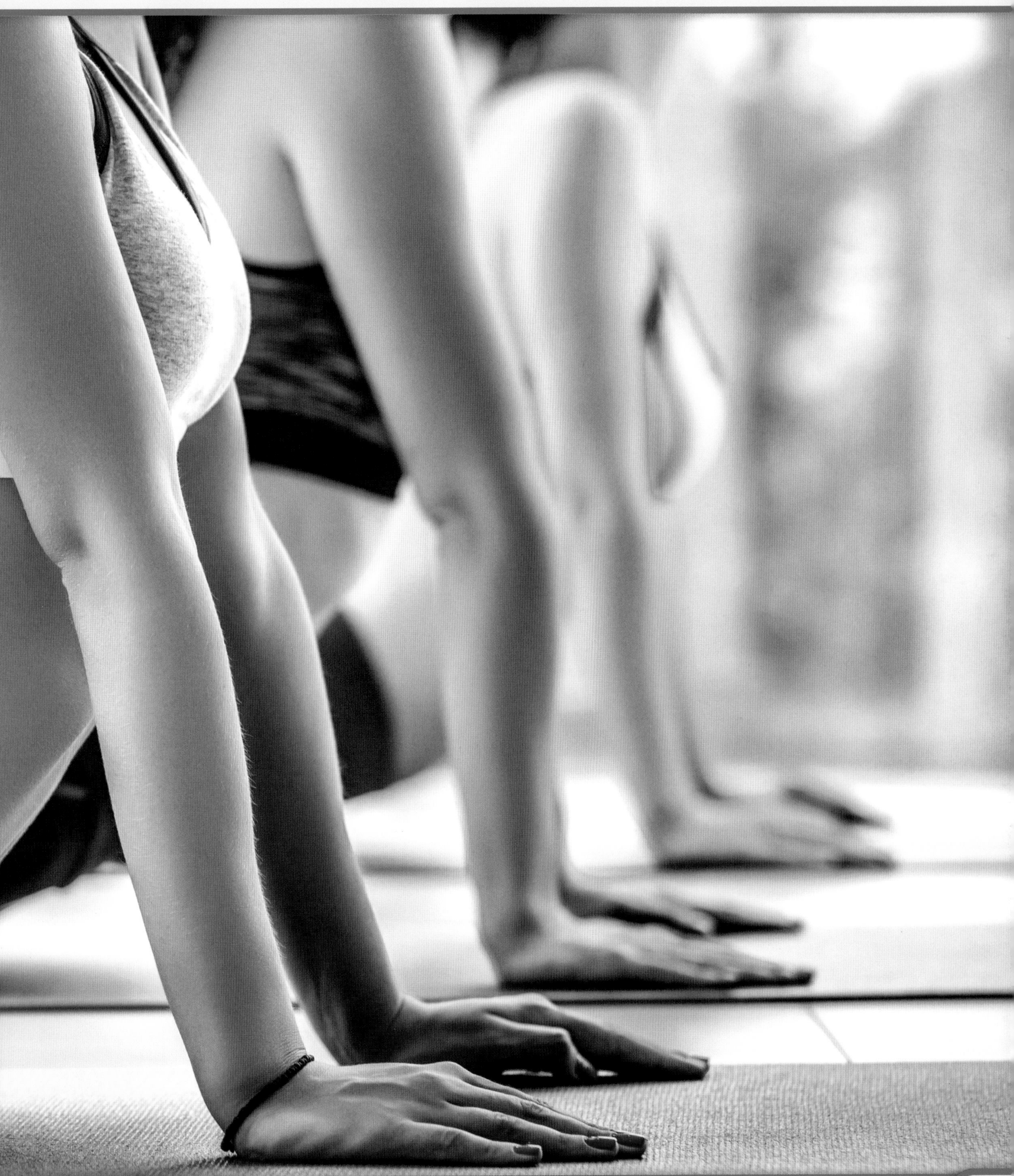

Push-Up Walkout

The Push-Up Walkout is a powerful combination exercise that builds upper-body strength and increases core endurance.

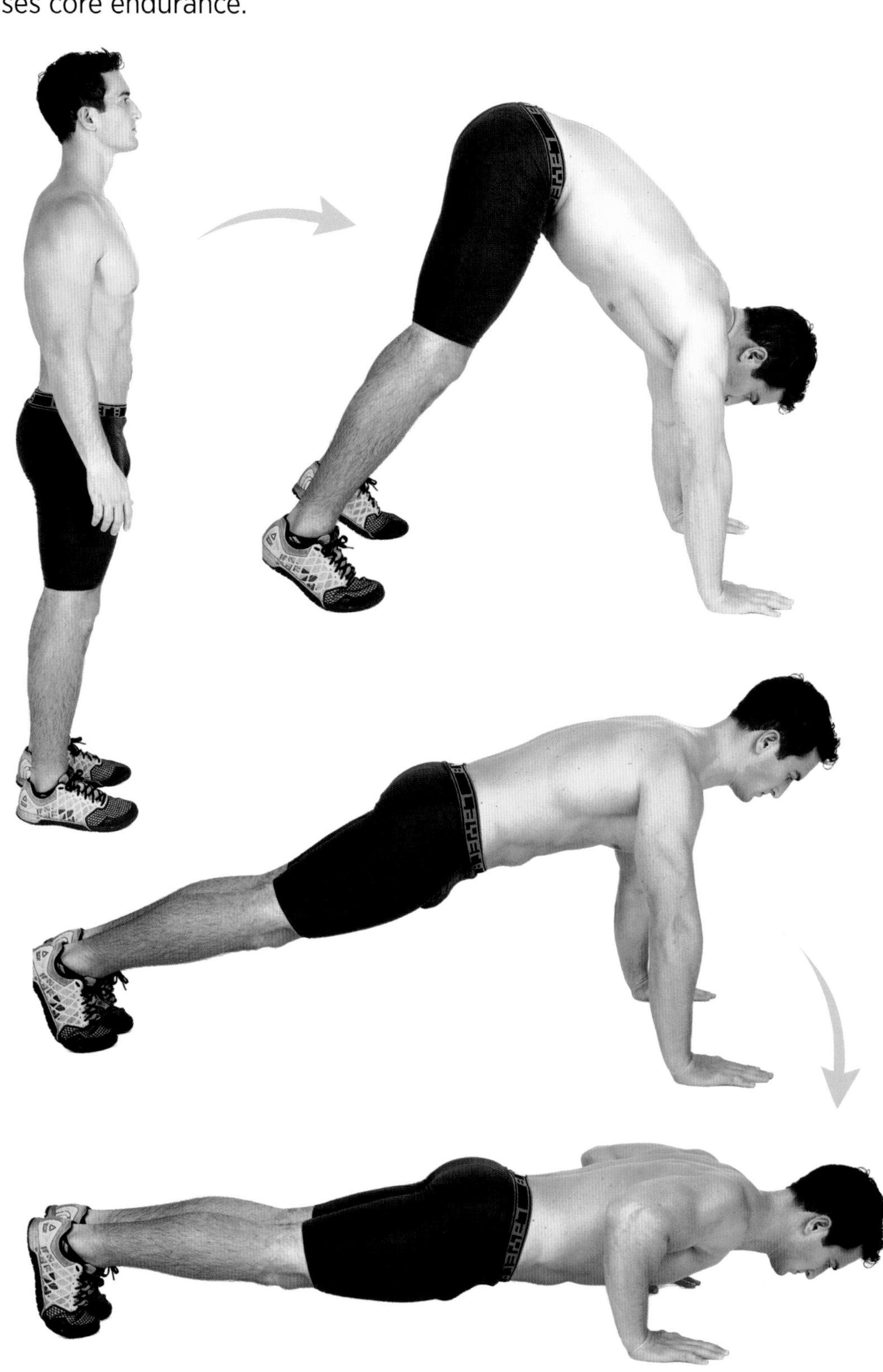

HOW TO DO IT

- Stand with your feet hip-width apart and your hands on your hips or at your sides.
- Bend forward until your hands reach the floor, and then walk your hands out as far in front of you as possible.
- Press your palms into the floor, and tuck your toes so that you are in a high plank position. Perform a push-up.
- Walk your hands back toward your feet.
- Perform the recommended repetitions, and then roll back up to the starting position.

DO IT RIGHT

- Keep your feet planted on the floor as you walk your hands forward and back.
- Keep your back in a neutral position while performing the push-up.
- Pull your stomach in and engage your abdominals.
- Avoid arching your back or hunching forward.
- Avoid going too far forward at first; instead, build up to the full walkout.
- Avoid tensing your neck.

MODIFICATION

EASIER: To make the push-up less strenuous, bend your legs and rest your knees on the floor.

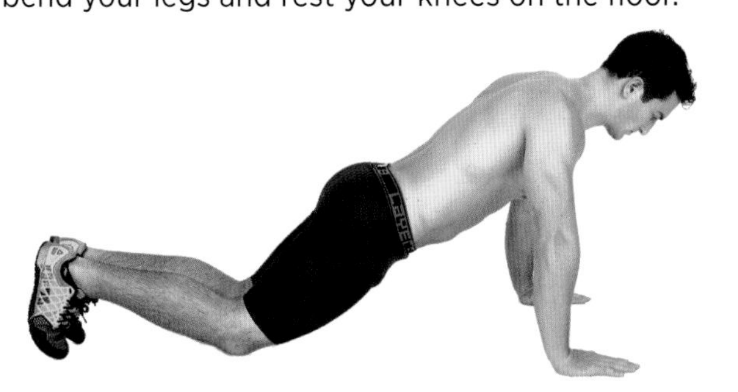

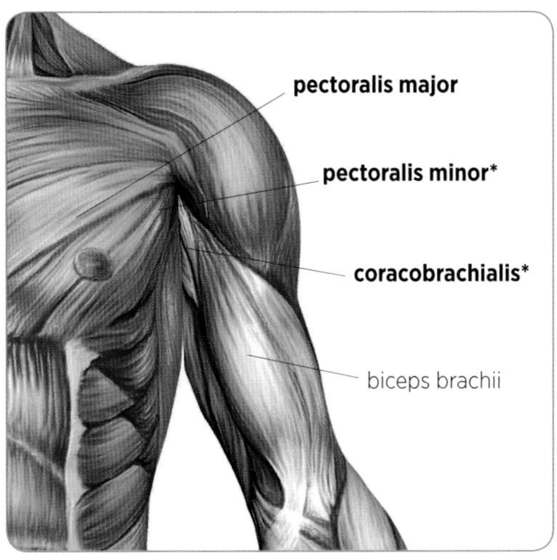

gluteus maximus

gluteus minimus*

tensor fasciae latae

quadratus lumborum*

tractus iliotibialis

erector spinae*

biceps femoris

latissimus dorsi

trapezius

rectus abdominis

serratus anterior

pectoralis major

brachialis

triceps brachii

Annotation Key

Bold text indicates target muscles
Light text indicates other working muscles
* indicates deep muscles

FACT FILE

TARGETS
- Abdominals
- Latissimus dorsi
- Pectorals
- Deltoids

EQUIPMENT
- None

BENEFITS
- Warms up muscles
- Improves coordination
- Strengthens and tones core, chest, and back muscles

CAUTIONS
- Shoulder issues
- Wrist issues
- Lower-back issues

Twisting Knee Raise

Work your abdominals—especially your obliques—while developing leg strength and endurance with Twisting Knee Raise. It will also burn calories as you prepare for a rigorous HIIT workout.

HOW TO DO IT

- Stand with your feet hip-width apart and your arms at your sides. Raise both arms and bend your elbows so that each arm forms a right angle, palms facing forward.
- Raise your left knee toward your abdomen. At the same time, bring your right elbow toward the knee. Aim for your knee and elbow to touch.
- Return to starting position. Repeat on the opposite side, alternating sides for the recommended repetitions.

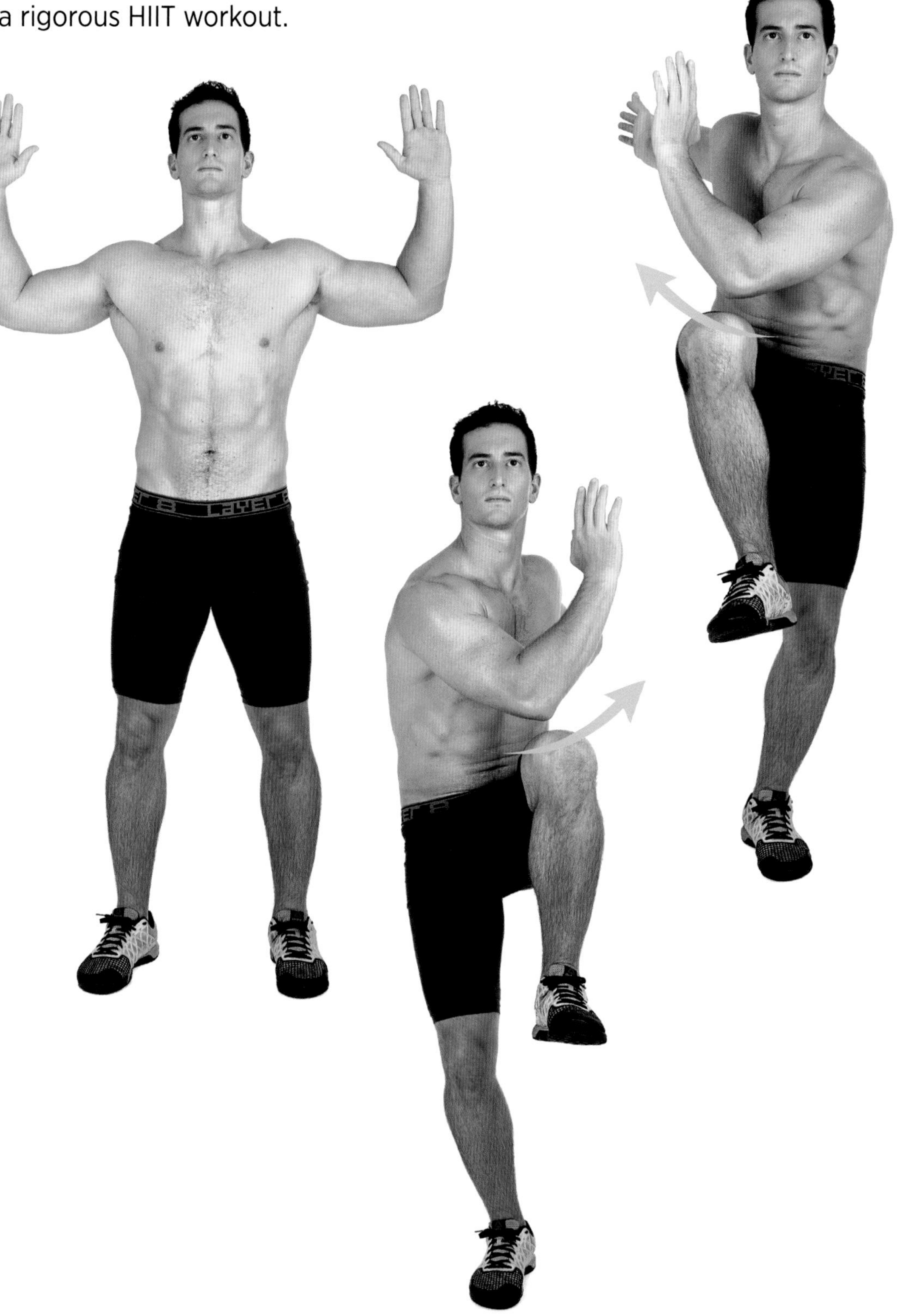

DO IT RIGHT

- Keep your abs engaged and contracted.
- Maintain a quick, consistent pace.
- Face forward as you perform the twist.
- Avoid hyperextending your back.
- Don't excessively twist your hips.

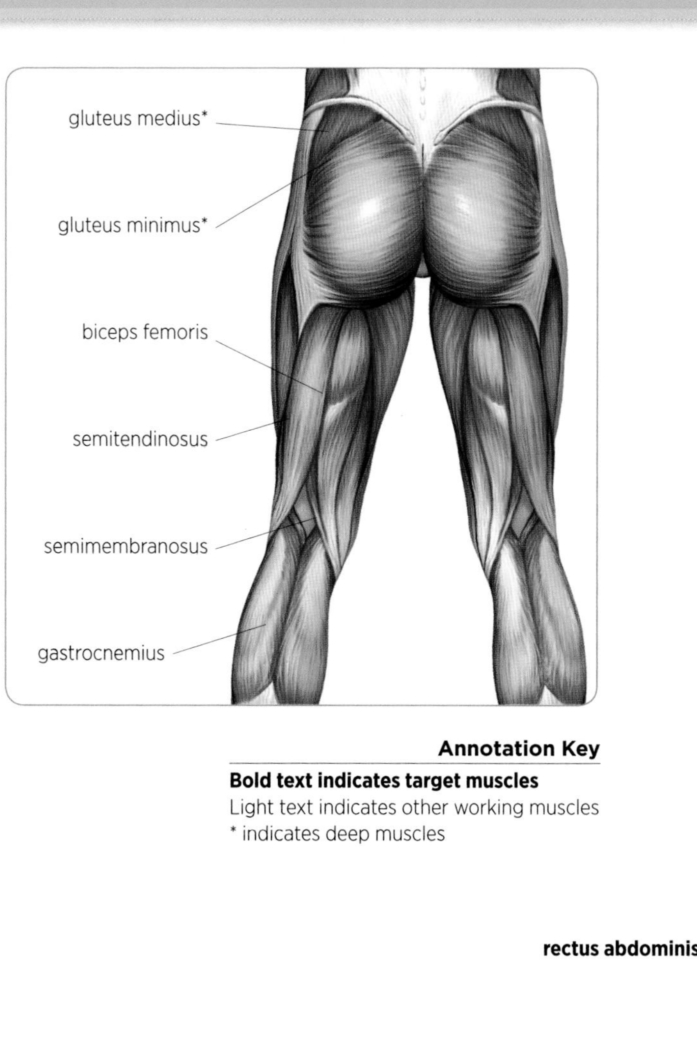

Annotation Key

Bold text indicates target muscles
Light text indicates other working muscles
* indicates deep muscles

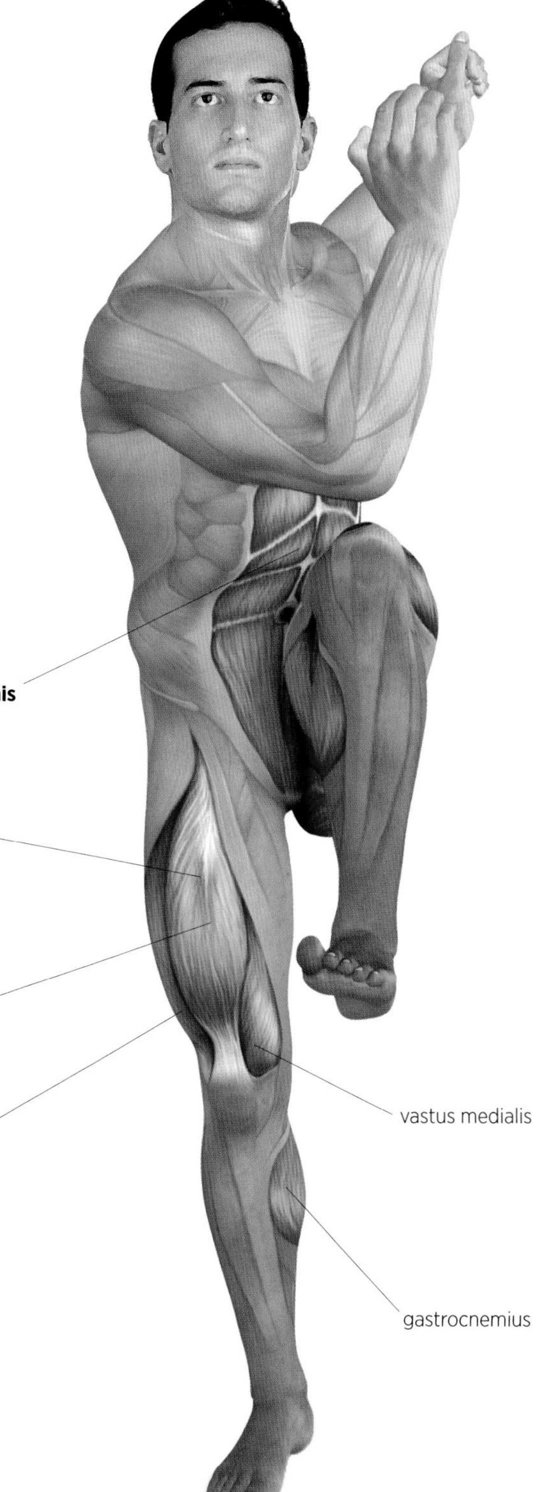

FACT FILE

TARGETS
- Abdominals
- Legs

EQUIPMENT
- None

BENEFITS
- Improves balance and coordination
- Improves agility and power
- Burn calories
- Elevates heart rate
- Strengthens and tones core muscles and calves

CAUTIONS
- Lower-back issues
- Knee issues

Piriformis Bridge

HIIT workouts can be hard on your gluteal muscles. To avoid tight, sore buttocks, keep these muscles, along with the piriformis (a deep muscle lying under the glutes) strong and flexible. Any bridging is great for the glutes, but this homes in on the piriformis.

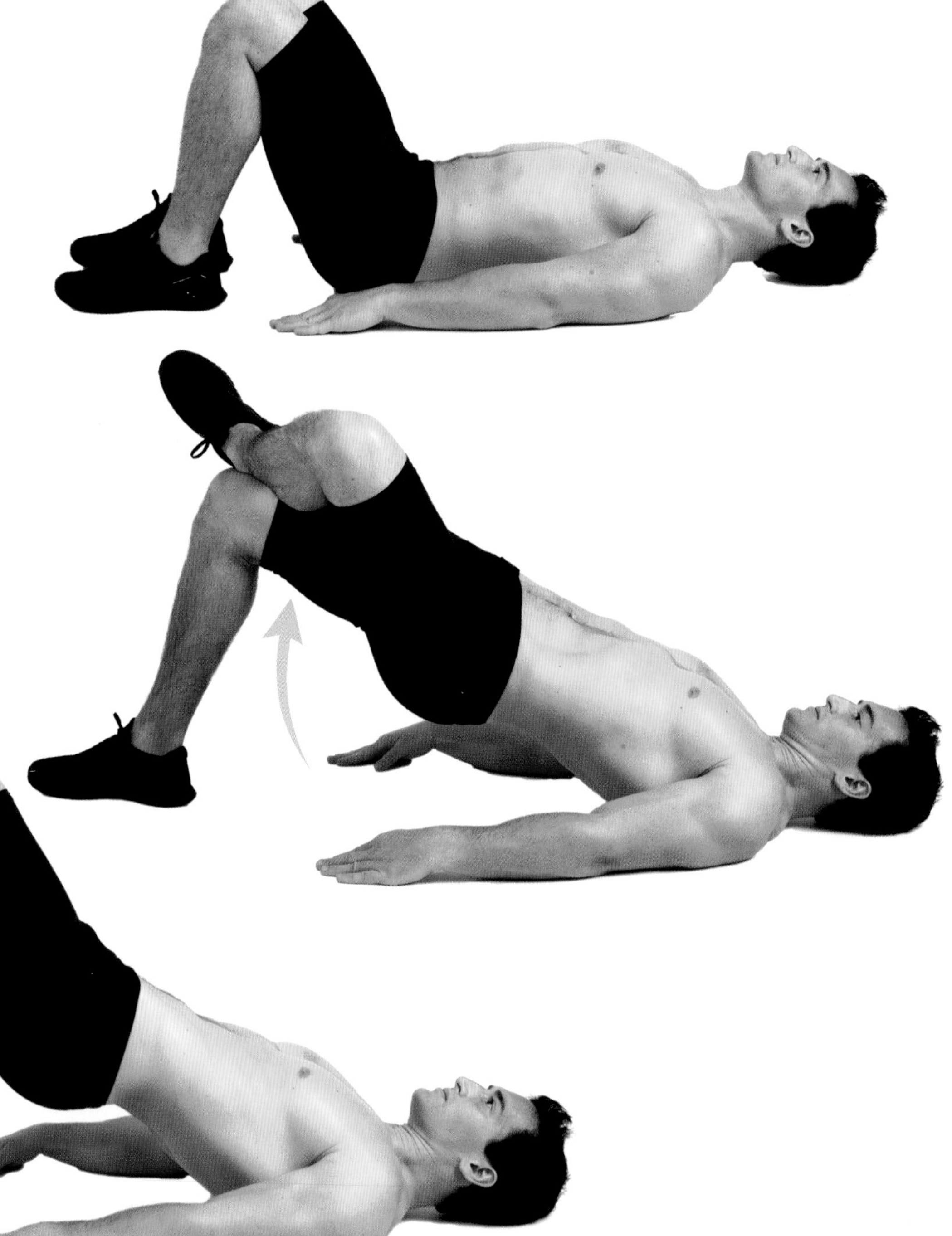

HOW TO DO IT

- Lie on your back, arms extended at your sides. Bend your knees, and plant your feet on the floor.

- Keeping the rest of your body still, raise your left leg to rest the ankle on your right knee.

- Press your palms into the floor, and engage your abdominal muscles to lift your body. Your body should form a diagonal line from shoulders to knees.

- Slowly and with control, return to the starting position. Switch legs, and repeat for the recommended repetitions on each side.

FACT FILE

TARGETS
- Glutes
- Hamstrings
- Quadriceps

EQUIPMENT
- None

BENEFITS
- Stretches piriformis
- Strengthens thigh muscles and glutes
- Stabilizes core

CAUTIONS
- Neck issues
- Lower-back issues

DO IT RIGHT
- Squeeze your buttocks as you lift and lower.
- Draw your navel in toward your spine.
- Press your shoulders down toward your back.
- Anchor your arms to the floor.
- Relax your neck.
- Avoid lifting your shoulders toward your ears.

erector spinae*
multifidus spinae*
quadratus lumborum*
gluteus medius*
gluteus minimus*
gluteus maximus
piriformis*
biceps femoris
semitendinosus
semimembranosus

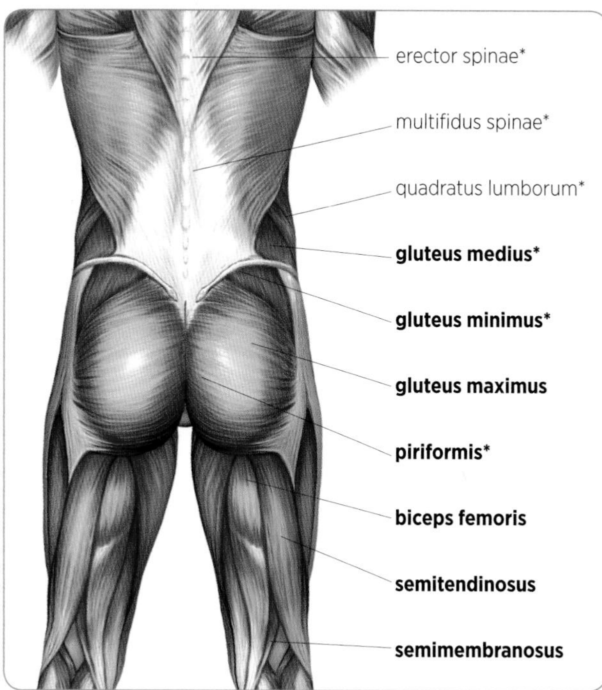

Annotation Key
Bold text indicates target muscles
Light text indicates other working muscles
* indicates deep muscles

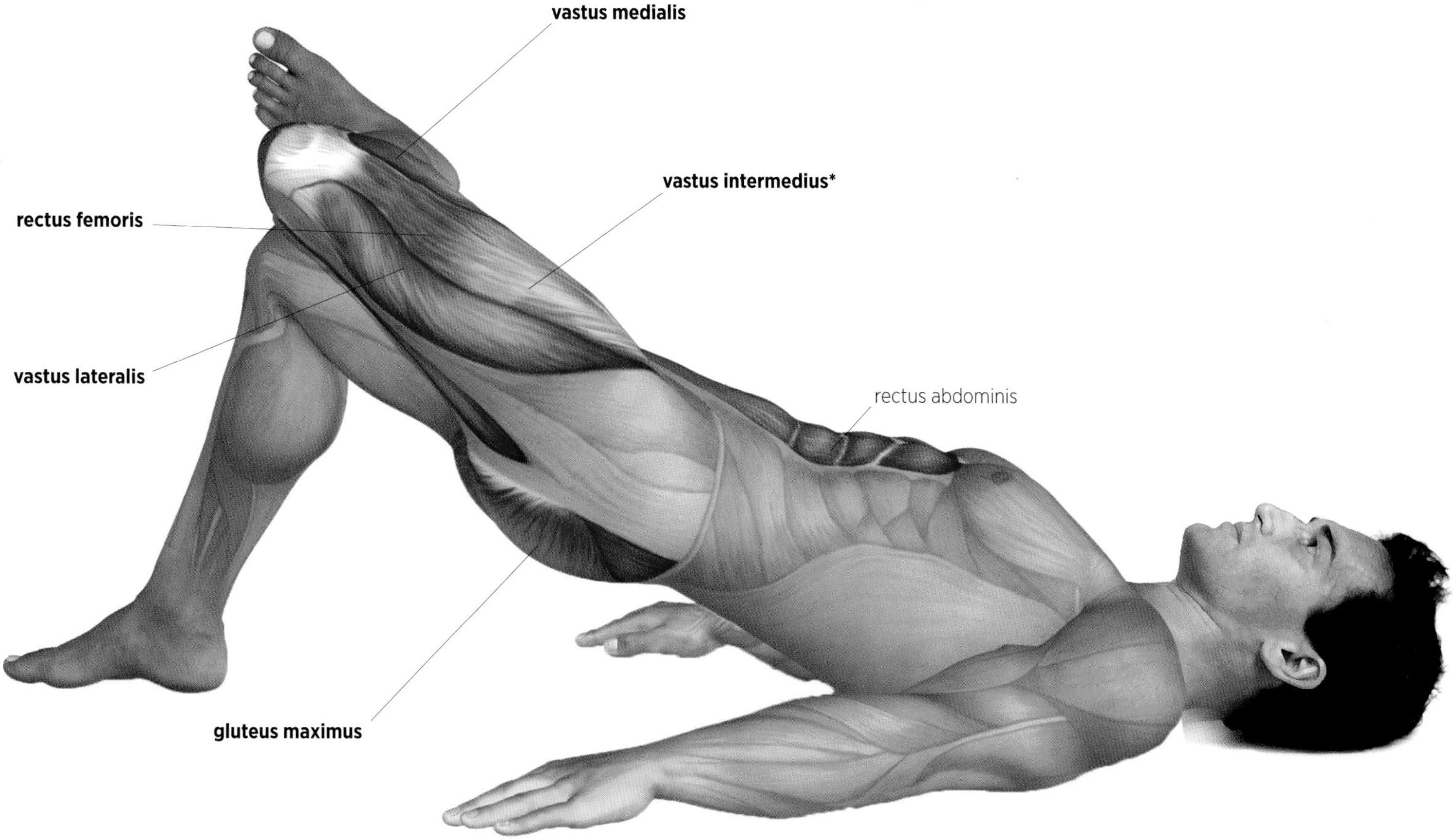

vastus medialis
vastus intermedius*
rectus femoris
vastus lateralis
rectus abdominis
gluteus maximus

Warm-Up Obstacle Course

The Warm-Up Obstacle Course exercise will get your heart pumping and test your agility and coordination. This fun exercise prepares you for complicated HIIT workouts.

HOW TO DO IT

- Set up seven small objects on the floor to form a triangle and a square.
- Taking small, quick steps, step around all of the objects in the triangle.
- Stand in front of the square, and jump forward to land in the middle of the square. Complete a Jumping Jack (see box on opposite page).
- Jump forward to land outside the square. Jog back to the beginning of the course, and repeat for the recommended time or repetitions.

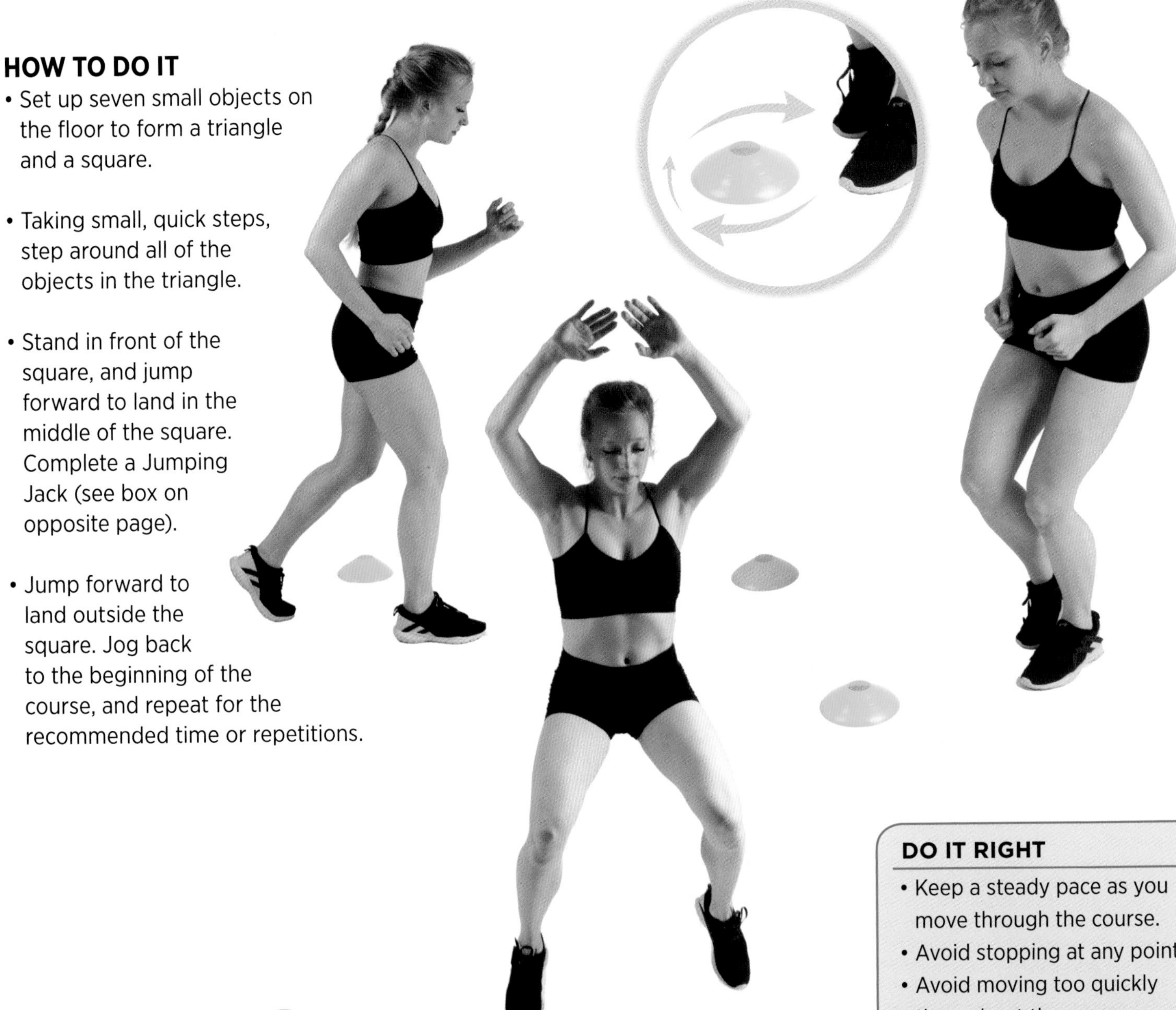

DO IT RIGHT

- Keep a steady pace as you move through the course.
- Avoid stopping at any point.
- Avoid moving too quickly throughout the course.
- Take small steps, focusing on coordination.
- Stand upright.
- Keep your abdominal muscles engaged.

FACT FILE

TARGETS
- Abdominals
- Glutes
- Hamstrings
- Quadriceps

EQUIPMENT
- Small cones

BENEFITS
- Warms up muscles
- Improves agility

CAUTIONS
- Knee issues

multifidus spinae*
gluteus minimus*
vastus lateralis
biceps femoris
semitendinosus
semimembranosus

rectus abdominis
vastus intermedius*
rectus femoris
vastus medialis
gluteus medius*
tensor fasciae latae
biceps femoris
gastrocnemius

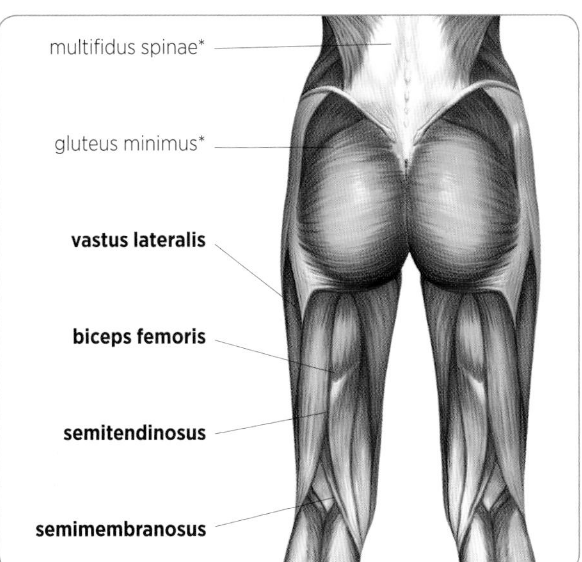

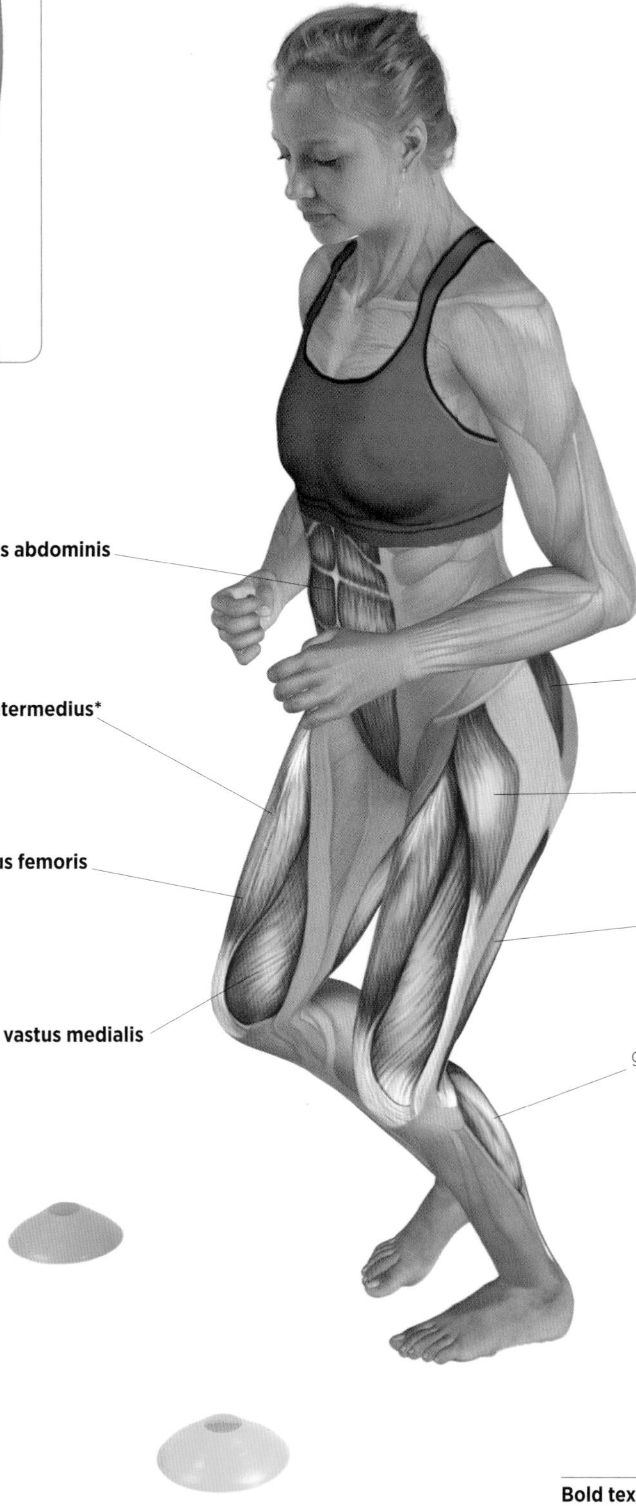

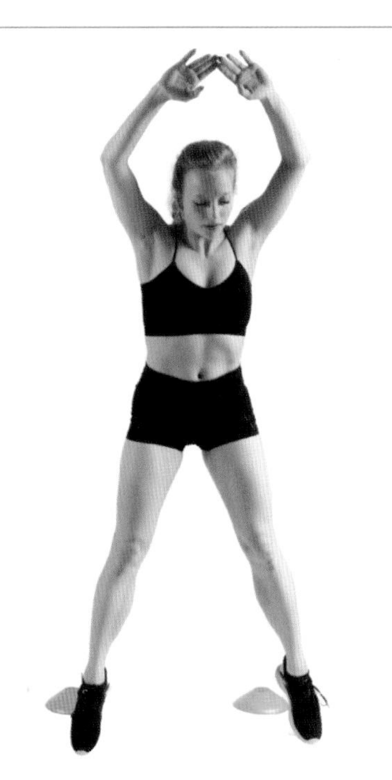

MODIFICATION

EASIER: To perform a Jumping Jack, stand with your arms at your sides and with your feet together and knees slightly bent. Keeping your knees bent, jump up, spreading your legs and bringing your arms up to touch overhead. Return to the starting position.

Annotation Key

Bold text indicates target muscles
Light text indicates other working muscles
* indicates deep muscles

Single-Leg Crossover

This multipurpose move has both strengthening and stretching benefits. It will tone and tighten your core muscles while keeping your glutes and lower back limber.

DO IT RIGHT

- Keep your abdominal muscles, especially your obliques, engaged as you roll.
- Keep your legs straight.
- Move at a steady pace
- Avoid rushing through the movement.

HOW TO DO IT

- Lie on your back, with your arms extended at your sides and your legs extended on the floor.
- Raise your right leg straight upward so that it is perpendicular to the floor.
- Turn your head to the right, and slowly rotate your lower body to the left, lowering your right leg until your foot is just above the floor.
- Roll your lower body and leg back, and then lower your leg to the starting position.
- Repeat, alternating sides for the recommended repetitions.

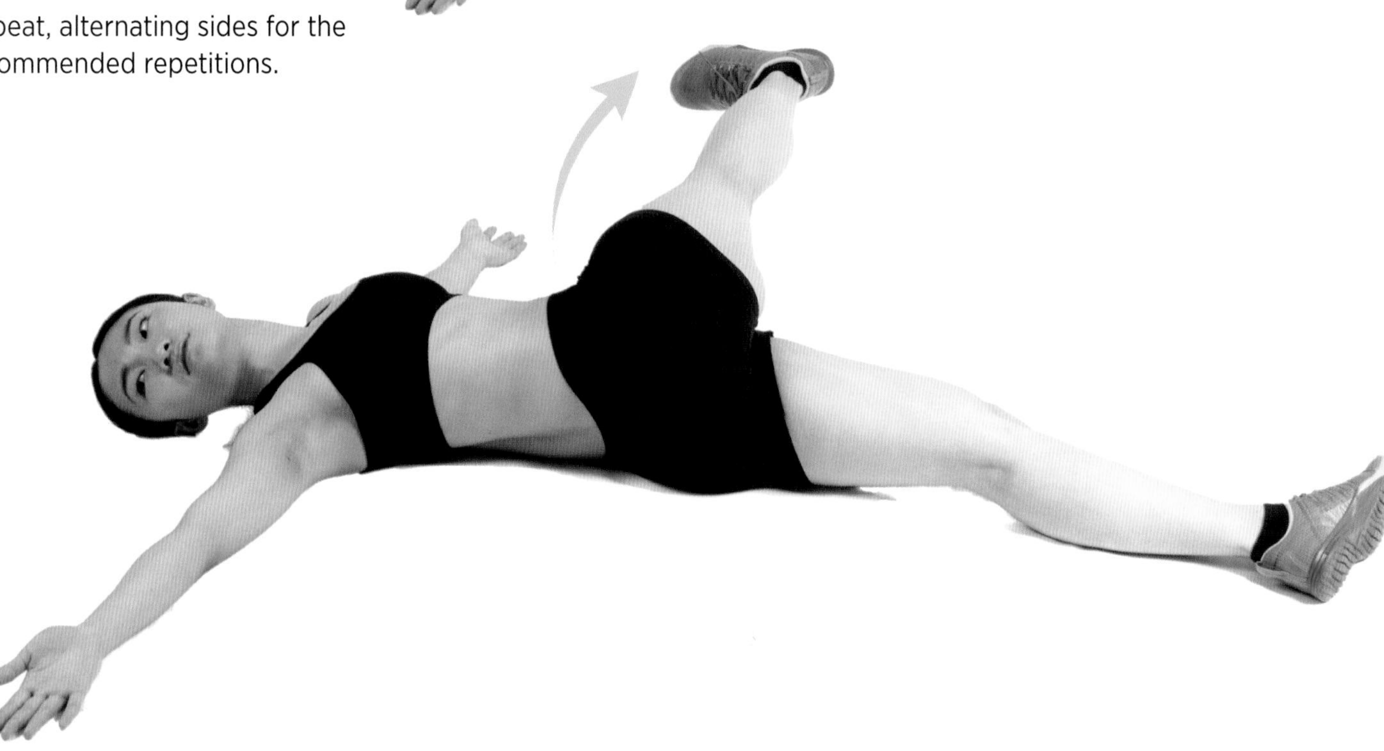

FACT FILE

TARGETS
- Obliques
- Abdominals
- Hamstrings
- Glutes
- Hip flexors
- Lower back

EQUIPMENT
- None

BENEFITS
- Tones cores muscles
- Increases lower-back flexibility
- Stretches glutes

CAUTIONS
- Severe lower-back pain

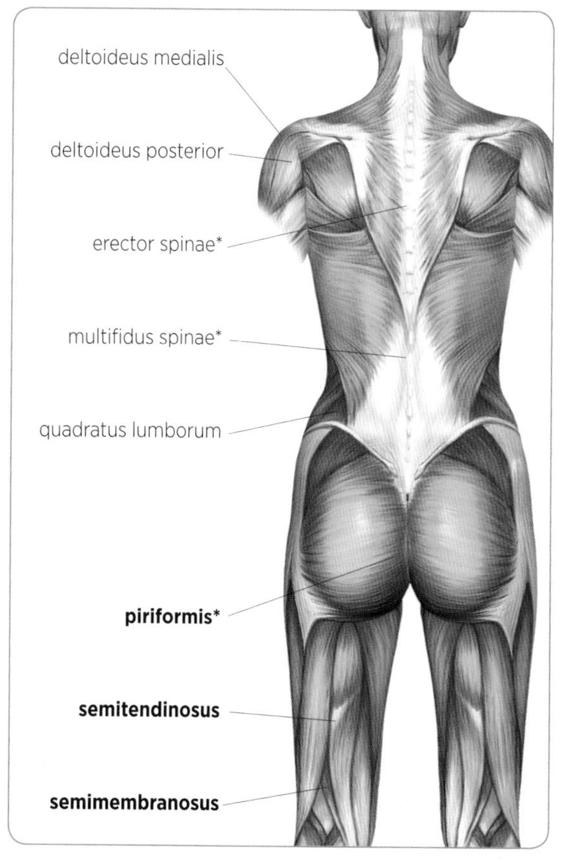

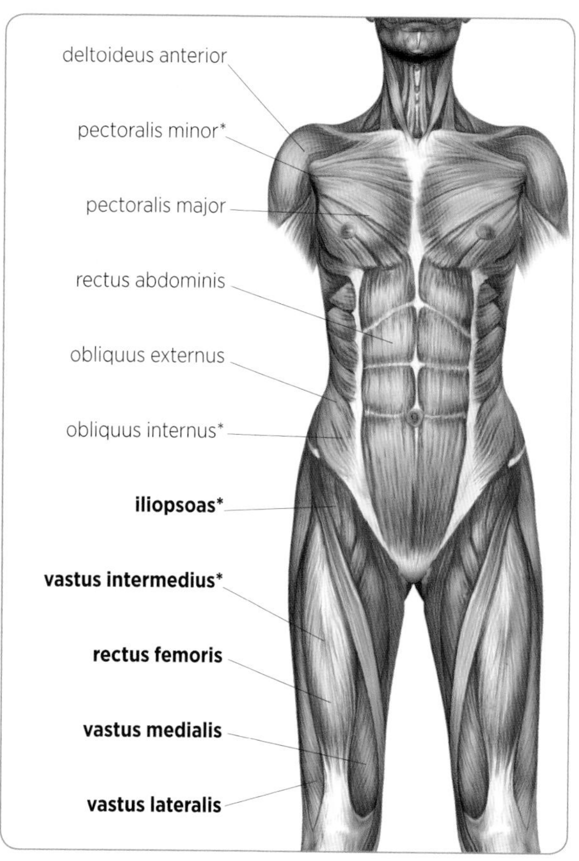

Annotation Key

Bold text indicates target muscles

Light text indicates other working muscles

* indicates deep muscles

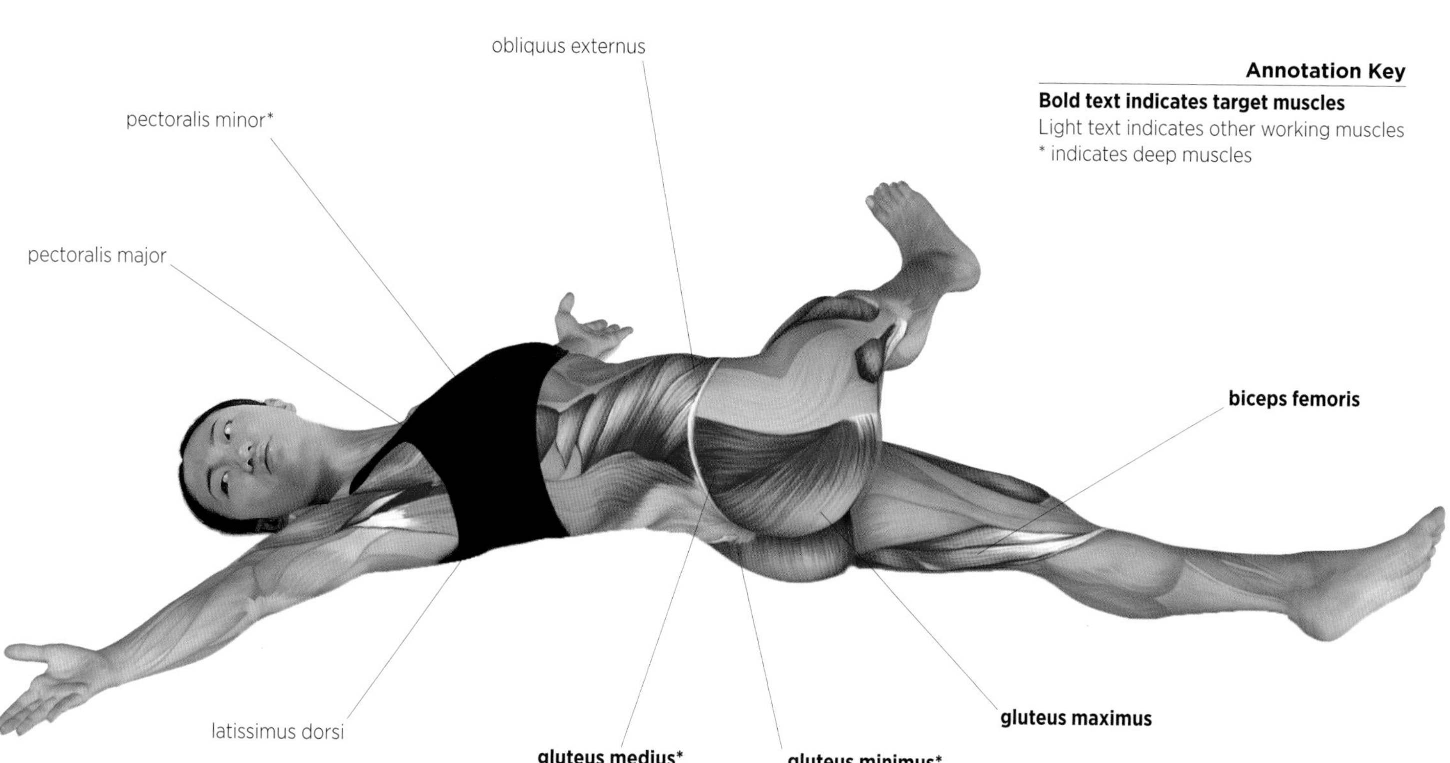

Adductor Stretch

The hip adductors are a group of muscles that bring the femur—the long bone of your thigh—toward the midline of your body. Keep these muscles lithe and flexible with this standing stretch.

FACT FILE

TARGETS
- Hip adductors

EQUIPMENT
- None

BENEFITS
- Stretches and strengthens hip flexor muscles

CAUTIONS
- Knee issues

HOW TO DO IT

- Stand with your feet wider than shoulder-width apart so that you are in a straddle position. Bend your knees.

- Place your hands on your knees, and bend at your hips, keeping your spine in a neutral position and your shoulders and your shoulders slightly forward.

- Keeping your torso in the same position and your hips behind your heels, shift your weight to the right, bending your knee while extending your left leg. Hold for a few moments, and then repeat on the opposite side. Continue alternating sides for the recommended repetitions.

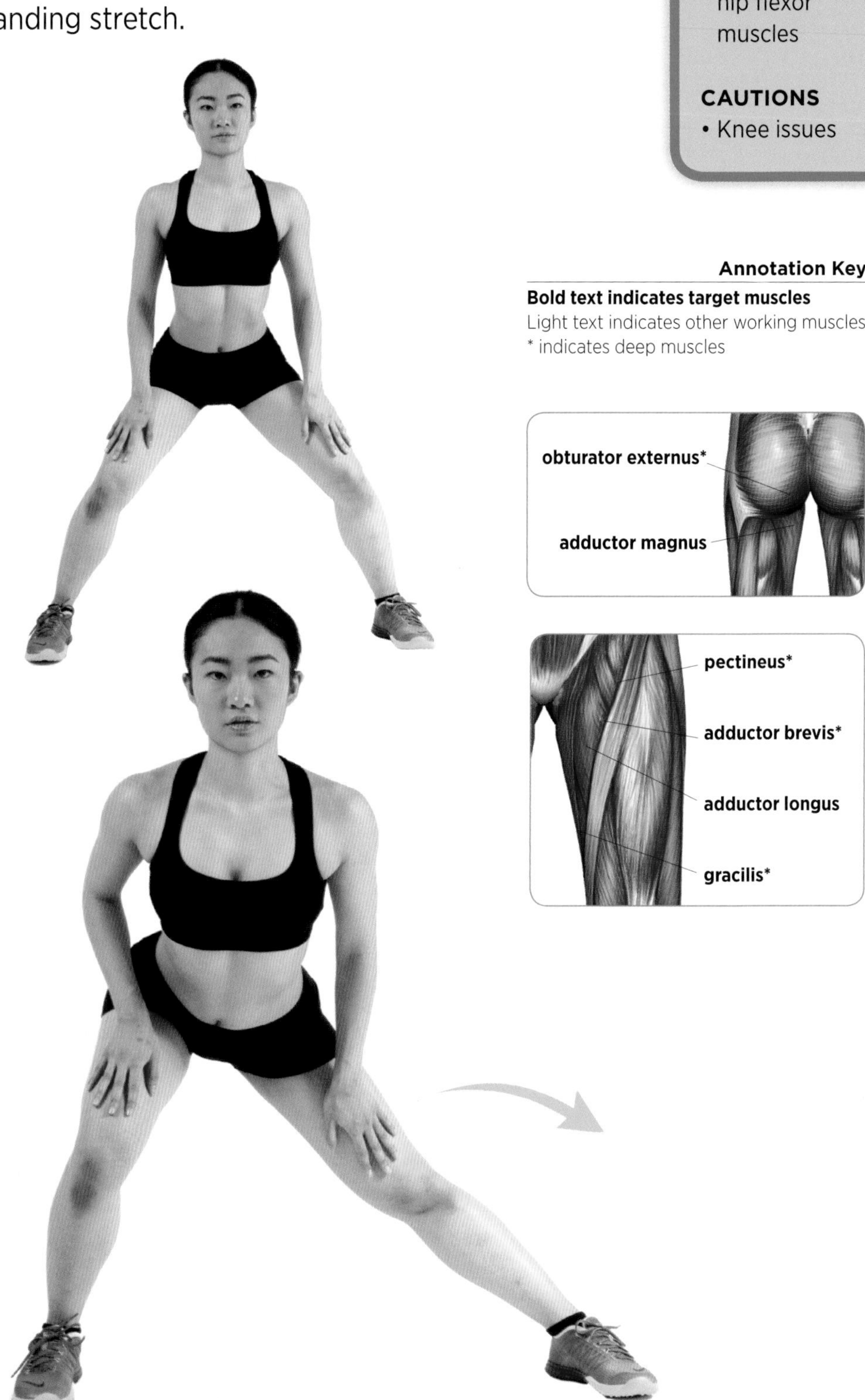

Annotation Key

Bold text indicates target muscles
Light text indicates other working muscles
* indicates deep muscles

DO IT RIGHT

- Keep your trunk aligned as you move from side to side.
- Keep your neck and shoulders relaxed.
- Use the hand placement on your thighs to assist your posture.
- Avoid rounding your spine.
- Keep your feet planted; avoid shifting or lifting them.
- Avoid extending your knees over your toes while bending.

Hip Flexor Stretch

The hip flexors are a group of muscles around the upper and inner thighs and pelvic region that draw together the bones of the leg and the hip or spine at the hip joint. Running, jumping, and standing call on these muscles, so keep them toned and supple with this targeted stretch.

FACT FILE

TARGETS
- Hip flexors

EQUIPMENT
- None

BENEFITS
- Strengthens and stretches the hip flexors
- Conditions hips for running and jumping

CAUTIONS
- Hip issues
- Knee issues

HOW TO DO IT

- Kneel on the floor, and then place your right foot in front of you so that your knee is bent less than 90 degrees.
- Bring your torso forward, bending your right knee so that it shifts toward your toes.
- Keeping your torso in neutral position, press your left hip forward and downward to create a stretch over the front of your thigh. Raise your arms toward the ceiling, keeping your shoulders relaxed.
- Bring your arms down, and move your hips backward. Straighten your right leg, and bring your torso forward. Place your hands on either side of your right leg for support.
- Hold for a few moments, and then repeat for the recommended repetitions on each leg.

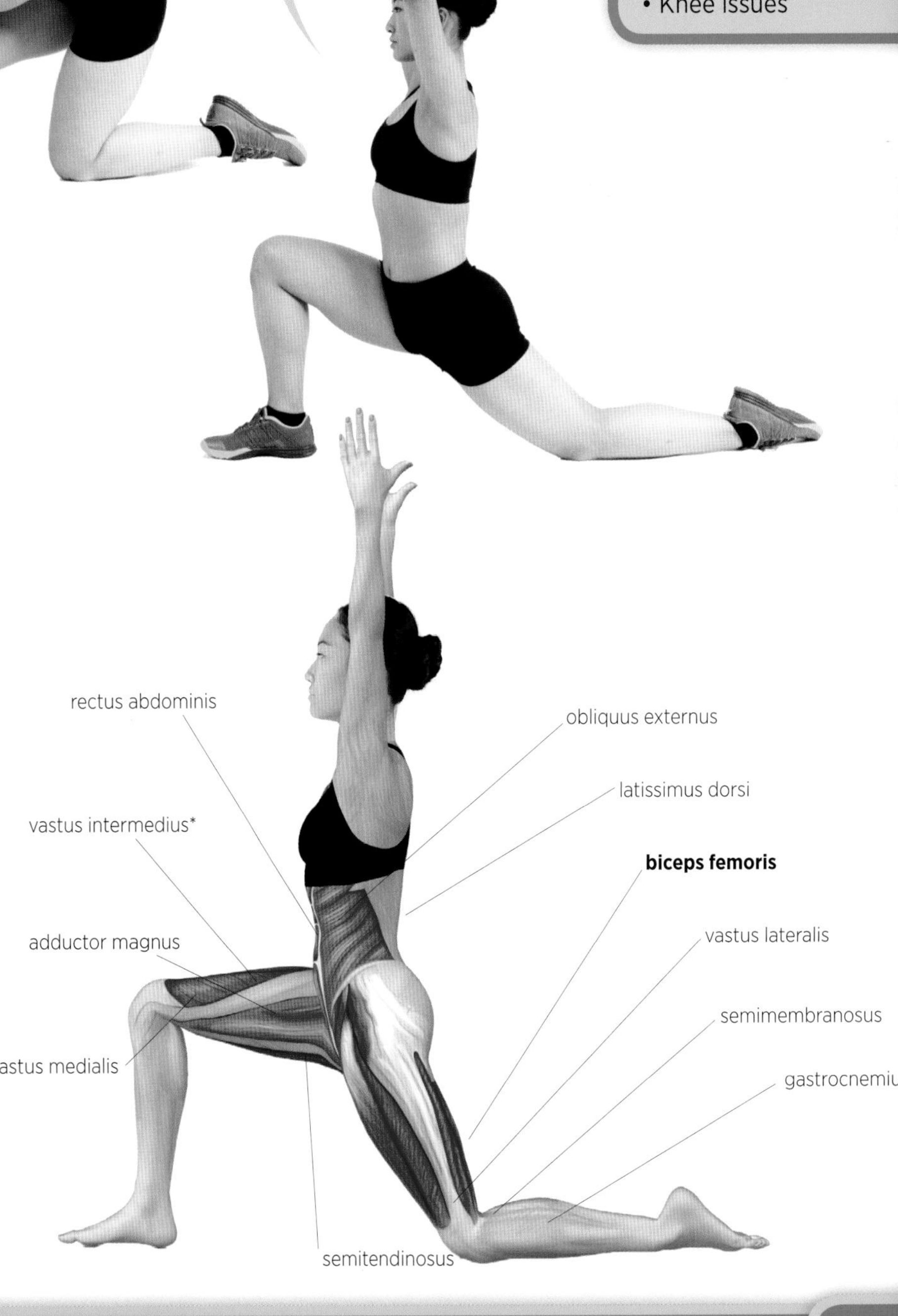

DO IT RIGHT

- Keep your shoulders and neck relaxed.
- Move your entire body as one unit as you go into the stretch.
- Avoid extending your front knee too far over the planted foot.

Annotation Key
Bold text indicates target muscles
Light text indicates other working muscles
* indicates deep muscles

High Lunge

An essential exercise in many disciplines, the High Lunge is an effective thigh strengthener. It also targets the hips and glutes, stabilizing and strengthening these muscles.

HOW TO DO IT

- Stand with your feet together and your arms at your sides.
- Move your left leg forward, and bend at hips while bringing your hands down to either side of your feet.
- Step back with your right foot, keeping your legs in line with your hips. Keep the ball of your left foot in contact with the floor.
- Press the ball of your left foot into the floor, contract your thigh muscles, and press up to maintain your left leg in a straight position.
- Hold for a few moments, and then slowly return to the starting position. Repeat on the opposite side, and then continue alternating legs for the recommended repetitions.

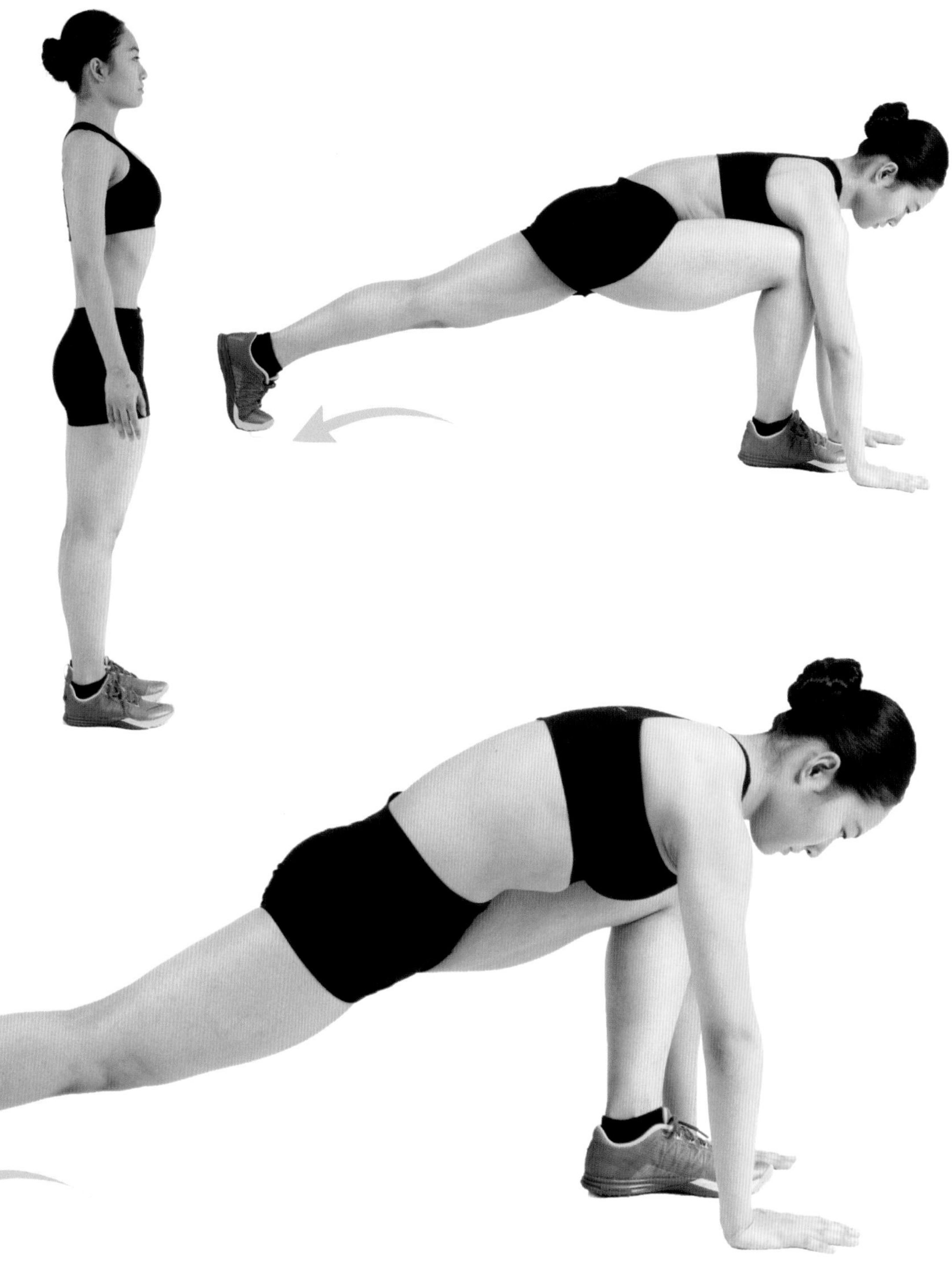

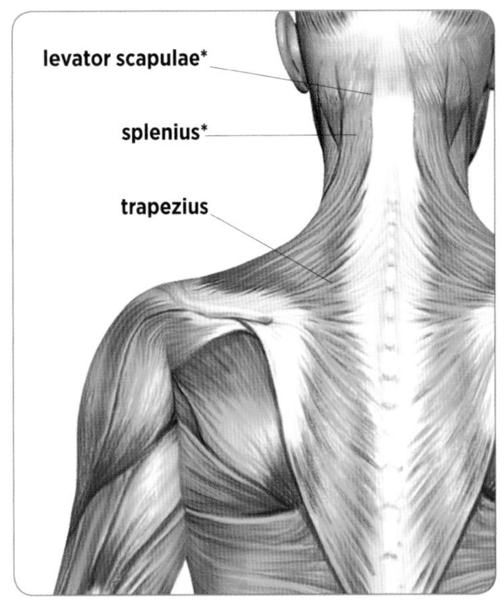

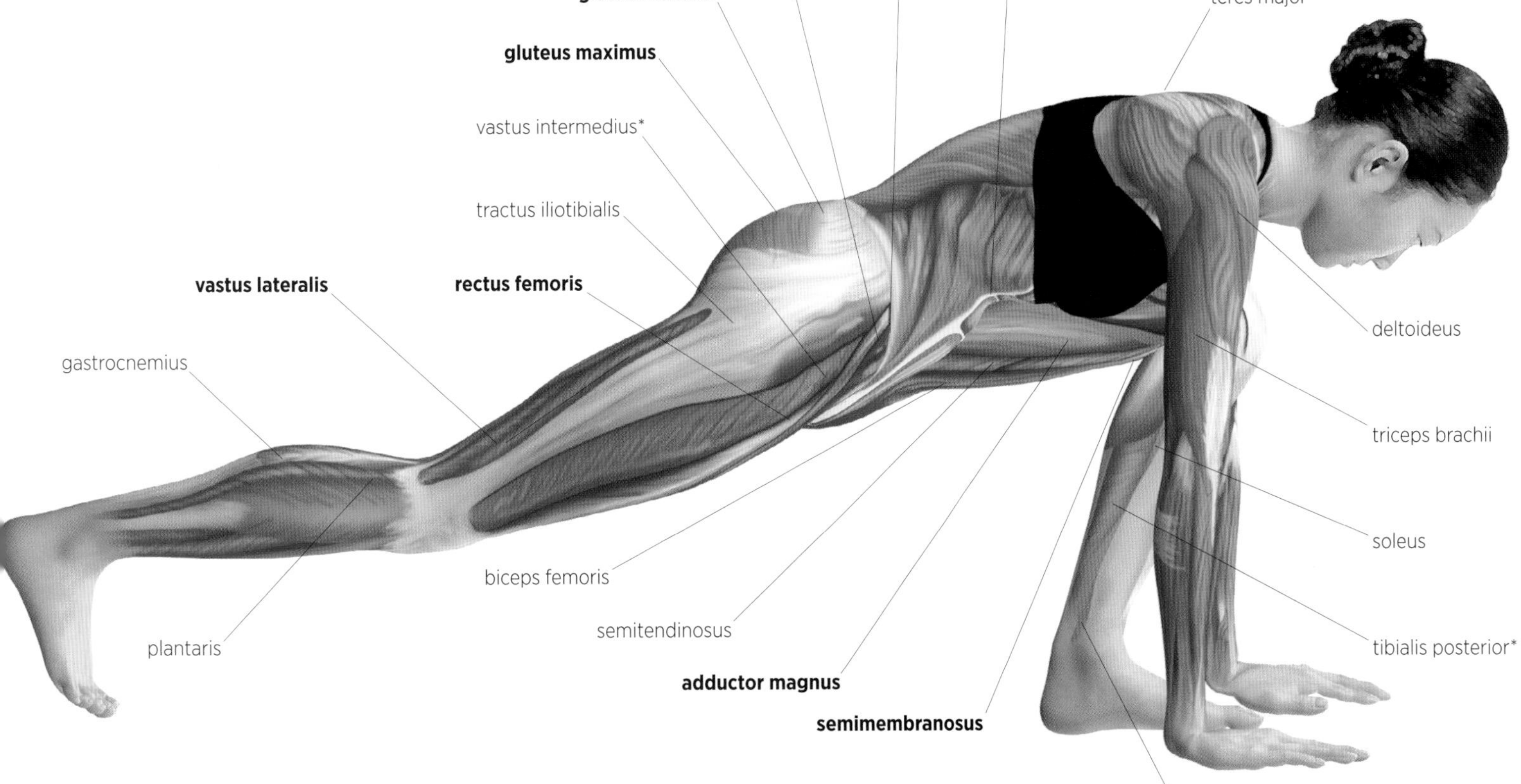

FACT FILE

TARGETS
- Quadriceps
- Gluteal area
- Hip flexors
- Hip adductors
- Hamstrings

EQUIPMENT
- None

BENEFITS
- Stretches groins
- Strengthens abdominals, legs, and arms
- Stretches hip flexors, shoulders, and chest

CAUTIONS
- Hip issues
- Knee issues

DO IT RIGHT
- Avoid dropping your back-extended knee to the floor.
- Bring your abdominals in, away from your thigh.
- Keep your hips firm as you stretch.
- If your back begins rounding when your fingertips touch the floor, bring your hands onto blocks to help elongate your spine.
- Avoid extending your front knee too far over your ankle.

levator scapulae*
splenius*
trapezius

Annotation Key
Bold text indicates target muscles
Light text indicates other working muscles
* indicates deep muscles

iliopsoas*
pectineus*
tensor fasciae latae
gluteus medius*
gluteus maximus
teres major
vastus intermedius*
tractus iliotibialis
vastus lateralis
rectus femoris
deltoideus
gastrocnemius
triceps brachii
soleus
biceps femoris
plantaris
semitendinosus
tibialis posterior*
adductor magnus
semimembranosus
flexor hallucis longus*

Cobra Stretch

Inspired by the Cobra Pose of yoga, this version also stretches and strengthens the spine. Do not try to lift your chest and shoulders too high at first; with this stretch, there is power in small movement.

HOW TO DO IT

- Lie facedown, legs extended behind you with toes pointed. Position the palms of your hands on the floor, slightly above your shoulders, and rest your elbows on the floor. 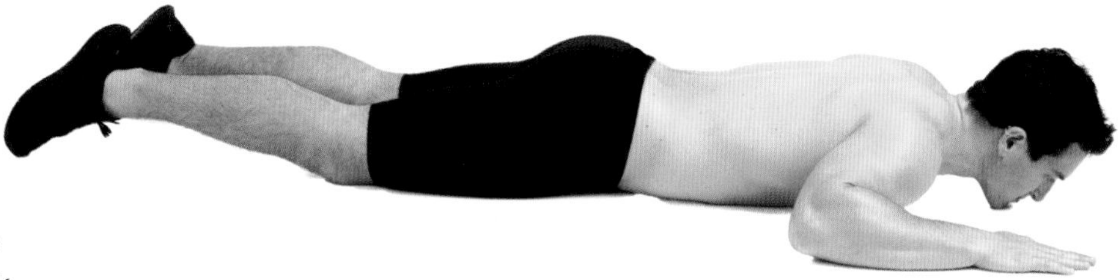
- Push down into the floor, and slowly lift through the top of your chest as you straighten your arms.
- Pull your tailbone down toward your pubis as you push your shoulders down and back.

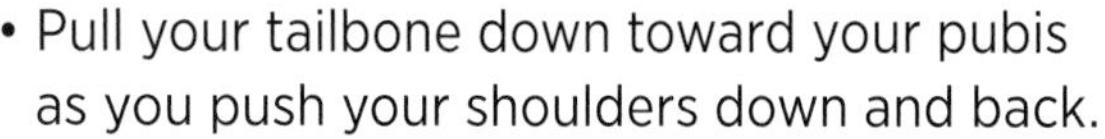

- Elongate your neck and gaze forward.

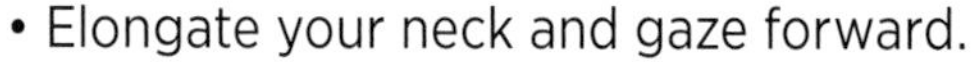

- Hold for a few moments, and then lower yourself to the floor. Repeat for the recommended repetitions.

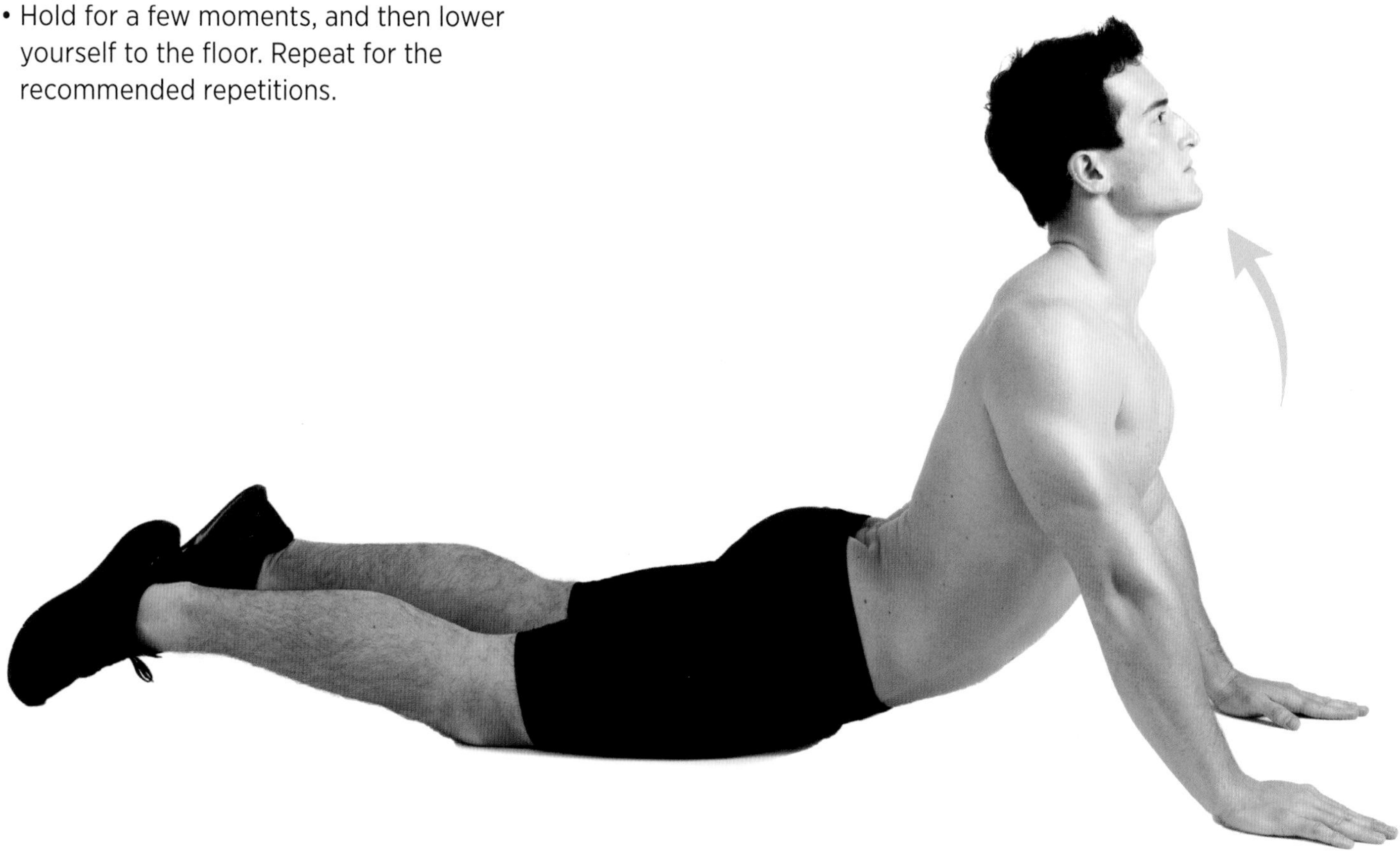

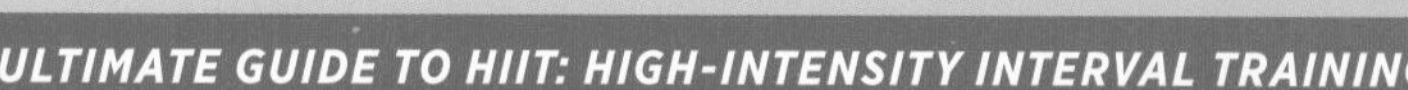

FACT FILE

TARGETS
- Abdominals
- Spine

EQUIPMENT
- None

BENEFITS
- Stretches chest, abdominals, and shoulders
- Strengthens spine

CAUTIONS
- Severe lower-back pain

MODIFICATION

EASIER: Follow the first two steps, only rising to rest on your forearms.

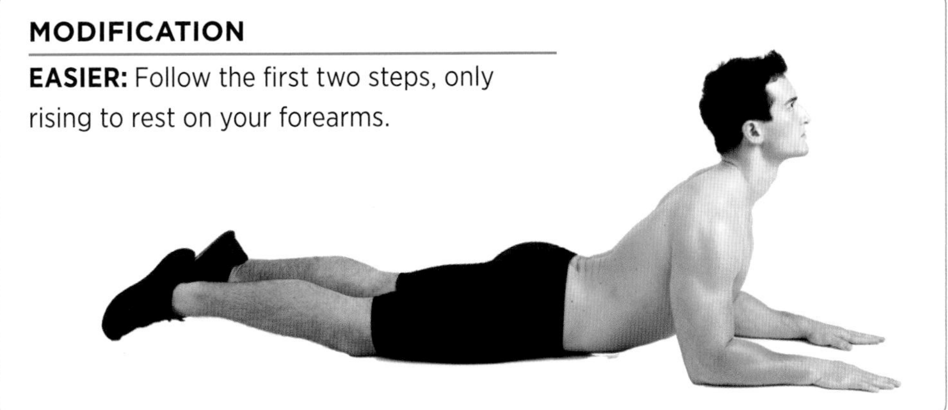

DO IT RIGHT

- Maintain pressure between the floor and your hips.
- Relax your shoulders, and keep them down and away from your ears.
- Avoid tipping your head too far backward; gaze forward.
- Keep your elbows pulled in toward your body.
- Lift from your chest and back, rather than depending too much on your arms to create the arch in your back.
- Avoid splaying your elbows out to the sides.
- Avoid lifting your hips off the floor.
- Avoid twisting your neck.

Annotation Key

Bold text indicates target muscles

Light text indicates other working muscles

* indicates deep muscles

obliquus externus

obliquus internus*

transversus abdominis*

rectus abdominis

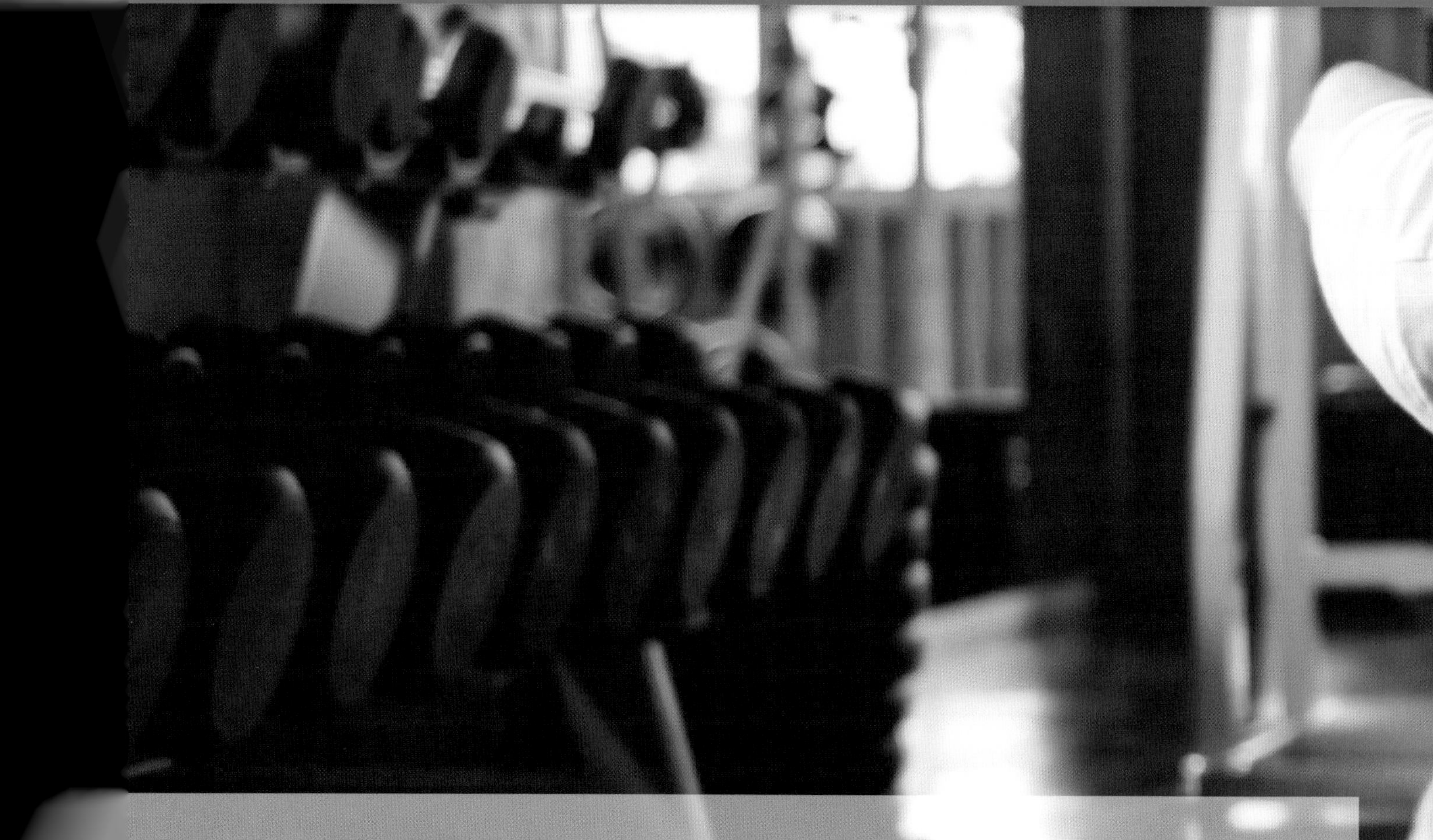

CHAPTER TWO

BODY-WEIGHT EXERCISES

Bring the gym with you—no equipment needed! This chapter will introduce and go over a multitude of high-intensity exercises that you can perform with little to no equipment at all. But don't be fooled, some of the hardest and most effective exercises utilize your body weight. The human body is amazing in its potential, and these exercises are here to bring that potential out. Demanding coordination, stabilization, strength, endurance, and motivation, this chapter contains exercises that are perfect for those who travel or who exercise at home.

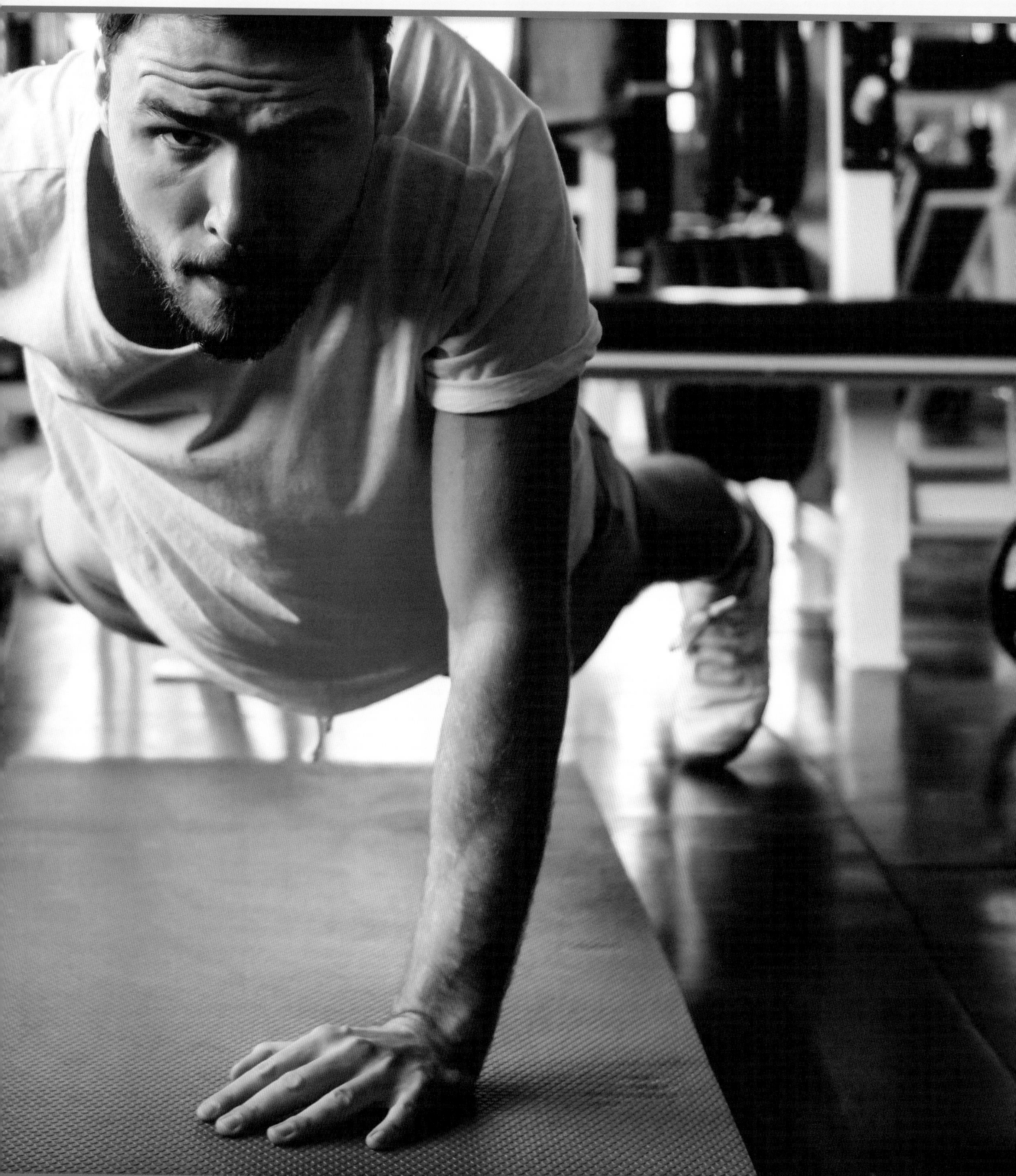

Pull-Up

The Pull-Up—also known as a Neutral-Grip Pull-Up—is a foundational upper-body strength exercise often used as a gauge of overall fitness. The neutral-grip hand position places emphasis on your latissimus dorsi, the broad, flat muscle of your upper back.

HOW TO DO IT

- Standing in front of a pull-up bar, either reach up or step on a stool. Place your hands shoulder-width apart on the bar, and hang until your arms are straight.

- Pull yourself up until your chest touches the bar. Hold for a slight pause, and then lower yourself slowly to the hanging position. Repeat for the recommended repetitions.

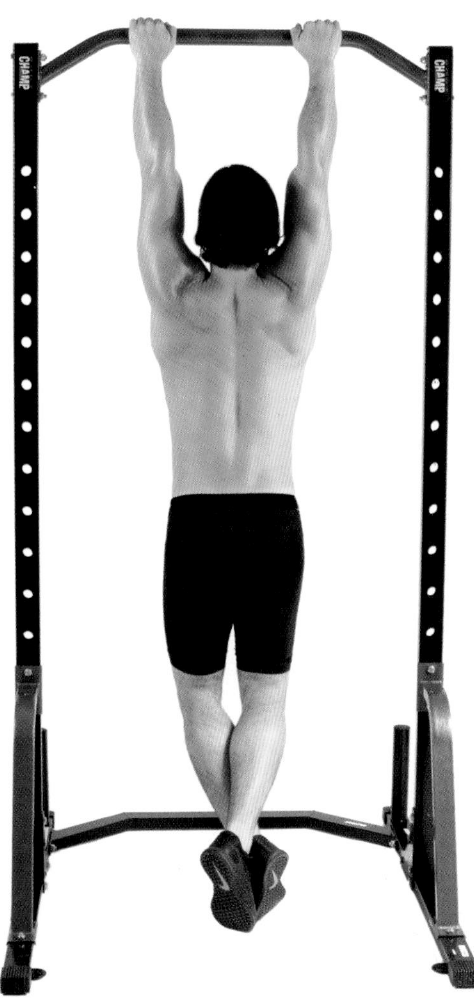

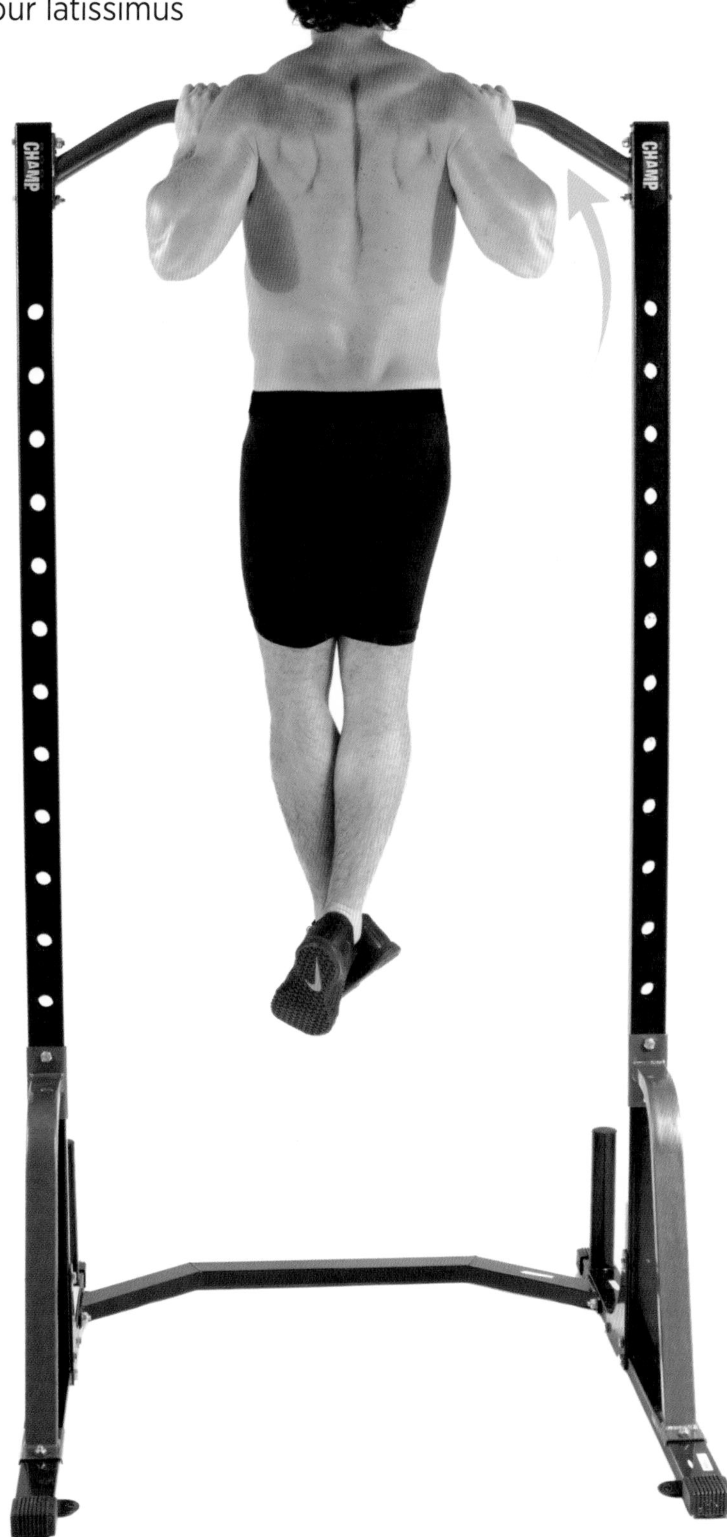

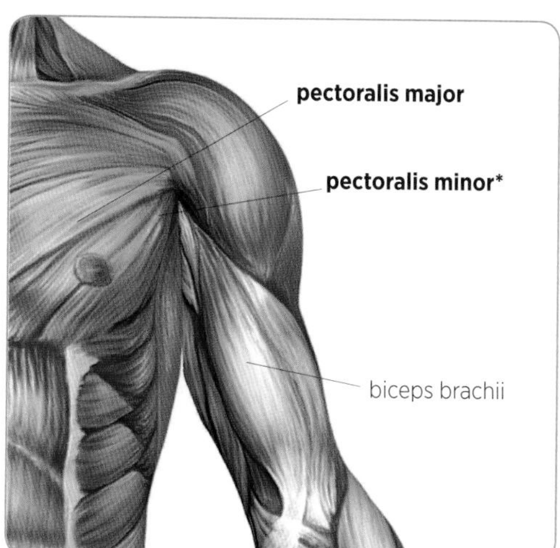

Annotation Key

Bold text indicates target muscles

Light text indicates other working muscles

* indicates deep muscles

levator scapulae*

trapezius

rhomboideus*

teres major

brachialis

triceps brachii

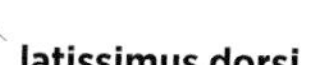

FACT FILE

TARGETS
- Latissimus dorsi

EQUIPMENT
- Pull-up bar

BENEFITS
- Strengthens back and arms

CAUTIONS
- Shoulder issues
- Wrist issues

MODIFICATION

EASIER: To perform a Close-Grip Pull-Up, grasp the bar with a firm overhand grip with your hands touching or separated by no more than 6 inches. Continue as you would for the Neutral-Grip Pull-Up. The narrow separation between your hands in this variation ensures a greater emphasis on your lower lats.

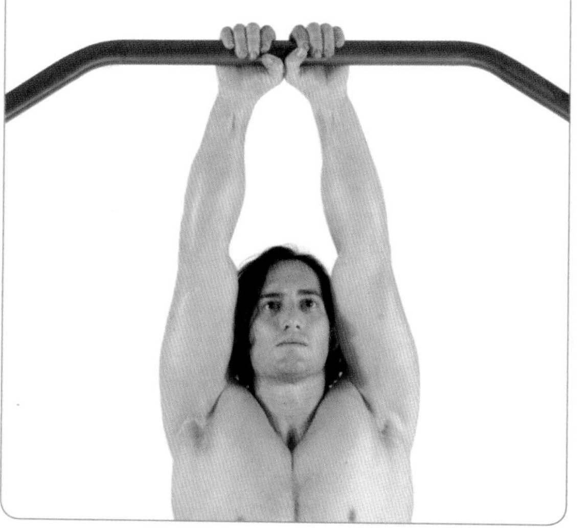

DO IT RIGHT

- Make sure your arms are straight in the hanging position, or the rep does not count.
- To strengthen your grip while performing pull-ups, grip your thumb over the top of the bar rather than wrapping it around the bar.
- Avoid kipping, or swinging, your body—a kipping movement can injure your rotator cuffs.

Chin-Up

Also known as a Reverse-Grip Pull-Up, this exercise places more emphasis on your biceps than other pull-ups. The reverse grip means that you grasp the bar with an underhand grip.

HOW TO DO IT

- Standing in front of a pull-up bar, either reach up or step on a stool. Place your hands shoulder-width apart, and take a close underhand grip on the bar, and hang until your arms are straight.
- Cross your legs at the ankles, and pull yourself up until your chin is as close to the bar as possible. With control, lower yourself to the hanging position. Repeat for the recommended repetitions.

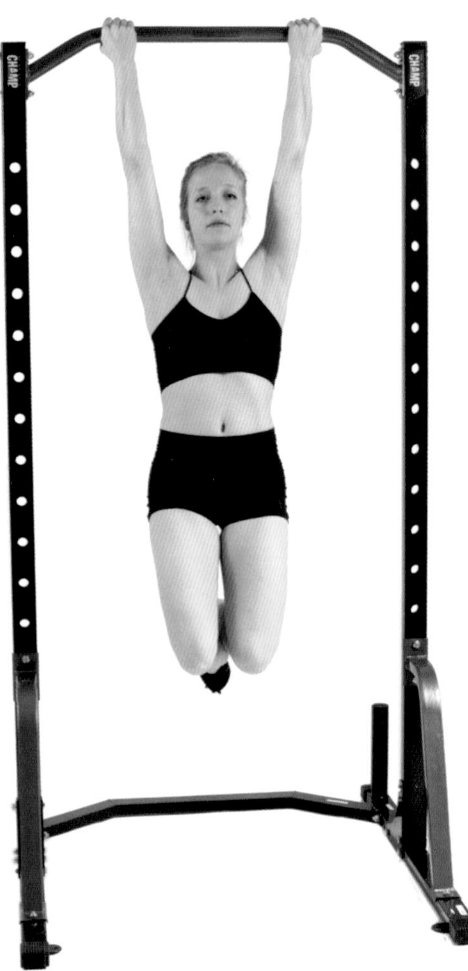

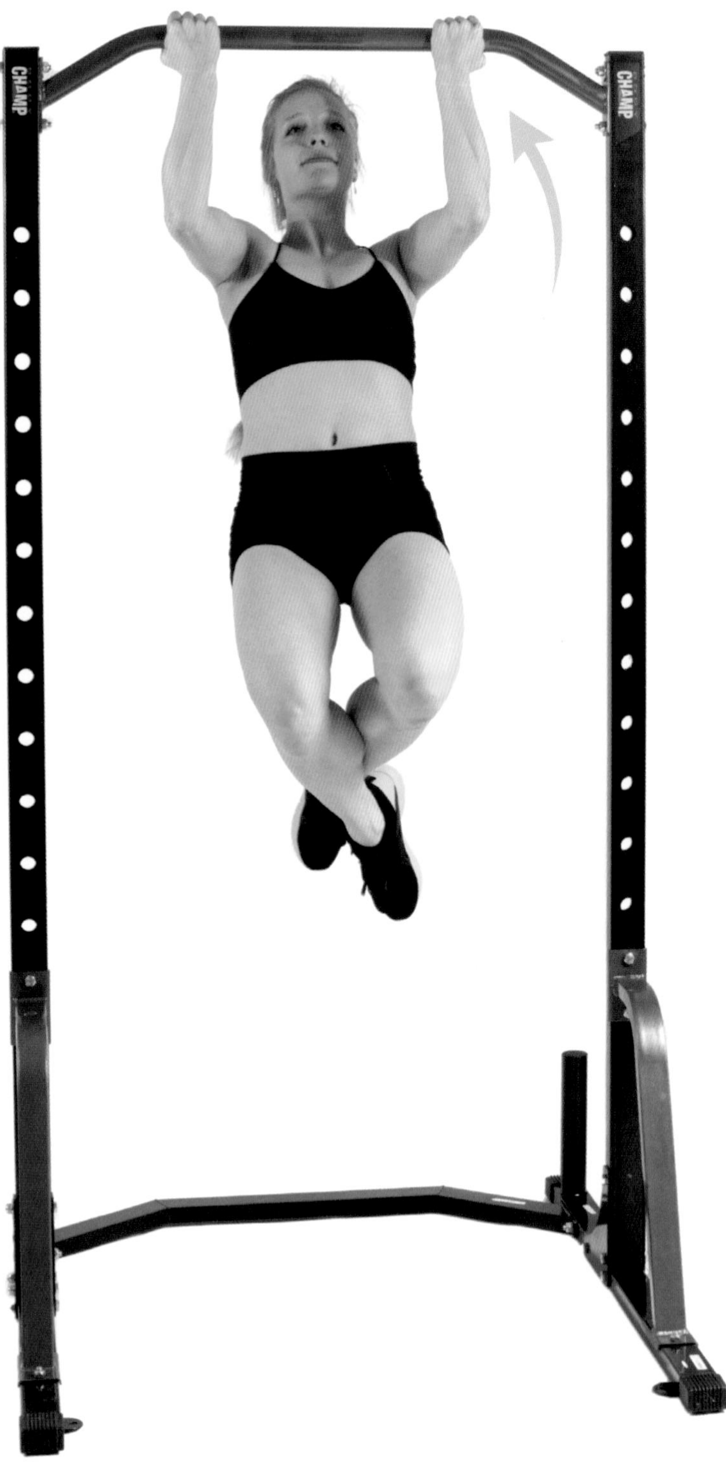

DO IT RIGHT

- Make sure your arms are straight in the hanging position, or the rep does not count.
- Avoid suddenly dropping your body weight.
- Avoid kipping, or swinging, your body—a kipping movement can injure your rotator cuffs.

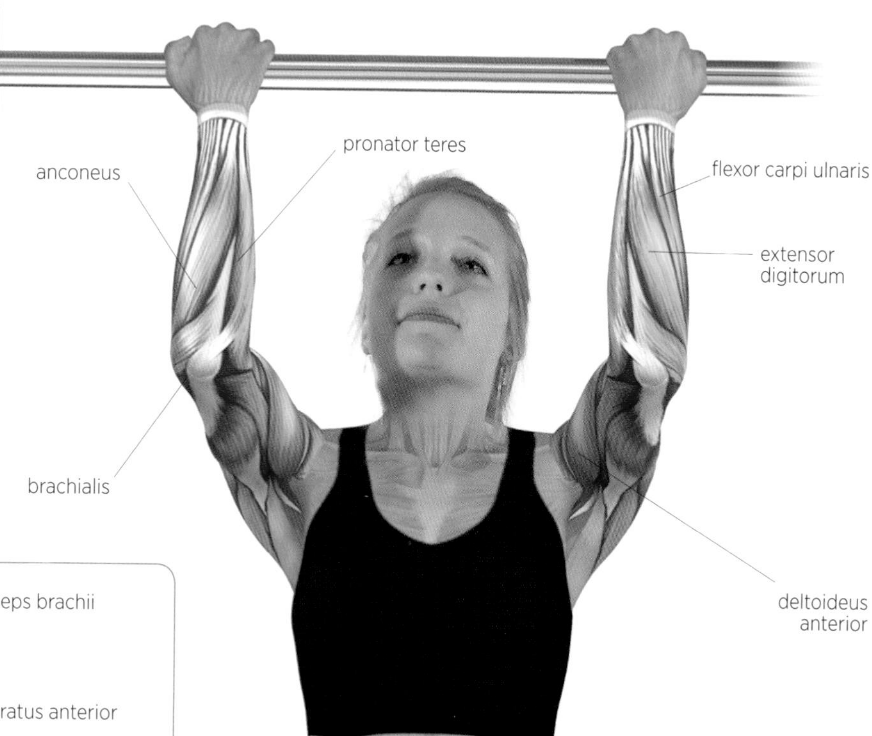

FACT FILE

TARGETS
- Latissimus dorsi
- Biceps brachii

EQUIPMENT
- Pull-up bar

BENEFITS
- Strengthens back and arms

CAUTIONS
- Shoulder issues
- Wrist issues

Annotation Key

Bold text indicates target muscles
Light text indicates other working muscles
* indicates deep muscles

Arm Hauler

A go-to exercise of special forces teams, the Arm Hauler builds upper-back and rear-shoulder strength. It is also an effective stabilizing exercise that can help prevent shoulder injuries.

HOW TO DO IT

- Lie facedown, and spread your arms wide, keeping them level with your shoulders.
- Lift your head, keeping your chin up while arching your lower back. Bring your arms off the floor, and reach as far behind you as possible.
- Without letting your hands touch the floor, bring your arms forward in front of you, touching your fingers together.
- Bring your hands back to the starting position, and repeat for the recommended repetitions.

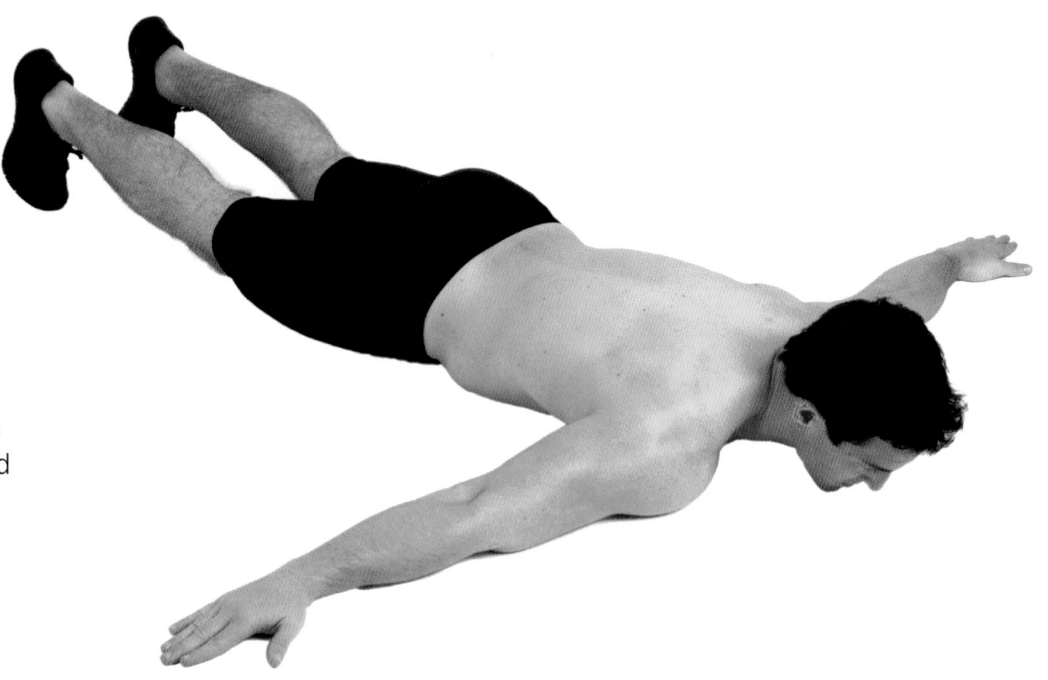

DO IT RIGHT

- Keep your chin up.
- Keep your lower back arched.
- Avoid dropping your head so that your chin touches the floor.

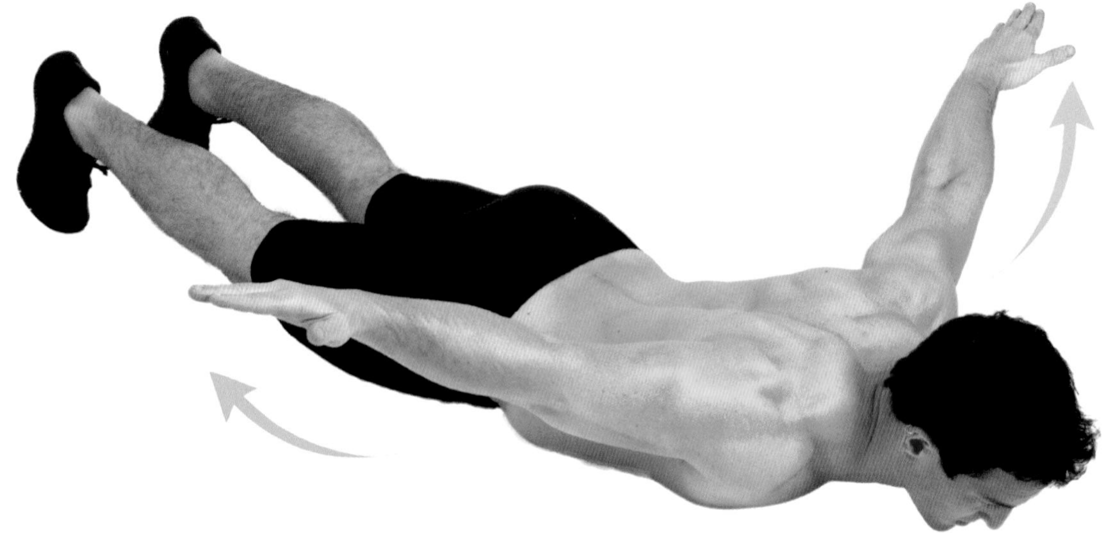

FACT FILE

TARGETS
- Upper back
- Shoulders

EQUIPMENT
- None

BENEFITS
- Strengthens and stabilizes back and shoulders

CAUTIONS
- Shoulder issues

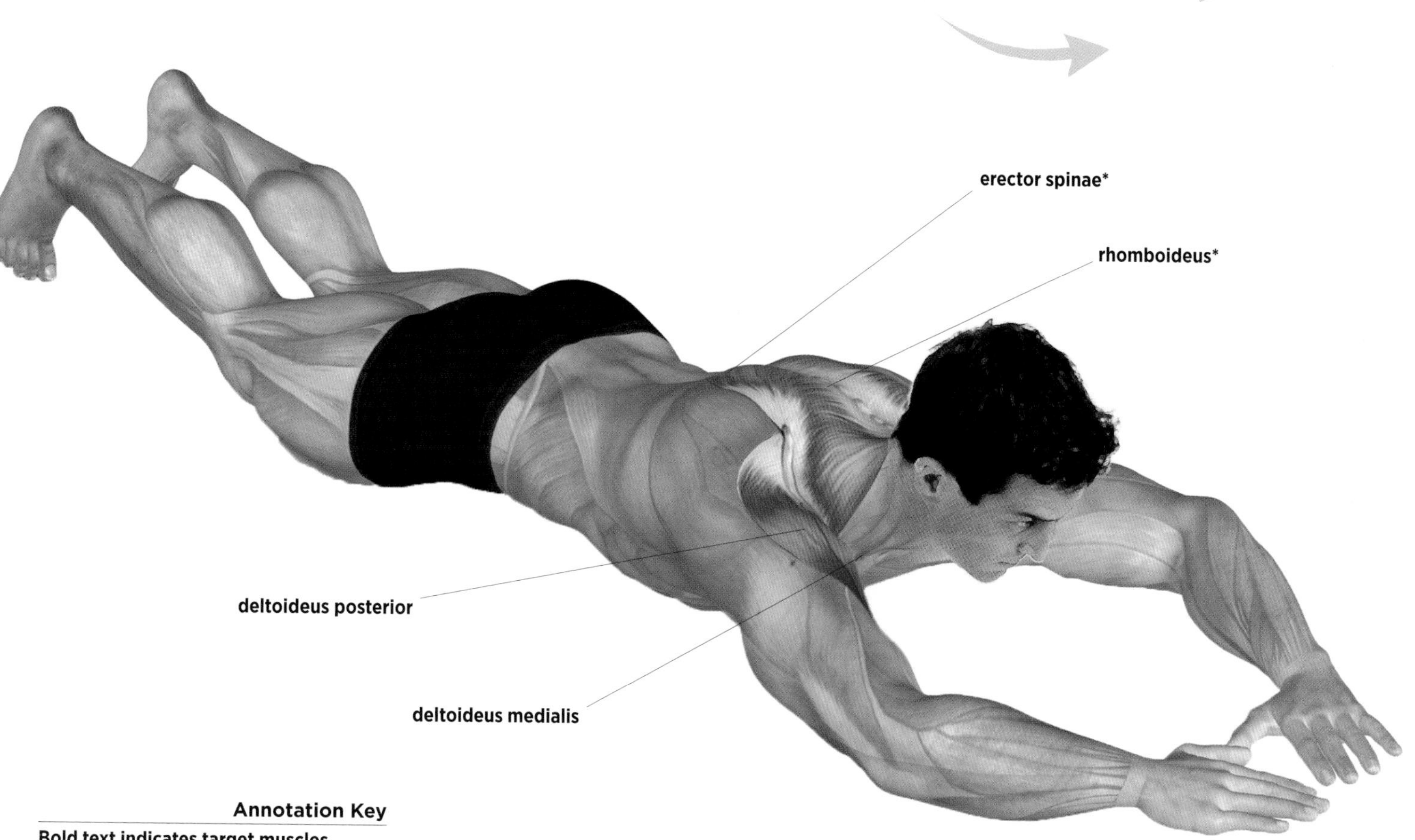

Annotation Key

Bold text indicates target muscles

Light text indicates other working muscles

* indicates deep muscles

Swimmer

An exercise that looks simple, the Swimmer is actually difficult to perform correctly. It engages just about every muscle in your body, but it especially targets your hip extensors, both stretching and strengthening them. It is also an effective back exercise for your back, strengthening the muscles that support your spine.

HOW TO DO IT

- Lie facedown with your legs hip-width apart. Stretch your arms upward beside your ears on the floor. Engage your pelvic floor, and draw your navel into your spine.
- Extend through your upper back as you lift your left arm and right leg simultaneously. Lift your head and shoulders off the floor.
- Lower your arm and leg to the starting position, maintaining a stretch in your limbs throughout.
- Extend your opposite arm and leg off the floor, lengthening and lifting your head and shoulders.
- Elongate your limbs as you return to the starting position. Repeat, alternating sides for the recommended repetitions.

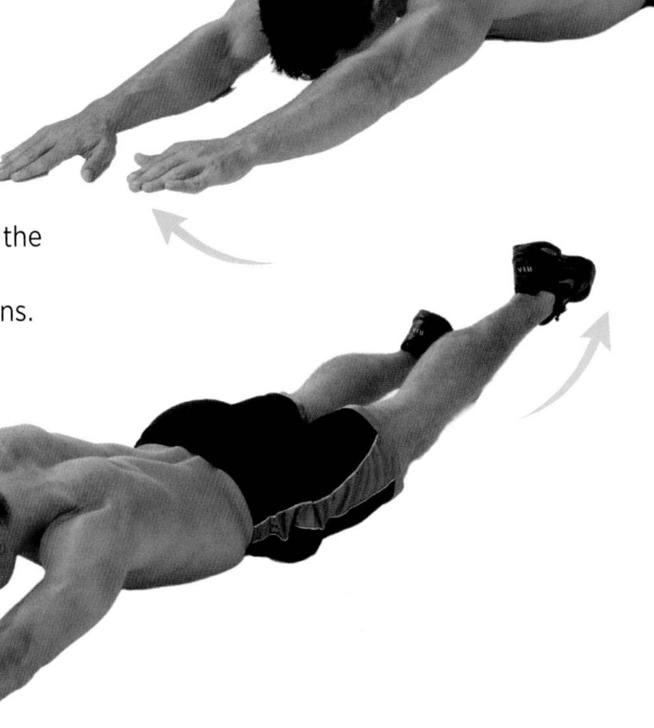

DO IT RIGHT

- Extend your limbs as long as possible in opposite directions.
- Keep your glutes tightly squeezed and your navel drawn in.
- Keep your neck long and relaxed.
- Avoid allowing your shoulders to lift toward your ears.

MODIFICATION

HARDER: Instead of lifting the opposite leg and arm, lift both arms and legs simultaneously, continuing to draw your navel into your spine. This version of the exercise is known as the Superman.

Annotation Key

Bold text indicates target muscles

Light text indicates other working muscles

* indicates deep muscles

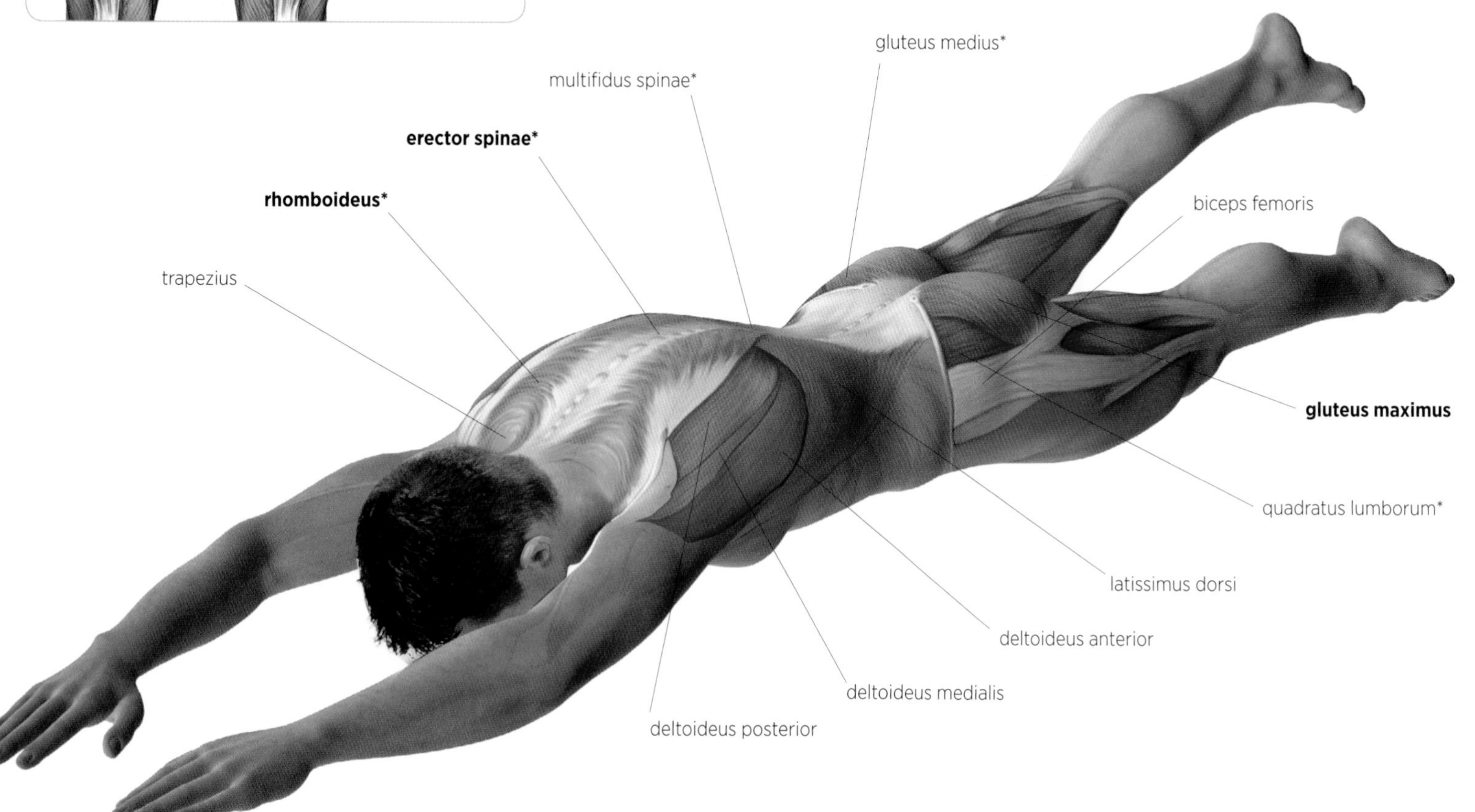

FACT FILE

TARGETS
- Hips
- Spine

EQUIPMENT
- None

BENEFITS
- Strengthens hip and spine extensors
- Challenges stabilization of the spine against rotation

CAUTIONS
- Lower-back pain
- Extreme curvature of upper spine
- Curvature of lower spine

Advanced Superman

The Advanced Superman builds on the Swimmer (pages 50–51), creating a medium-intensity exercise that strengthens your core and lower-back muscles.

FACT FILE

TARGETS
- Core
- Lower back

EQUIPMENT
- None

BENEFITS
- Strengthens core and lower back

CAUTIONS
- Wrist pain
- Shoulder issues
- Lower-back pain

HOW TO DO IT

- Lie facedown, and bend your elbows, placing your hands behind your ears. Extend your legs, and press down into the floor with your thighs and the tops of your feet.

- Lift your chest and legs off the floor. Hold for a few moments, and then lower yourself to the floor. Repeat for the recommended repetitions.

DO IT RIGHT
- Keep your body in a straight line.
- Avoid bending your knees.
- Avoid overarching your back.

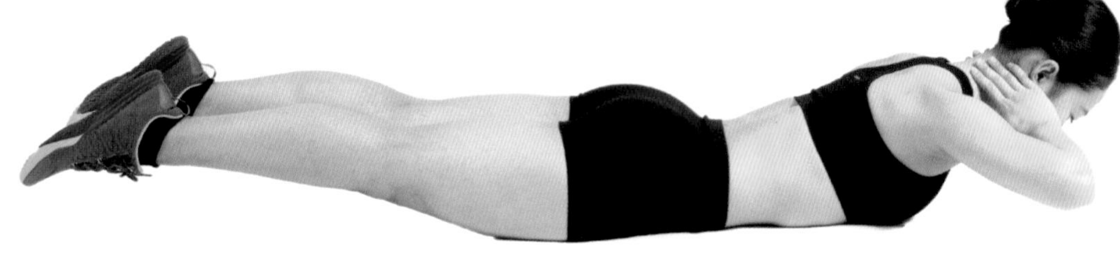

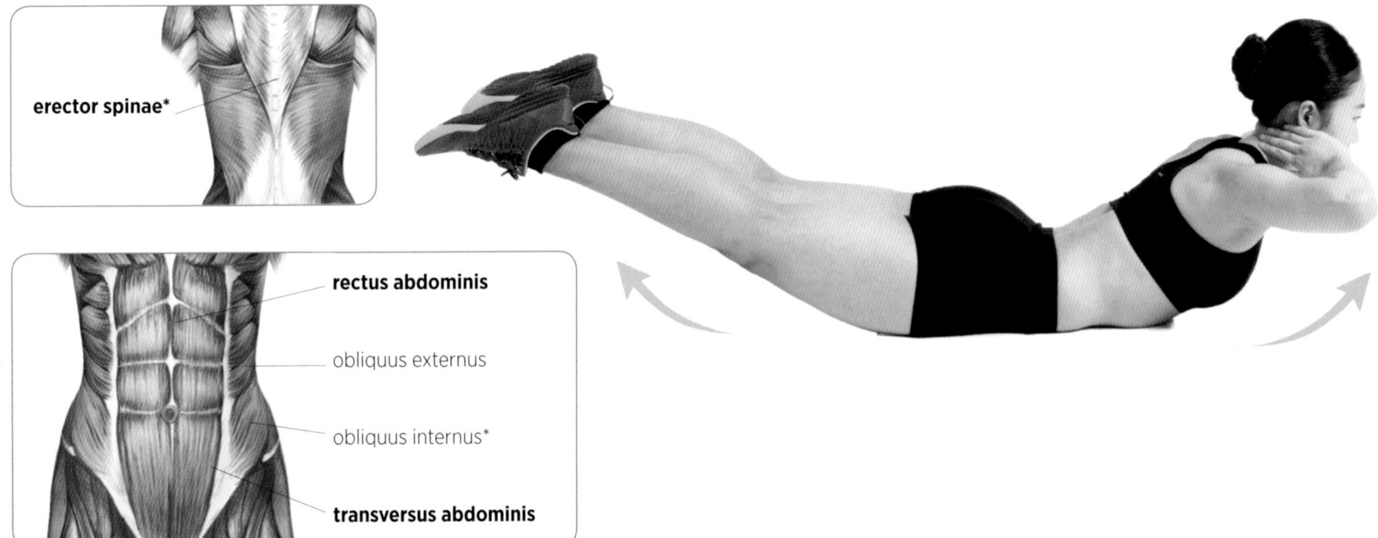

The Y

Named for the shape your body takes while performing it, The Y is a great body-weight exercise that develops your postural muscles. If you want a healthier back, this strengthener is one of the essentials you'll need to keep in your toolbox.

HOW TO DO IT

- Lie facedown on the floor with arms extended front and above you, placing your body in the shape of a Y.
- Keeping your lower body and torso planted on the floor, lift both arms. Lead with your thumbs and reach as high as possible.
- Return your arms to the floor, and repeat for the recommended repetitions.

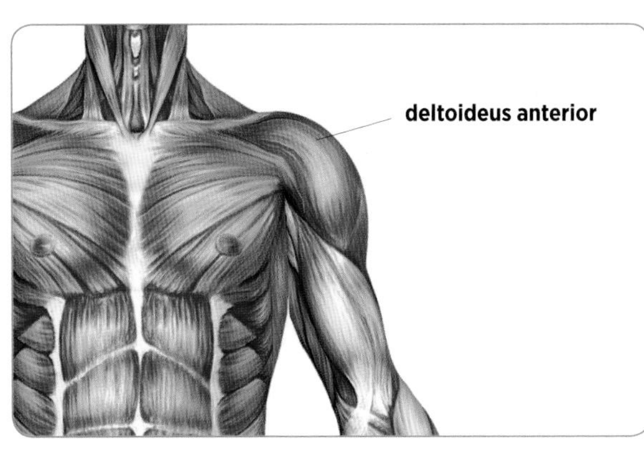

FACT FILE

TARGETS
- Deltoids
- Middle back

EQUIPMENT
- None

BENEFITS
- Warms up muscles
- Promotes proper scapular-humeral movement
- Strengthens and tones midscapular muscles

CAUTIONS
- Lower-back pain
- Extreme curvature of upper spine
- Curvature of lower spine

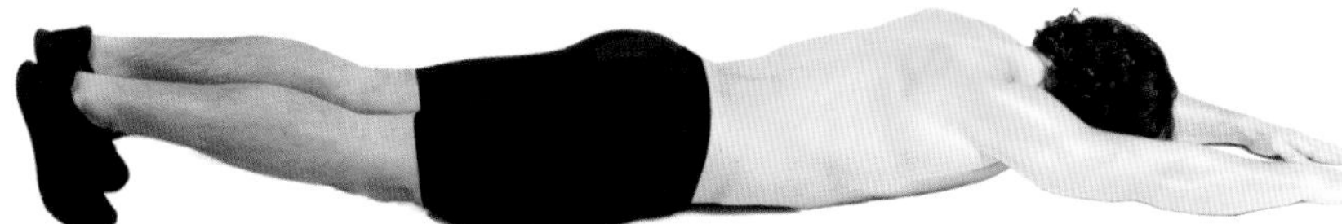

DO IT RIGHT

- Keep your torso on the floor.
- Avoid excessive trunk movement during exercise.
- Flare your hands out to ease shoulder stress.

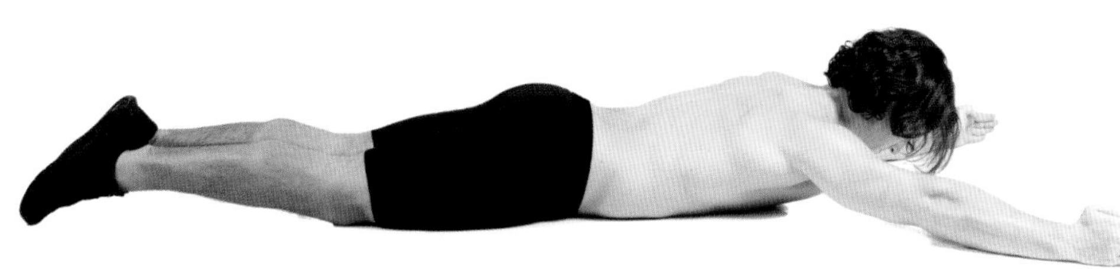

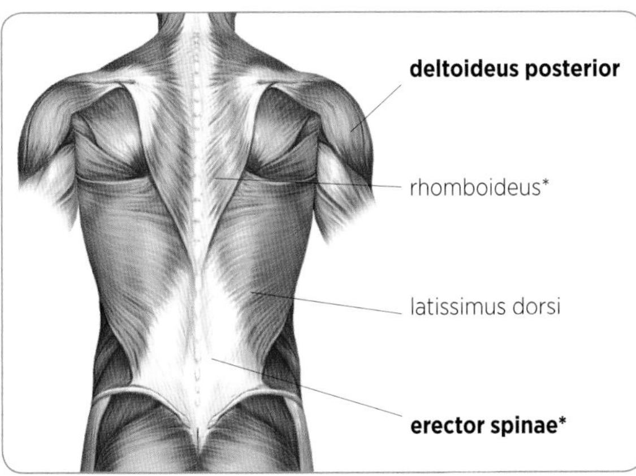

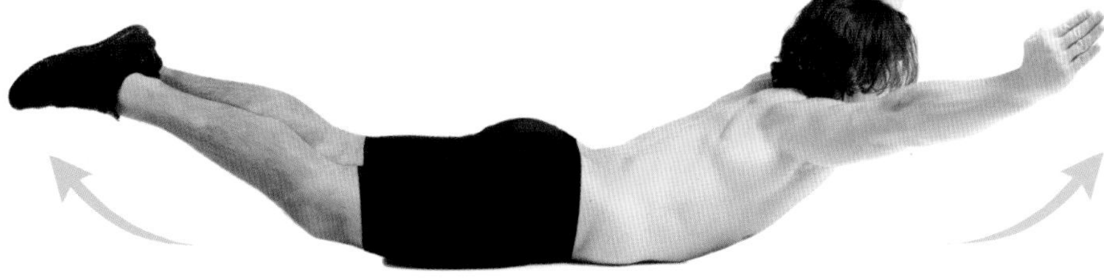

Annotation Key
Bold text indicates target muscles
Light text indicates other working muscles
* indicates deep muscles

Bird-Dog

The Bird-Dog is an effective exercise for building back, abdominal, and glute strength and developing core body strength. It has the added bonus of improving balance and smooth coordination.

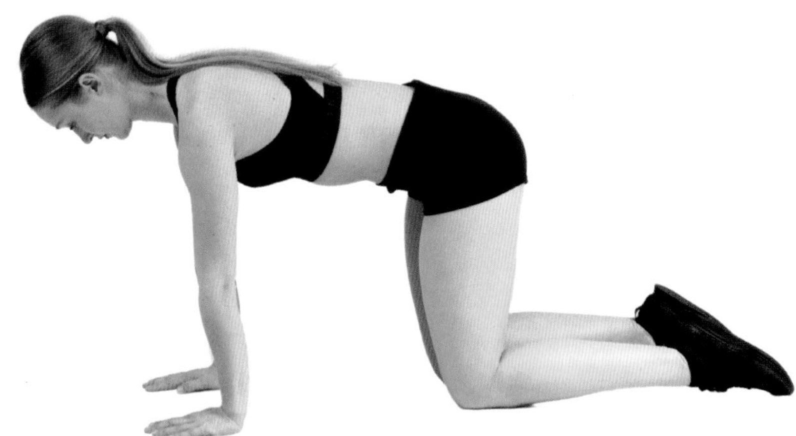

HOW TO DO IT

- Kneel on all fours with your back straight and your abdominals pulled in.
- Keeping your torso stable and your abdominals engaged, contract your right arm and your left leg into your body.
- Extend your right arm and left leg outward. Hold the extended position for the recommended time.
- Return to the starting position, and repeat on the opposite side.

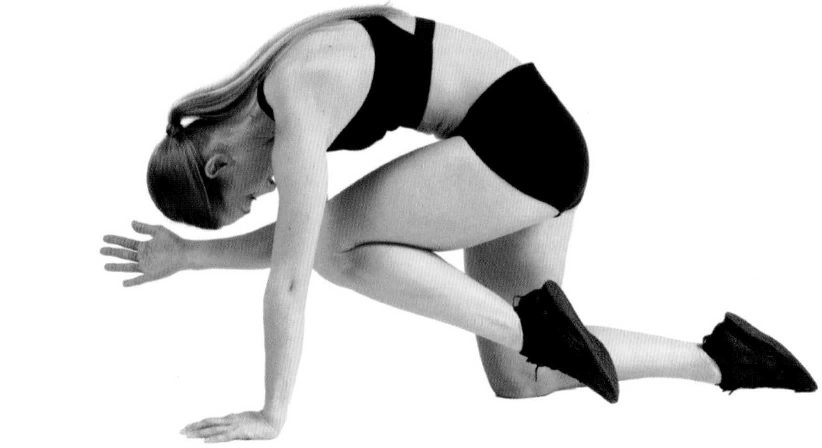

DO IT RIGHT

- Move slowly and with control.
- Keep your neck relaxed and your gaze toward the floor.
- Tuck your chin slightly while contracting your arm and leg inward.
- Keep your abs pulled.
- Avoid twisting your torso.
- Avoid arching your back while your arm and leg are extended.

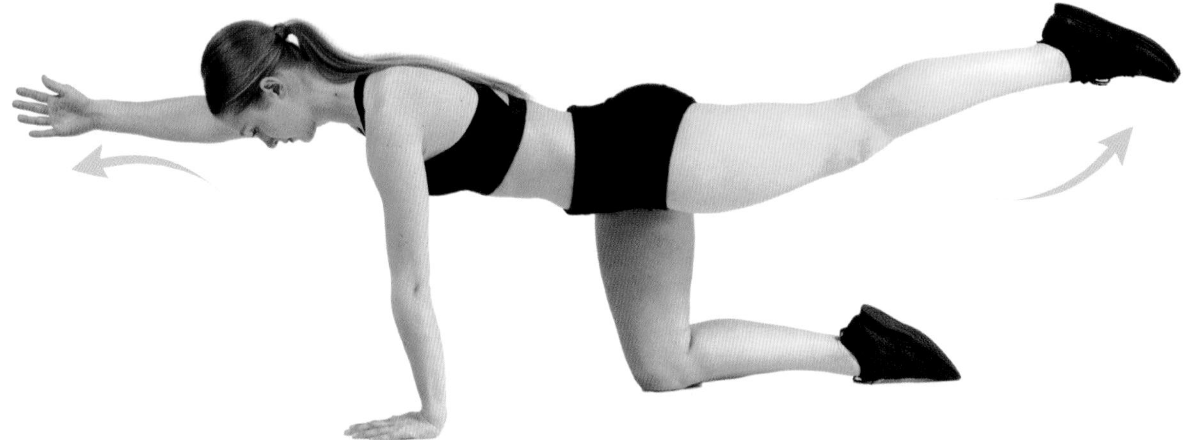

FACT FILE

TARGETS
- Abdominals
- Back
- Glutes

EQUIPMENT
- None

BENEFITS
- Stretches and tones abdominals, arms, and legs
- Hones balance and coordination

CAUTIONS
- Wrist pain
- Lower-back pain
- Knee injury

MODIFICATION

HARDER: Instead of kneeling, press into a plank position to begin, and then raise the opposite arm and leg.

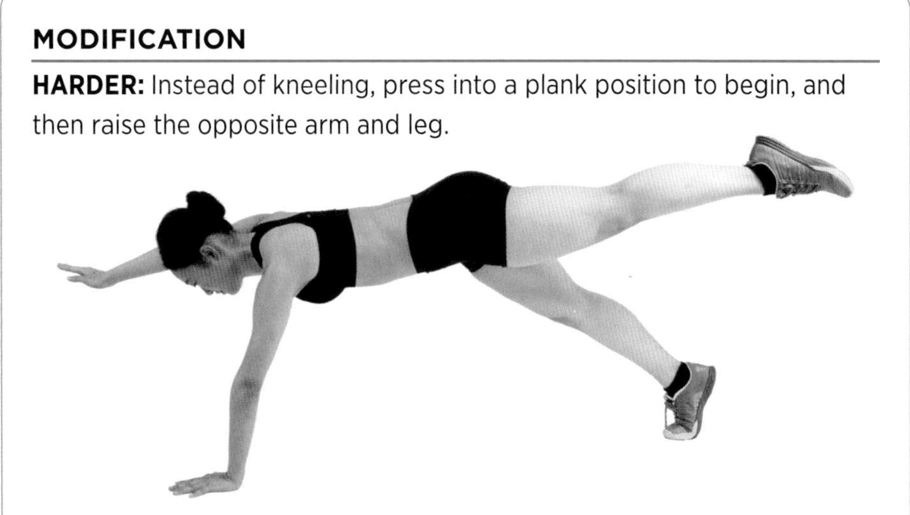

gluteus medius*
gluteus maximus
gluteus minimus*
semitendinosus
latissimus dorsi
biceps femoris
semimembranosus
deltoideus anterior
vastus lateralis
deltoideus medialis
rectus femoris
vastus intermedius
deltoideus posterior
serratus anterior
rectus abdominis
erector spinae*
adductor magnus
adductor longus
vastus medialis
transversus abdominis*

trapezius
infraspinatus*
supraspinatus*
teres minor
subscapularis*

Annotation Key
Bold text indicates target muscles
Light text indicates other working muscles
* indicates deep muscles

Swiss Ball Hyperextension

If you do not have access to a gym's hyperextension machine, performing this exercise on a Swiss ball is a great way to work your lower-back muscles. It also strengthens you abdominals and glutes.

HOW TO DO IT

- Lie facedown on top of a Swiss ball, with your abdominals covering most of the ball, your legs spread with toes on the floor, and your arms behind your head. Push your toes into the floor for stability.
- Raise your torso so that it forms a line with the lower half of your body.
- Squeeze your glutes as you lower your upper body, and then raise it back to the starting position.
- Continue lowering and raising, for the recommended repetitions.

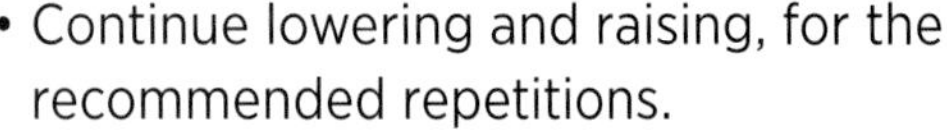

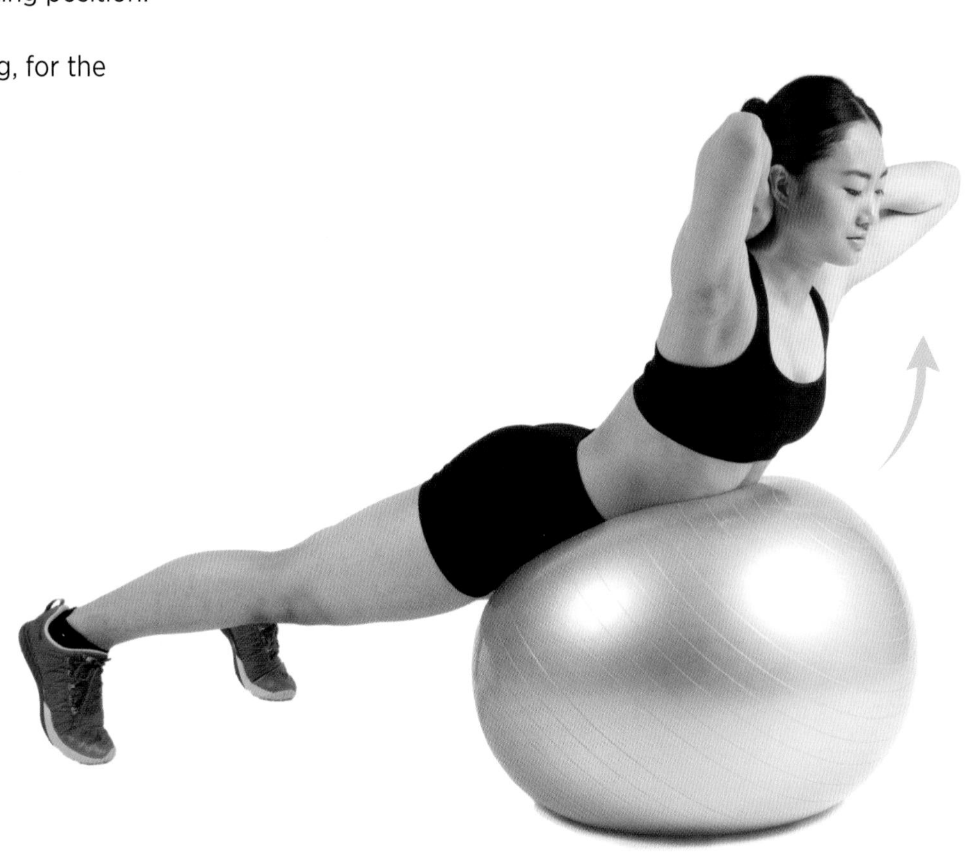

DO IT RIGHT

- Complete the full range of motion in both the negative (the downward stretch) and positive (the upward motion) movements of the exercise.
- Avoid overcontracting or hyperextending your back at the top of the movement.

FACT FILE

TARGETS
- Lower back
- Abdominals
- Glutes

EQUIPMENT
- Swiss ball

BENEFITS
- Strengthens abdominals, lower back and glutes

CAUTIONS
- Lower-back issues
- Neck issues

rectus abdominis
obliquus internus*
transversus abdominis*
iliopsoas*

trapezius
deltoideus medialis
deltoideus posterior
infraspinatus*
supraspinatus*
subscapularis*
rhomboideus*
erector spinae*

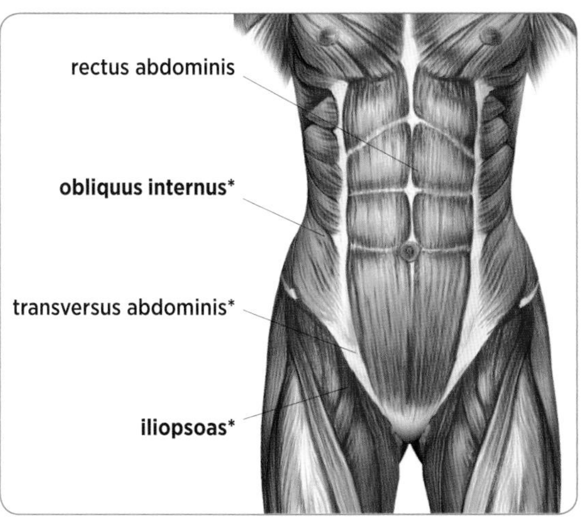

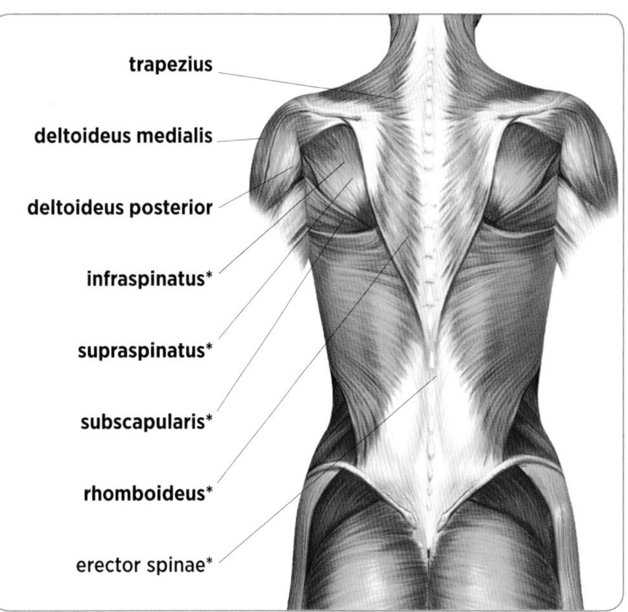

Annotation Key

Bold text indicates target muscles

Light text indicates other working muscles

* indicates deep muscles

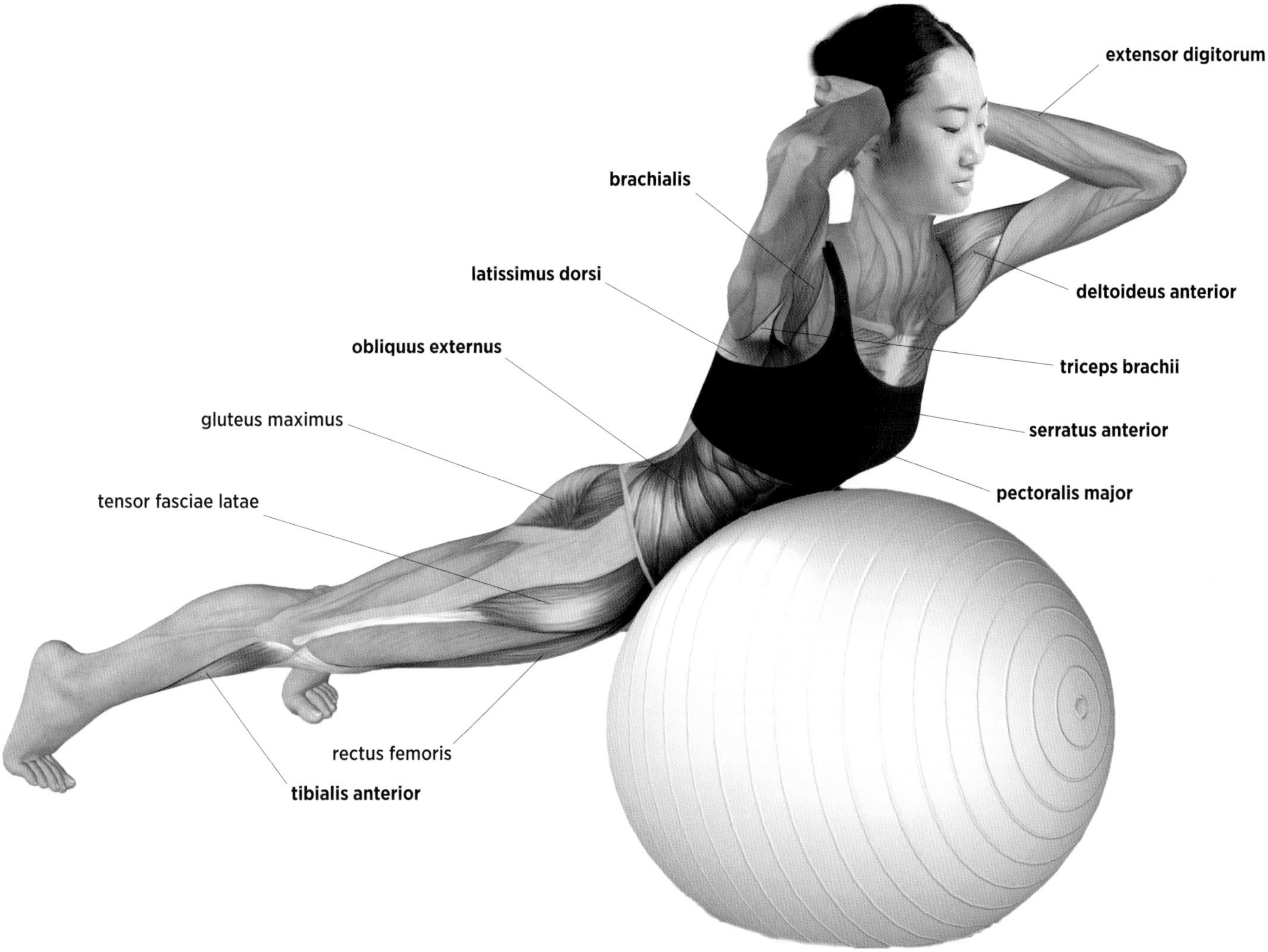

extensor digitorum
brachialis
latissimus dorsi
deltoideus anterior
obliquus externus
triceps brachii
gluteus maximus
serratus anterior
pectoralis major
tensor fasciae latae
rectus femoris
tibialis anterior

Rotated Back Extension

The Rotated Back Extension, performed on a Swiss ball, engages your abdominals to make it a great core exercise. It also provides your back and sides with a significant stretch.

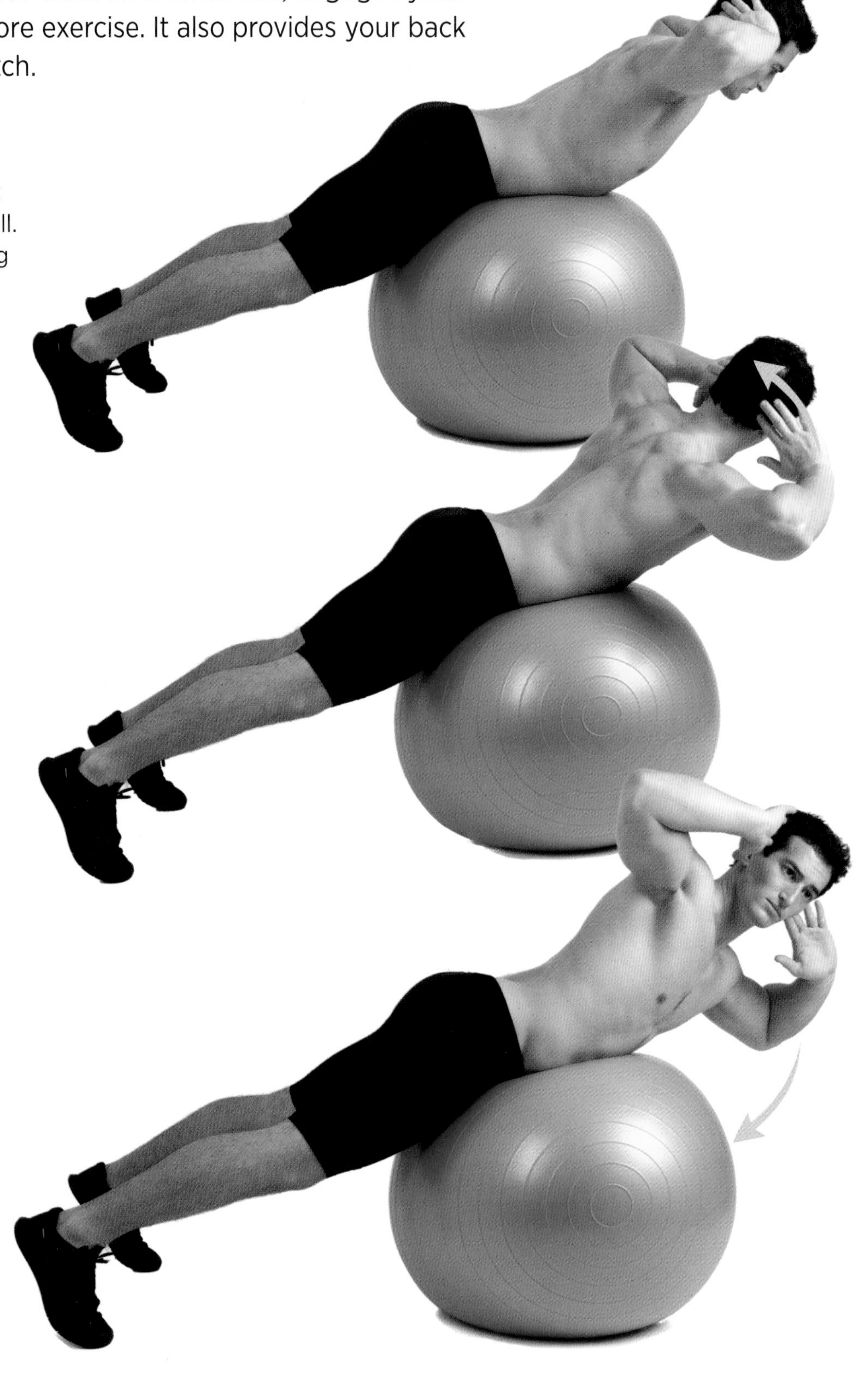

HOW TO DO IT

- Lie facedown on a Swiss ball so that your navel is on the center of the ball. Extend your legs behind you, resting on your toes.
- Place your hands behind your head, with your elbows out.
- Extend your back, lifting your chest away from the ball, and rotate your torso to the right.
- Hold for a few moments, and then return to the starting position.
- Repeat on the opposite side, alternating sides for the recommended repetitions.

DO IT RIGHT

- Keep your toes firmly planted on the floor.
- Keep your arms out at a 90-degree angle to your body with your elbows bent.
- Widen your feet for increased stability.
- Avoid shifting your hips as you rotate—hold them square to the ball throughout the movement.

FACT FILE

TARGETS
- Middle Back
- Lower Back
- Obliques

EQUIPMENT
- Swiss ball

BENEFITS
- Stretches lower back and obliques
- Strengthens core and back

CAUTIONS
- Neck issues
- Lower-back pain

pectoralis major
deltoideus anterior
rectus abdominis
obliquus externus
serratus anterior
transversus abdominis*
obliquus internus*
sartorius
iliopsoas*

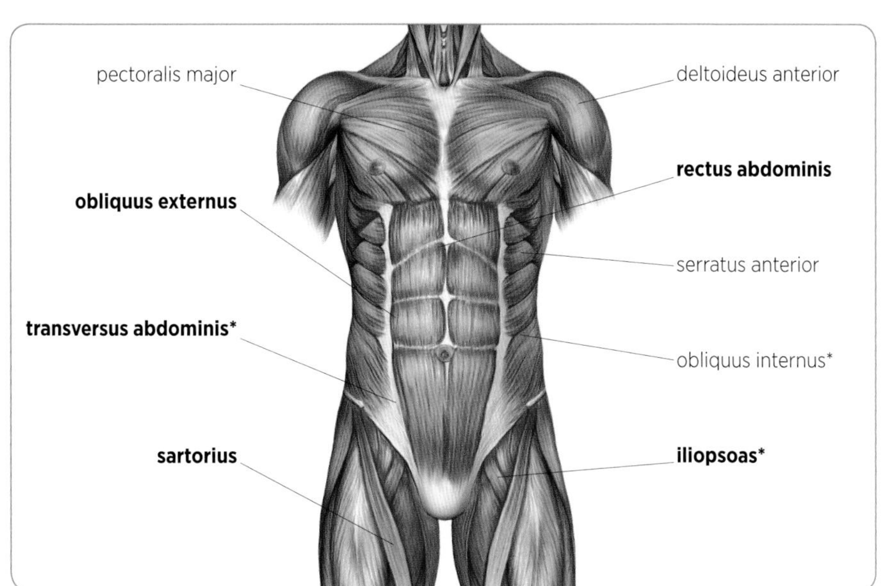

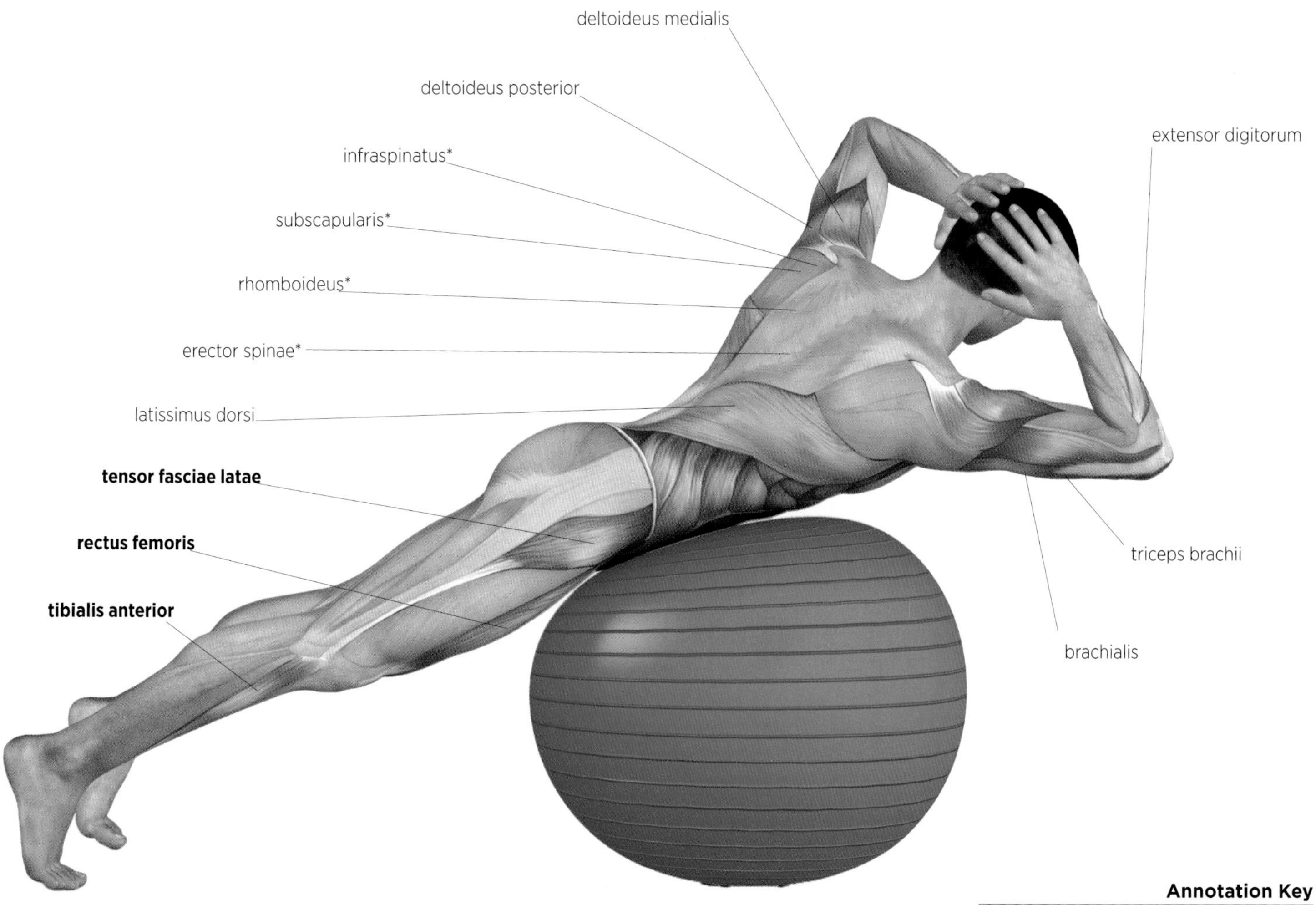

deltoideus medialis
deltoideus posterior
extensor digitorum
infraspinatus*
subscapularis*
rhomboideus*
erector spinae*
latissimus dorsi
tensor fasciae latae
rectus femoris
triceps brachii
tibialis anterior
brachialis

Annotation Key

Bold text indicates target muscles
Light text indicates other working muscles
* indicates deep muscles

Good Morning

Good Mornings are a healthy back essential to keep in your toolbox. This simple exercise specifically focuses on your erector spinae, a bundle of deep muscles also known as your lumbar extensors. By strengthening these muscles, you can avoid lower back pain.

FACT FILE

TARGETS
- Lumbar extensors
- Hamstrings
- Glutes
- Core

EQUIPMENT
- None

BENEFITS
- Warms up muscles
- Strengthens back, core, legs, and glutes

CAUTIONS
- Severe lower-back pain

HOW TO DO IT

- Stand with your feet hips-width apart, arms positioned behind your head.
- Keeping your lower back in a neutral position and your legs straight, hinge at the hip to 90 degrees, or as far down as flexibility will allow.
- Return to upright position, by engaging your hip extensors, pushing your hips forward until you have assumed the starting position.

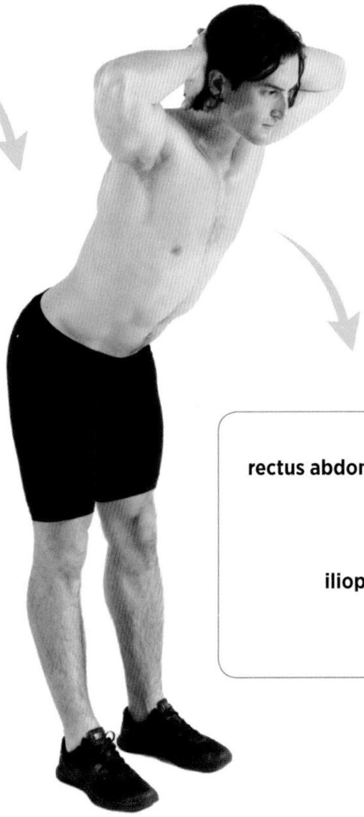

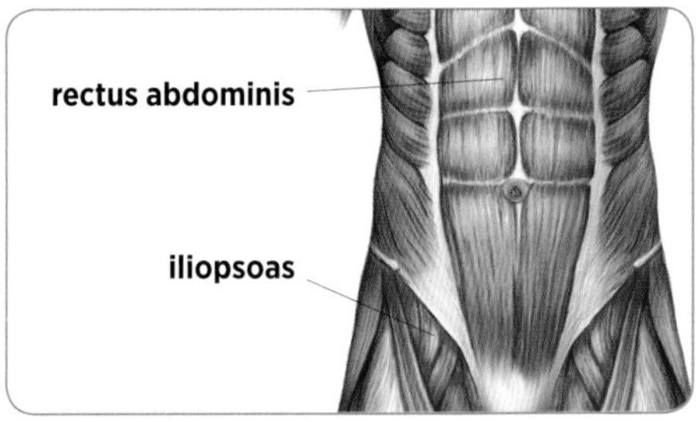

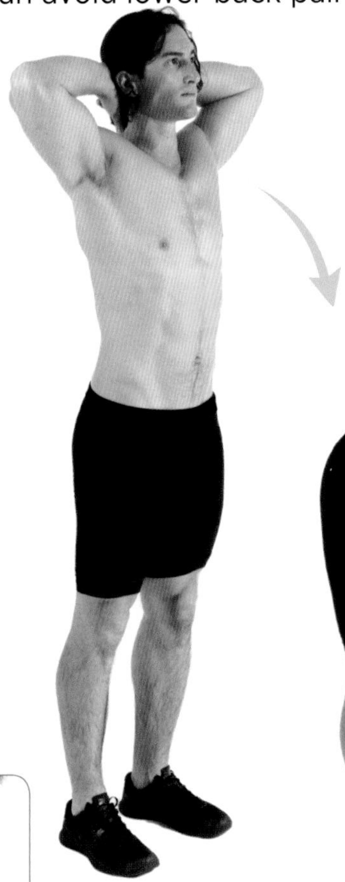

rectus abdominis

iliopsoas

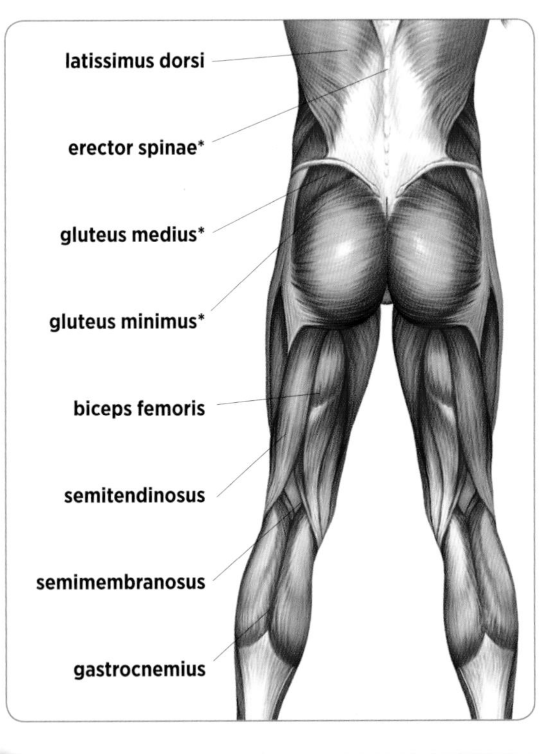

Annotation Key

Bold text indicates target muscles
Light text indicates other working muscles
* indicates deep muscles

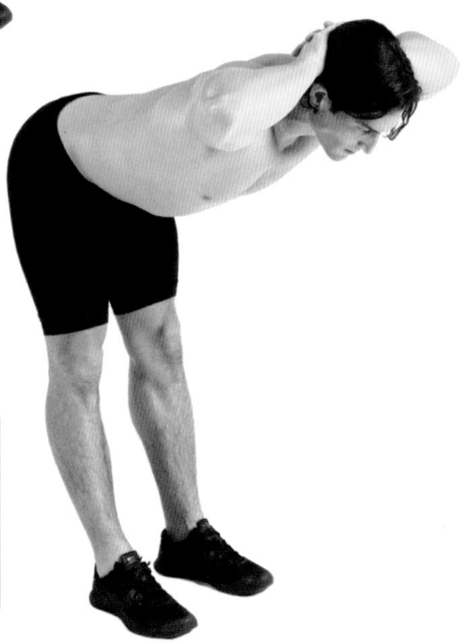

DO IT RIGHT

- Keep your back and legs straight.
- Keep your shoulder blades pulled back and down.
- Avoid slumping.

Layout Push-Up

The Layout Push-Up is an advanced movement requiring intense effort from your back and core musculature. Don't let the "push-up" name fool you because this is not your average gym class exercise—rather than your pectorals, it mainly focuses on your triceps and lats.

HOW TO DO IT

- Lie facedown with your feet together. Stretch your arms upward beside your ears on the floor. Engage your pelvic floor, and draw your navel into your spine.
- While keeping your core engaged, lift your body up and away from the floor.
- Lower yourself back to the starting position, and repeat for the recommended repetitions.

DO IT RIGHT

- Keep your core engaged.
- Avoid excessive arching of your spine.

Annotation Key

Bold text indicates target muscles

Light text indicates other working muscles

* indicates deep muscles

pectoralis minor

pectorailis major

rectus abdominis

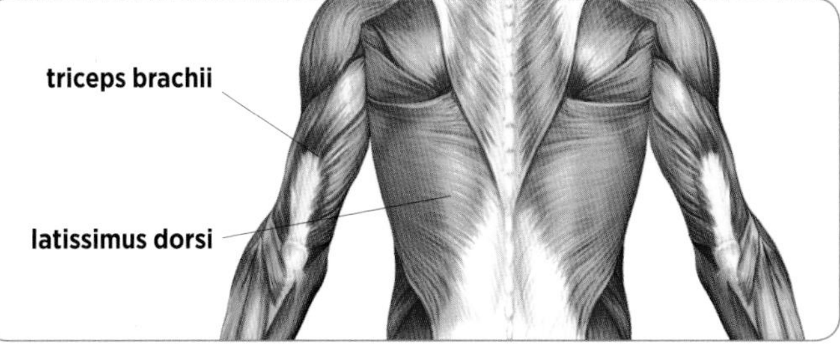

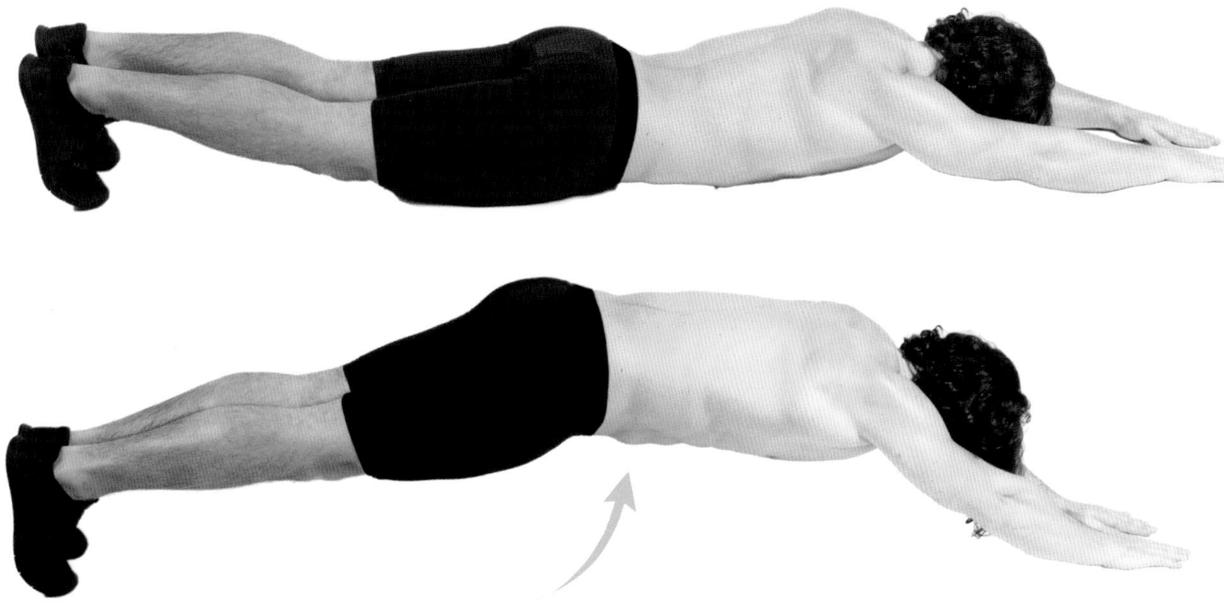

FACT FILE

TARGETS
- Latissimus dorsi
- Triceps
- Pectorals
- Abdominals

EQUIPMENT
- None

BENEFITS
- Strengthens triceps, lats, abdominals, and pectorals
- Increases core stability

CAUTIONS
- Shoulder or rotator cuff issues

Bench Dip

The Bench Dip is a classic body-weight exercise that targets your hard-to-isolate triceps. This version replaces a weight bench with an ordinary chair.

HOW TO DO IT

- Sit up tall near the front of a sturdy chair. Place your hands beside your hips, wrapping your fingers over the front edge of the chair.
- Extend your legs in front of you slightly, and place your feet flat on the floor. Scoot off the edge of the chair until your knees align directly above your feet and your torso will be able to clear the chair as you dip down.
- Bend your elbows directly behind you without splaying them out to the sides, and lower your torso until your elbows make a 90-degree angle.
- Press into the chair, raising your body back to the starting position. Repeat for the recommended repetitions.

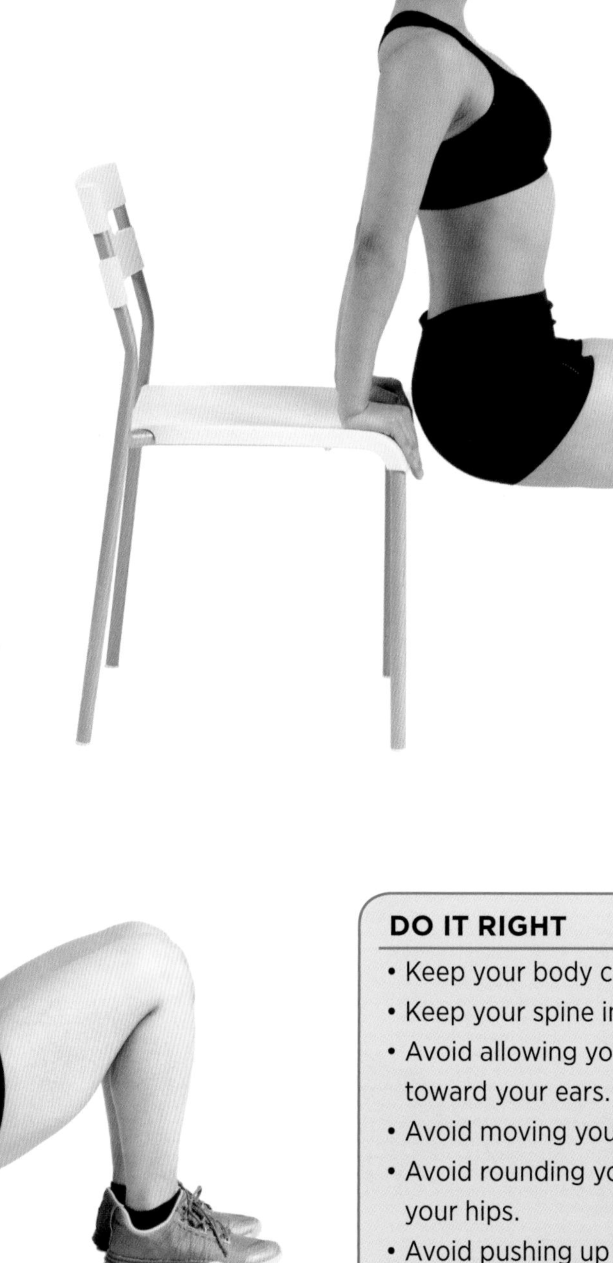

DO IT RIGHT

- Keep your body close to the chair.
- Keep your spine in a neutral position.
- Avoid allowing your shoulders to lift toward your ears.
- Avoid moving your feet.
- Avoid rounding your back as you lower your hips.
- Avoid pushing up solely with your feet. Instead use your arm strength.

FACT FILE

TARGETS
- Triceps
- Shoulders
- Core

EQUIPMENT
- Bench or chair

BENEFITS
- Tones triceps
- Strengthens shoulder girdle

CAUTIONS
- Shoulder issues
- Wrist issues

MODIFICATION

HARDER: Perform the exerise with one leg raised and stretched out in front, continuing to draw your navel into your spine. Repeat with the other leg.

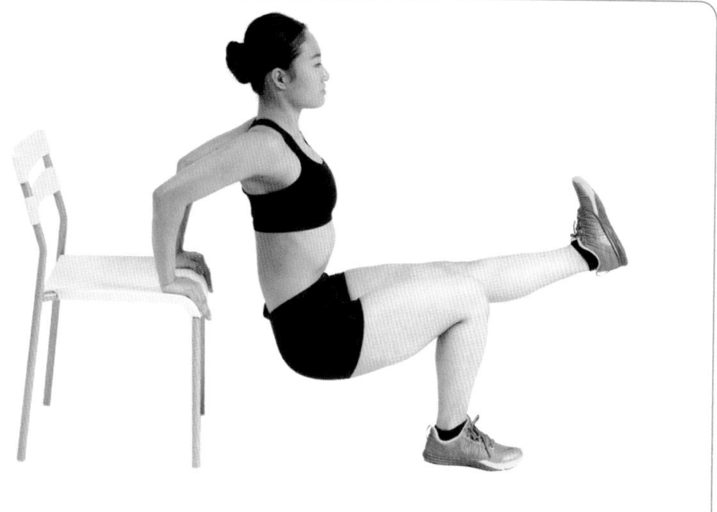

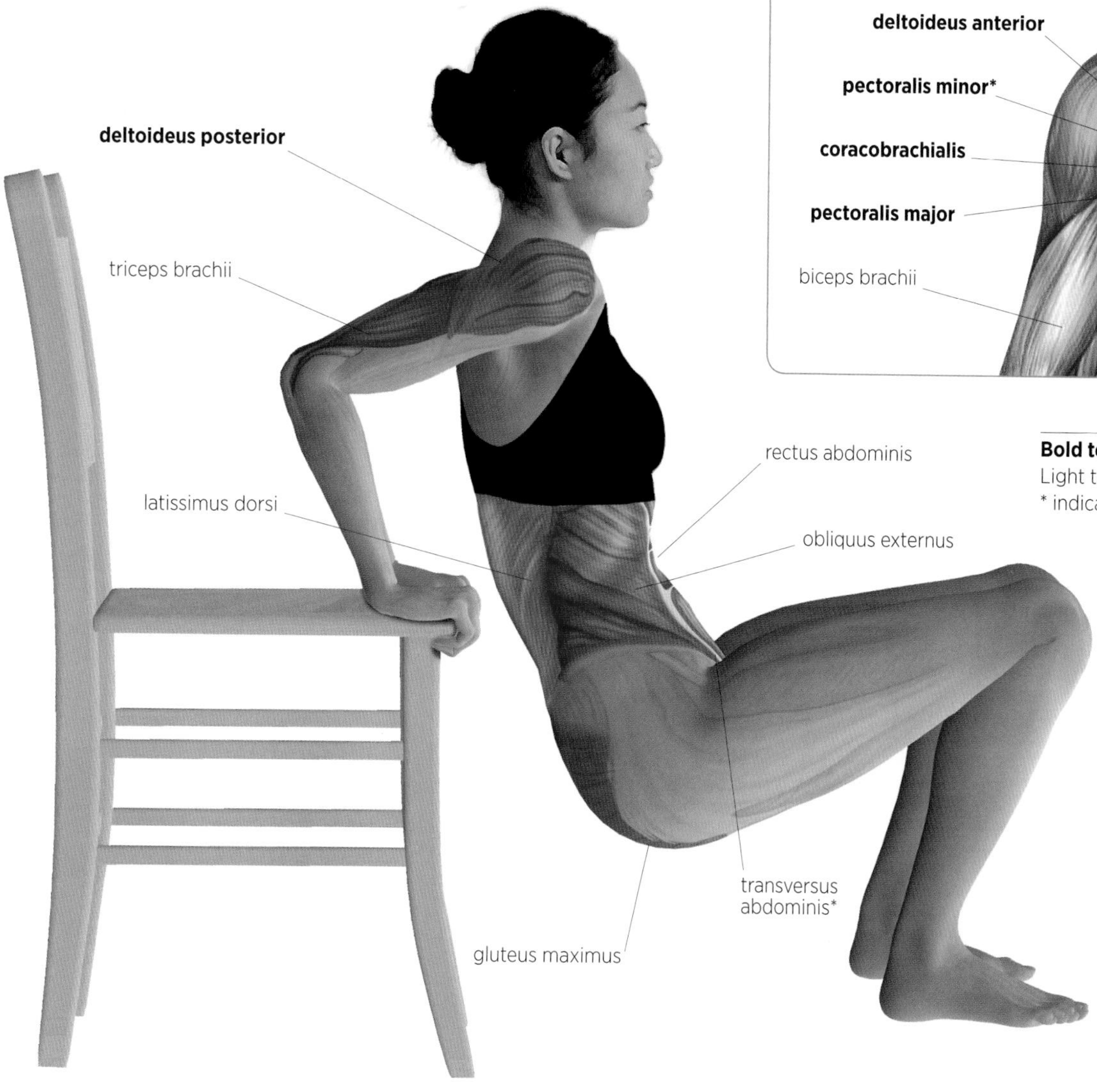

deltoideus anterior

pectoralis minor*

coracobrachialis

pectoralis major

biceps brachii

deltoideus posterior

triceps brachii

latissimus dorsi

rectus abdominis

obliquus externus

transversus abdominis*

gluteus maximus

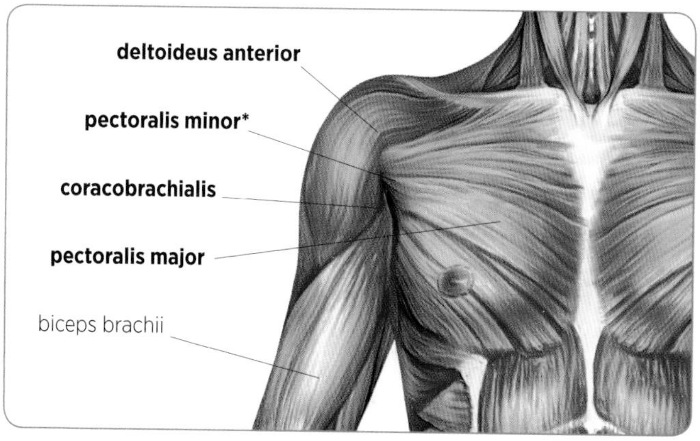

Annotation Key

Bold text indicates target muscles
Light text indicates other working muscles
* indicates deep muscles

Triceps Push-Up

Hand position has a significant impact on which muscles work hardest. In a basic push-up, your pectorals are the primary movers. In this version, you plant your hands closer together to place greater emphasis on your shoulders and triceps.

HOW TO DO IT

- With your hands close together, place your palms on the floor and assume a plank position with your weight on the balls on your feet. Your wrists should be directly beneath your shoulders, with your arms straight and your fingers pointing forward.
- Bend your arms, and lower your torso until your chest touches the floor.
- Straighten your arms to rise back to the starting position. Repeat for the recommended repetitions.

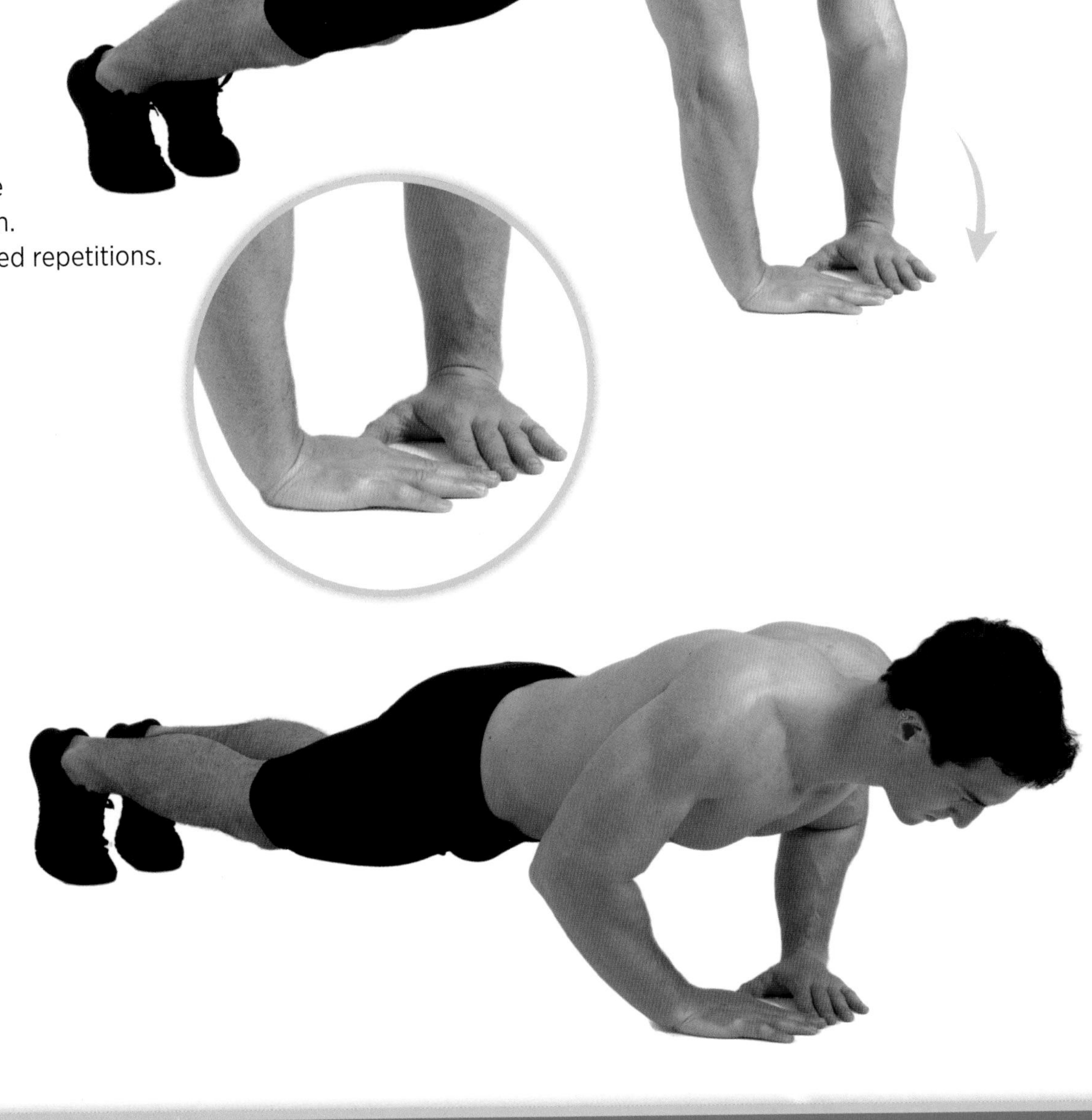

DO IT RIGHT

- Keep your elbows close to your rib cage as you lower your chest to the floor.
- Avoid pushing your hips into the air.
- Avoid pointing your elbows to the side during the down movement; this places undue stress on your front deltoids.

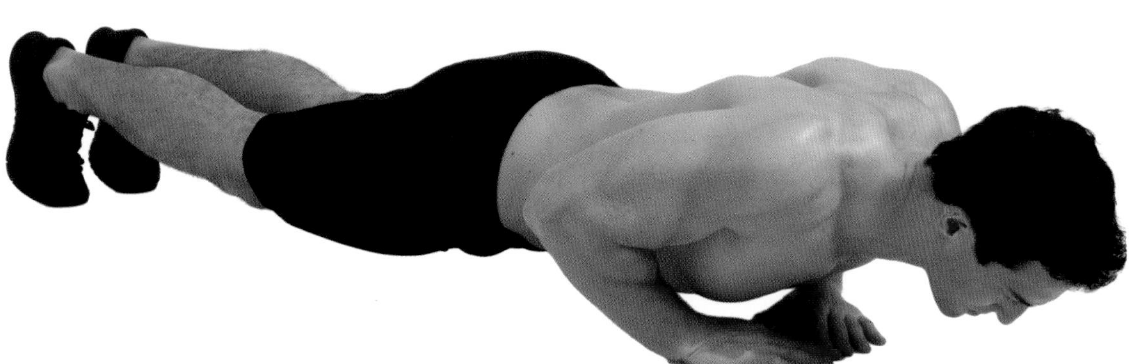

FACT FILE

TARGETS
- Triceps
- Shoulders
- Core

EQUIPMENT
- None

BENEFITS
- Tones triceps
- Strengthens upper body and abdominals
- Stabilizes core

CAUTIONS
- Shoulder issues
- Wrist issues
- Lower-back pain

Annotation Key

Bold text indicates target muscles

Light text indicates other working muscles

* indicates deep muscles

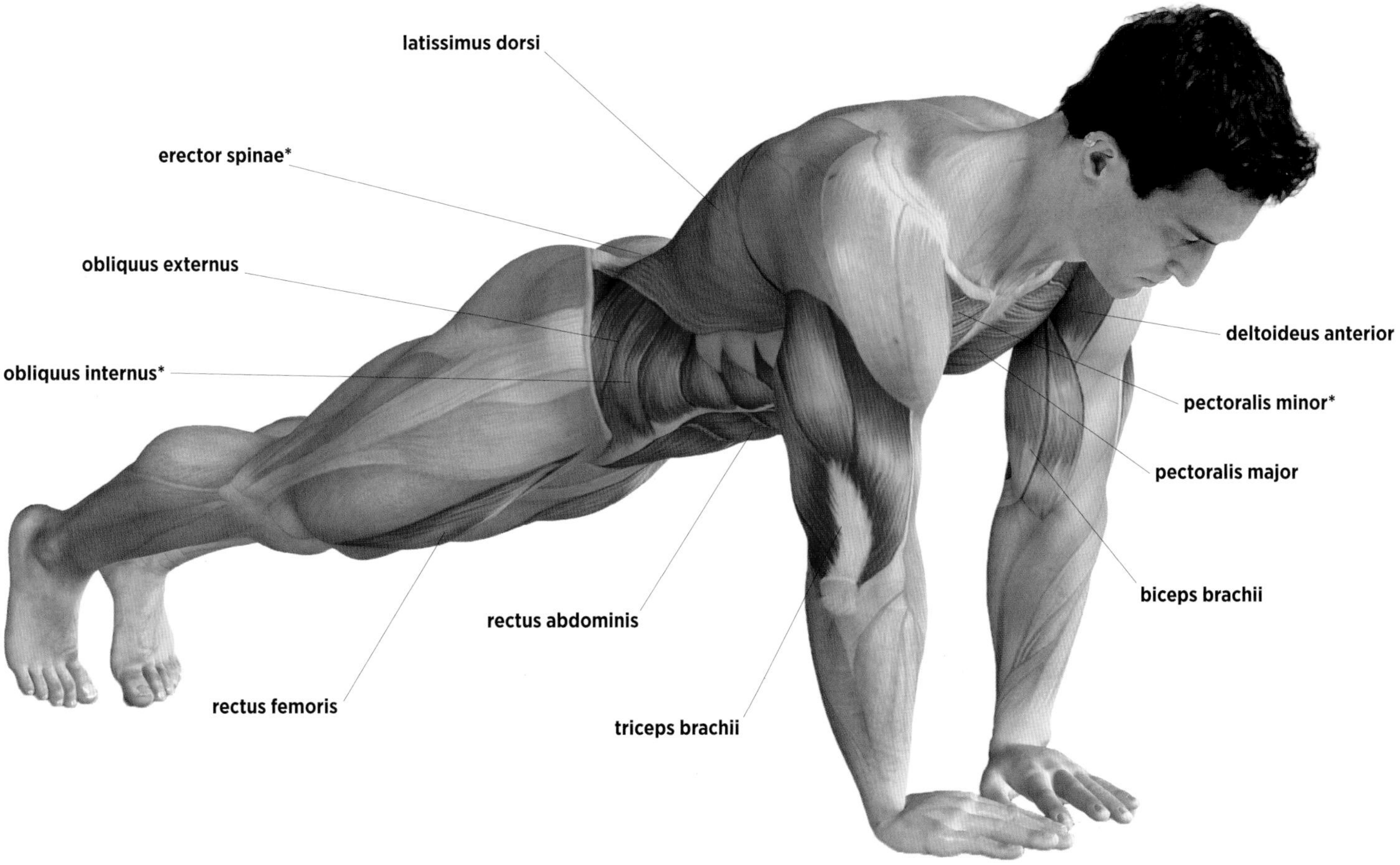

latissimus dorsi

erector spinae*

obliquus externus

obliquus internus*

deltoideus anterior

pectoralis minor*

pectoralis major

biceps brachii

rectus abdominis

rectus femoris

triceps brachii

Inchworm

The Inchworm, also known as Monkey Walk, is a good gauge of overall fitness. It requires core and upper-body strength, and this full-body stretch really tests the limits of your flexibility.

HOW TO DO IT

- Stand tall, and then carefully bend forward toward the floor until your palms are flat on the floor in front of you.
- Slowly walk your hands out to a plank position with your wrists directly under your shoulders. Keep your body parallel to the floor, legs hip-width apart, navel pressing toward your spine and shoulders pressing down your back.
- Pop your hips upward, and push your weight back onto your heels. Your body should be in the shape of an upside-down V. Hold for a few moments before slowly walking your hands back toward your legs.
- Carefully rise back to a standing position. Pause, and then repeat for the recommended repetitions.

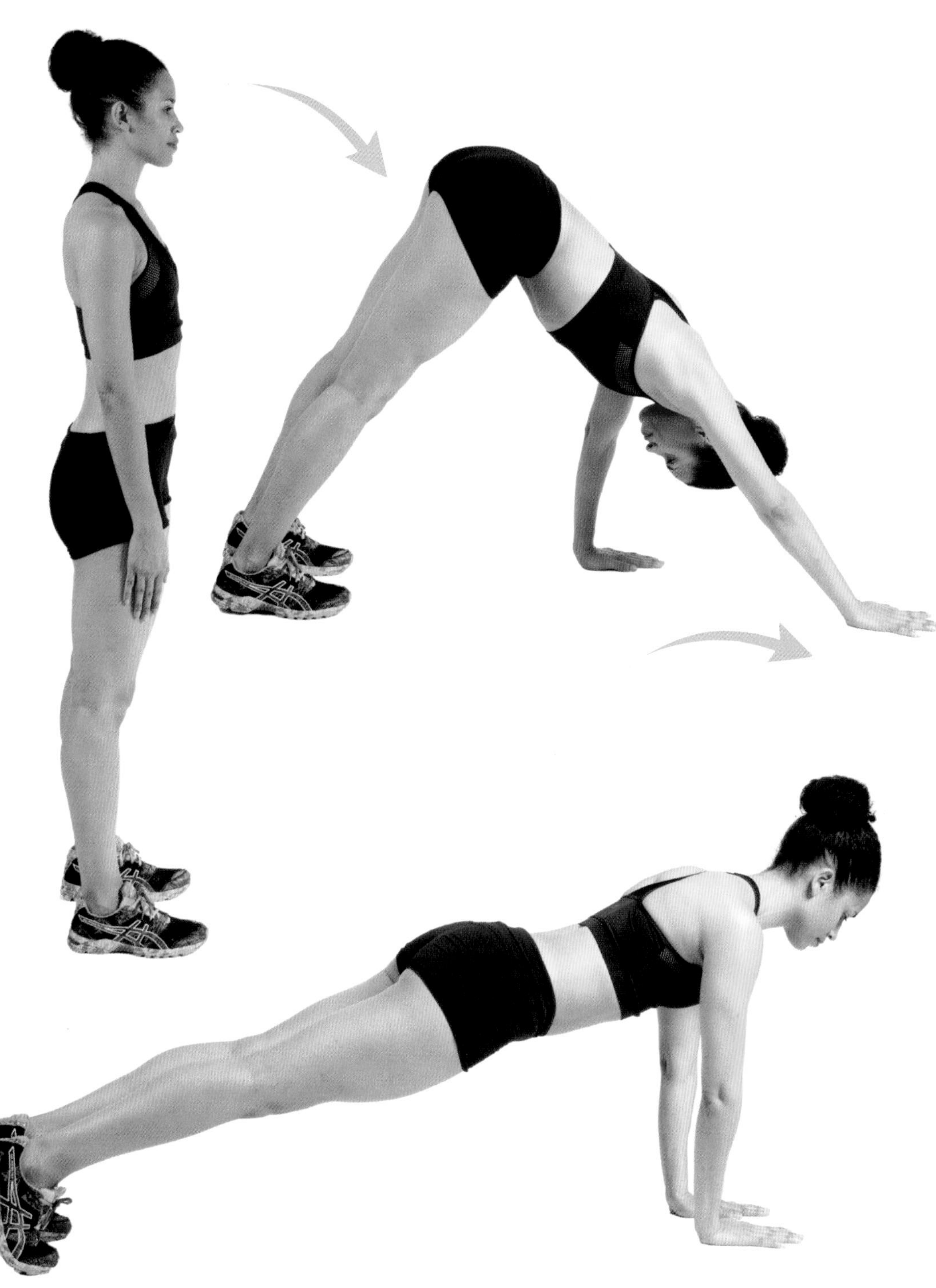

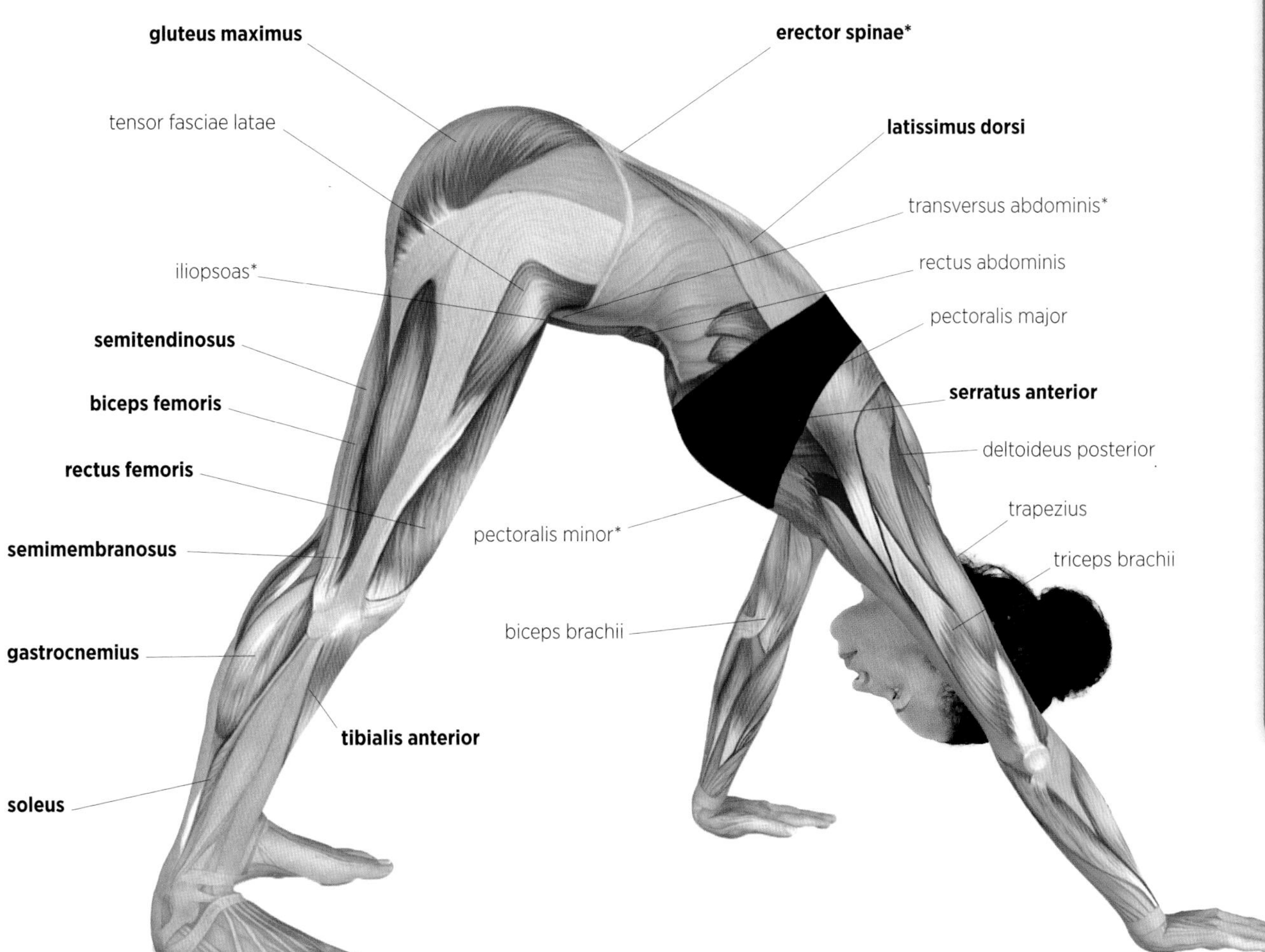

FACT FILE

TARGETS
- Upper arms
- Back
- Legs
- Glutes

EQUIPMENT
- None

BENEFITS
- Warms up muscles
- Stretches back and legs
- Tones arms, glutes, and back

CAUTIONS
- Lower-back issues
- Shoulder issues
- Wrist issues

Annotation Key

Bold text indicates target muscles
Light text indicates other working muscles
* indicates deep muscles

DO IT RIGHT

- Widen your stance if you have trouble reaching the floor with your hands.
- Keep your abdominals sleek and compact.
- Avoid rushing through the exercise.
- Avoid letting your stomach and spine sag while in the plank position.

Plank-Up

Plank-Up is an effective exercise to strengthen your abdominals and arms. Focus on your form, keeping your core fully engaged as you move from low to high and back again.

HOW TO DO IT

- Begin in a forearm plank position with your weight evenly distributed on your forearms and the balls of your feet. Take a moment to stabilize your hips and fully engage your abdominals.

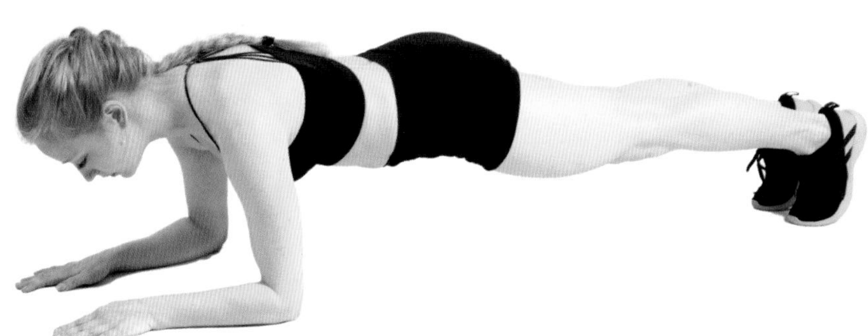

- Reposition your left arm and then the right so that your hands are planted beneath your shoulders, lifting your body into a high plank position.

- Return to the forearm plank, repositioning your left arm and then the right.

- Repeat for the recommended repetitions, alternating leading with one arm and then the other.

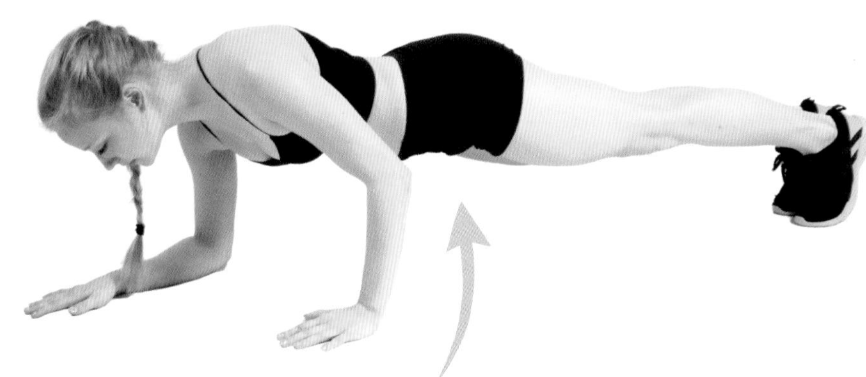

DO IT RIGHT

- Pull your navel in toward your spine to engage your abdominals.
- Avoid letting your stomach or ribcage sag.
- Avoid lifting your shoulders up or forward.
- Avoid shifting your weight when you change levels.

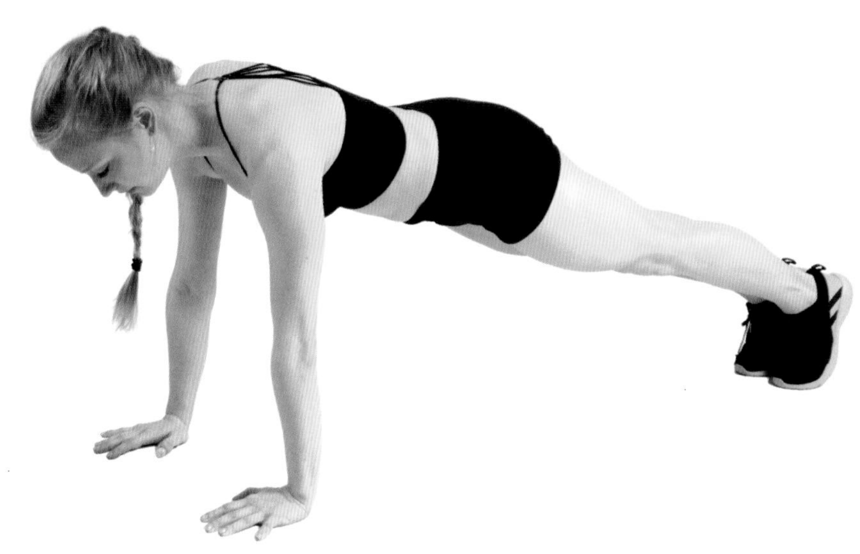

Annotation Key

Bold text indicates target muscles

Light text indicates other working muscles

* indicates deep muscles

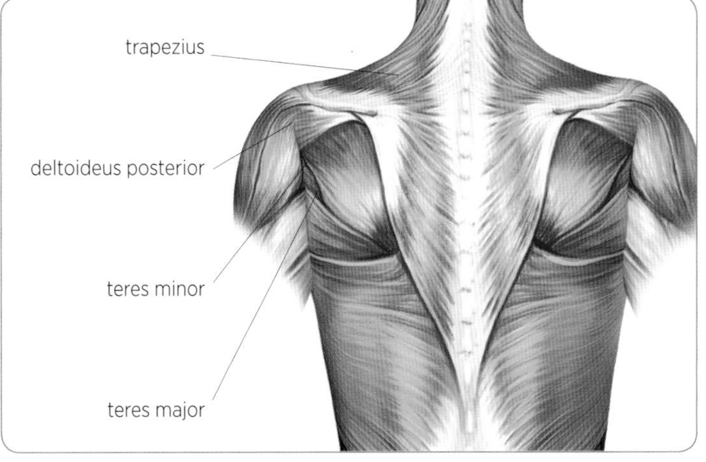

serratus anterior

obliquus externus

vastus lateralis

gastrocnemius

pectoralis major

triceps brachii

rectus abdominis

rectus femoris

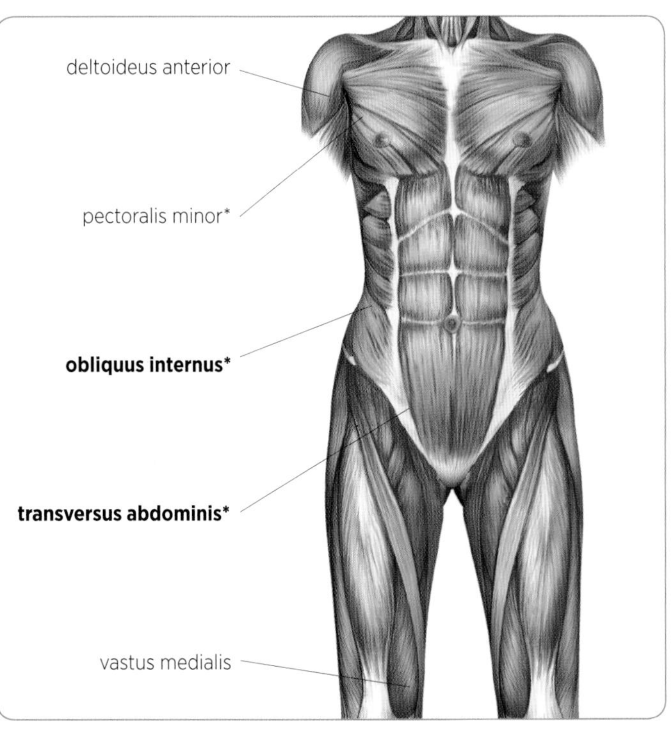

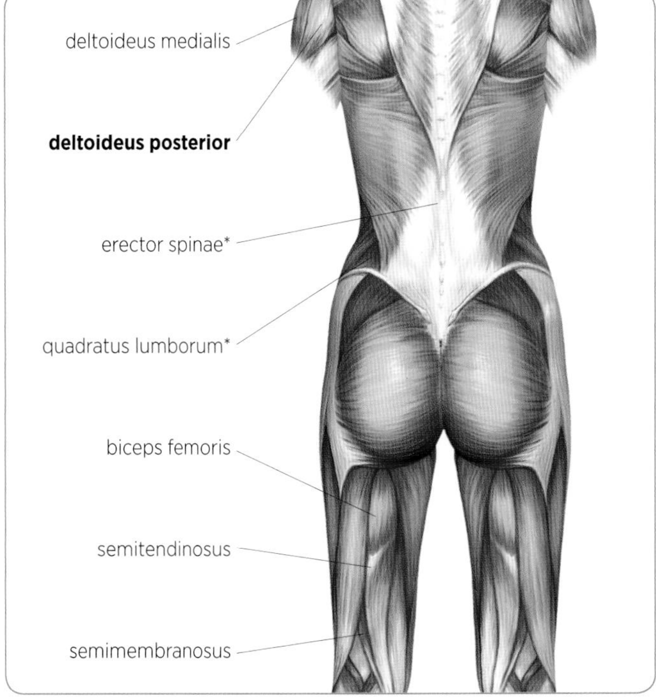

FACT FILE

TARGETS
- Triceps
- Abdominals

EQUIPMENT
- None

BENEFITS
- Stabilizes core
- Strengthens abdominals
- Strengthens triceps

CAUTIONS
- Shoulder issues
- Back issues
- Wrist issues

Power Punch

The Power Punch gives you a great upper-body workout, strengthening and toning big muscles, such as the deltoids. It works as a cardio exercise, helping to raise your heart rate and burn calories.

HOW TO DO IT

- Stand with your feet shoulder-width apart and your left leg placed slightly in front of the other, putting most of your weight on your back leg. Keep your elbows in, and raise your fists up.

- Transferring your weight to your front leg, punch straight in front of you with your right fist as you turn your torso in to lend power to the punch.

- Punch for the recommended repetitions, and then switch arms and legs to repeat on the opposite side. Continue alternating sides for the recommended repetitions.

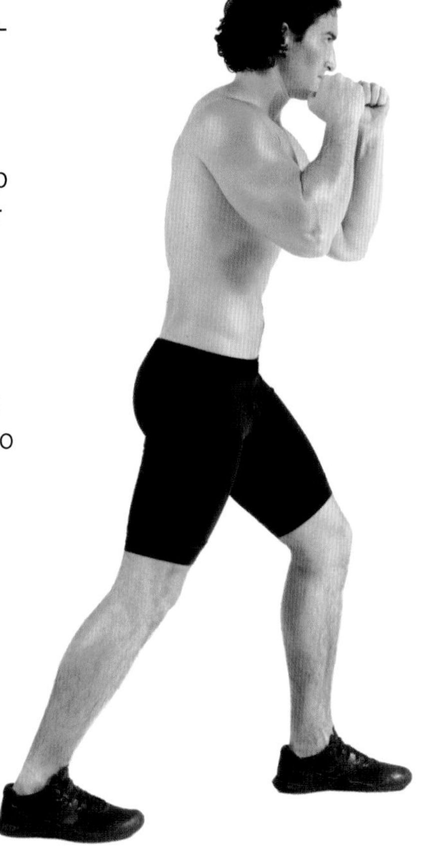

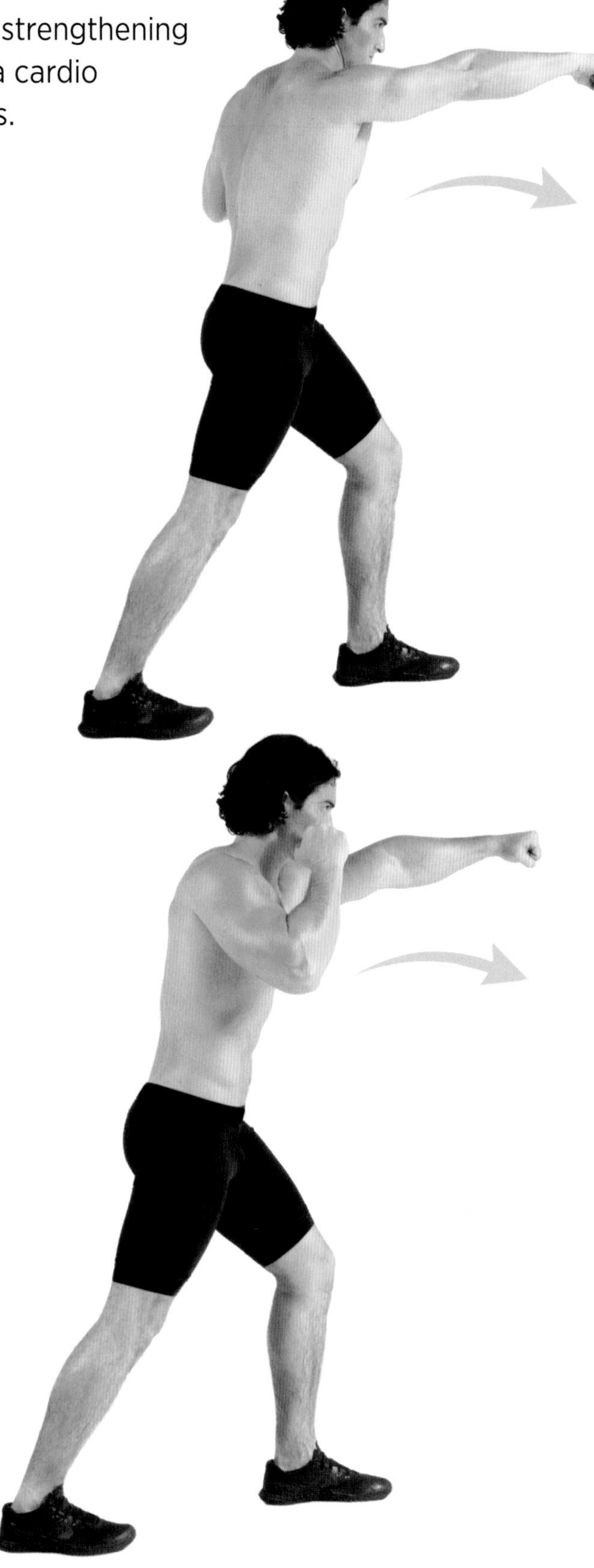

DO IT RIGHT

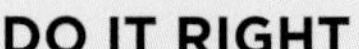

- Maintain a steady, even—but modest—pace.
- Rotate your torso to drive the movement.
- Keep your fists up.
- Avoid excessive speed.
- Avoid sloppy form.

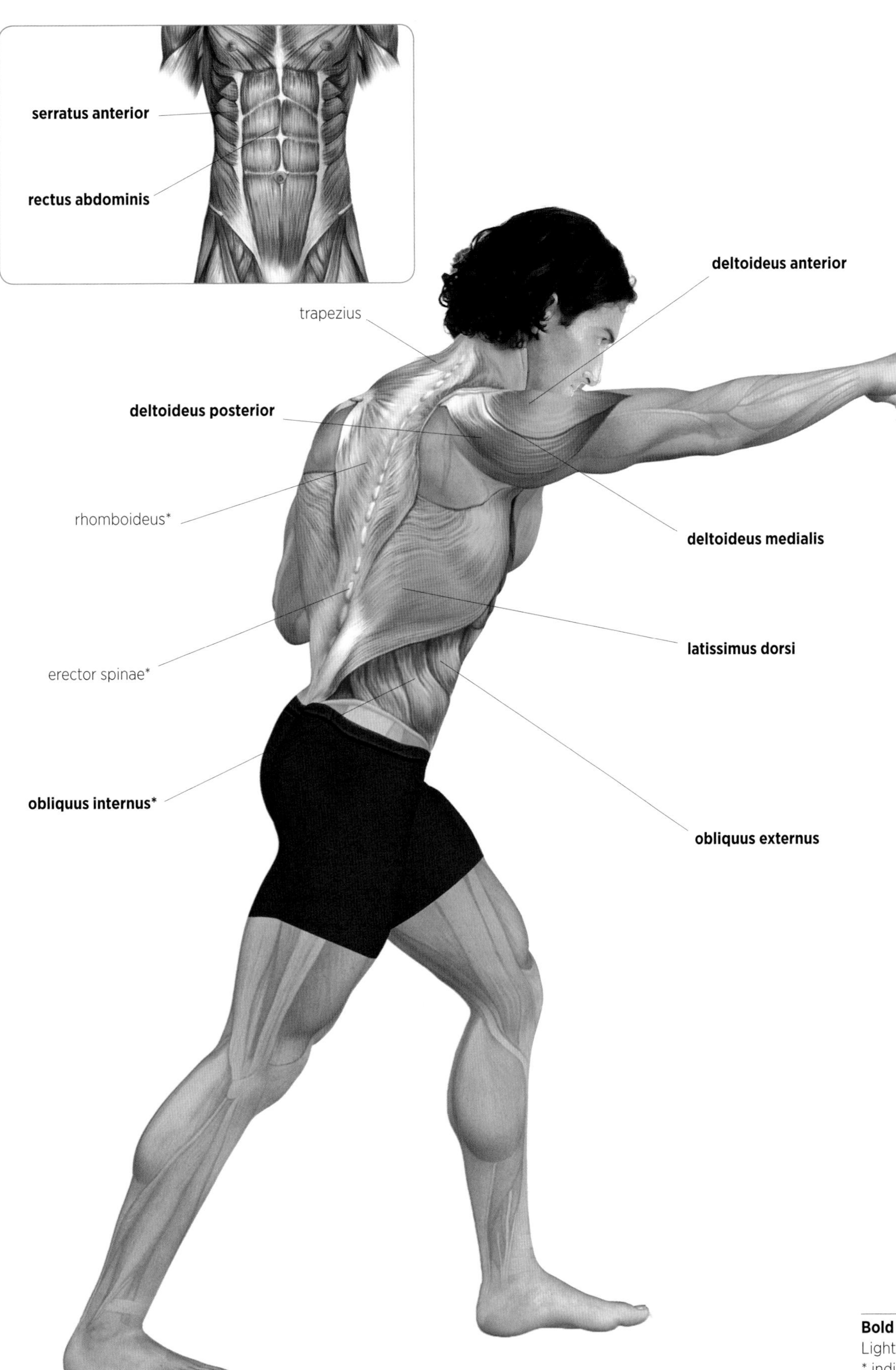

FACT FILE

TARGETS
- Back
- Shoulders
- Abdominals

EQUIPMENT
- None

BENEFITS
- Strengthens back and shoulders
- Builds endurance

CAUTIONS
- Shoulder issues

Annotation Key

Bold text indicates target muscles

Light text indicates other working muscles

* indicates deep muscles

Supine Reverse-Grip Back Row

This exercise uses your body weight to blast your arms. Focusing on your biceps, this exercise also requires a good amount of mid-scapular strength, as well as core stability.

FACT FILE

TARGETS
- Biceps
- Back
- Abdominals
- Glutes

EQUIPMENT
- Bar

BENEFITS
- Strengthens and tones abdominals, back, arms, and legs

CAUTIONS
- Wrist issues
- Shoulder issues

HOW TO DO IT
- Place yourself beneath a bar with your legs extended, resting on your heels to create a straight line from your heels to shoulders. Grasp the bar underhand with each hand about shoulder-width apart.

- With your core engaged, draw your elbows back behind your torso to pull your body upward until your chest makes contact with the bar.

- Extend your elbows until your arms are straight to lower your body back to the starting position. Repeat for the recommended repetitions.

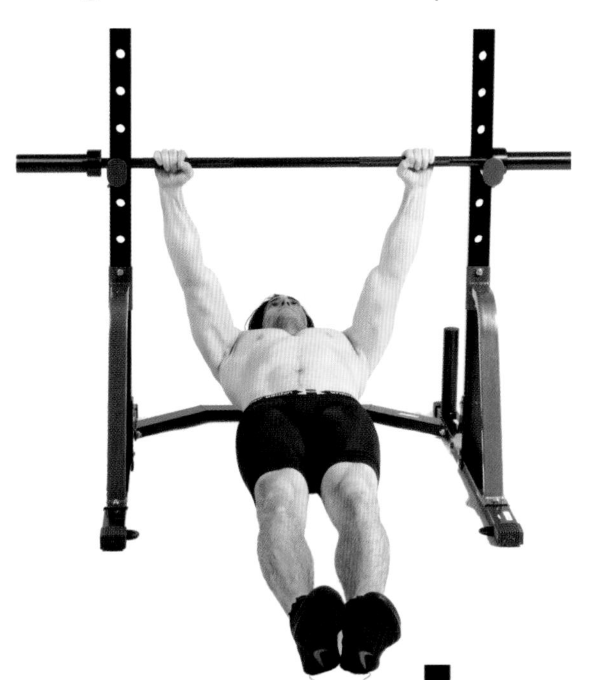

DO IT RIGHT
- Keep your back and legs straight.
- Rest your flexed feet on your heels; do not place feet flat on the floor.

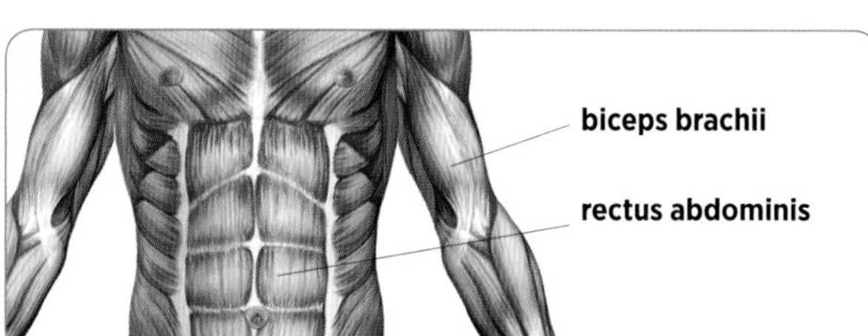

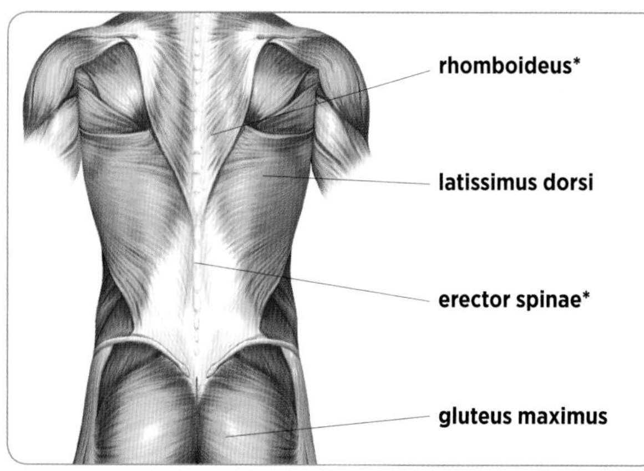

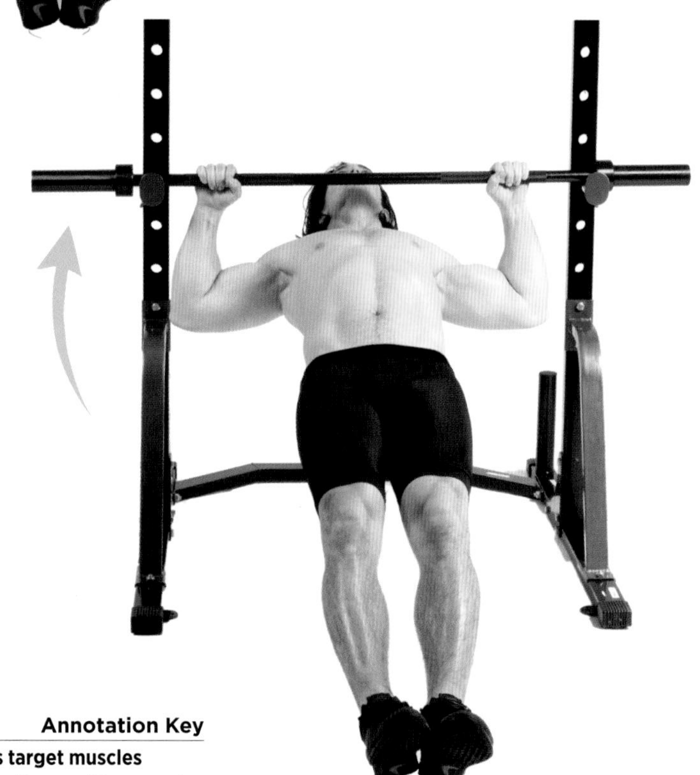

Annotation Key

Bold text indicates target muscles

Light text indicates other working muscles

* indicates deep muscles

Bar Dip

The Bar Dip is a fantastic gymnastic exercise that develops your upper body. With its focus on the lower pectorals and triceps, it will develop the posterior aspect of your arms in a way no other exercise can.

FACT FILE

TARGETS
- Triceps
- Pectorals

EQUIPMENT
- Pull-up bar

BENEFITS
- Strengthens and tones chest and arms

CAUTIONS
- Wrist issues

HOW TO DO IT

- Begin with your upper body over the bar, grasping the bar with each hand approximately shoulder-width apart and your legs directly beneath you.

- Extend your arms downward to press your body up and away from the bar, supporting your body weight on your hands.

- Bend your elbows to lower your body back to the starting position. Repeat for the recommended repetitions.

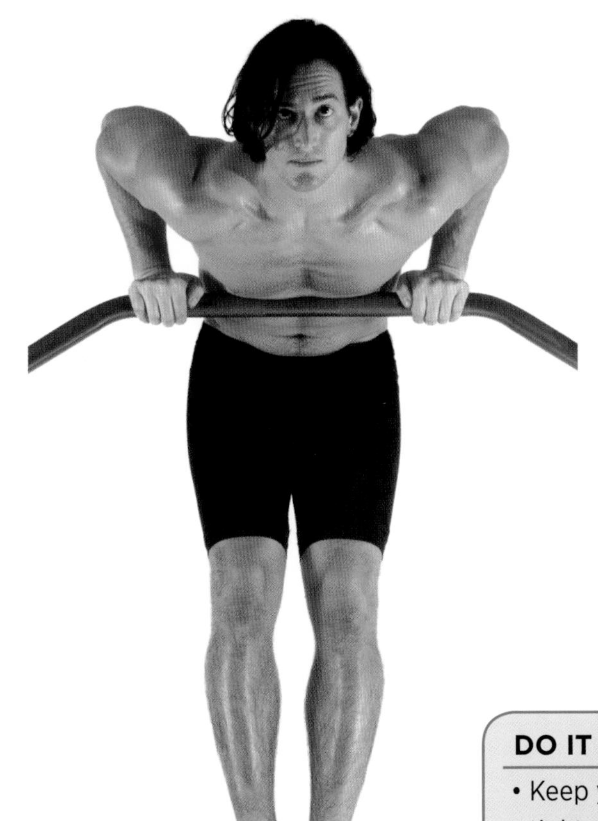

DO IT RIGHT
- Keep your elbows close and tight against your torso.
- Avoid movement in your lower extremities.

Annotation Key

Bold text indicates target muscles
Light text indicates other working muscles
* indicates deep muscles

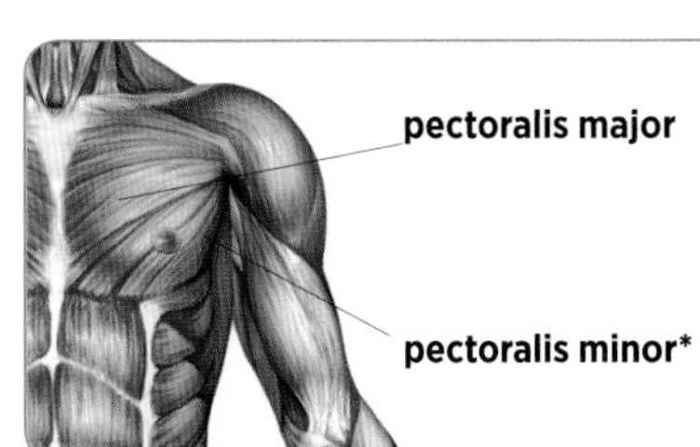

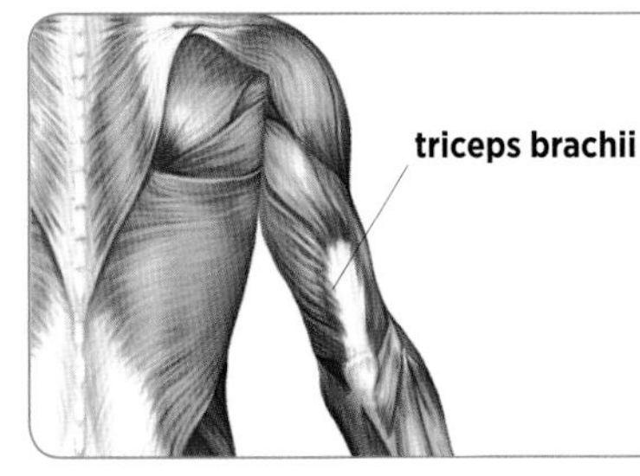

Handstand Push-Up

The Handstand Push-Up is an advanced movement requiring an immense amount of upper-body strength, specifically from your shoulders and triceps, as well as midline stability from your core. Make sure you are strong and stable enough before attempting this exercise.

HOW TO DO IT

- Begin in a tripod position, with your head and hands on the floor, your head located between your hands and slightly forward making a triangle or tripod.
- Draw your legs above you, extending your hips and knees to stabilize your body in a single line, stacking your lower extremities above your trunk.
- Keeping your legs pointed toward the ceiling and your core engaged, press into the floor, extending your elbows, lifting your head and body up and away from the floor.
- Bending your elbows until your head makes contact with the mat. Repeat for the recommended repetitions.

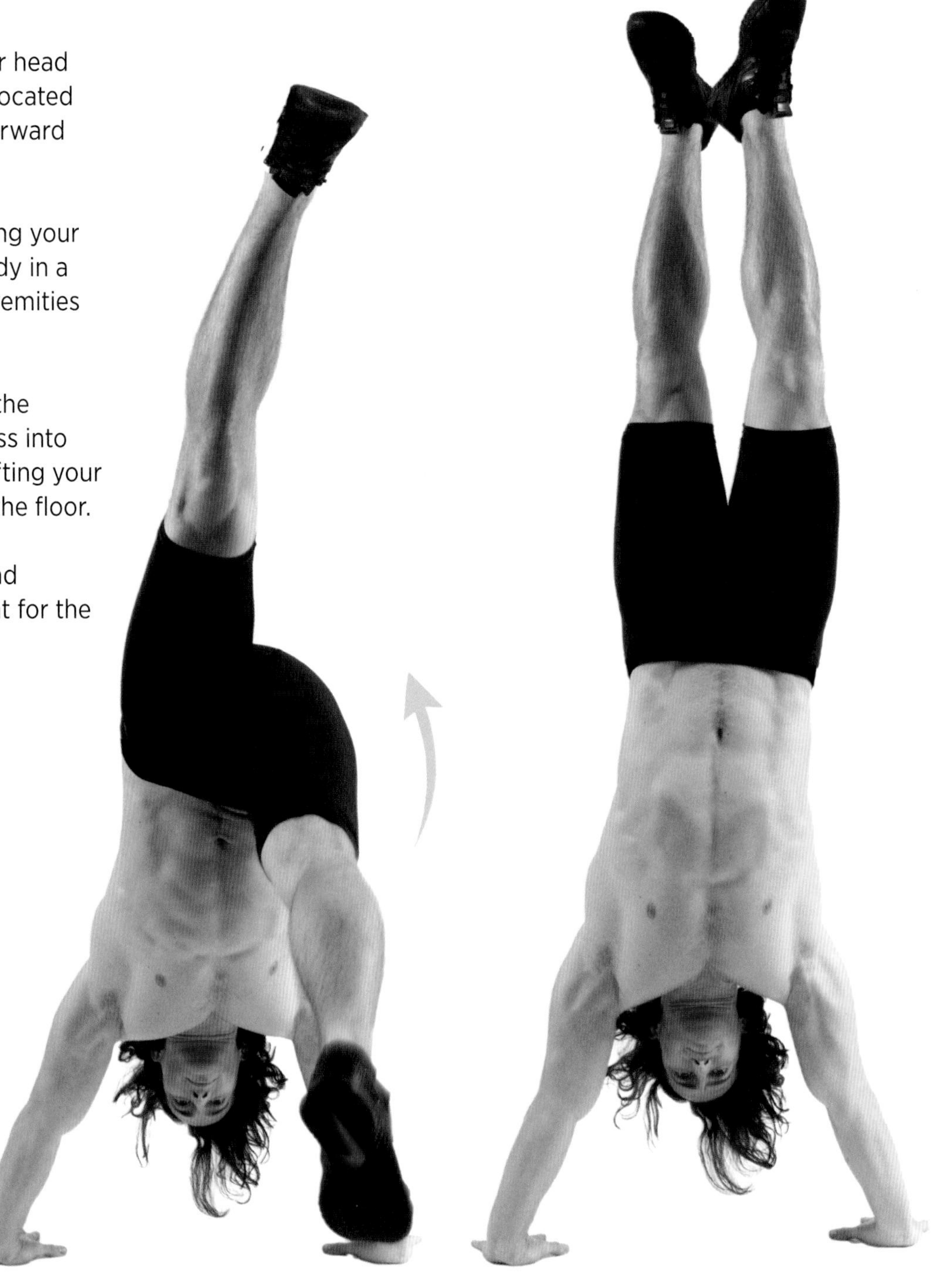

DO IT RIGHT

- Keep your back straight.
- Flare your hands out to ease stress on your wrists.
- Utilize a towel or pad underneath your head for safety and comfort.
- Avoid excessive trunk sway.
- As you master this exercise, perform it against a wall for added support.
- Use a spotter for safety.

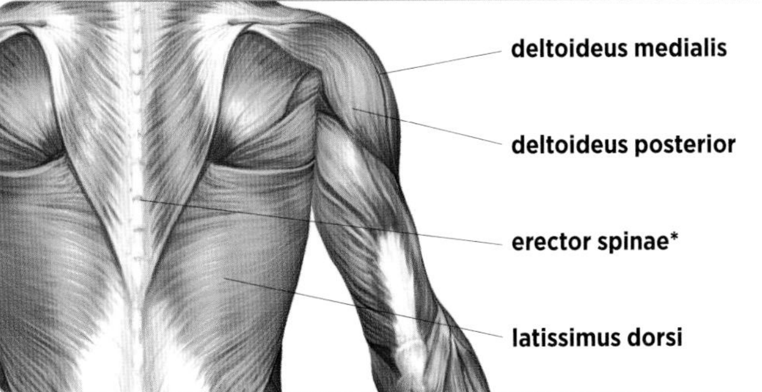

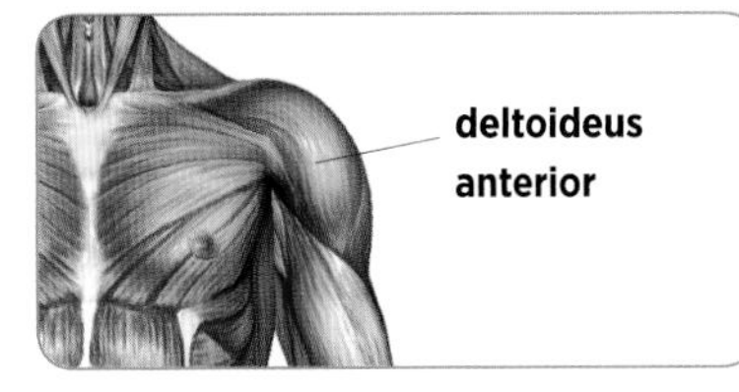

Annotation Key

Bold text indicates target muscles
Light text indicates other working muscles
* indicates deep muscles

FACT FILE

TARGETS
- Triceps
- Deltoids
- Abdominals
- Back

EQUIPMENT
- None

BENEFITS
- Warms up muscles
- Improves coordination
- Strengthens and tones abdominals, chest, arms, and legs
- Increases cardiovascular endurance

CAUTIONS
- Wrist issues
- Shoulder issues

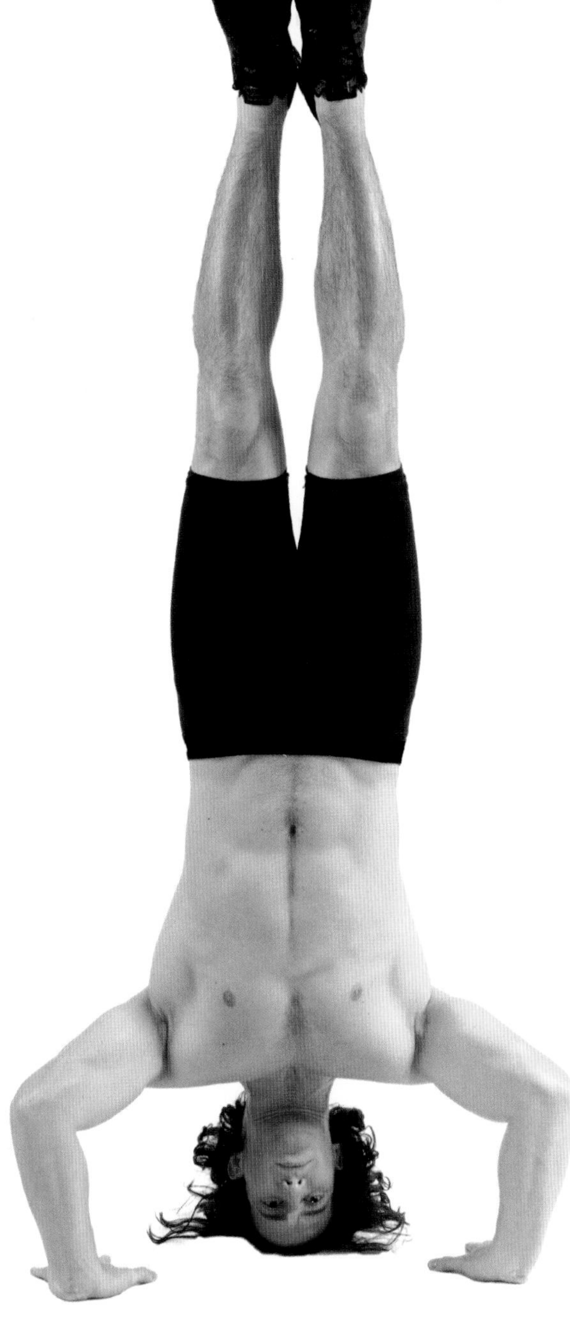

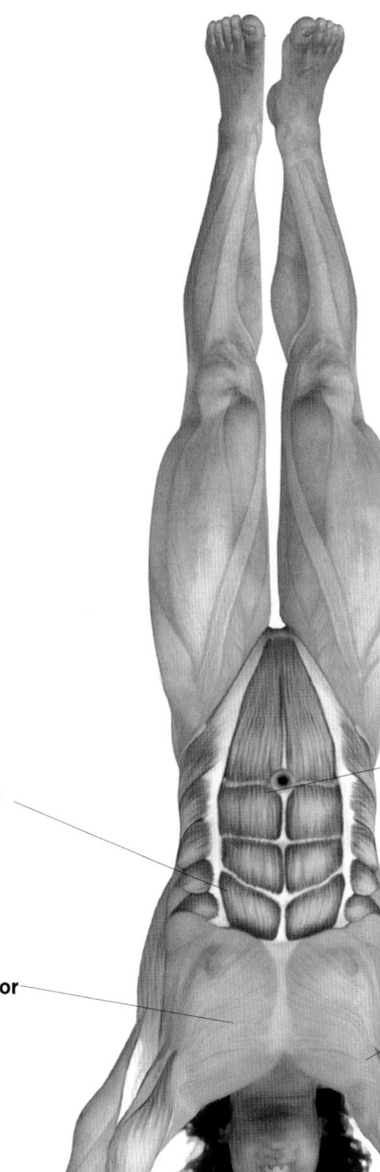

Push-Up

From military boot camps to high school gyms, you will find people performing the Push-Up. This proven calisthenics exercise works your chest, shoulders, arms, back, and core.

HOW TO DO IT

- Begin on your hands and knees, with your hands planted slightly wider than shoulder-width apart. Extend your legs back to come into a high plank position.
- With control, slowly lower the full length of your body toward the floor, bending your elbows.
- Straighten your elbows to return to the high plank position. Repeat for the recommended repetitions.

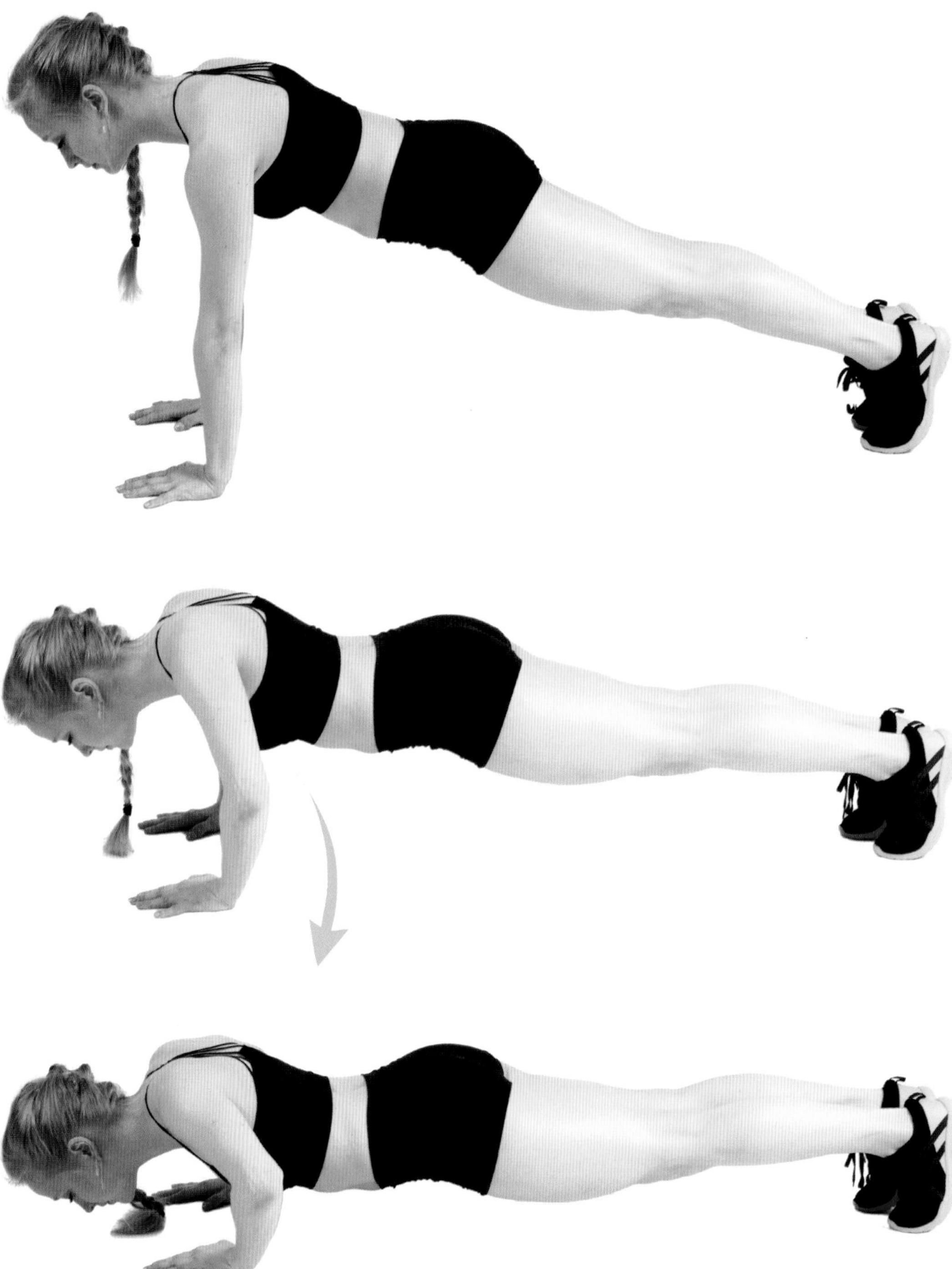

DO IT RIGHT

- Keep your shoulders pressed down your back.
- Imagine a straight line running from the top of your head to your heels.
- Avoid compromising the neutral alignment of your pelvis or spine.

FACT FILE

TARGETS
- Pectorals
- Biceps
- Deltoids
- Abdominals
- Back

EQUIPMENT
- None

BENEFITS
- Strengthens biceps, shoulders, chest, back, and core
- Tones abdominals

CAUTIONS
- Shoulder issues
- Wrist issues

MODIFICATION

EASIER: Kneel on all fours with your hands planted slightly wider than shoulder-width apart. Lift your feet toward your buttocks until your calves and thighs form a 90-degree angle. Perform as you would a basic push-up.

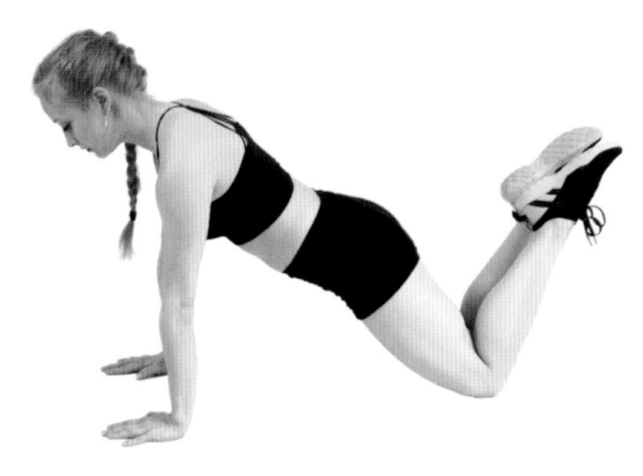

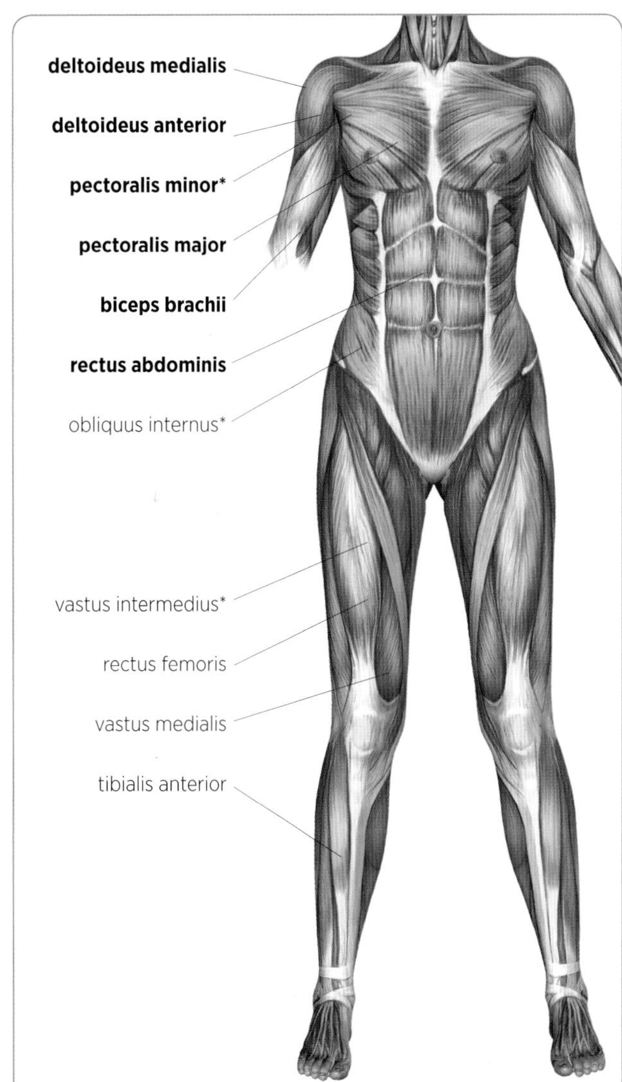

Annotation Key

Bold text indicates target muscles

Light text indicates other working muscles

* indicates deep muscles

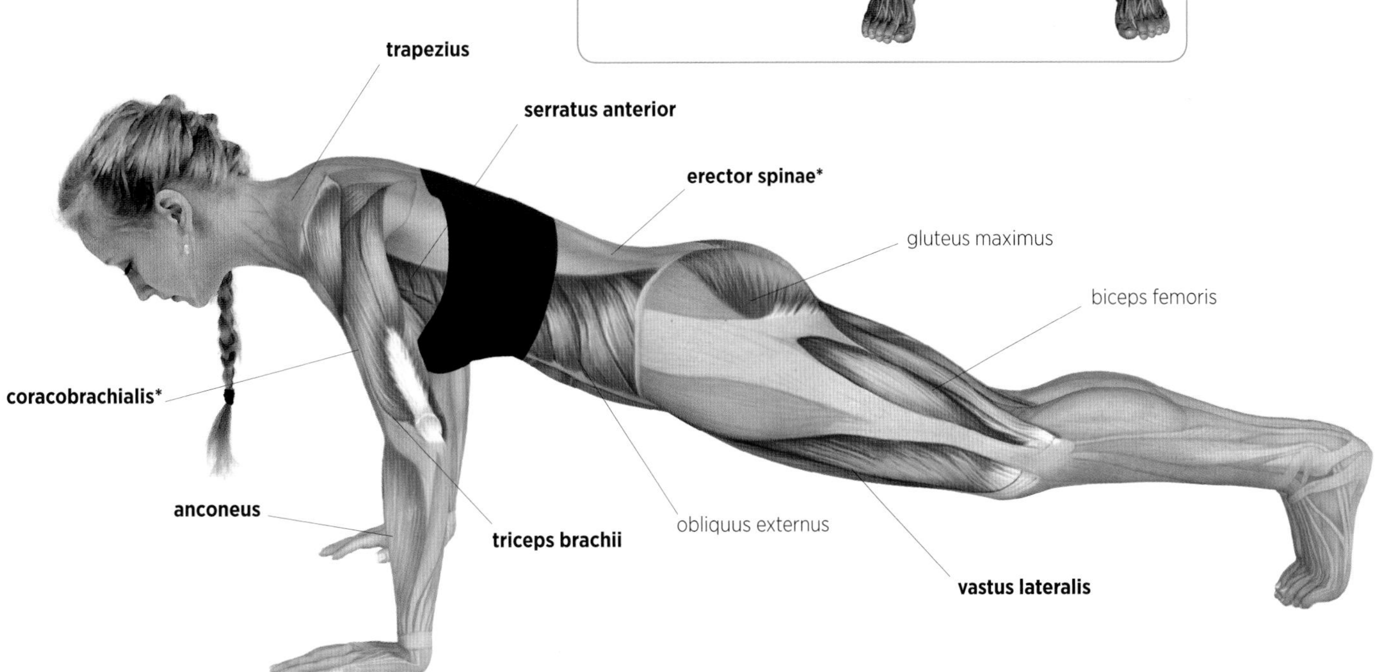

Shoulder-Tap Push-Up

The Shoulder-Tap Push-Up takes the standard push-up exercise to the next level, shifting your body weight from side to side, which further strengthens your arms. It requires good midline stability, dexterity, and chest and triceps strength.

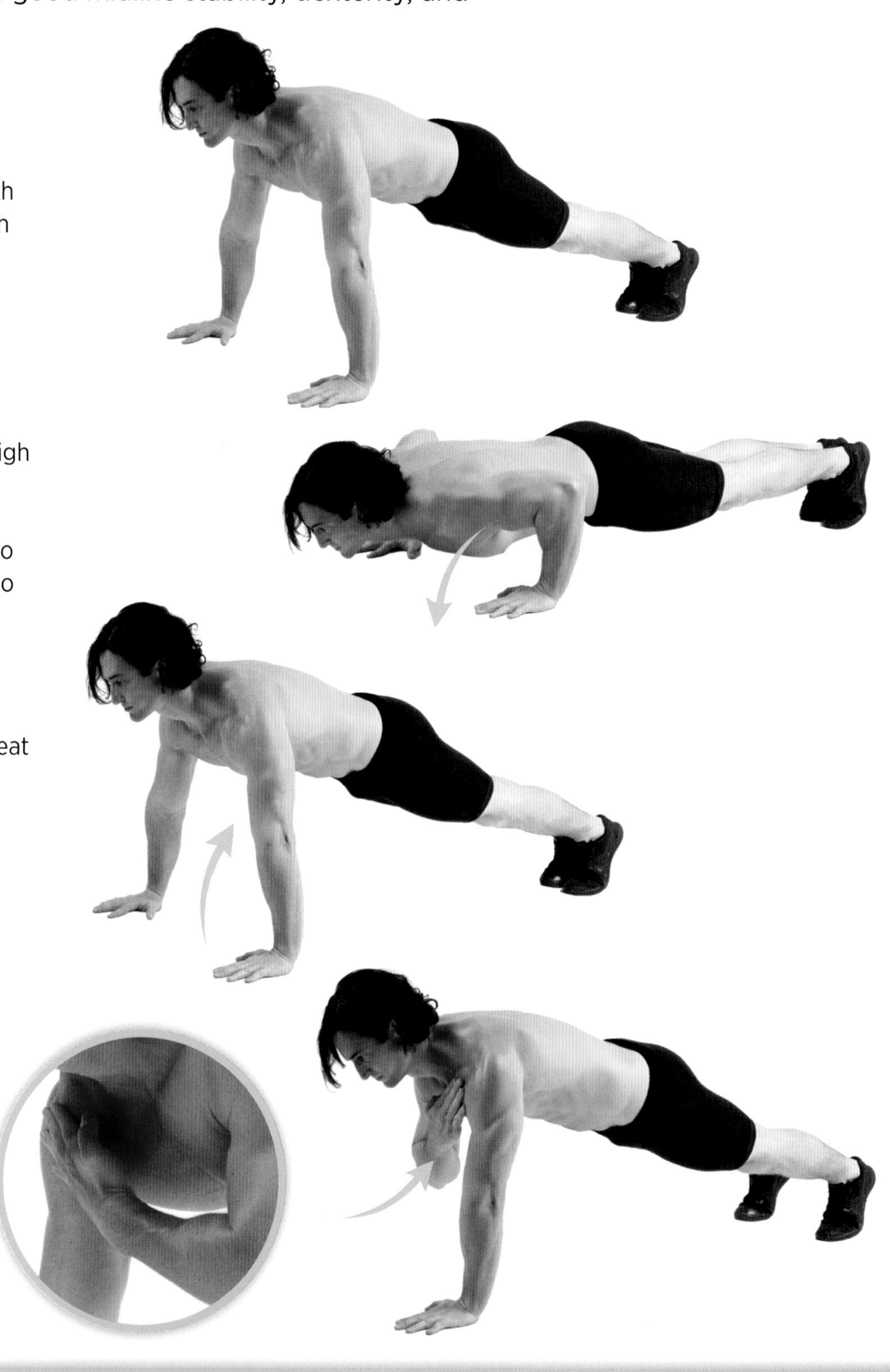

HOW TO DO IT

- Begin in a high plank position with your feet spread wider than hips-width apart and your hands planted beneath your shoulders.
- Perform a push-up, lowering yourself until your chest reaches the floor.
- While engaging your core, press your palms into the floor to return to the high plank position.
- Shift your weight onto your left arm so that you are able lift your right hand to tap your opposite (left) shoulder.
- Return your hand back to the floor.
- Repeat the entire exercise again. Repeat for the recommended repetitions, alternating arms with every rep.

DO IT RIGHT

- Keep your core engaged and your back straight.
- Completely shift your body weight before removing a hand from the ground.
- Keep your hips square to the floor, avoiding too much movement in your pelvis, even during the weight shift.

deltoideus anterior
pectoralis minor*
pectoralis major
rectus abdominis

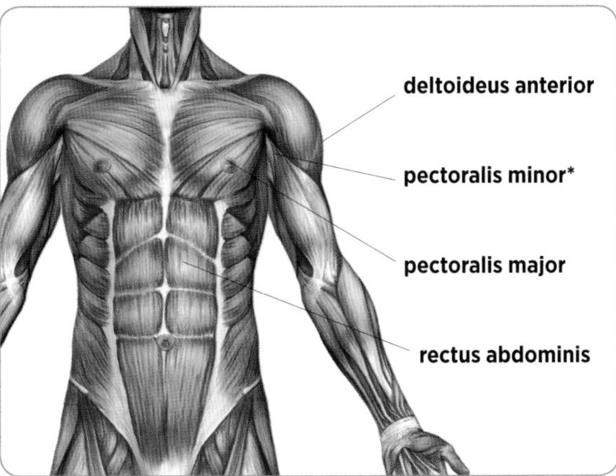

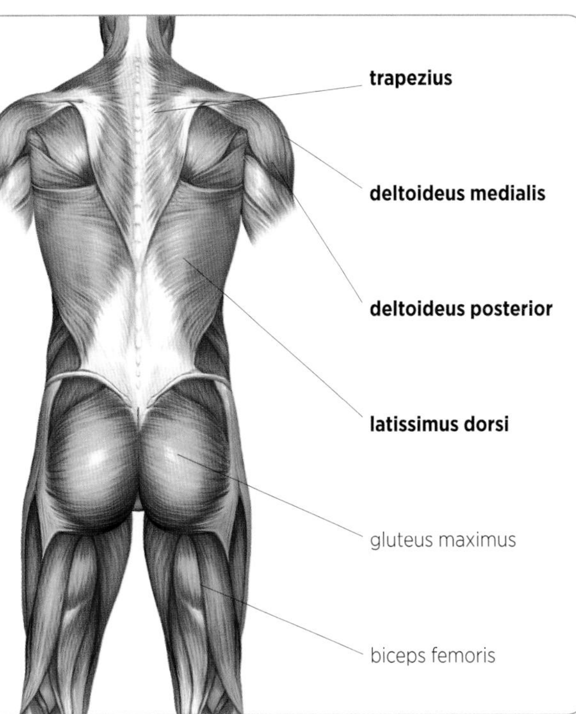

Annotation Key

Bold text indicates target muscles

Light text indicates other working muscles

* indicates deep muscles

trapezius
deltoideus medialis
deltoideus posterior
latissimus dorsi
gluteus maximus
biceps femoris

FACT FILE

TARGETS
- Pectorals
- Triceps
- Deltoids
- Abdominals

EQUIPMENT
- None

BENEFITS
- Improves balance
- Improves coordination
- Strengthens and tones abdominals, chest, arms, and legs
- Increases midline stability

CAUTIONS
- Wrist issues
- Back issues

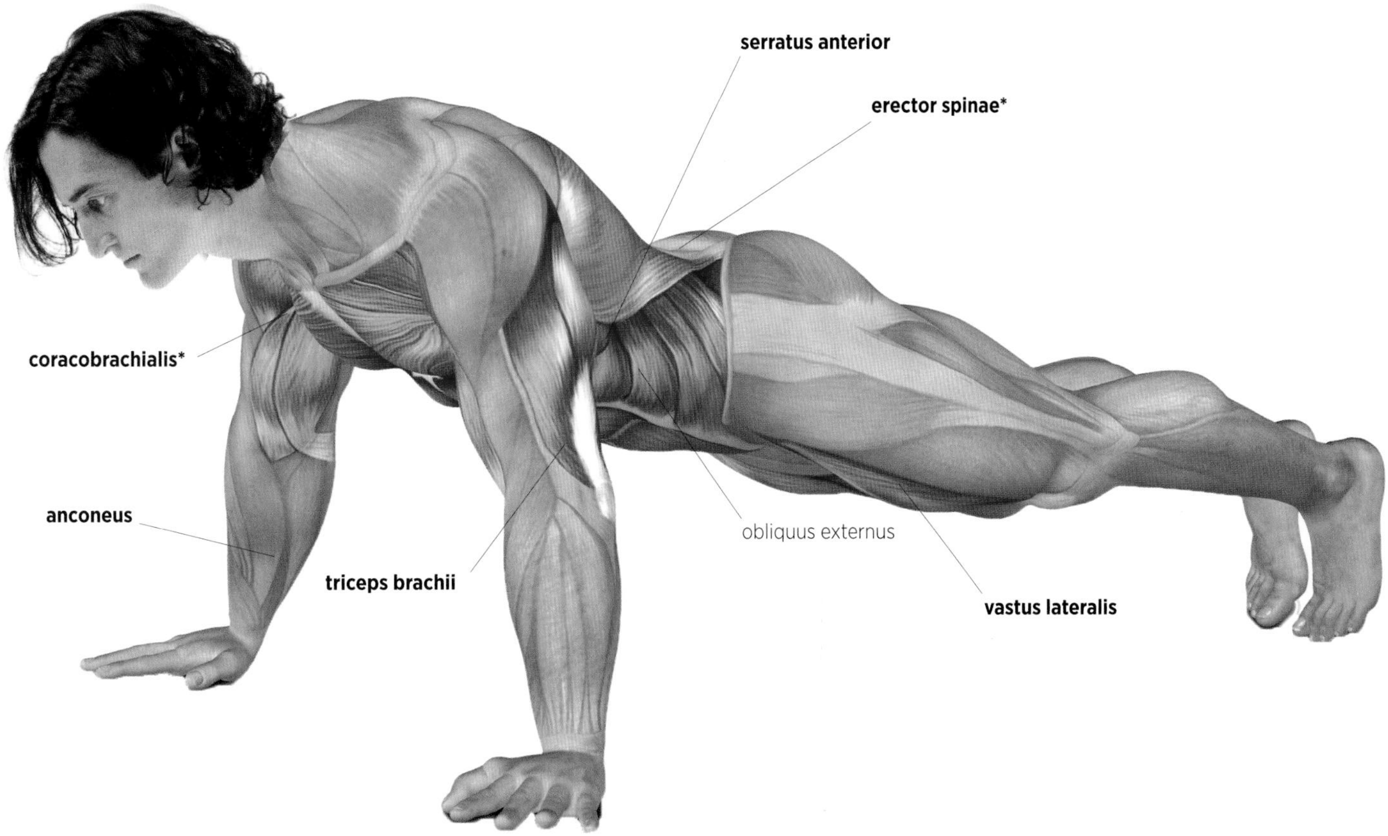

serratus anterior
erector spinae*
coracobrachialis*
anconeus
triceps brachii
obliquus externus
vastus lateralis

Alternating Single-Arm Push-Up

The Alternating Single-Arm Push-Up is an advanced, dynamically engaging chest exercise. It focuses on your pectorals, but it doesn't leave much untouched. With your triceps and deltoids engaged, as well as your core and legs providing a stable base, it will strengthen your entire body.

HOW TO DO IT

- Begin in a high plank position with your feet spread wider than hips-width apart and your hands planted beneath your shoulders.
- Place your right hand on the small of your back.
- Keeping your core engaged, bend your left elbow to bring your chest toward the floor.
- Press your left hand into the floor, and extend your elbow to return to the starting position.
- Repeat for the recommended repetitions, alternating arms with every rep.

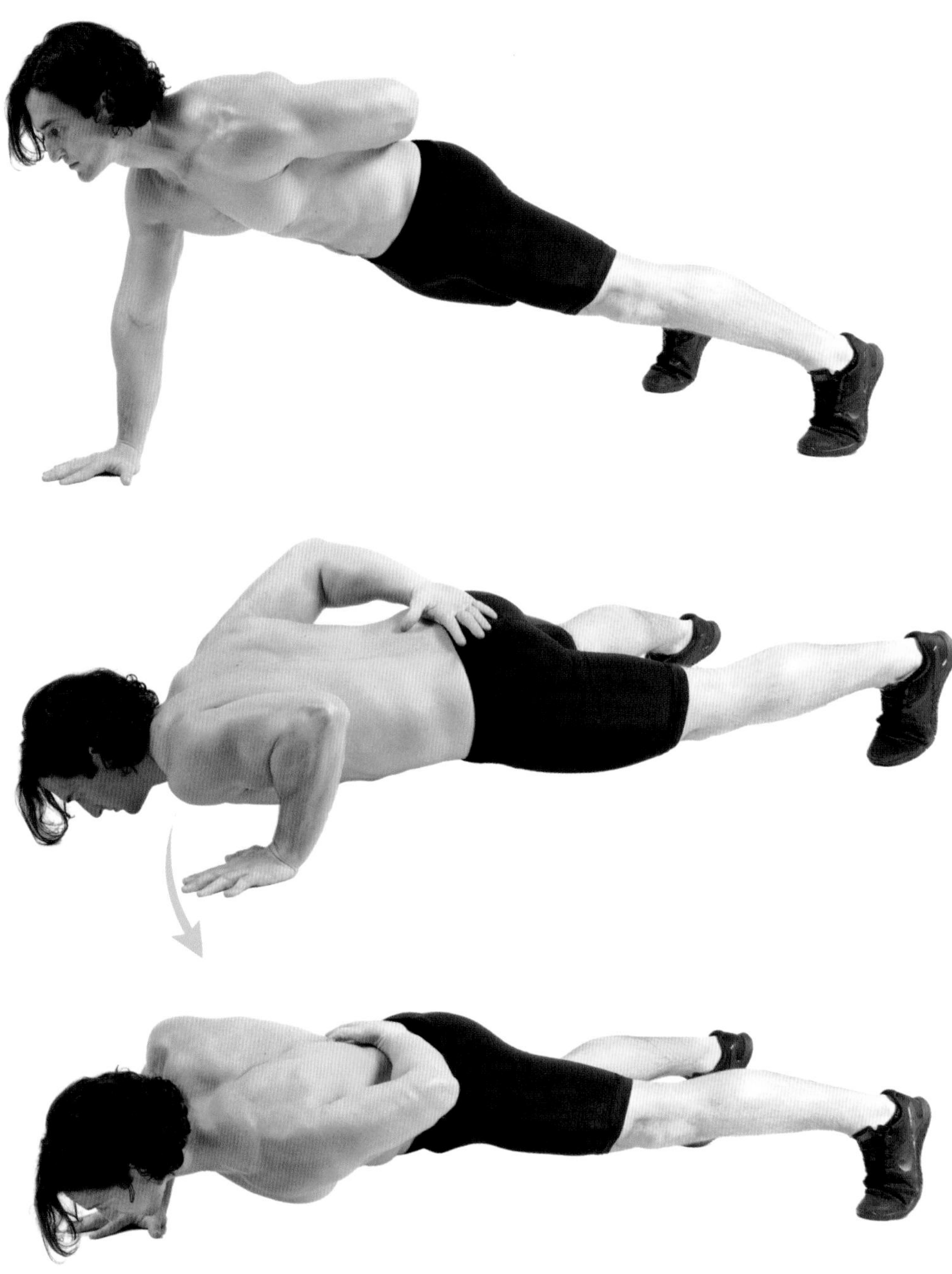

DO IT RIGHT

- Keep your back straight and hips square to the floor.
- Move with control.
- Avoid excessive arching of the spine.

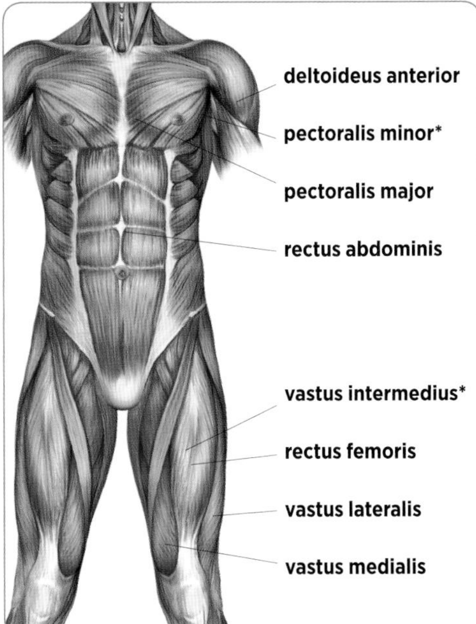

Annotation Key
Bold text indicates target muscles
Light text indicates other working muscles
* indicates deep muscles

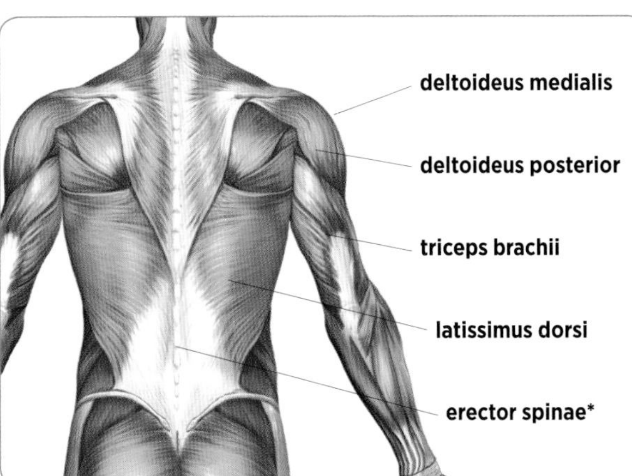

FACT FILE

TARGETS
- Pectorals
- Triceps
- Deltoids
- Abdominals
- Quadriceps

EQUIPMENT
- None

BENEFITS
- Improves balance
- Improves coordination
- Strengthens and tones chest, arms, abdominals, and legs

CAUTIONS
- Wrist issues
- Shoulder issues

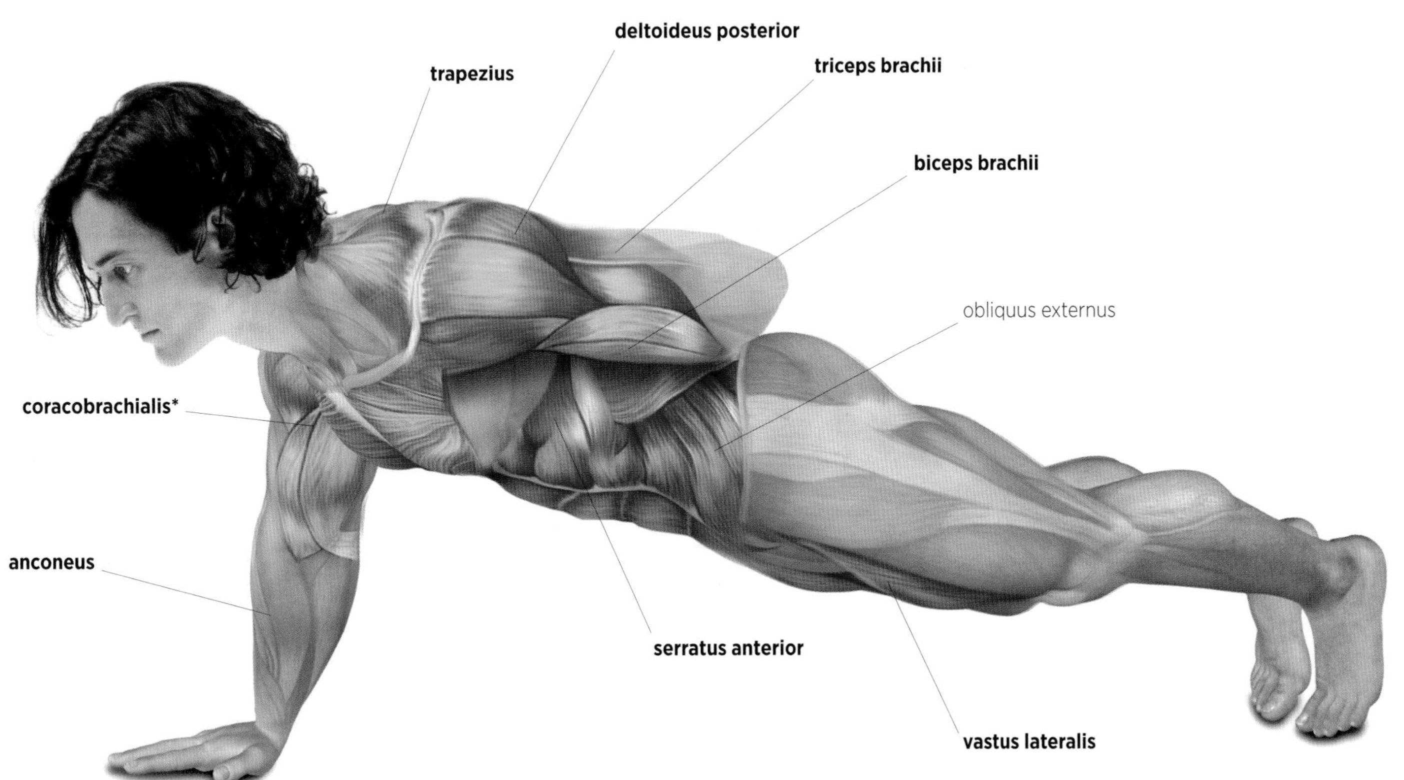

Dive-Bomber Push-Up

This upper-body and core exercise gets its name from the swooping movement you make as you move though the exercise. It will effectively strengthen your arms, shoulders, chest, back, and abdominals.

HOW TO DO IT

- Stand with your feet shoulder-width apart. Bend forward to place your hands on the floor, also shoulder-width apart. Raise your hips so that your body forms an inverted V.
- With a controlled movement, swoop your hips toward the floor while simultaneously raising your chest.
- Continue rising upward until you're looking toward the ceiling and your back is arched.
- Swoop back down, and then repeat the entire sequence for the recommended repetitions.

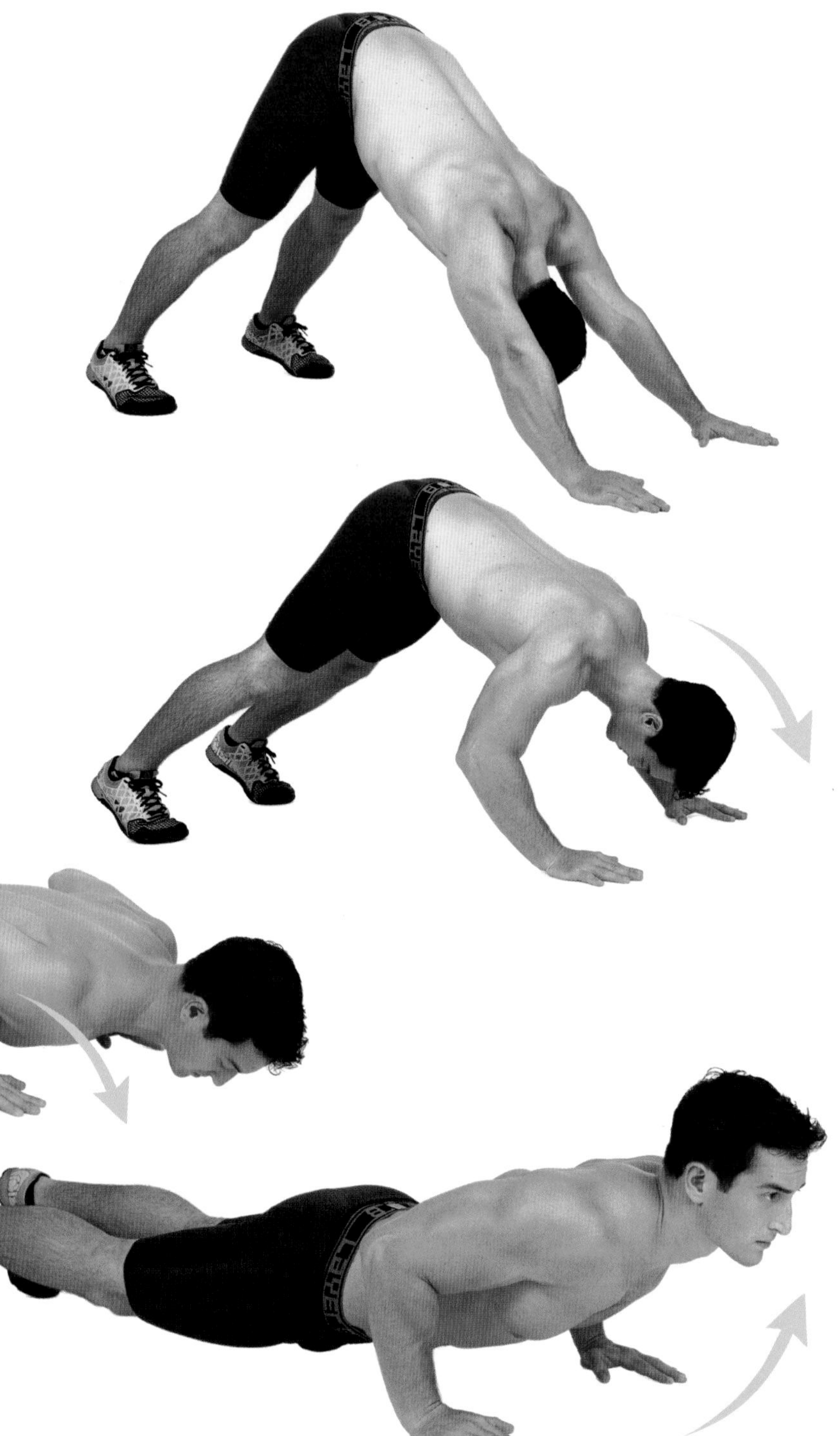

DO IT RIGHT

- Plant your hands firmly on the floor, securely grounding your fingers.
- Move with control.

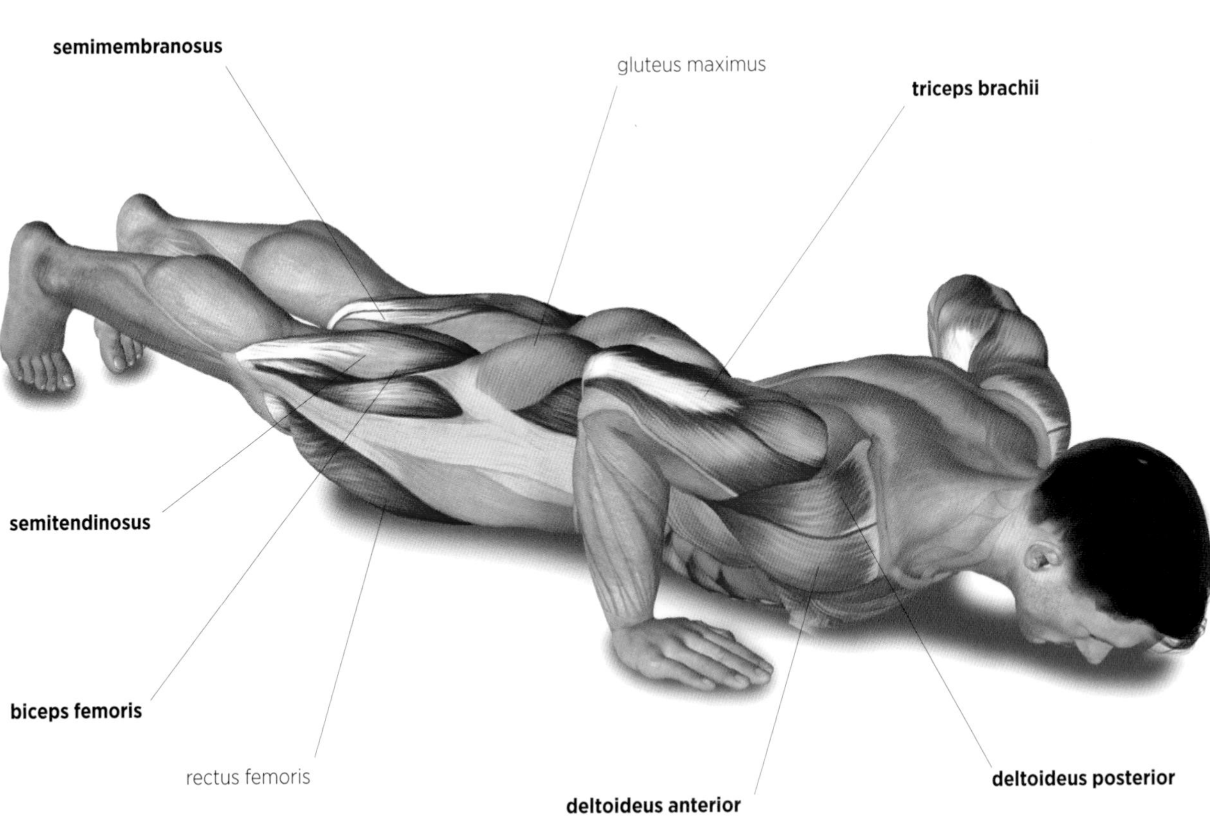

FACT FILE

TARGETS
- Pectorals
- Deltoids
- Hamstrings
- Back
- Abdominals

EQUIPMENT
- None

BENEFITS
- Strengthens legs, wrists, arms, and spine
- Stretches chest, shoulders, thighs, and abdomen
- Improves posture

CAUTIONS
- Back injury
- Wrist injury or carpal tunnel syndrome

Annotation Key

Bold text indicates target muscles

Light text indicates other working muscles

* indicates deep muscles

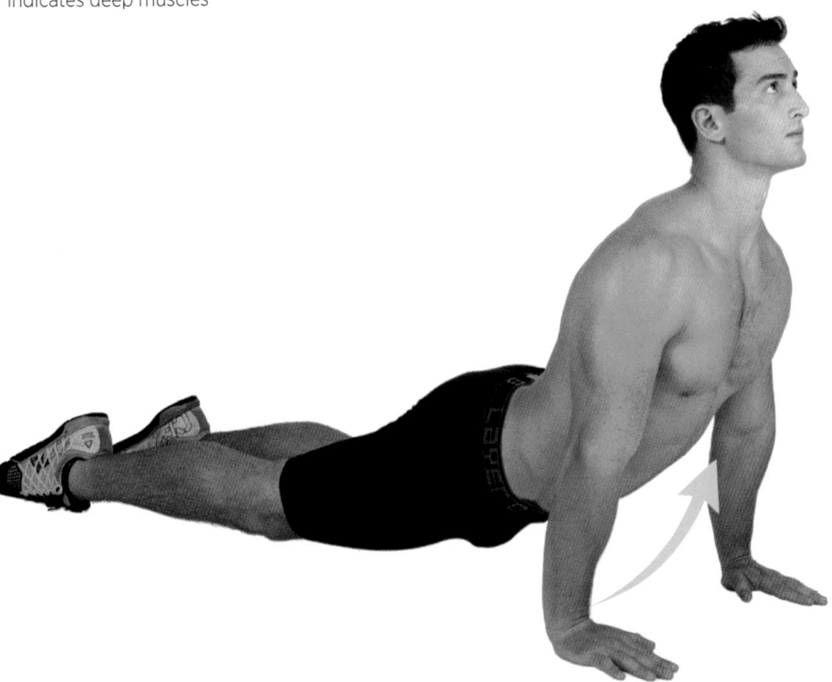

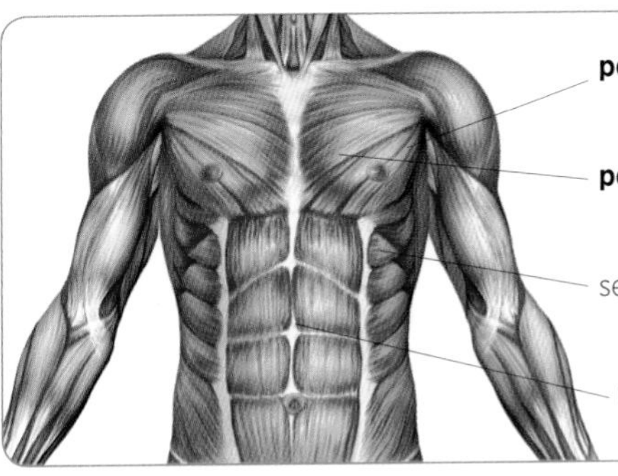

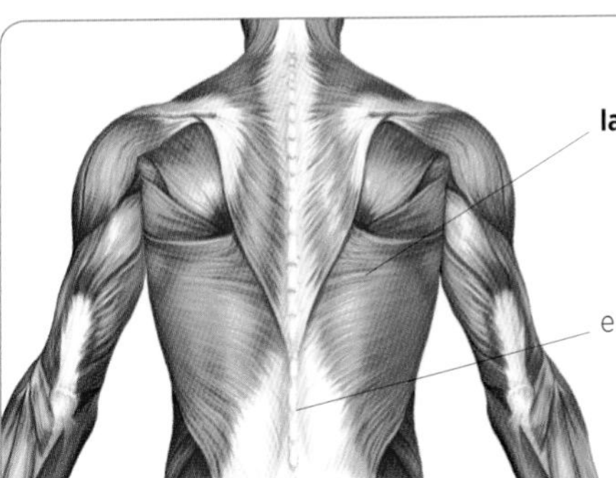

Towel Fly

The Towel Fly is a great addition to your chest workout. Its in-out movement not only engages your chest muscles but also recruits numerous other muscles, including those of the arms, back, hips, and abdomen, to keep your body stabilized.

HOW TO DO IT

- Place a towel on the floor in front of you. Assume a high plank position, with your elbows fully extended and the towel under your hands.
- Maintaining a rigid plank position and putting your weight into your heels, move your hands together. The towel should bunch together below your sternum.
- Straighten out the towel by pressing outward with your arms, returning to the starting position. Repeat for the recommended repetitions.

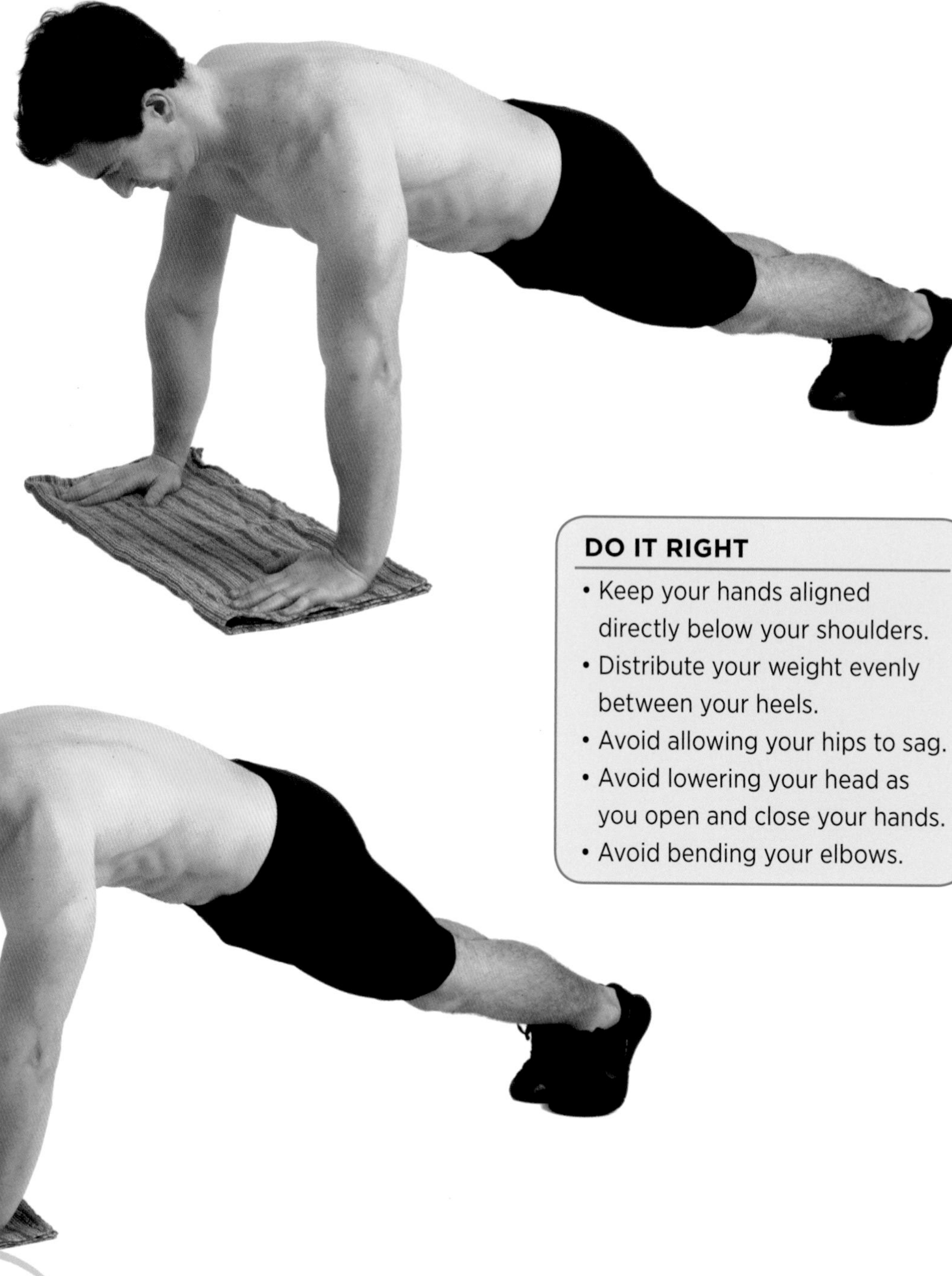

DO IT RIGHT

- Keep your hands aligned directly below your shoulders.
- Distribute your weight evenly between your heels.
- Avoid allowing your hips to sag.
- Avoid lowering your head as you open and close your hands.
- Avoid bending your elbows.

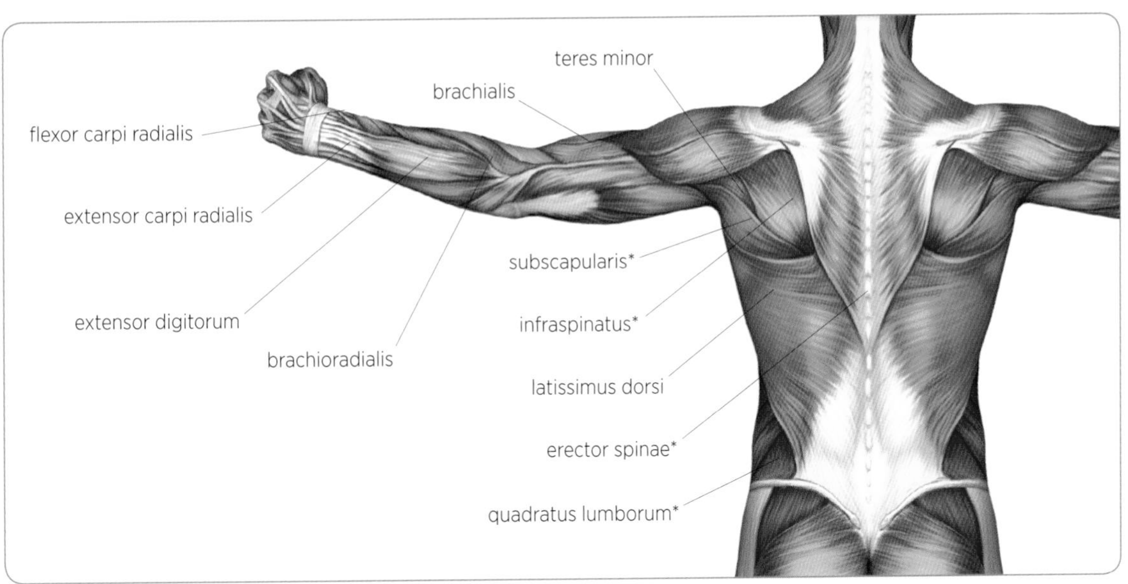

FACT FILE

TARGETS
- Pectorals
- Deltoids
- Hamstrings
- Back
- Abdominals

EQUIPMENT
- None

BENEFITS
- Strengthens chest and upper arm muscles
- Develops trunk and pelvic stability

CAUTIONS
- Shoulder issues
- Wrist issues
- Neck pain
- Lower-back pain

Annotation Key

Bold text indicates target muscles
Light text indicates other working muscles
* indicates deep muscles

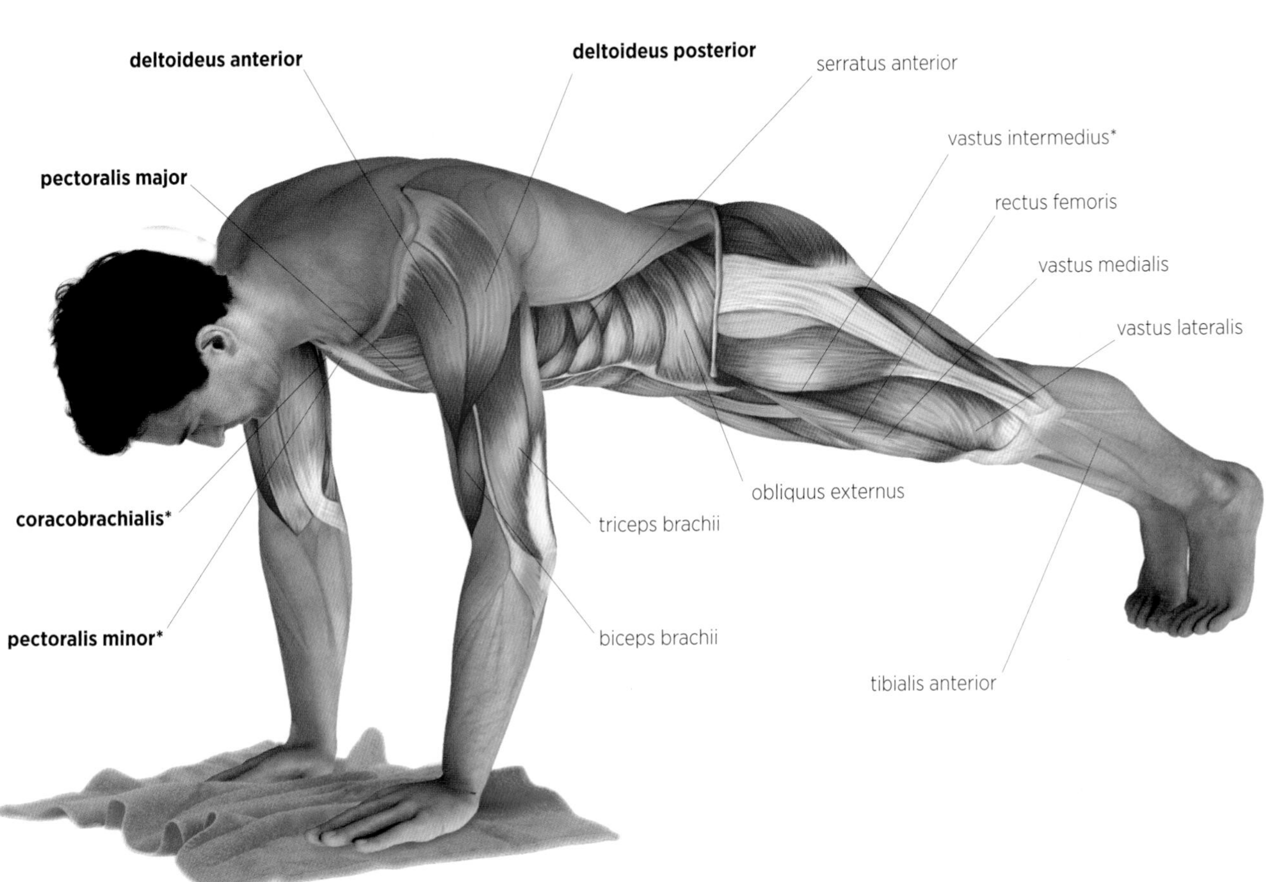

Sprawl Push-Up

Try the Sprawl Push-Up for a cardio-intensive version of the basic Push-Up. Perform this exercise as quickly as possible to increase the demand on your cardiovascular system.

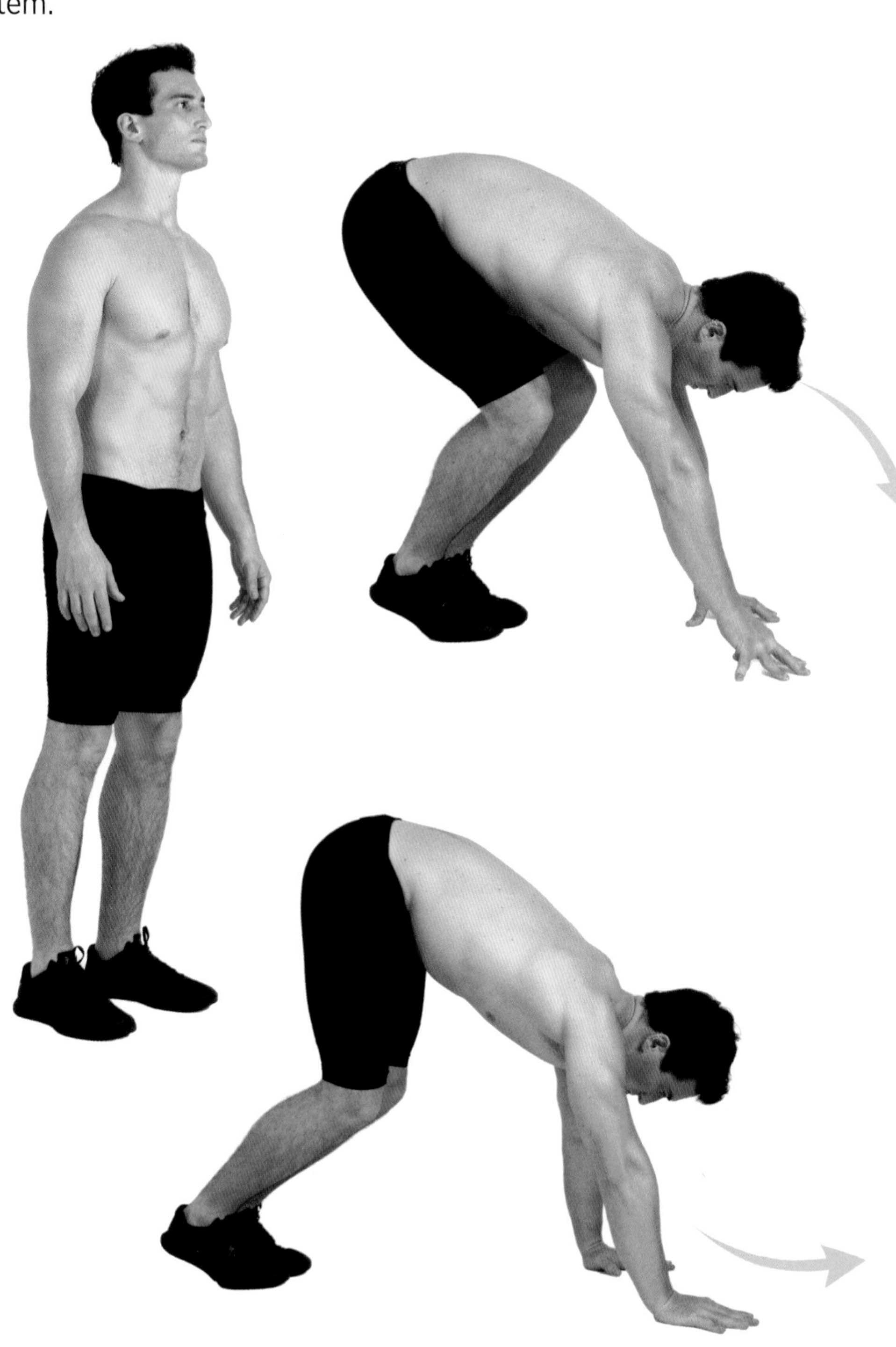

HOW TO DO IT

- Stand with your feet together.
- Bend forward from your hips, and place your hands on the floor, walking them forward.
- Continue walking your hands forward until you are in a flat Push-Up position.
- Raise your body to a high plank position with your feet spread wider than hips-width apart and your hands planted beneath your shoulders.
- Lower your chest back to floor. This is one repetition.
- Walk your hands back to your feet to return to a standing position. Perform as many repetitions as possible in the recommended time.

DO IT RIGHT

- Keep your legs and back straight during the push-up portion.
- Perform this exercise as quickly as possible to increase the demand on your cardiovascular system.
- Avoid pointing your elbows to the side during the down movement; this places undue stress on the anterior deltoids.

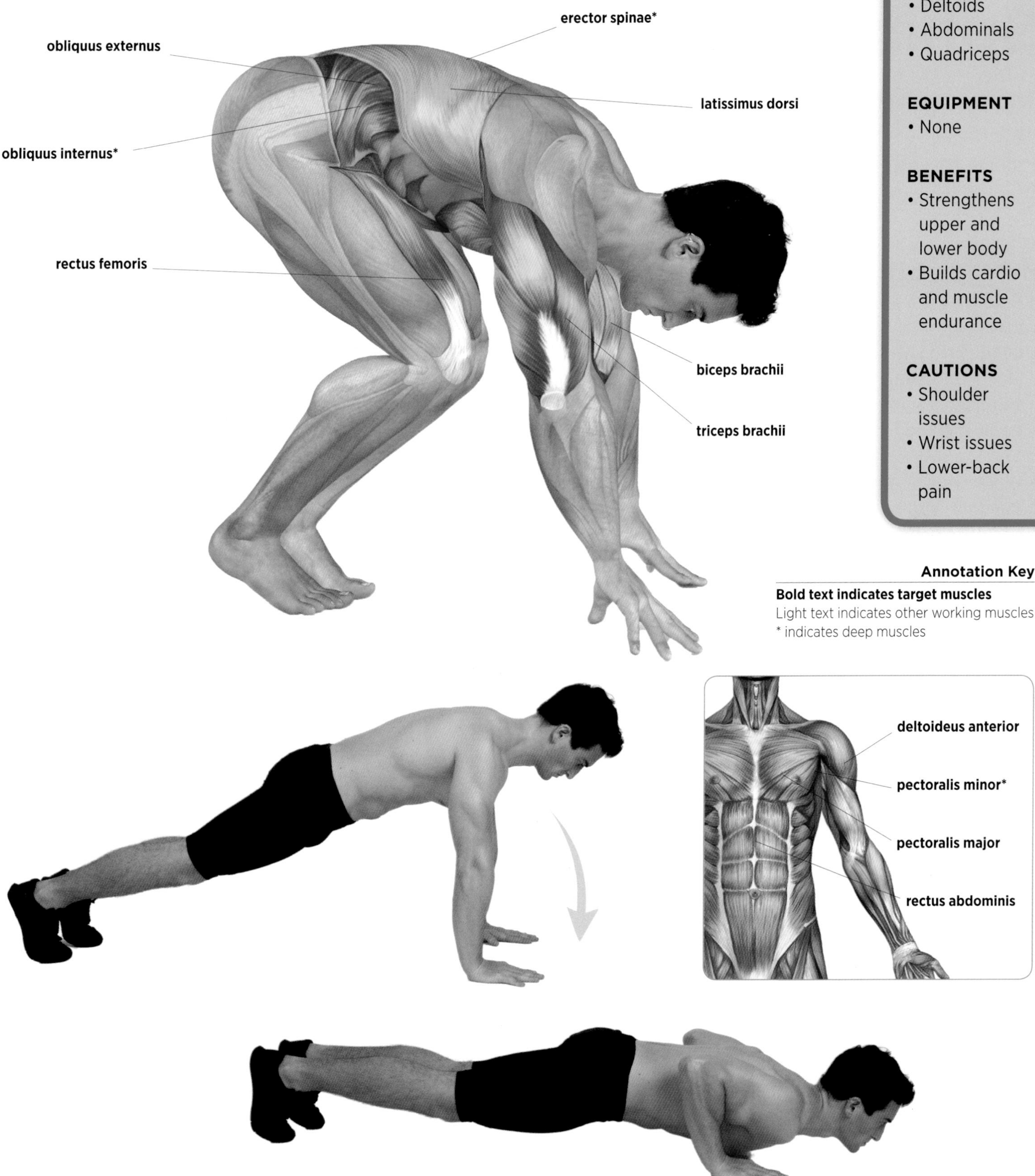

FACT FILE

TARGETS
- Pectorals
- Triceps
- Deltoids
- Abdominals
- Quadriceps

EQUIPMENT
- None

BENEFITS
- Strengthens upper and lower body
- Builds cardio and muscle endurance

CAUTIONS
- Shoulder issues
- Wrist issues
- Lower-back pain

Annotation Key

Bold text indicates target muscles

Light text indicates other working muscles

* indicates deep muscles

Sphinx Push-Up

Inspired by the statuesque Egyptian figure, this exercise will give you rock-hard muscles that will stand the test of time. With a focus on the triceps, this intermediate exercise combines the best benefits of planks and push-ups into one high-intensity movement.

FACT FILE

TARGETS
- Triceps
- Pectorals
- Abdominals

EQUIPMENT
- None

BENEFITS
- Strengthens and tones arms, abdominals, and chest
- Improves core stability

CAUTIONS
- Wrist issues

HOW TO DO IT

- Assume a low plank position with your forearms positioned directly under your shoulders, your palms facing downward, your legs extended behind you, and your feet firmly planted.
- While engaging your core, press into the floor with both hands, extending at your elbows to lift your body away from the floor until your arms are straight and you are in a high plank position.
- Bend your elbows until you are again resting on your forearms to return to the starting position.

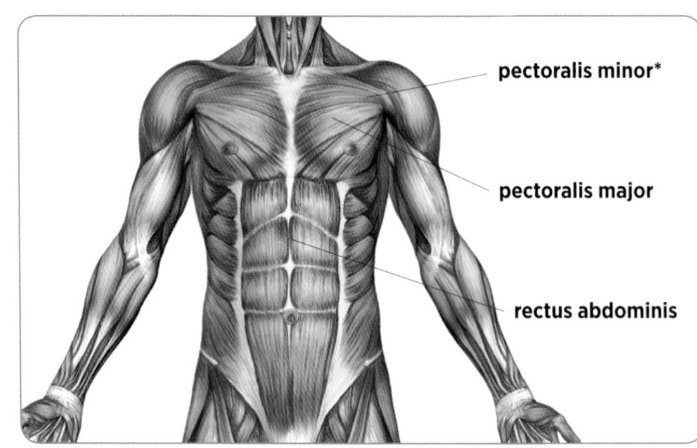
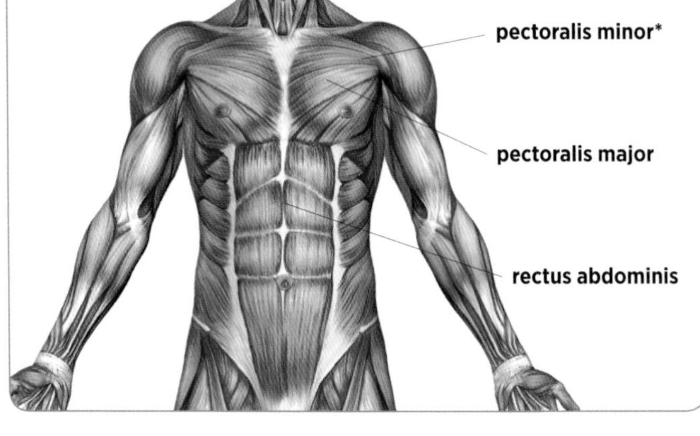

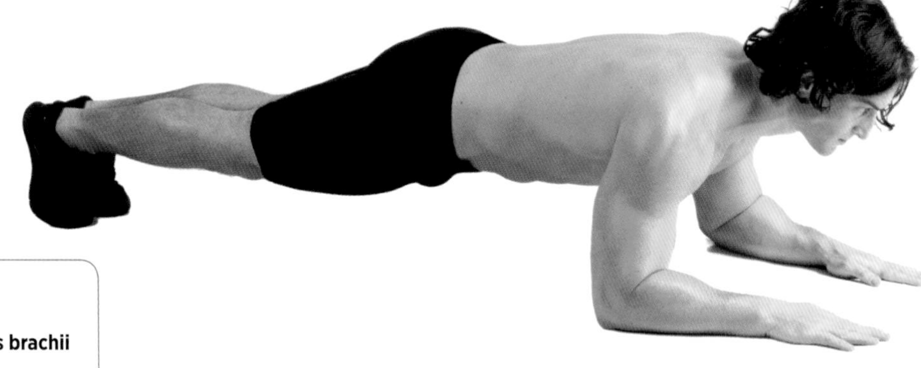

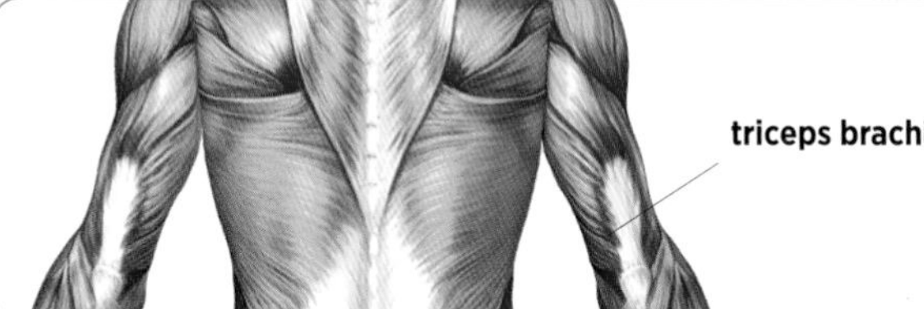

Annotation Key
Bold text indicates target muscles
Light text indicates other working muscles
* indicates deep muscles

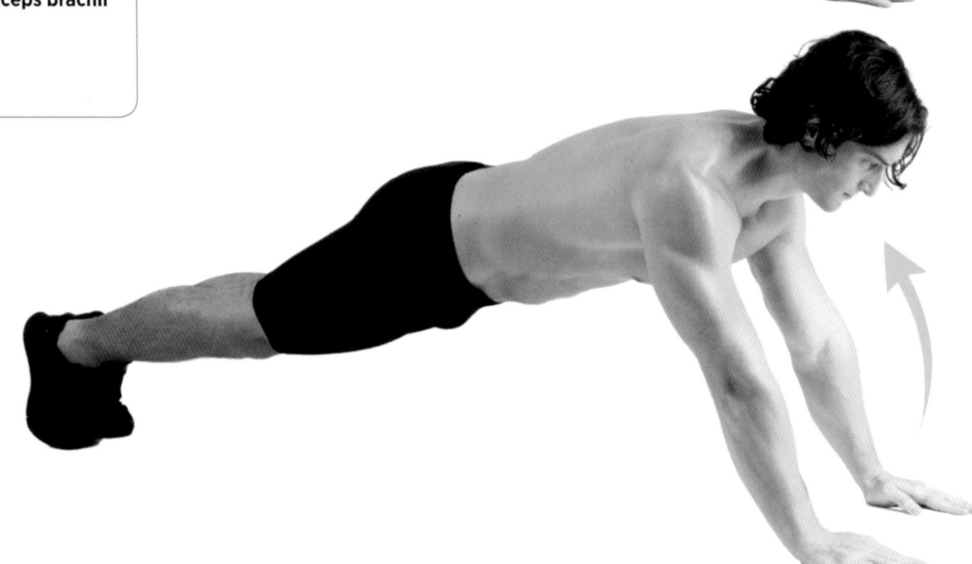

DO IT RIGHT

- Keep your back straight.
- Keep your hands in line with your shoulders.
- Avoid excessive arching of your spine.

Star Push-Up

This stellar exercise says goodbye to the earthly confines of the basic push-up and will launch your workout to a higher level. The Star Push-Up places high stress on the pectorals, as well as the serratus anterior, core, quadriceps, and many other muscles.

FACT FILE

TARGETS
- Biceps
- Pectorals
- Abdominals
- Hip flexors
- Quadriceps

EQUIPMENT
- None

BENEFITS
- Strengthens and tones abdominal, chest, arms, and legs
- Improves core stability

CAUTIONS
- Lower-back issues

HOW TO DO IT

- Lie facedown with your arms and legs extended, creating a star shape with your body.
- Keeping your core engaged, simultaneously press your hands and feet into the floor to lift your body. Keep your arms and legs as straight as possible.
- Return to the starting position, and then repeat for the recommended repetitions.

DO IT RIGHT
- Keep your back straight.
- Keep your abdominals engaged.
- Avoid bending your arms or legs.

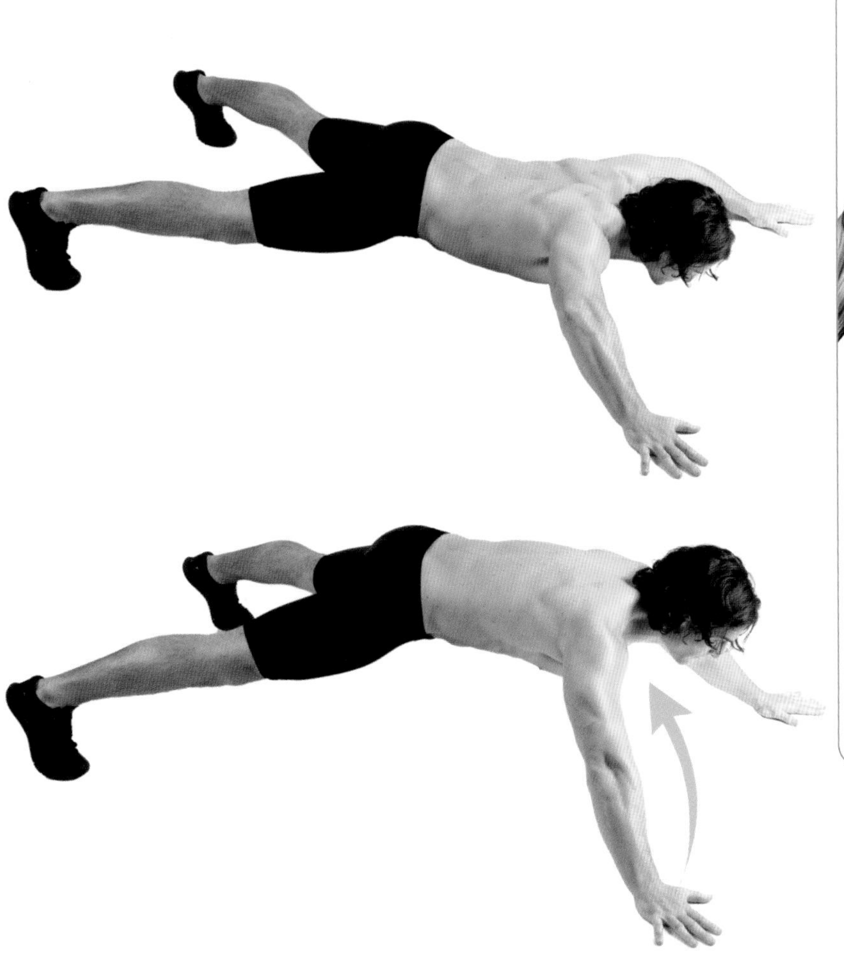

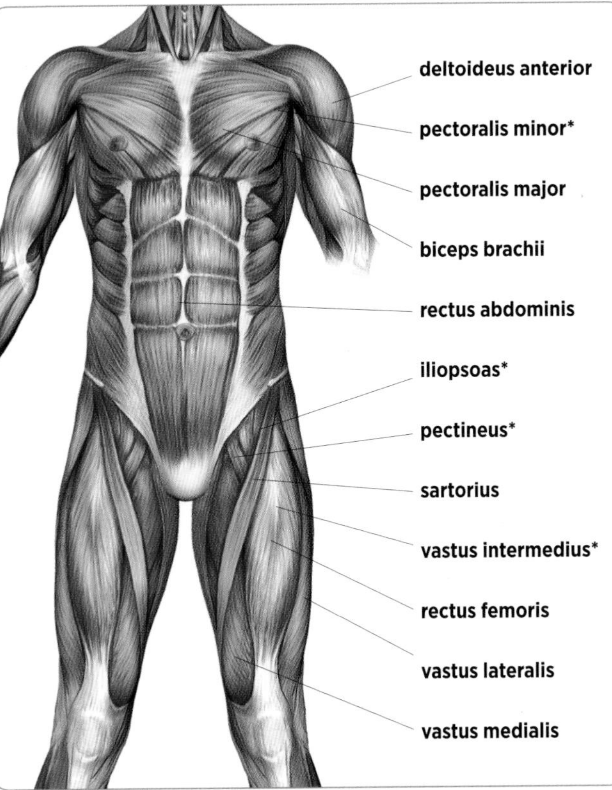

Annotation Key
Bold text indicates target muscles
Light text indicates other working muscles
* indicates deep muscles

Bent-Knee Sit-Up

Also called Crunches, Bent-Knee Sit-Ups are classic exercises for abdominal-endurance training, hitting both your abs and obliques.

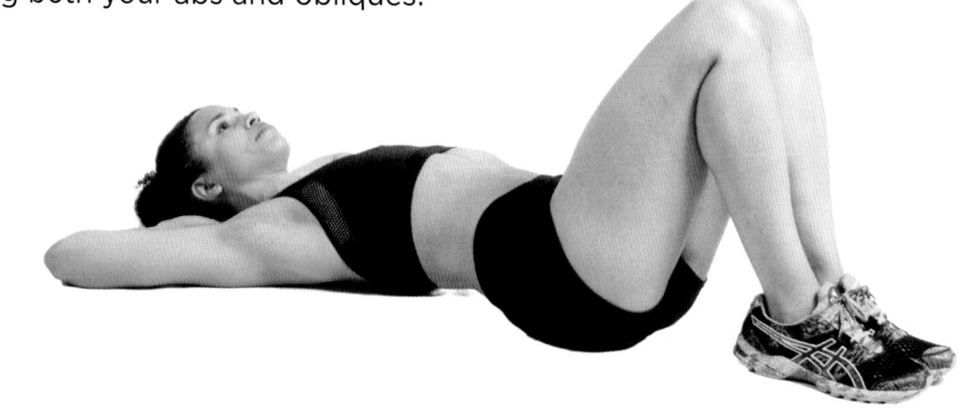

HOW TO DO IT

- Lie faceup with your legs bent so that your feet are tucked as close to your buttocks as possible. Either put your hands on your head or cross your arms over your chest.
- Flex your torso toward your thighs until your back is off the floor.
- Lower back down to the starting position, and then repeat for the recommended repetitions.

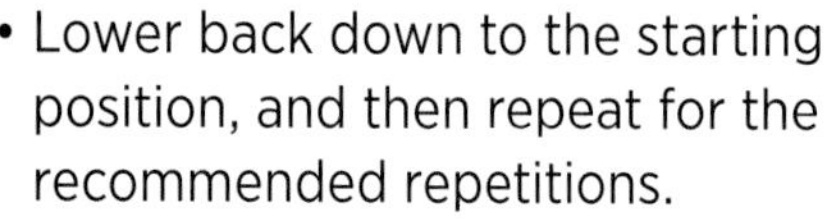

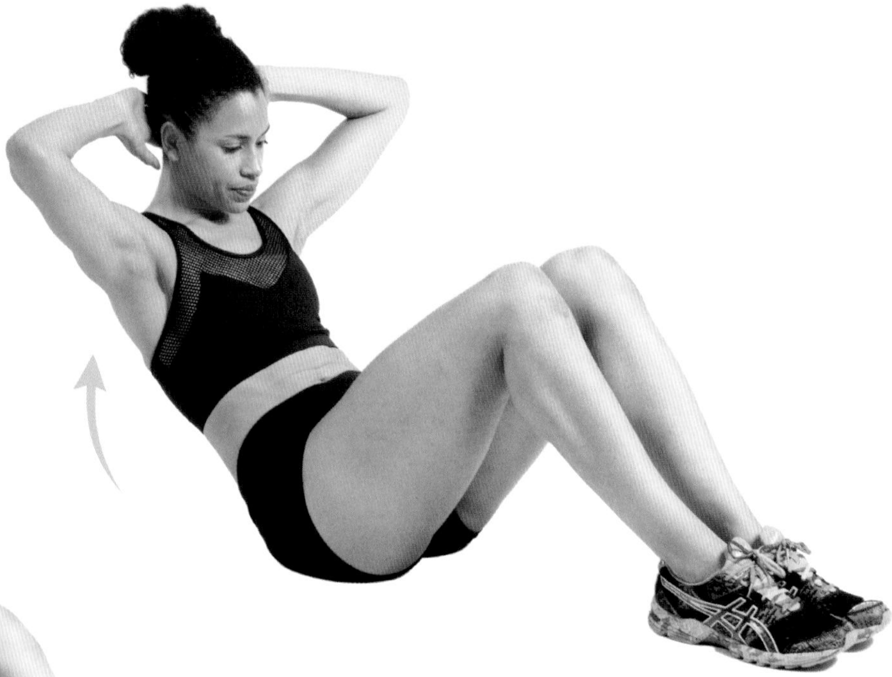

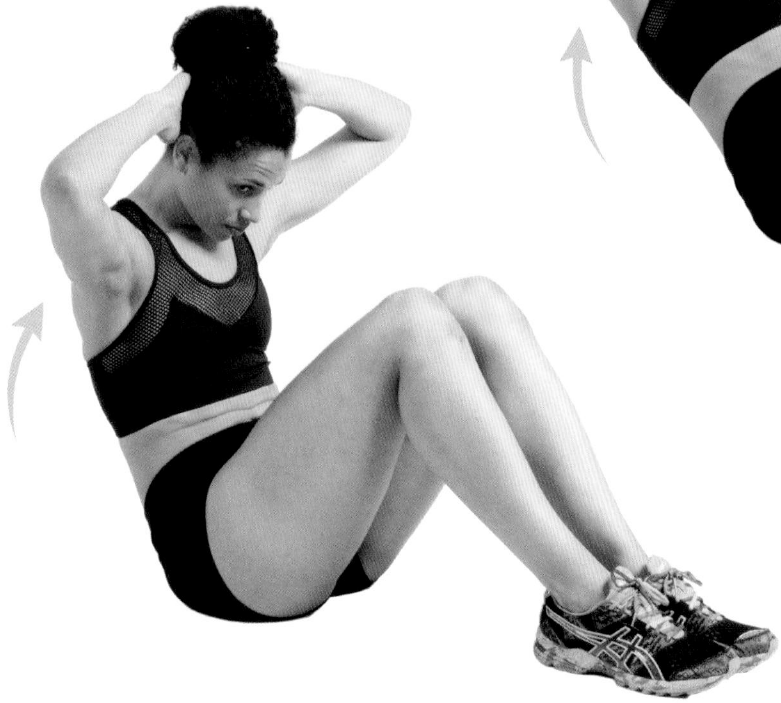

DO IT RIGHT

- Be sure to engage your core, not your neck.
- Avoid rounding your back.

deltoideus posterior
latissimus dorsi
erector spinae*
quadratus lumborum*
gluteus minimus*
semimembranosus

obliquus internus*
transversus abdominis*
iliopsoas*
sartorius
rectus femoris

FACT FILE

TARGETS
- Abdominals
- Obliques
- Hip flexors
- Spine

EQUIPMENT
- None

BENEFITS
- Strengthens abdominals, obliques, hip flexors, and spinal erectors

CAUTIONS
- Lower-back issues
- Neck issues

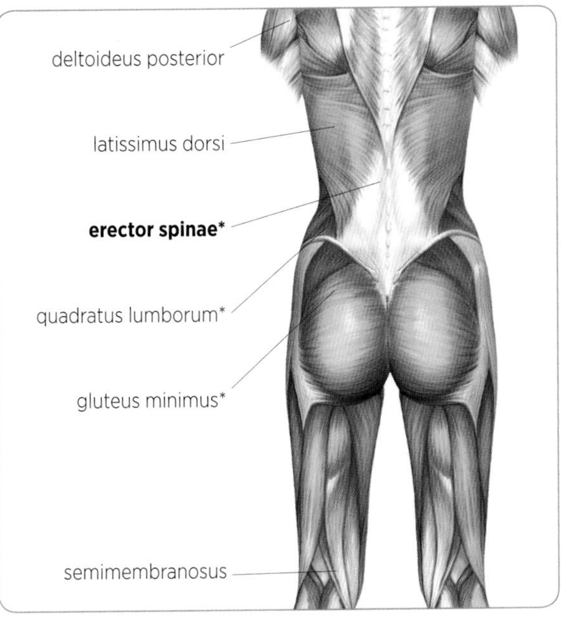

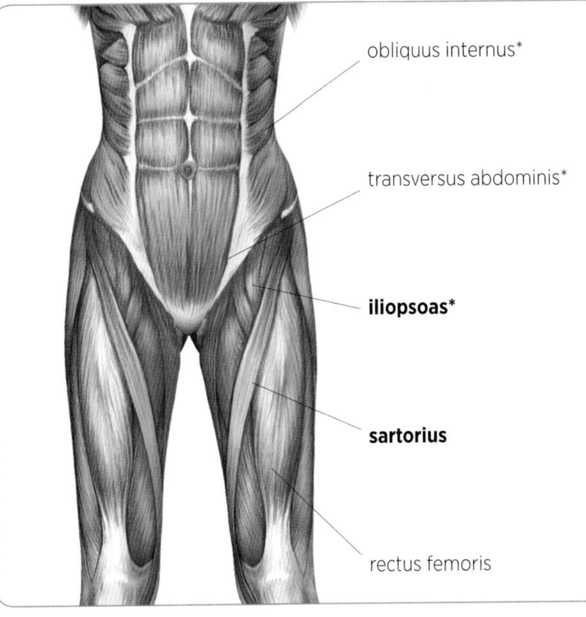

Annotation Key

Bold text indicates target muscles
Light text indicates other working muscles
* indicates deep muscles

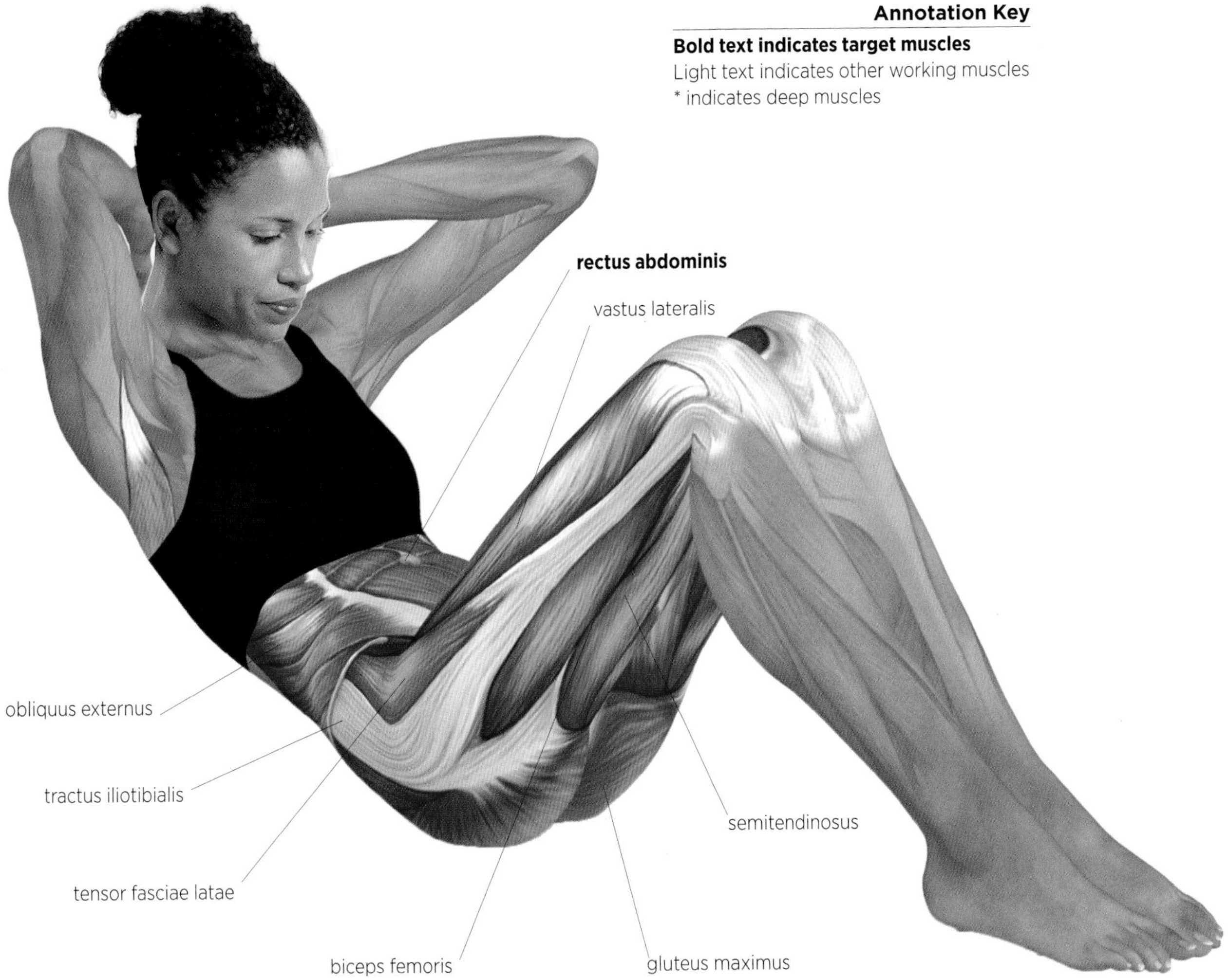

rectus abdominis
vastus lateralis
obliquus externus
tractus iliotibialis
tensor fasciae latae
biceps femoris
gluteus maximus
semitendinosus

Bicycle Crunch

The Bicycle Crunch targets your upper abdominals and your obliques, strengthening and toning these muscles. Resist the urge to "cycle" too quickly; a smooth, controlled pace is most effective.

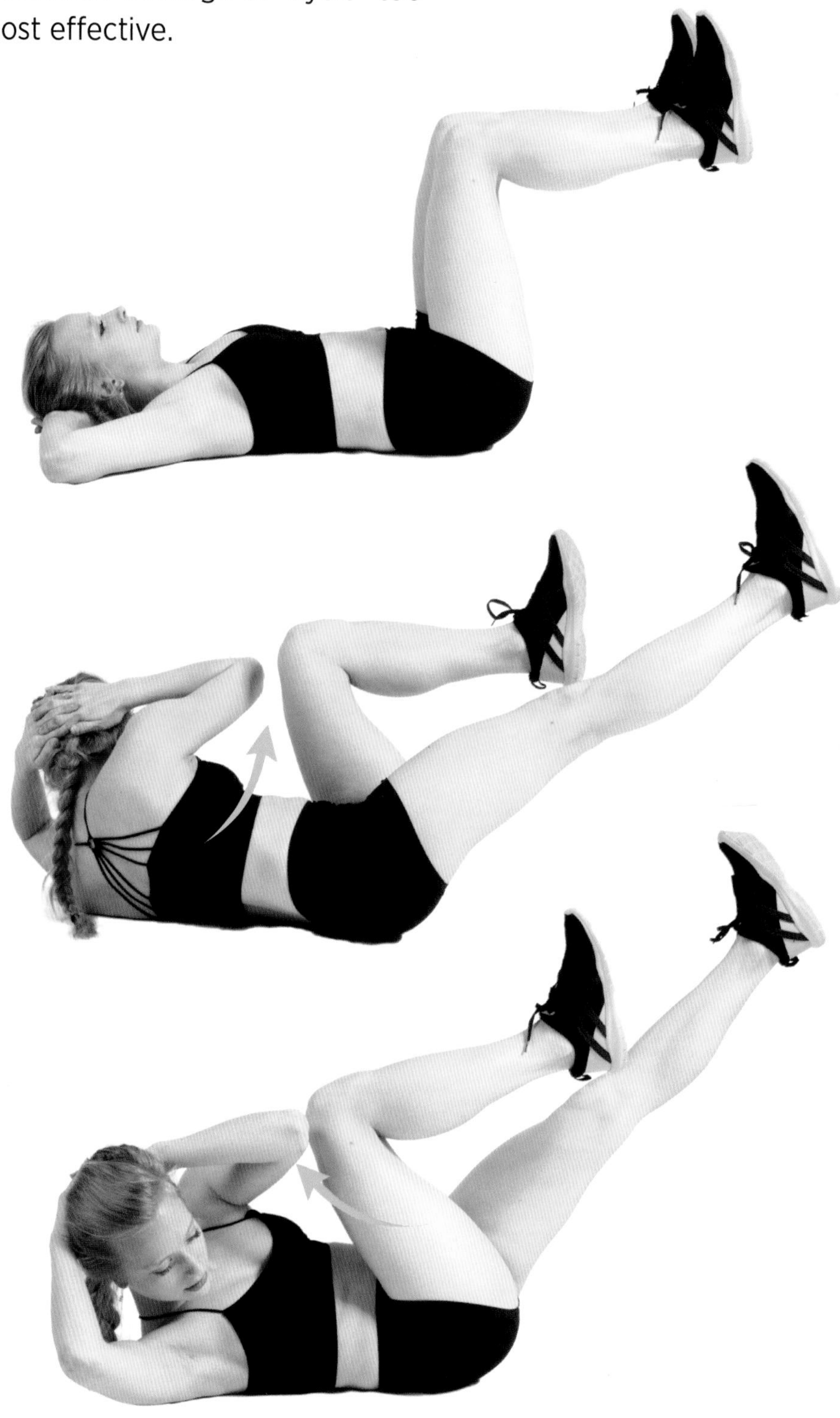

HOW TO DO IT

- Lie faceup with fingers at your ears, your elbows flared outward, and your legs bent to form a 90-degree angle.
- Begin to lift your shoulders and upper torso off the floor as your raise your right elbow diagonally. At the same time, bring your left knee toward your elbow and extend your right leg diagonally forward until your right elbow and left knee meet.
- Lower, and then repeat on the other side. Continue alternating sides for the recommended repetitions.

DO IT RIGHT

- Raise your elbow and opposite knee equally so that they meet in the middle.
- Avoid raising your lower back off the floor.
- Avoid rushing through the movement.

obliquus internus*
iliopsoas*
pectineus*
vastus intermedius*
rectus femoris
gracilis*
vastus medialis

biceps femoris
semitendinosus
semimembranosus

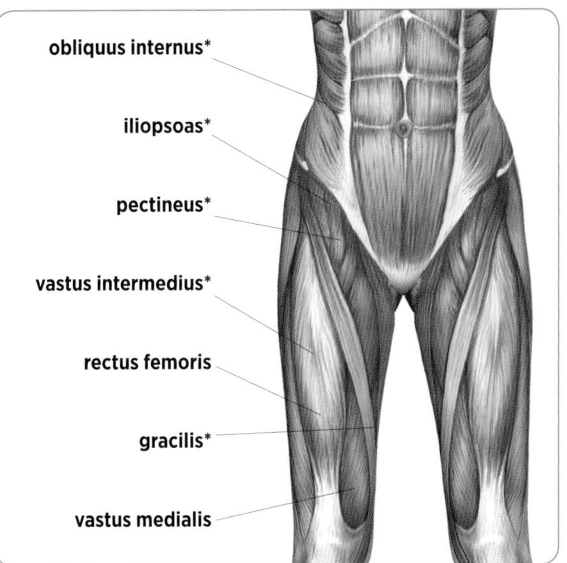

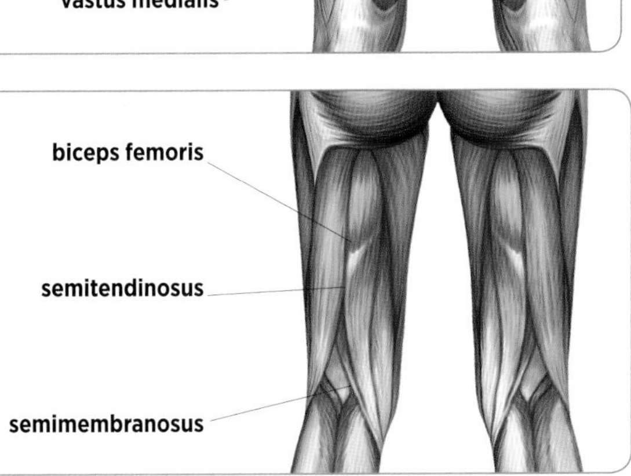

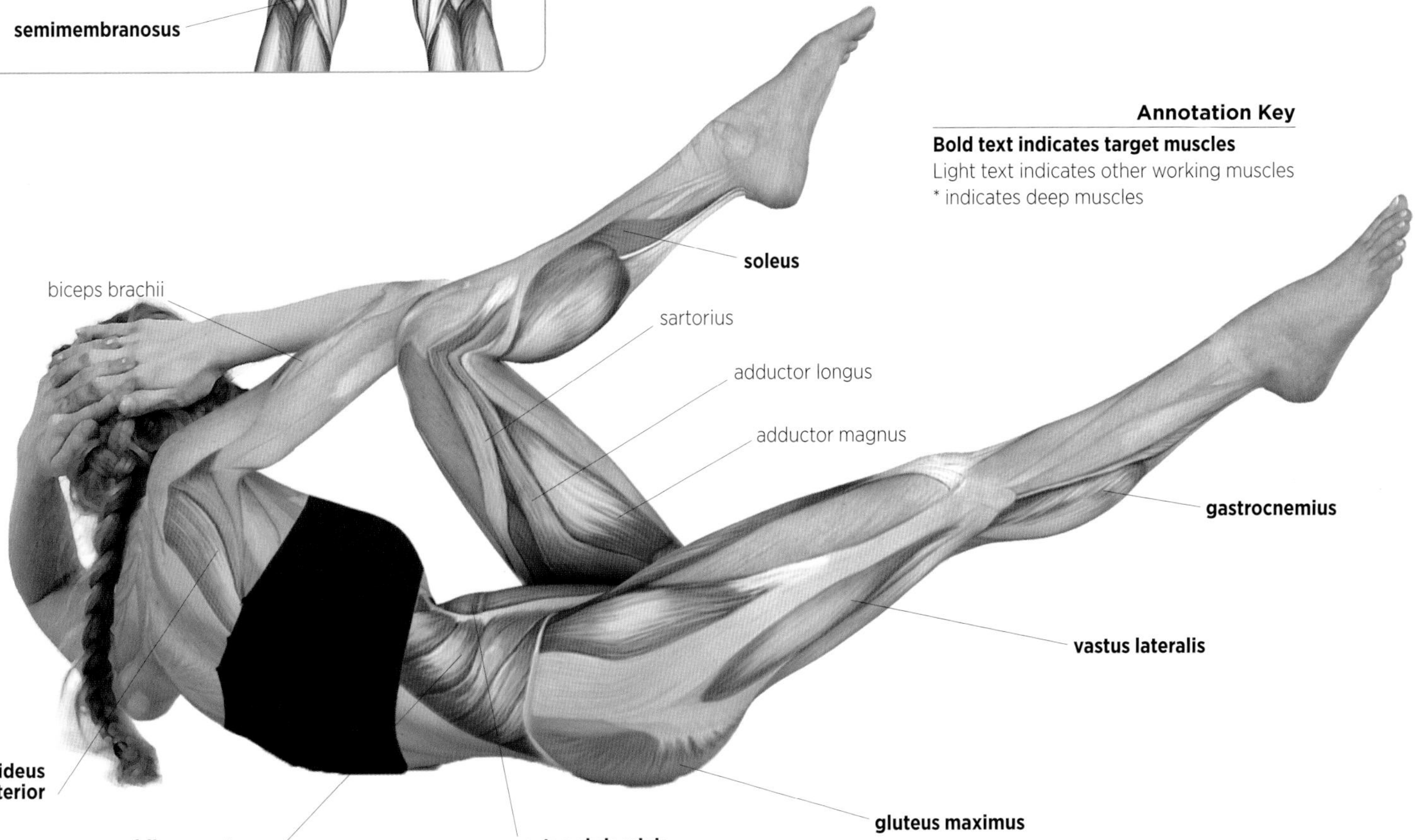

MODIFICATION

EASIER: Bend both knees and place both feet on the floor, keeping them anchored there throughout the exercise. Leading with your abdominals, raise your entire torso off the floor as you bring your left elbow to your right knee. Lower and repeat, alternating sides.

FACT FILE

TARGETS
- Abdominals
- Obliques
- Hip flexors
- Spine

EQUIPMENT
- None

BENEFITS
- Strengthens abdominals
- Stabilizes core
- Tones obliques and midsection

CAUTIONS
- Lower-back issues
- Neck issues

soleus
biceps brachii
sartorius
adductor longus
adductor magnus
gastrocnemius
vastus lateralis
deltoideus posterior
obliquus externus
rectus abdominis
gluteus maximus

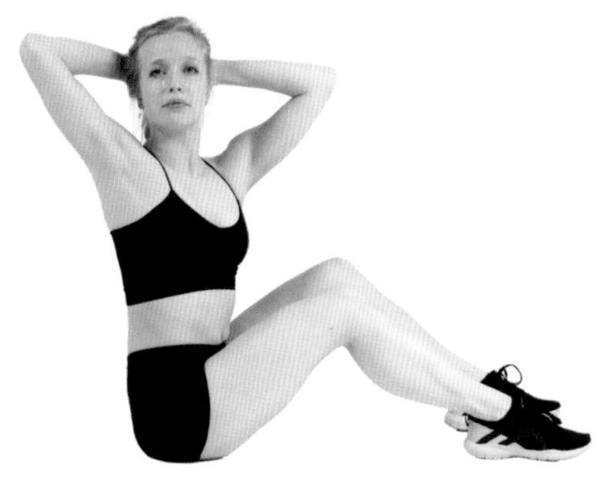

Annotation Key
Bold text indicates target muscles
Light text indicates other working muscles
* indicates deep muscles

High Knees

This simple exercise offers a high-intensity, calorie-burning cardiovascular workout that also strengthens your abdominals, thighs, calves, and glutes. You can perform High Knees while jogging over a distance or just running in place.

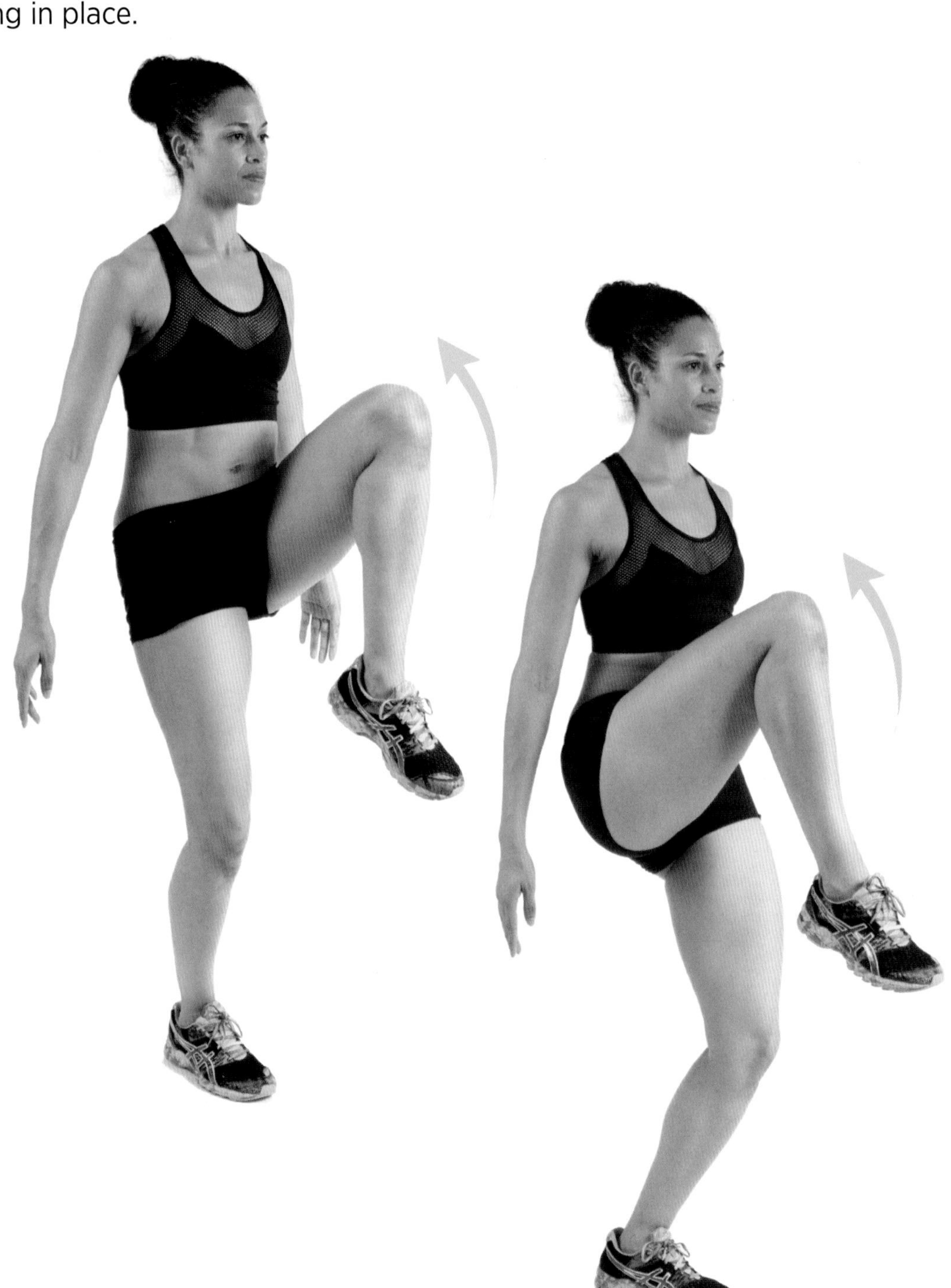

HOW TO DO IT

- Stand tall with your hands either on your hips or down by your sides.
- Raise your left knee as high as you are able, and then return to the starting position.
- Alternate legs while increasing your speed as you jog over distance or run in place. Continue for the recommended time or repetitions.

DO IT RIGHT

- Build up in speed as you go.
- Push off from your entire foot.
- Avoid pushing solely off your toes.

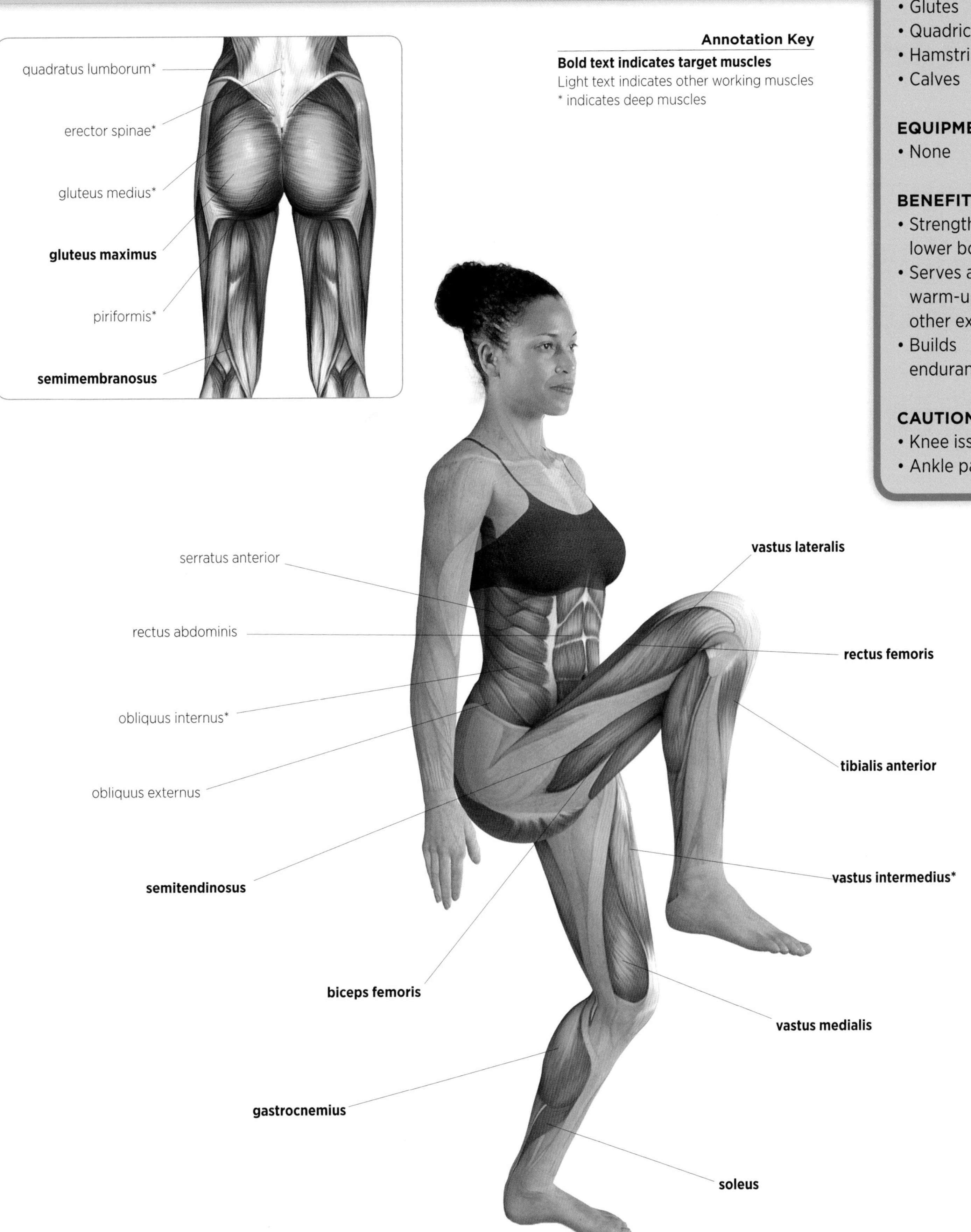

FACT FILE

TARGETS
- Abdominals
- Glutes
- Quadriceps
- Hamstrings
- Calves

EQUIPMENT
- None

BENEFITS
- Strengthens lower body
- Serves as a warm-up for other exercise
- Builds endurance

CAUTIONS
- Knee issues
- Ankle pain

V-Up

The challenging V-Up has multiple benefits. Its full range of motion targets both your upper and lower rectus abdominis, and it also works to strengthen your lower-back muscles and tighten your quads.

HOW TO DO IT

- Lie faceup with your legs straight and your arms extended behind your head.
- Simultaneously raise your arms and legs so that your fingertips are nearly touching your feet, while maintaining a flat back.
- Lower back down to the starting position, and then repeat for the recommended repetitions.

DO IT RIGHT

- Keep your arms and legs straight.
- Avoid using a jerking motion as you raise or lower your arms and legs.

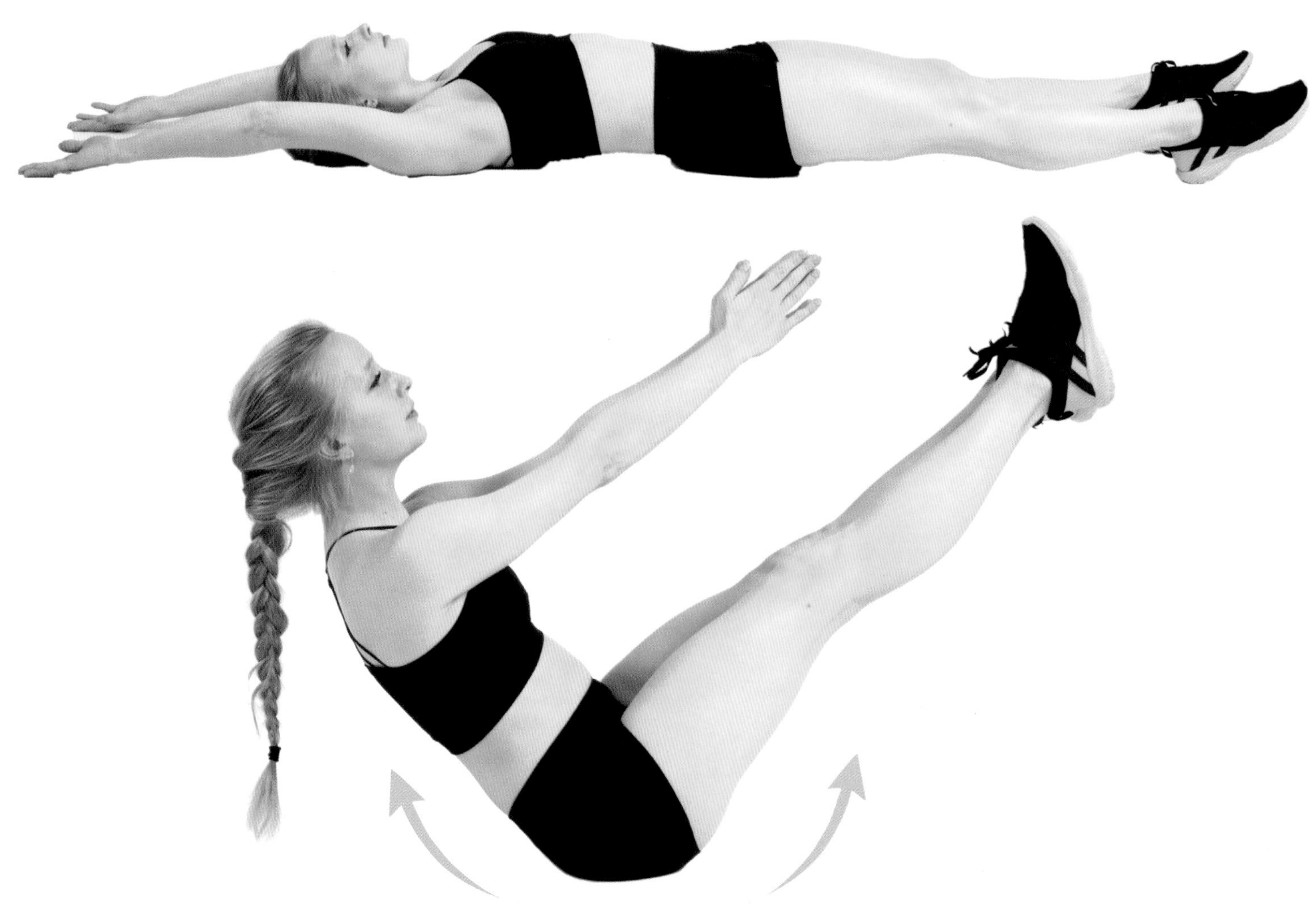

FACT FILE

TARGETS
- Abdominals
- Lower back

EQUIPMENT
- None

BENEFITS
- Strengthens core
- Increases spinal mobility

CAUTIONS
- Lower-back issues
- Neck issues

MODIFICATION

HARDER: Grasp a medicine ball in your hands, keeping it in place throughout the exercise.

transversus abdominis*
iliopsoas*
pectineus*
adductor longus
vastus intermedius*
rectus femoris
vastus medialis

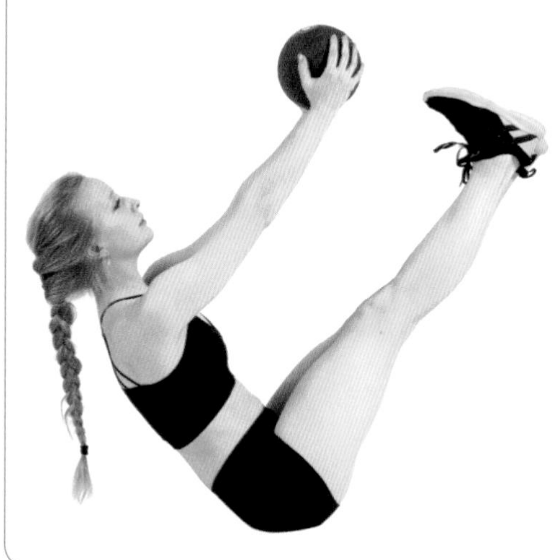

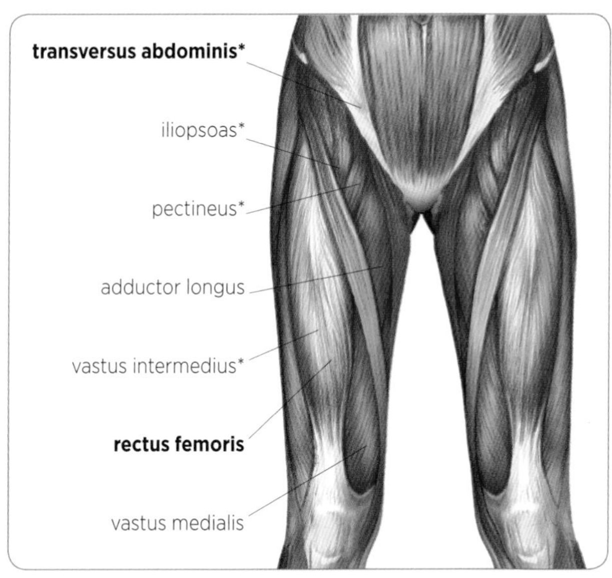

Annotation Key
Bold text indicates target muscles
Light text indicates other working muscles
* indicates deep muscles

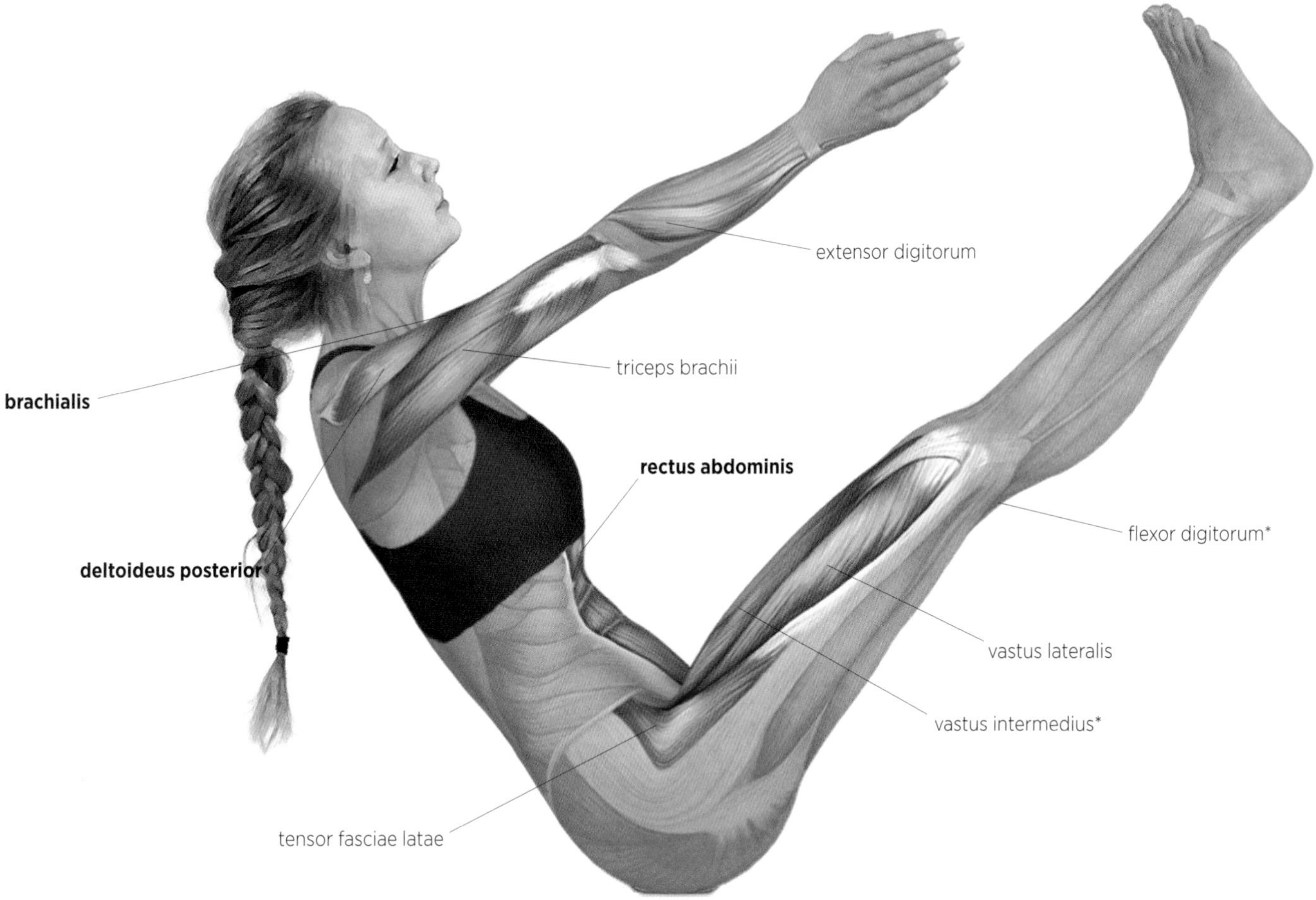

extensor digitorum
triceps brachii
brachialis
rectus abdominis
flexor digitorum*
deltoideus posterior
vastus lateralis
vastus intermedius*
tensor fasciae latae

Knees to Chest

Inspired by boot-camp training, Knees to Chest targets your lower abdominals and hip flexors. As with many military-style exercises, it is a multiphase exercise featuring four movements performed to a counting beat.

HOW TO DO IT

- Lie faceup with your legs straight and your head raised off the floor. Place both hands under your buttocks to straighten your lumbar spine, and then lift both legs so that your feet are about 6 inches off the floor. Your knees should be bent slightly.
- Keeping your feet together, bring both knees to your chest for count 1, and then straighten your legs for count 2.
- Repeat this movement for counts 3 and 4 to complete one rep. Repeat for the recommended repetitions.

DO IT RIGHT

- Keep your hands under your butt to protect your lower back from excess extension.
- Avoid resting your head on the floor.

FACT FILE

TARGETS
- Abdominals
- Hip flexors

EQUIPMENT
- None

BENEFITS
- Strengthens abdominals and hip flexors
- Increases endurance

CAUTIONS
- Lower-back pain

Annotation Key
Bold text indicates target muscles
Light text indicates other working muscles
* indicates deep muscles

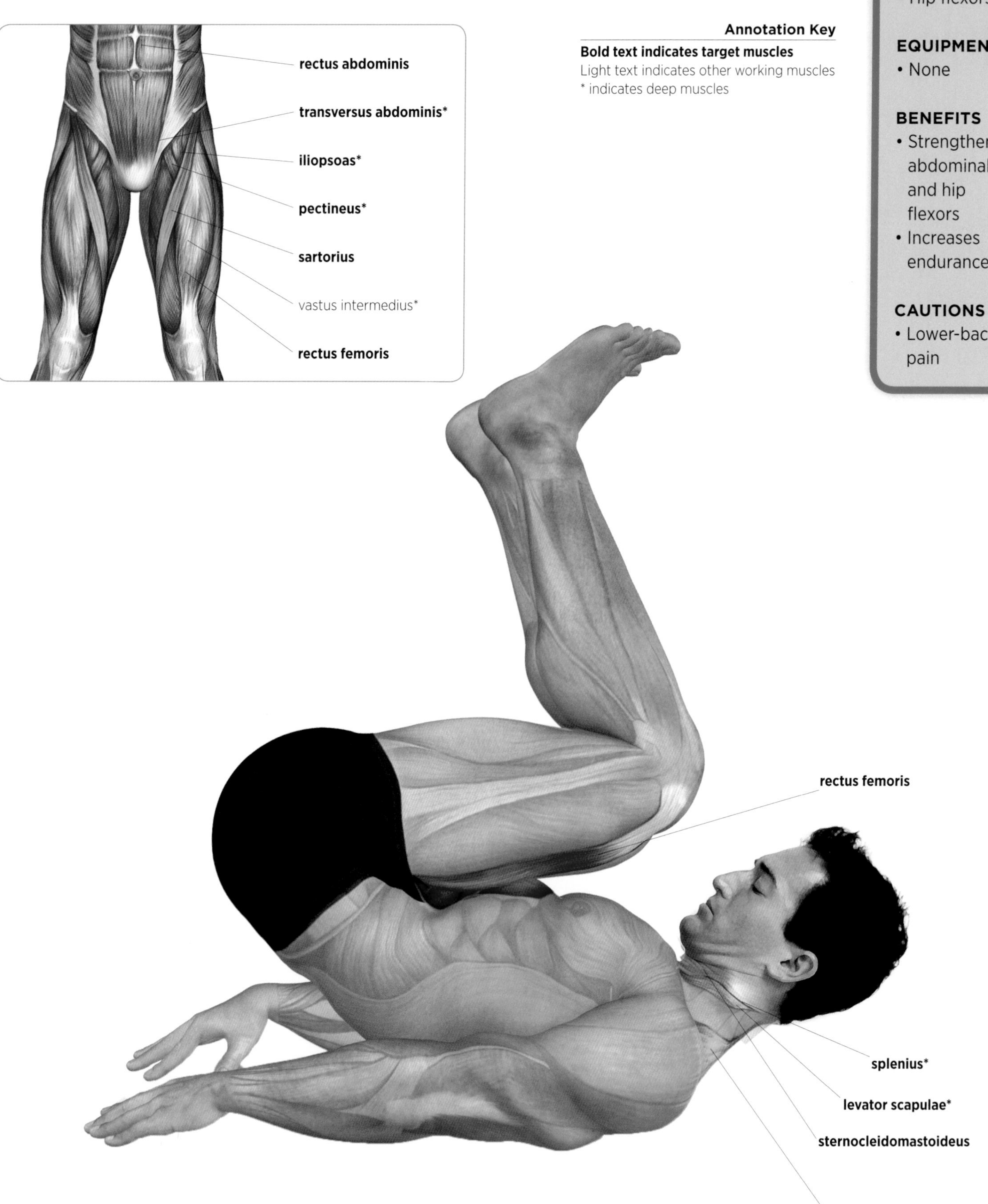

Abdominal Kick

This intense exercise strengthens and stabilizes your abdominals, particularly your lower abs. Perform the Abdominal Kick at a steady, controlled pace for the best results.

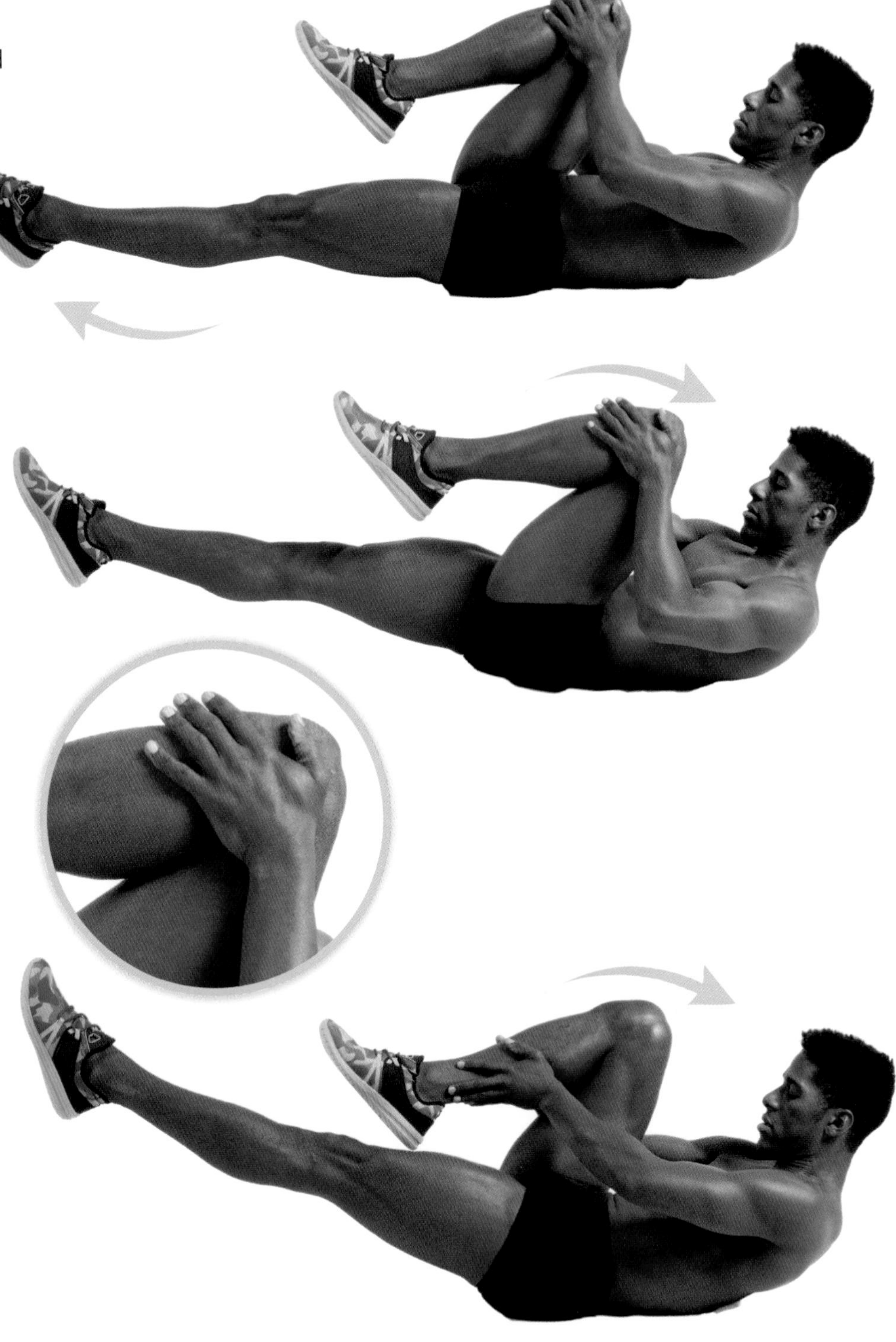

HOW TO DO IT

- Lie faceup with your legs straight and your head raised off the floor.
- Pull your right knee toward your chest, and straighten your left leg, raising it about 45 degrees from the floor. Place your left hand on the inside of your right ankle and your right hand on your bent knee.
- Switch your legs two times, switching your hand placement simultaneously.
- Switch your legs two more times, keeping your hands in their proper placement. Continue alternating sides for the recommended repetitions.

DO IT RIGHT

- Place your hand on the ankle of your bent leg and your inside hand on your bent knee.
- Lift the top of your sternum forward.
- Avoid allowing your lower back to rise up off the floor; use your abdominals to stabilize core while switching legs.

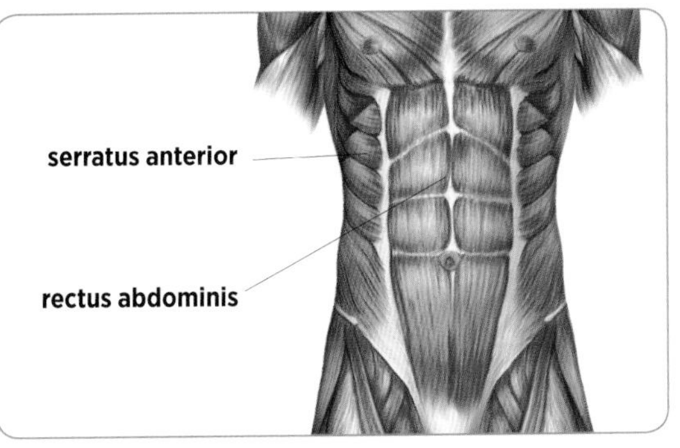

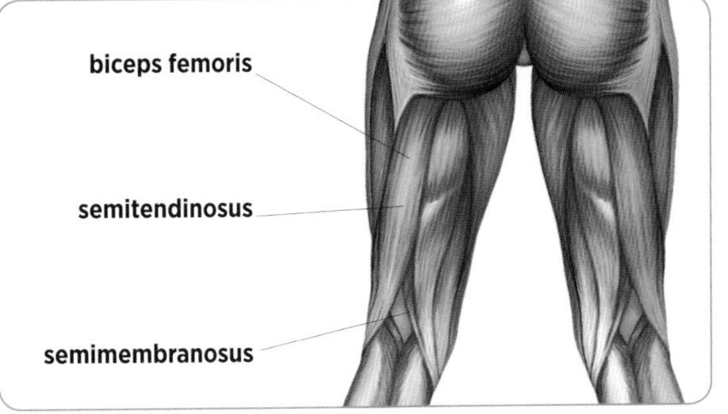

FACT FILE

TARGETS
- Abdominals

EQUIPMENT
- None

BENEFITS
- Strengthens abdominals
- Stabilizes core while extremities are in motion

CAUTIONS
- Neck issues
- Lower-back pain

serratus anterior
rectus abdominis

biceps femoris
semitendinosus
semimembranosus

Annotation Key

Bold text indicates target muscles
Light text indicates other working muscles
* indicates deep muscles

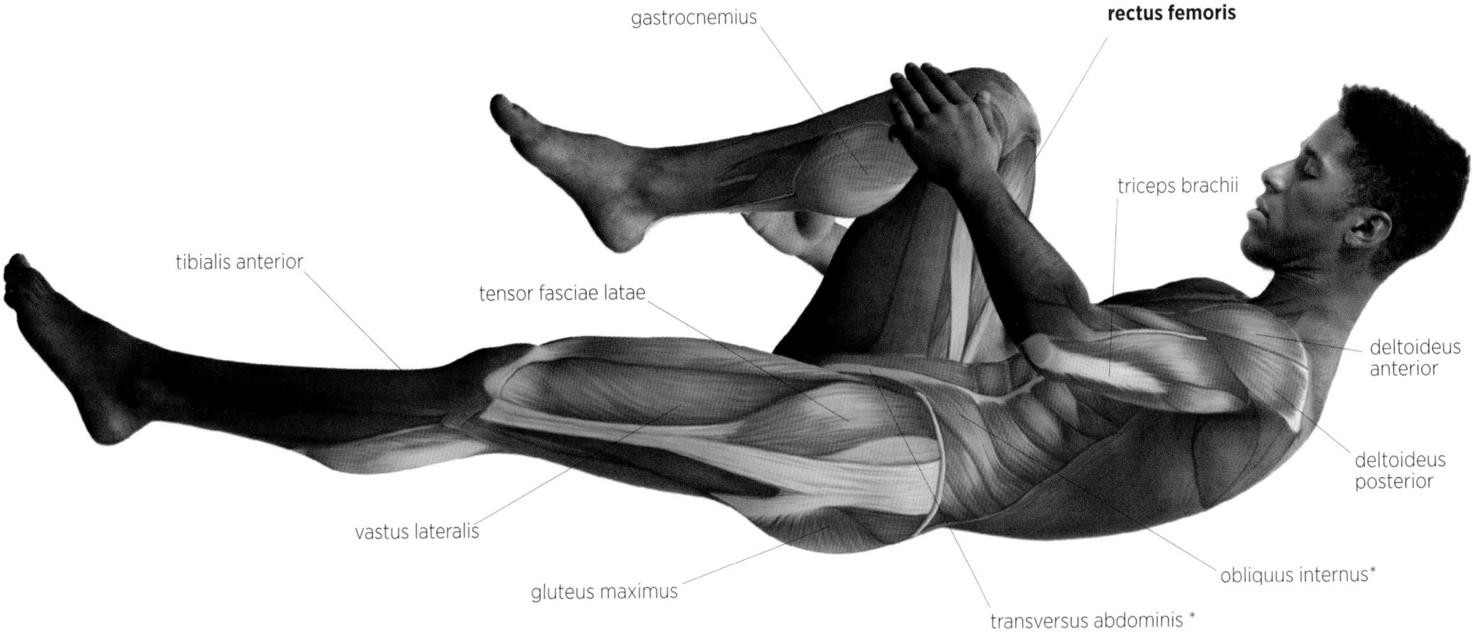

gastrocnemius
rectus femoris
triceps brachii
tibialis anterior
tensor fasciae latae
deltoideus anterior
deltoideus posterior
vastus lateralis
gluteus maximus
obliquus internus*
transversus abdominis *

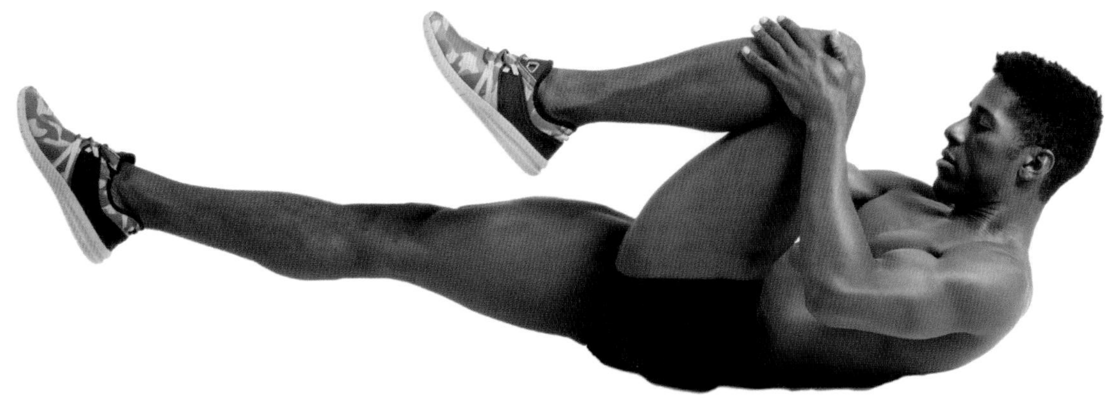

Double Leg Lift

It may look simple, but the Double Leg Lift challenges your hard-to-reach, inner-core muscles. Both strengthening and stabilizing, this Pilates exercise targets both your internal and external abdominals.

HOW TO DO IT

- Lie faceup with your legs together and your arms down at your sides. Lift your legs so that they form a 30-degree angle with the floor, and point your toes.

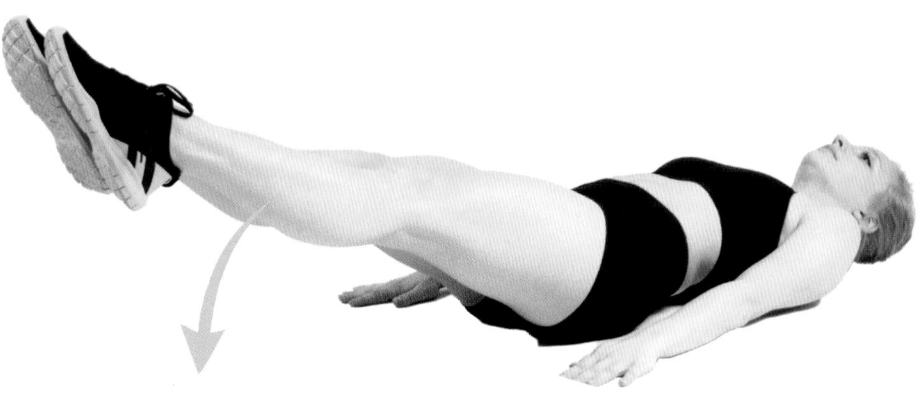

- Pull in your abdominals, and lower your legs to the floor.

- Keeping your back flat, pull your abdominals in again, and lift your legs back up. Continue lifting and lowering your legs for the recommended repetitions.

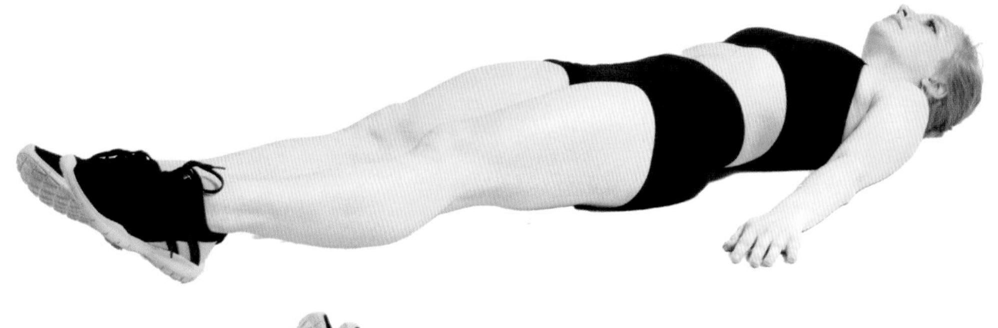

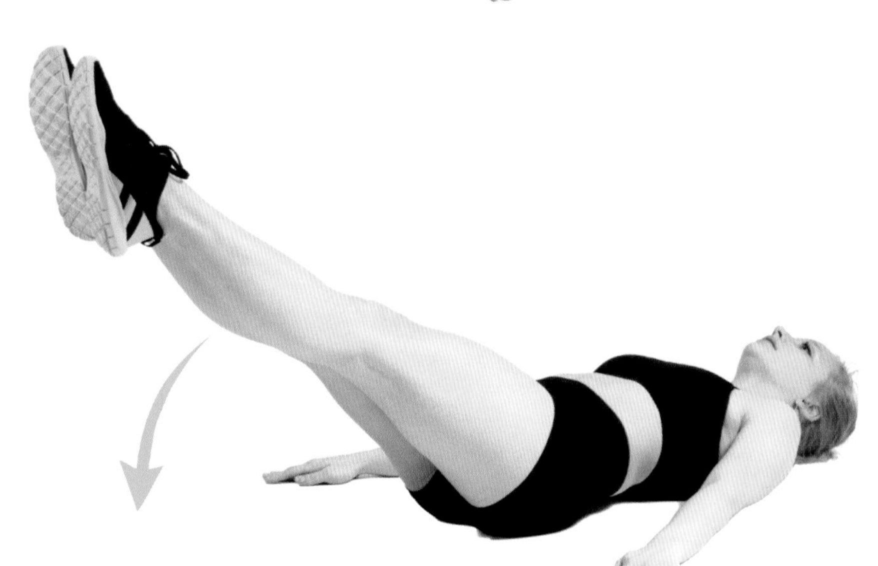

DO IT RIGHT

- Keep your back flat on the floor.
- Avoid dropping your legs; move slowly and with control.
- Use your abdominals to drive the movement.

FACT FILE

TARGETS
- Abdominals
- Hip flexors

EQUIPMENT
- None

BENEFITS
- Strengthens internal and external abdominals
- Stabilizes core

CAUTIONS
- Lower-back pain

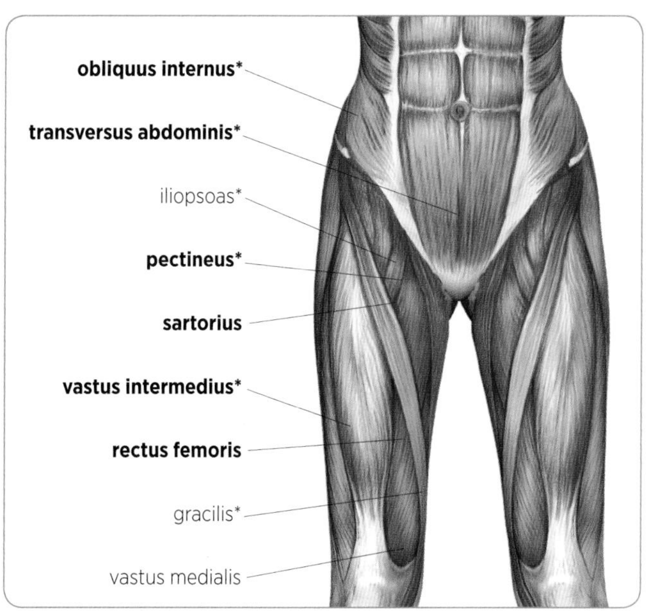

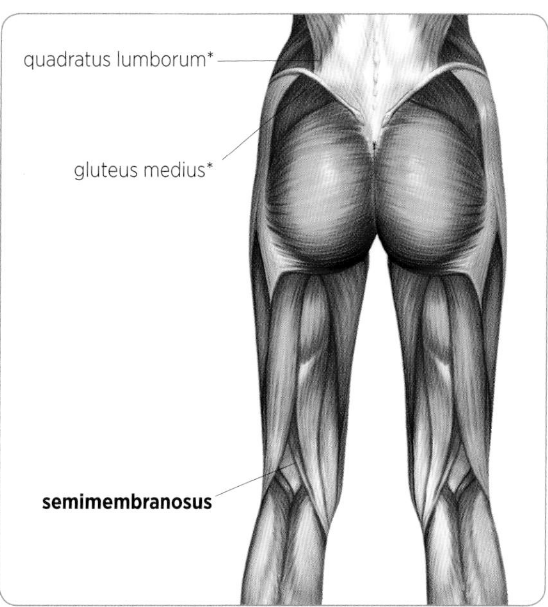

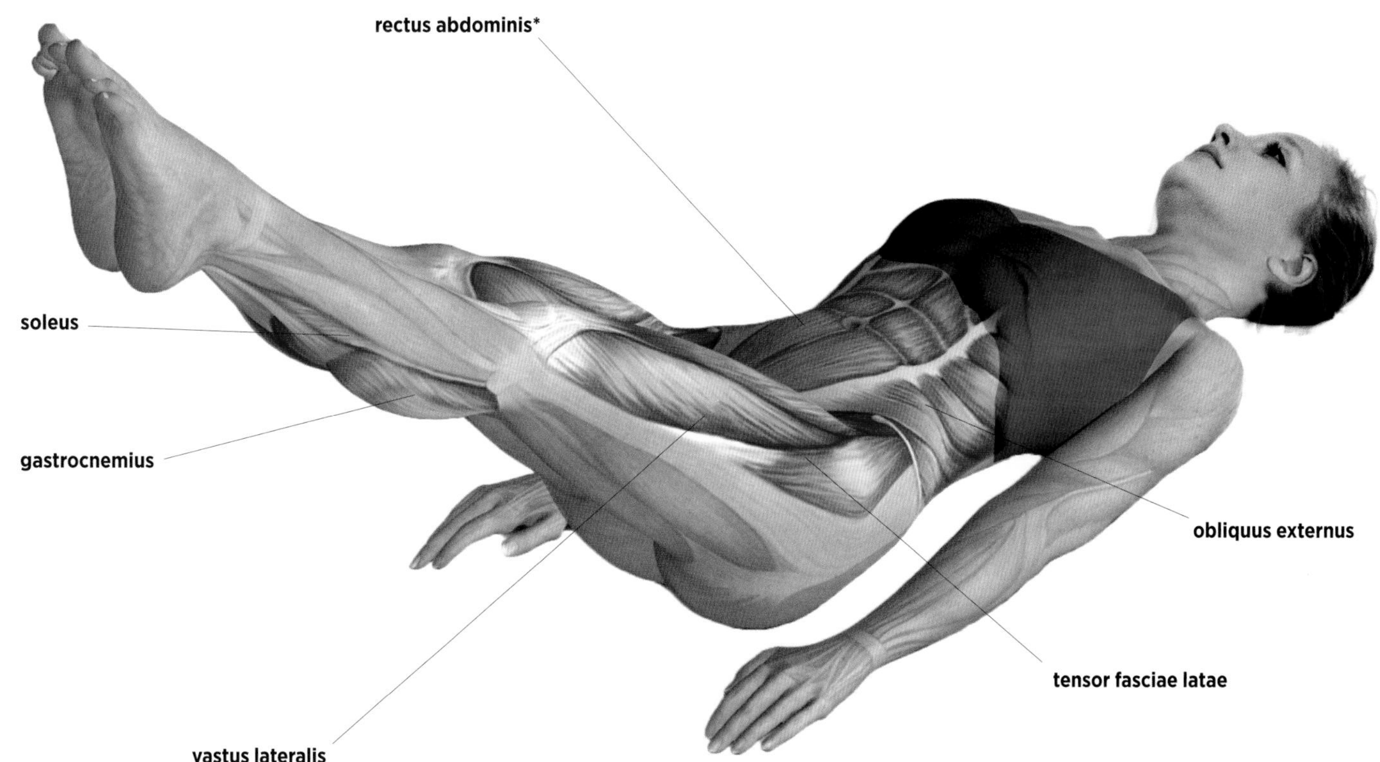

Metronome

Metronomes are wonderful for engaging your core musculature in a twisting motion. With its focus on your obliques, as well as your transverse abdominis, you will get a fantastic core workout.

HOW TO DO IT

- Lie faceup with your arms extended out from your sides to provide a good base of support. Keeping your legs together, lift them toward the ceiling so that your legs and form a 90-degree angle.
- Lower your legs to the right, twisting your torso and allowing your hips to turn while keeping your upper torso stationary. Control the motion so that your feet tap the floor.
- Reverse the motion, bringing the legs back to the starting position.
- Repeat on the other side. Continue alternating sides for the recommended repetitions.

FACT FILE

TARGETS
- Abdominals
- Hip flexors

EQUIPMENT
- None

BENEFITS
- Strengthens and tones abdominal muscles
- Engages several different abdominal fibers
- Improves flexibility

CAUTIONS
- Lower-back issues

DO IT RIGHT

- Keep your legs straight.
- Lower your legs only as far down as you can while still keeping both shoulders on the floor.
- Keeps your hips flexed to 90 degrees throughout hip rotation; don't allow your legs to drop.

rectus abdominis
obliquus internus*
obliquus externus
transversus abdominis*
iliopsoas*
pectineus*
sartorius
vastus intermedius*
rectus femoris

Annotation Key
Bold text indicates target muscles
Light text indicates other working muscles
* indicates deep muscles

Hollow Hold to Superman

This advanced exercise hits every core muscle group, making this the one-stop shop for a stronger core and well-defined abdominals. Combining the benefits of the Hollow Hold gymnastic exercise and the Superman back extension, it will engage your all your abdominal muscles, including your obliques, as well as the deep muscles in your back.

FACT FILE

TARGETS
- Abdominals
- Back
- Hip flexors
- Glutes

EQUIPMENT
- None

BENEFITS
- Strengthens and tones abdominals and back extensors
- Improves coordination

CAUTIONS
- Lower-back issues

HOW TO DO IT

- Lie faceup with your legs and arms extended.
- To perform the Hollow Hold, engage your core, pulling your navel toward your spine. Lift your legs off the floor, and elevate your shoulder blades. Keep your arms outstretched overhead.
- Using only your obliques, roll over so that you end up facing down, keeping your arms and legs elevated off the floor by engaging your lower-back extensor muscles. This is the Superman position.
- Using only your core, rotate back to the starting position. Repeat on the other side. Continue alternating sides for the recommended repetitions.

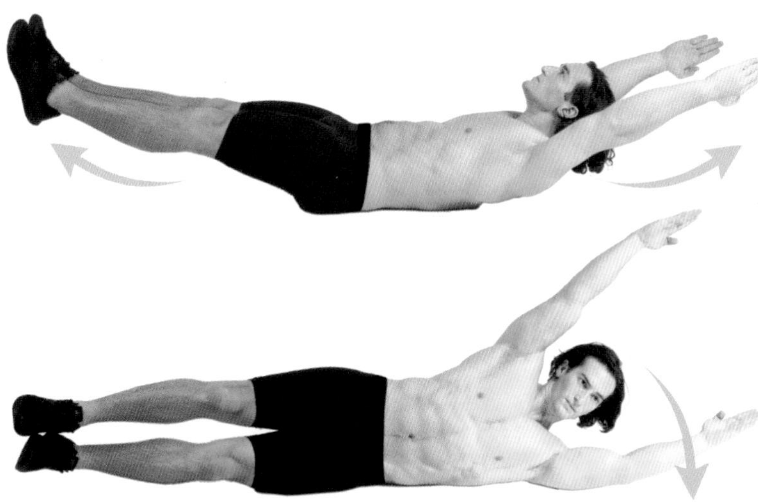

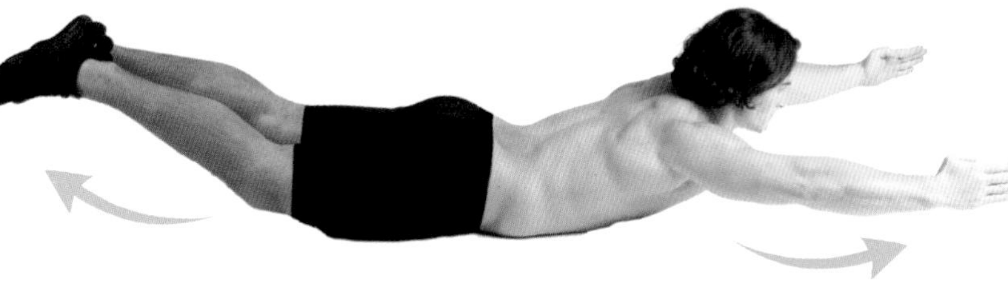

DO IT RIGHT

- Keep your core engaged.
- Press your lower back into the floor while in the Hollow Hold, avoiding excessive spinal arching.
- Perform in both directions to engage both sides symmetrically.

Annotation Key
Bold text indicates target muscles
Light text indicates other working muscles
* indicates deep muscles

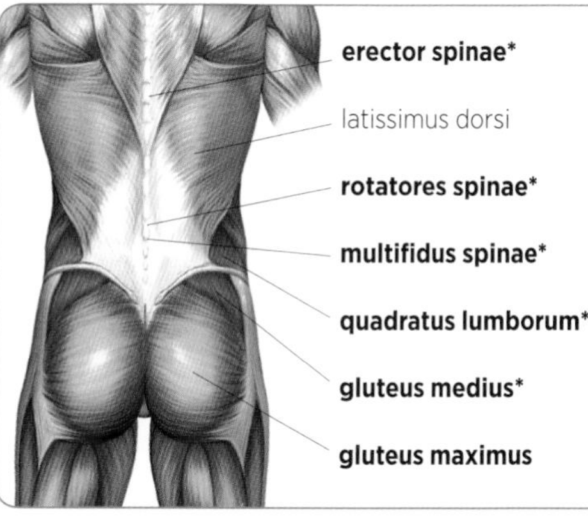

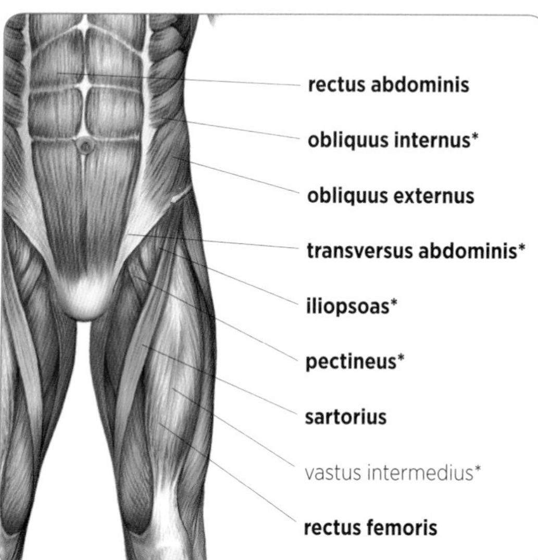

Squat

A powerful compound exercise, the Squat strengthens muscles from your hips to the arches of your feet. Form is essential, so while you build strength, lower only as far as you can without letting your knees just out past your toes.

HOW TO DO IT

- Stand with your legs and feet parallel and shoulder-width apart. Tuck your pelvis slightly forward, lift your chest, and press your shoulders down and back. Extend your arms in front of your body for stability, keeping them even with your shoulders. With your feet planted firmly on the floor, curl your toes slightly upward.
- Draw in your abdominals, and bend into a squat. Keep your heels planted on the floor and your chest as upright as possible, resisting the urge to bend too far forward.
- Rise back to the starting position, and then repeat for the recommended repetitions.

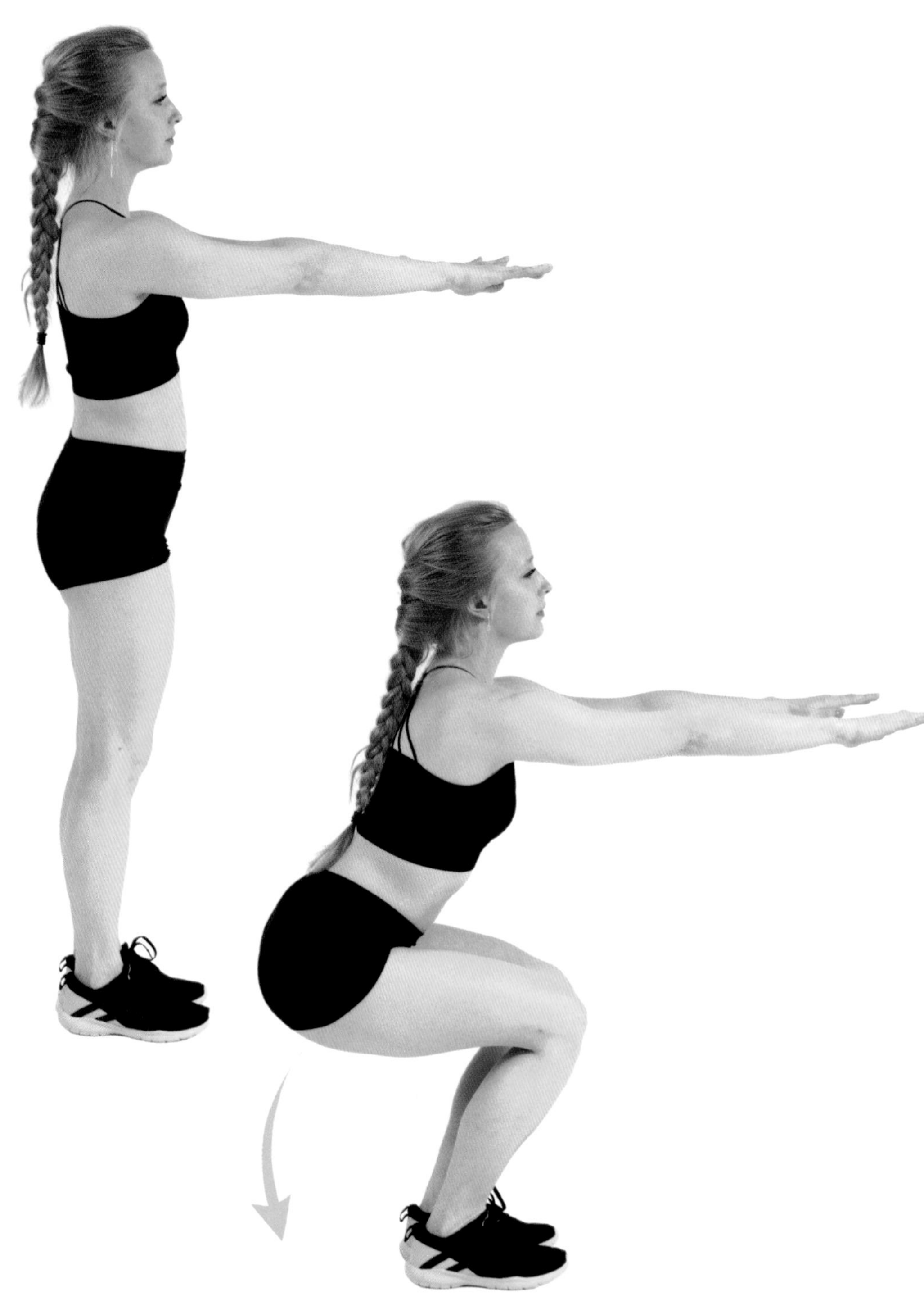

DO IT RIGHT

- Keep your chest upright.
- Pull your abdominals in toward your spine.
- Curl your toes upward.
- Imagine pressing into the floor as you rise from the squat, creating your body's own resistance in your leg muscles.
- Avoid allowing your heels to lift off the floor.
- Avoid rising too quickly to the standing position.

Annotation Key
Bold text indicates target muscles
Light text indicates other working muscles
* indicates deep muscles

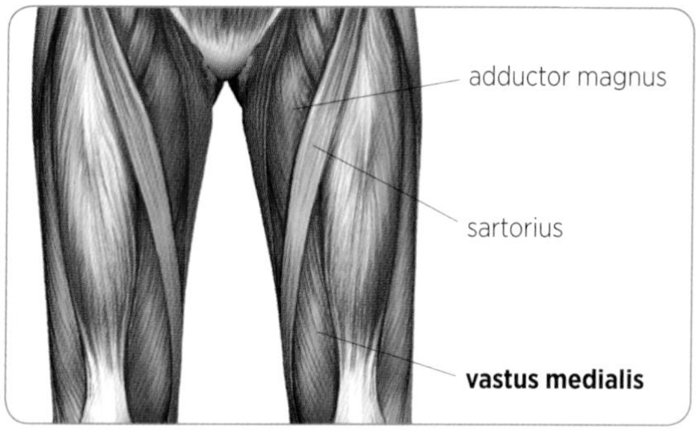

adductor magnus
sartorius
vastus medialis

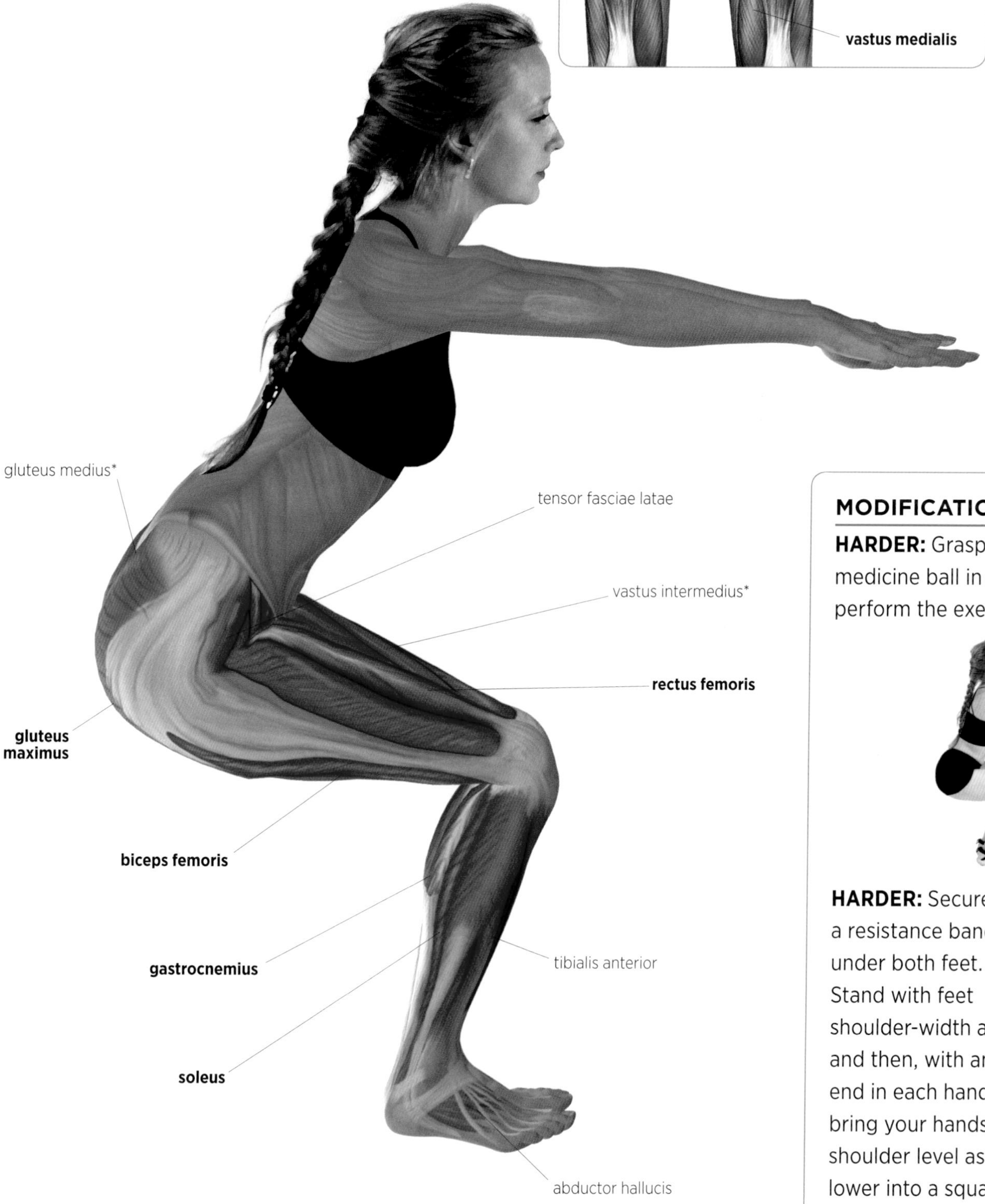

gluteus medius*
tensor fasciae latae
vastus intermedius*
rectus femoris
gluteus maximus
biceps femoris
gastrocnemius
tibialis anterior
soleus
abductor hallucis

FACT FILE

TARGETS
- Quadriceps
- Hamstrings
- Hip flexors
- Glutes
- Calves
- Arches of feet

EQUIPMENT
- None

BENEFITS
- Strengthens thighs, glutes, hips, and feet
- Lengthens calves
- Improves balance

CAUTIONS
- Knee issues
- Foot pain

MODIFICATIONS

HARDER: Grasp a weighted medicine ball in both hands as you perform the exercise.

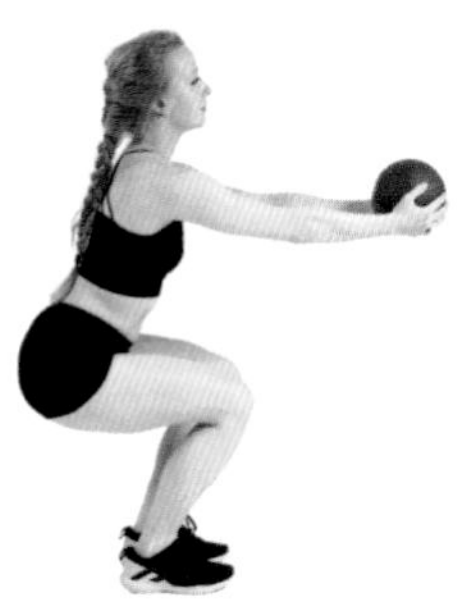

HARDER: Secure a resistance band under both feet. Stand with feet shoulder-width apart, and then, with an end in each hand, bring your hands to shoulder level as you lower into a squat.

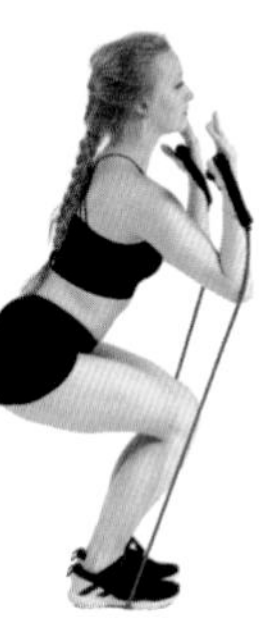

Switch Lunge

The dynamic Switch Lunge takes a basic lunge a step further, calling for you to jump upward to switch legs. It will stabilize your hips, knees, and ankles; stretch your hip flexors; and strengthen your hamstrings, quadriceps, and glutes.

HOW TO DO IT

- Stand with your left leg stepped out in front of your body. Keep a slight bend in your left knee.
- Drop your right knee, touching it lightly on the floor.
- Jump up, switching your legs in the air.
- Land with your right leg forward, and drop your left knee. Lunging and jumping once on each leg equals one repetition. Continue alternating sides for the recommended repetitions.

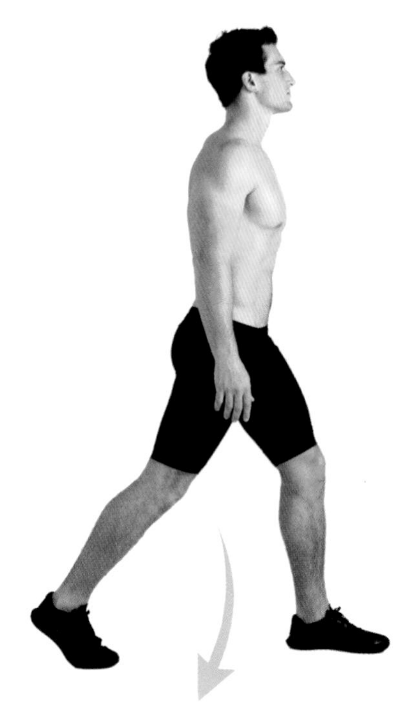

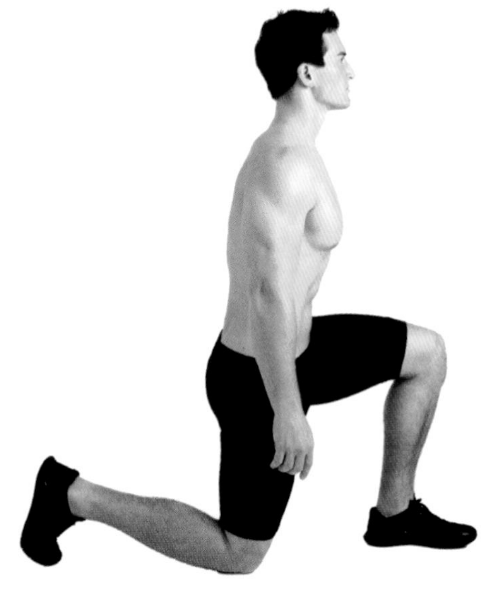

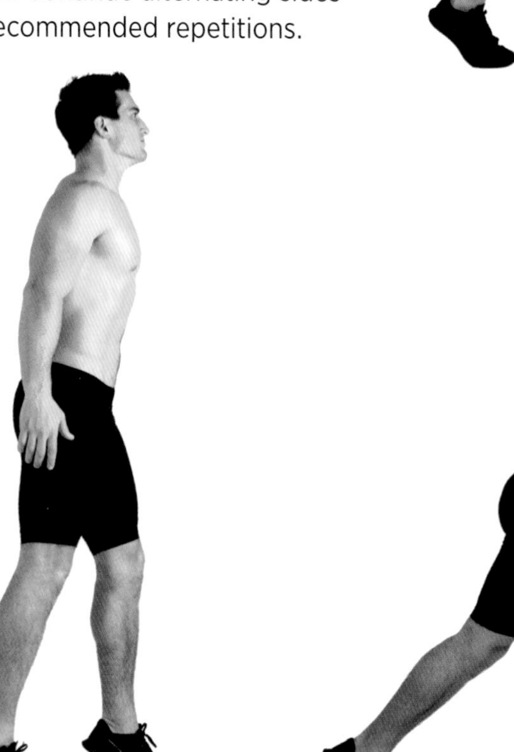

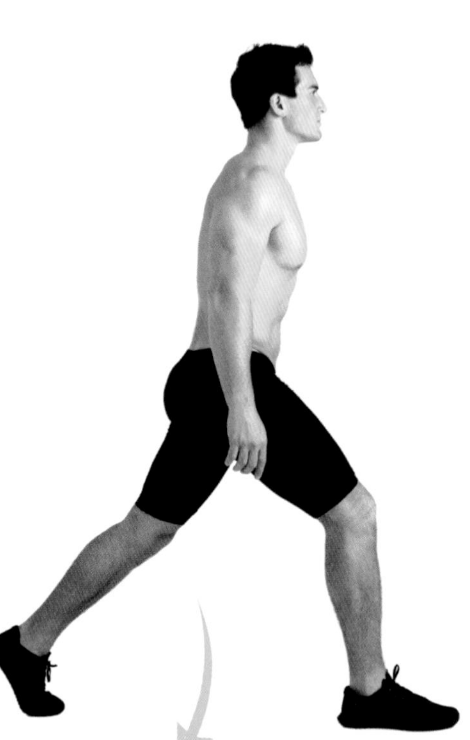

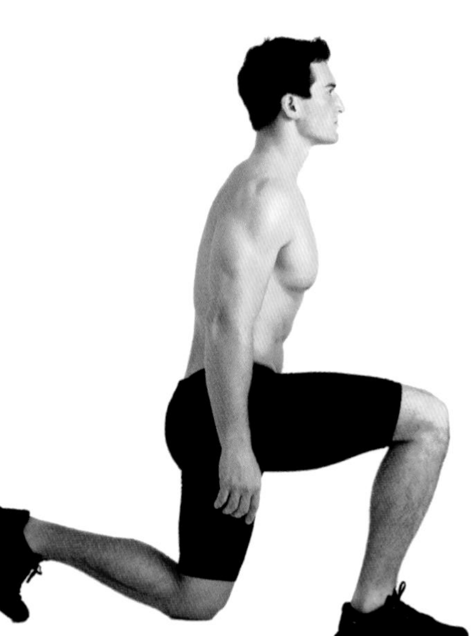

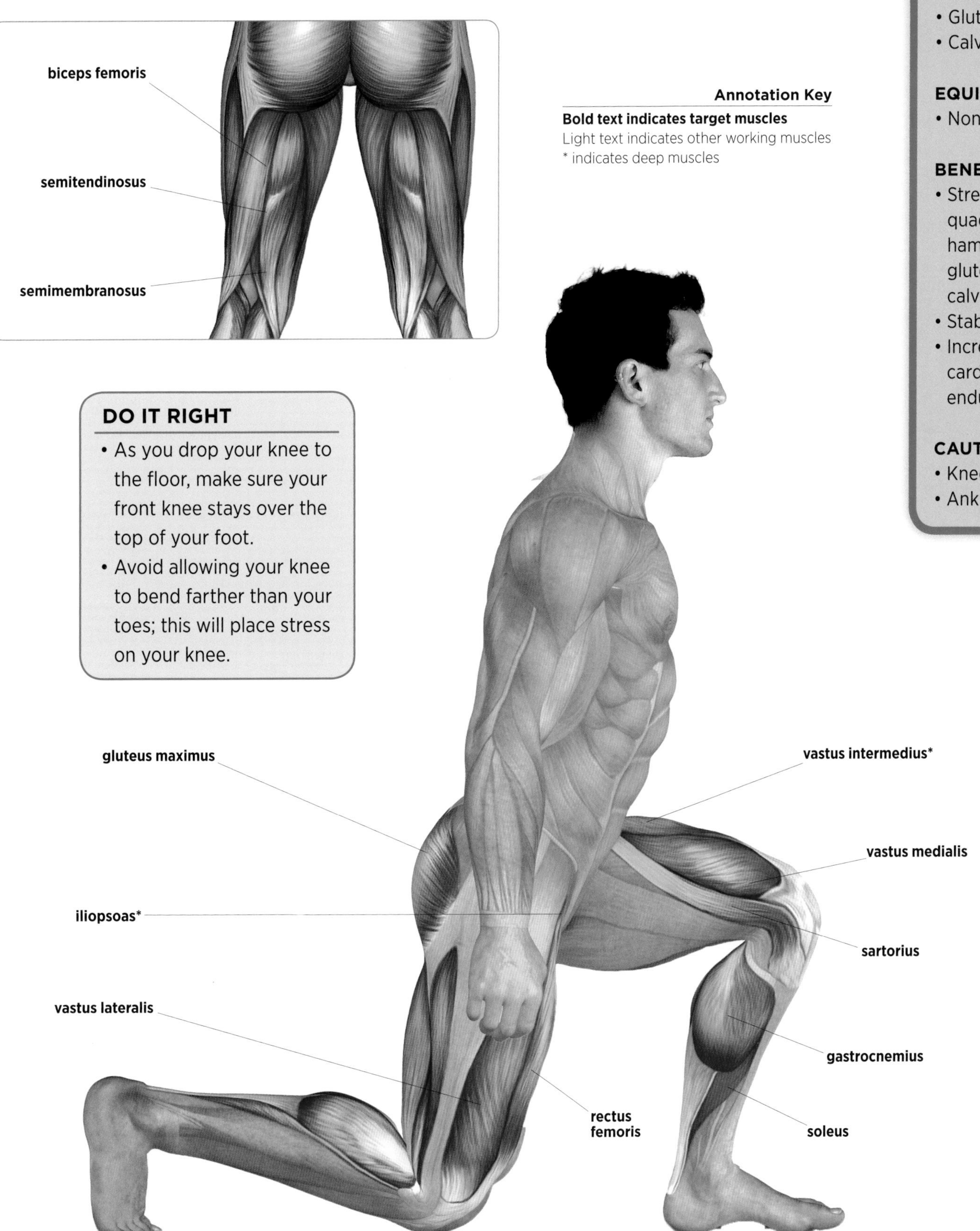

Annotation Key

Bold text indicates target muscles
Light text indicates other working muscles
* indicates deep muscles

DO IT RIGHT

- As you drop your knee to the floor, make sure your front knee stays over the top of your foot.
- Avoid allowing your knee to bend farther than your toes; this will place stress on your knee.

FACT FILE

TARGETS
- Quadriceps
- Hamstrings
- Glutes
- Calves

EQUIPMENT
- None

BENEFITS
- Strengthens quadriceps, hamstrings, glutes, and calves
- Stabilizes hips
- Increases cardiovascular endurance

CAUTIONS
- Knee issues
- Ankle pain

Lateral Lunge with Squat

The Lateral Lunge with Squat combines the benefits of two exercise mainstays: a sideways lunge and a squat. This isolation exercise targets the inner and outer thighs, which can help build strength and stability in the hip and lateral knee.

HOW TO DO IT

- Stand with your feet together and your hands on your hips.
- Contract your abdominals and glutes, and step out your right foot. Keeping your weight on your heels, bend your left knee and lower your hips as far as you can.
- Push off the ground with your right foot, and return to the starting position.
- Repeat on the opposite side, alternating sides for the recommended repetitions.

DO IT RIGHT

- Keep your spine in neutral position as you bend your hips.
- Relax your shoulders and neck.
- Align your knee with the toe of your bent leg.
- Lower as far as you are able, but not beyond your thighs parallel to the floor.
- Avoid lifting your heels—squat only as deeply as you can while keeping your feet flat on the floor.
- Avoid arching your back.

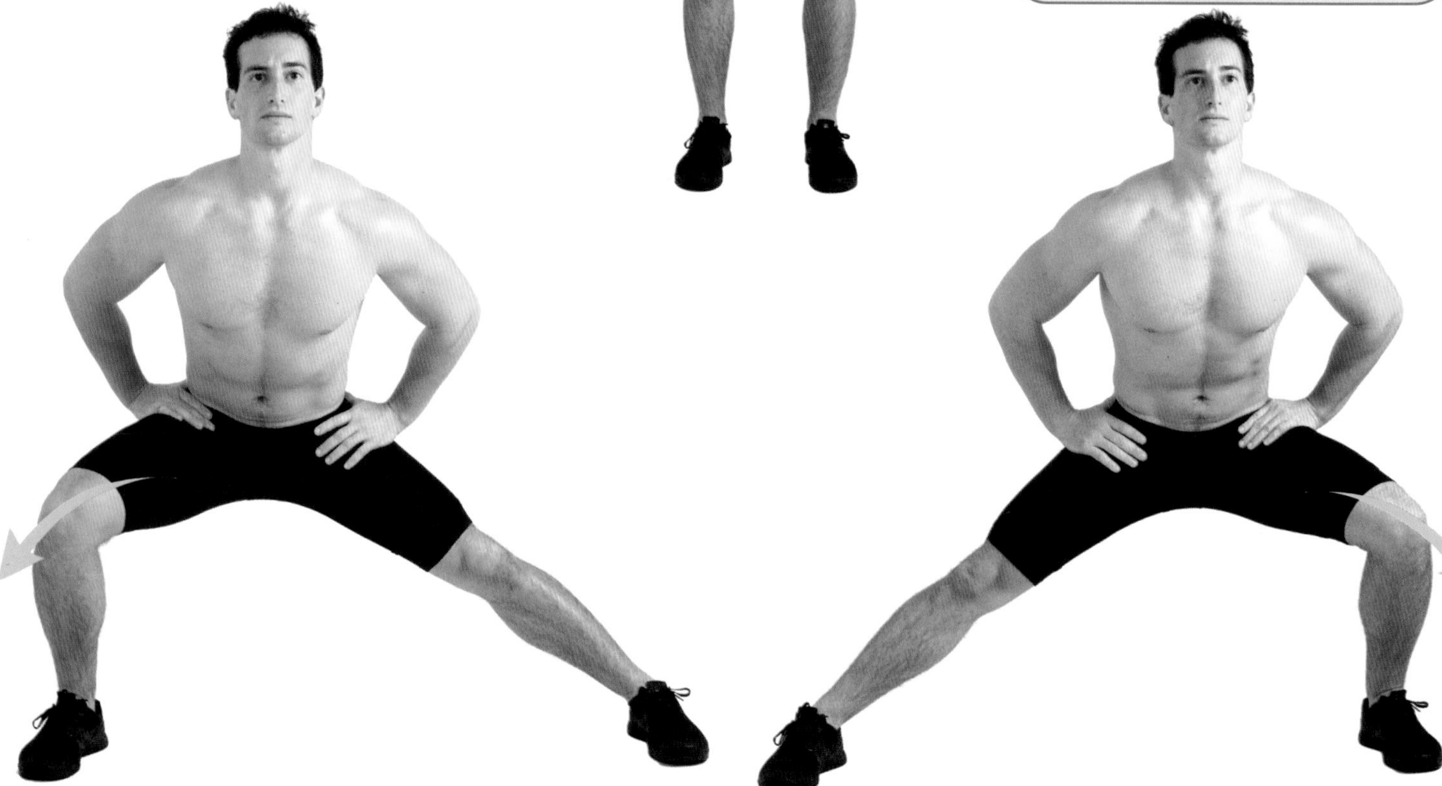

FACT FILE

TARGETS
- Thighs
- Hips
- Glutes
- Calves

EQUIPMENT
- None

BENEFITS
- Strengthens glutes, thighs, and calves
- Strengthens and stabilizes hip abductors and adductors
- Strengthens and stabilizes lateral knee muscles

CAUTIONS
- Knee pain
- Hip pain

Annotation Key

Bold text indicates target muscles

Light text indicates other working muscles

* indicates deep muscles

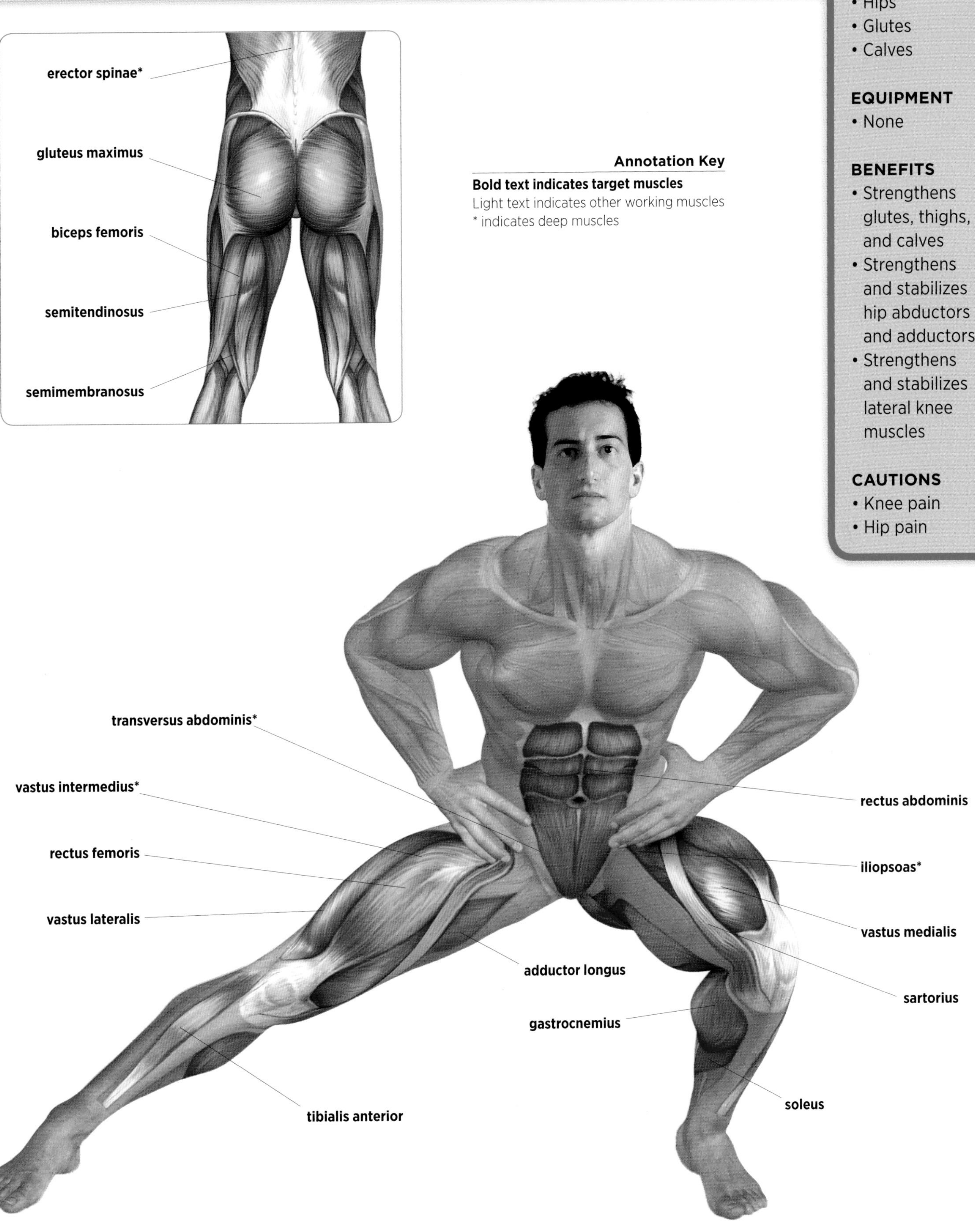

High Lunge with Twist

Like the basic High Lunge, this version is an effective strengthening exercise for your thighs, hips, and glutes. The added twist gives it a boost, stretching your obliques, chest, and shoulders.

HOW TO DO IT

- Begin in a High Lunge (pages 38–39) with your right leg forward.
- Balance your weight on your left hand, and carefully and slowly guide your right arm up toward the ceiling, twisting your torso to the right.
- Return to the center, and then repeat on the opposite side. Continue alternating sides for the recommended repetitions.

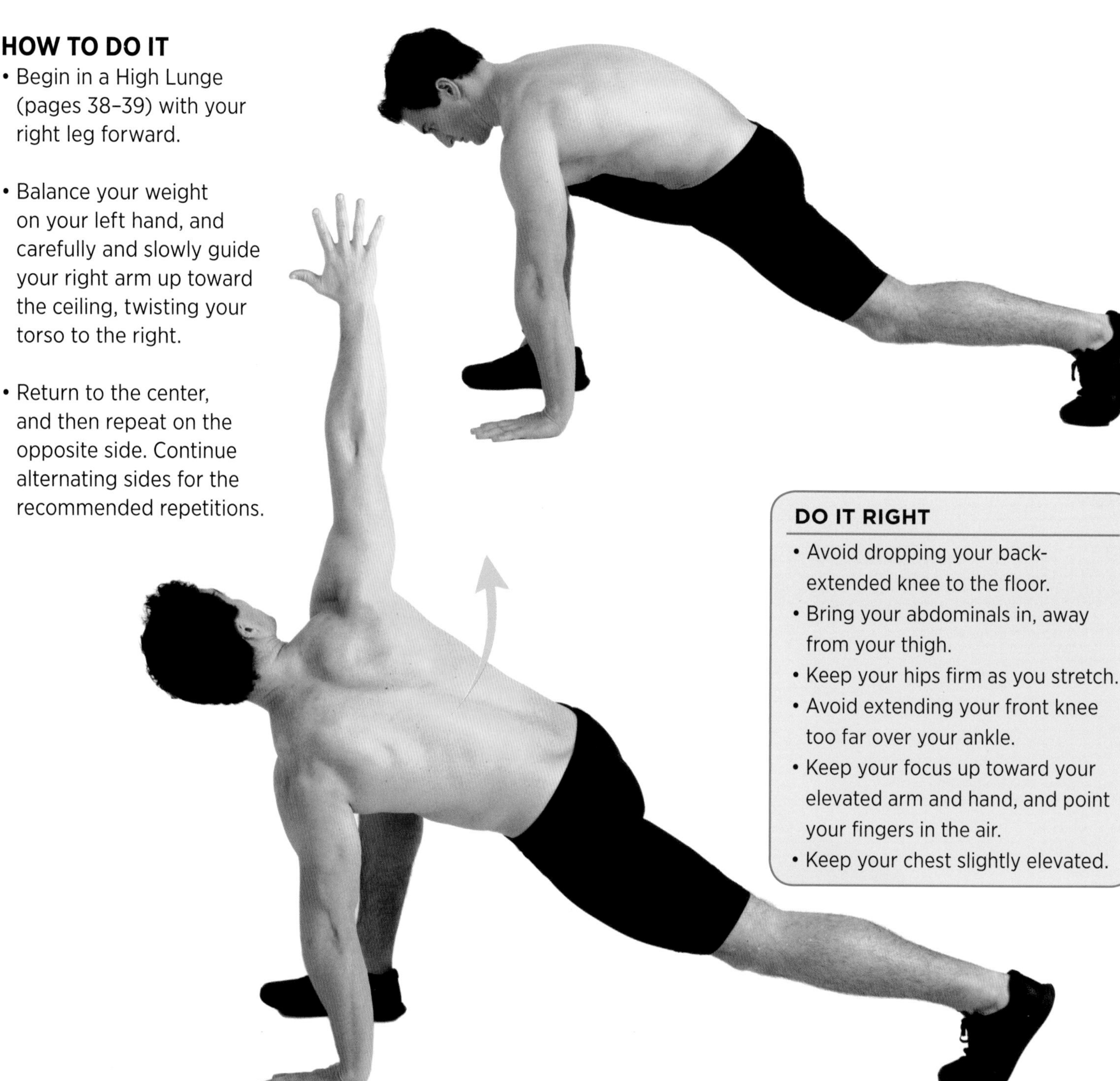

DO IT RIGHT

- Avoid dropping your back-extended knee to the floor.
- Bring your abdominals in, away from your thigh.
- Keep your hips firm as you stretch.
- Avoid extending your front knee too far over your ankle.
- Keep your focus up toward your elevated arm and hand, and point your fingers in the air.
- Keep your chest slightly elevated.

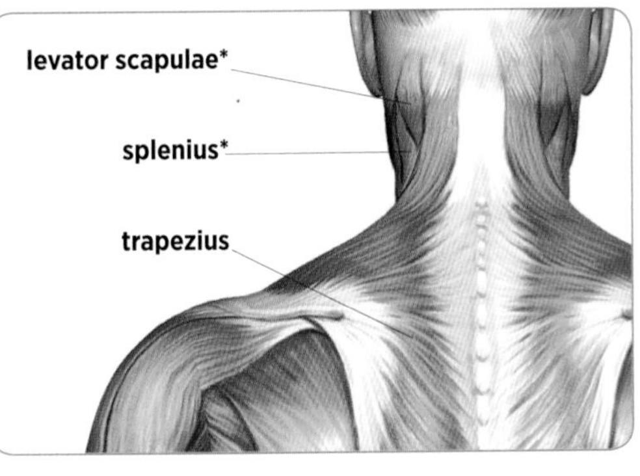

Annotation Key
Bold text indicates target muscles
Light text indicates other working muscles
* indicates deep muscles

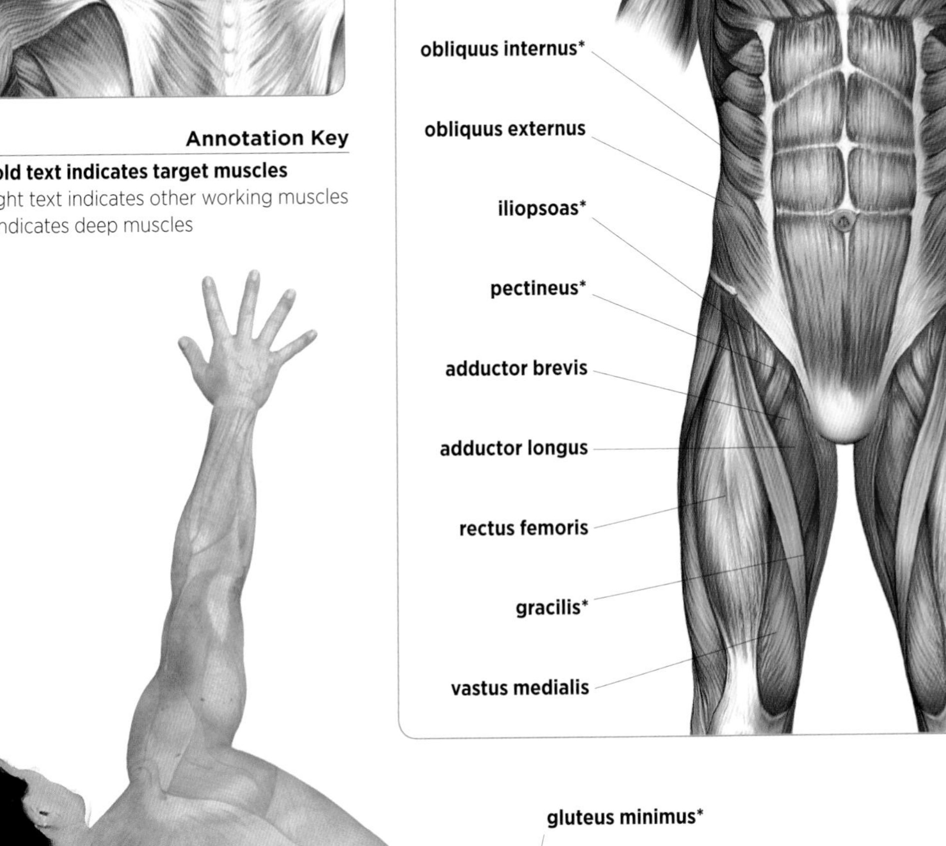

FACT FILE

TARGETS
- Quadriceps
- Gluteal area
- Hip flexors
- Hip adductors
- Hamstrings
- Obliques
- Rib cage
- Chest
- Shoulders

EQUIPMENT
- None

BENEFITS
- Stretches groins and obliques
- Strengthens abdominals, legs, and arms
- Stretches hip flexors, shoulders, and chest

CAUTIONS
- Hip issues
- Knee issues

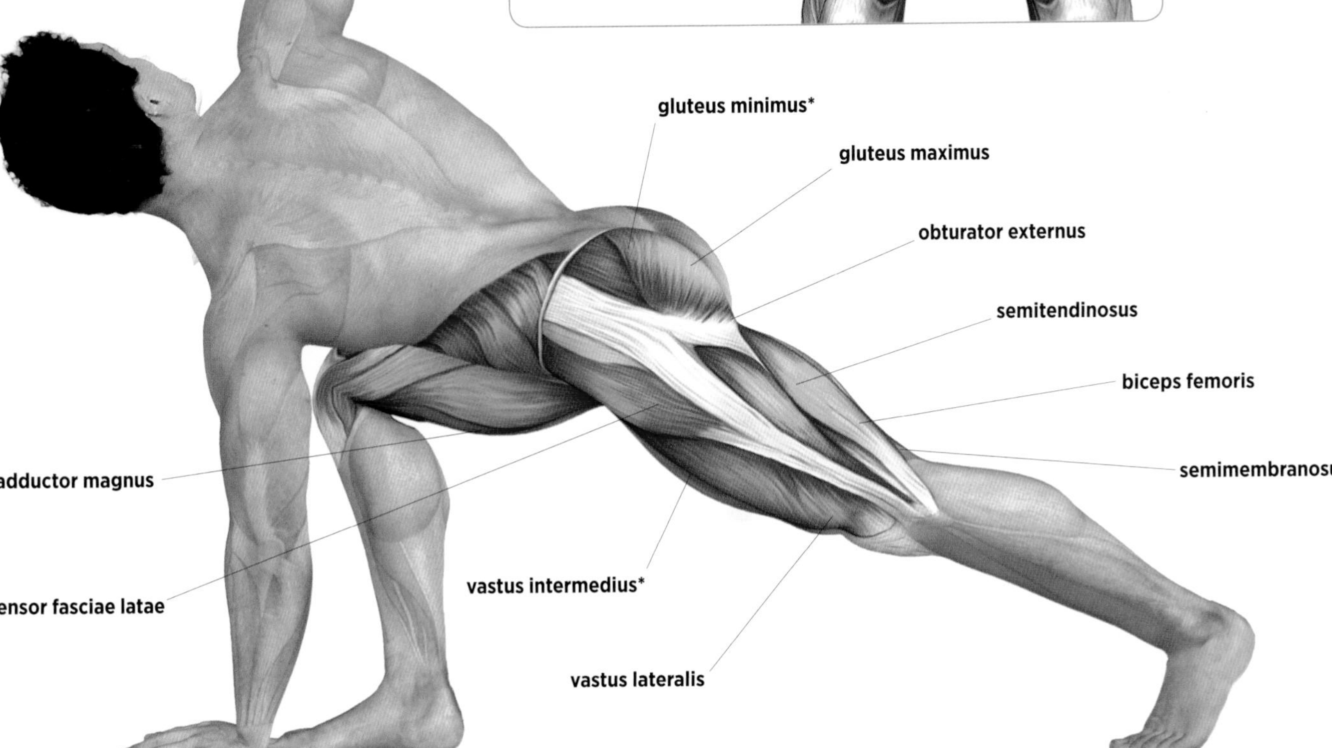

Box Jump

Jumping exercises have a lot to offer, providing strength and power benefits, as well as giving you a cardio boost. The Box Jump targets your lower body and promotes explosive power so that you can perform at top levels.

HOW TO DO IT

- Stand in front of a plyo box, aerobics step, or other low platform.
- Drop into a quarter-squat.
- Push through your heels, swing your arms, and spring up onto the box.
- Step back down, and then repeat for the recommended repetitions.

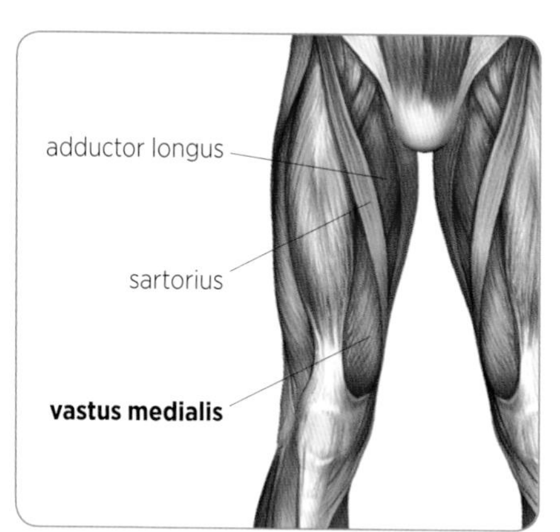

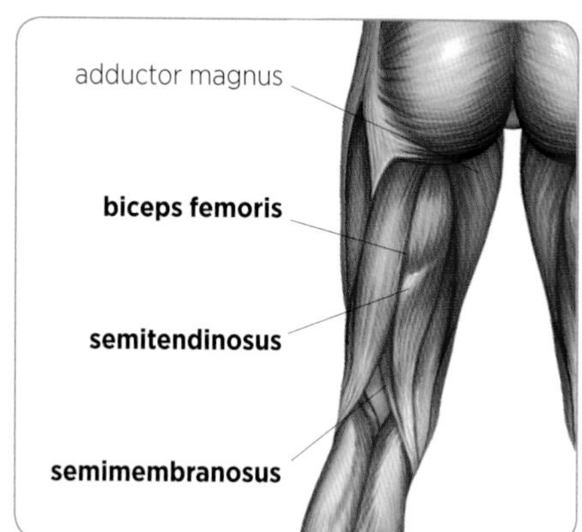

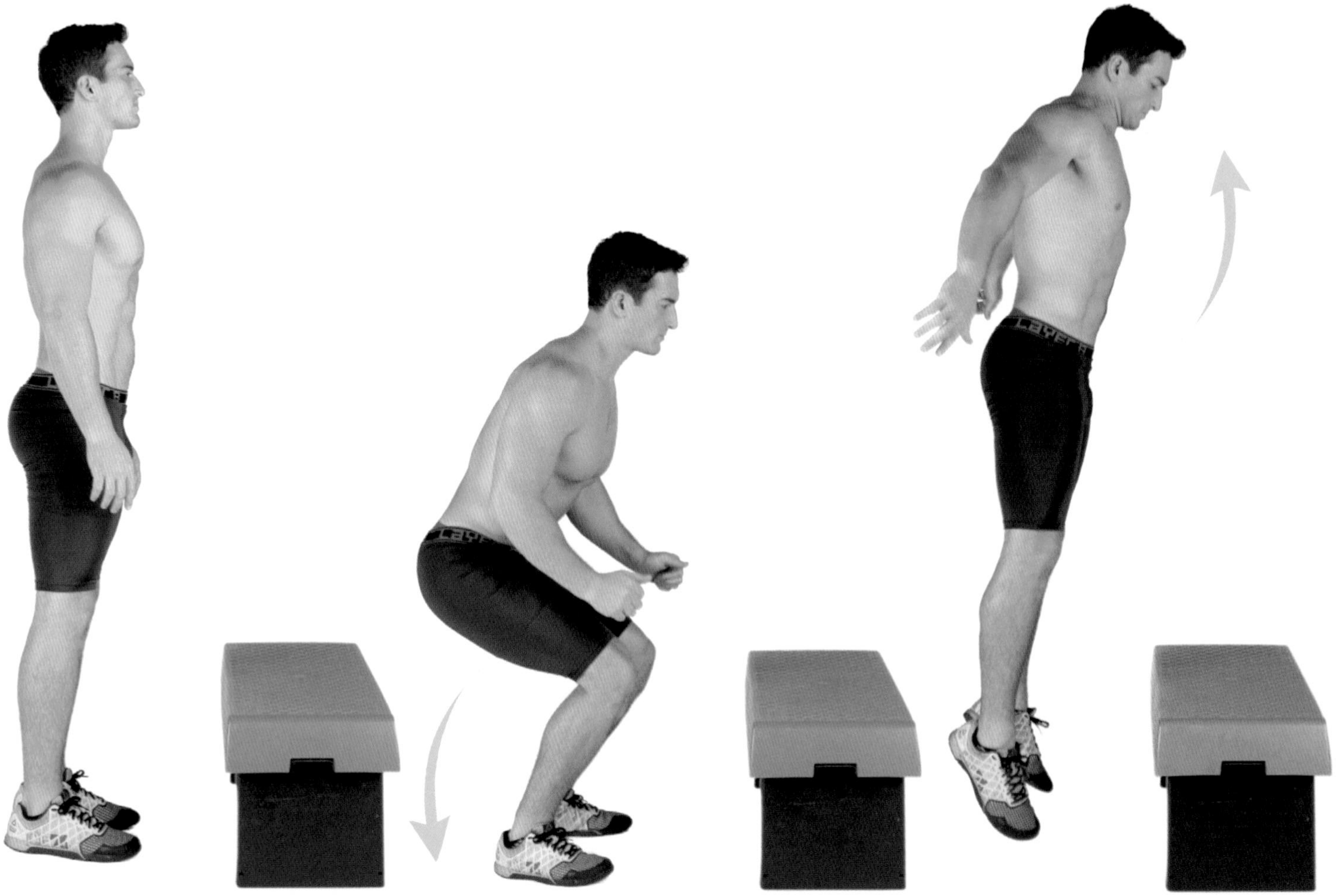

MODIFICATION

EASIER: Use a lower step.

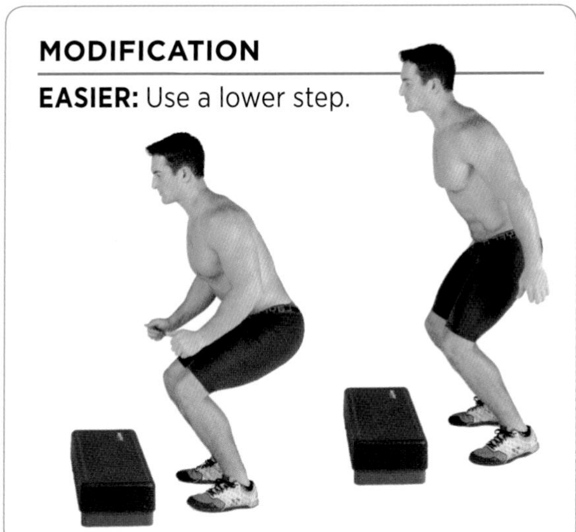

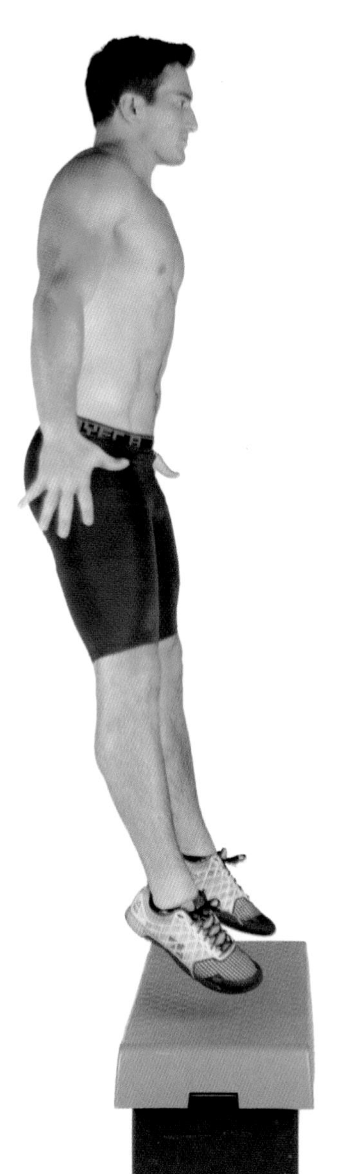

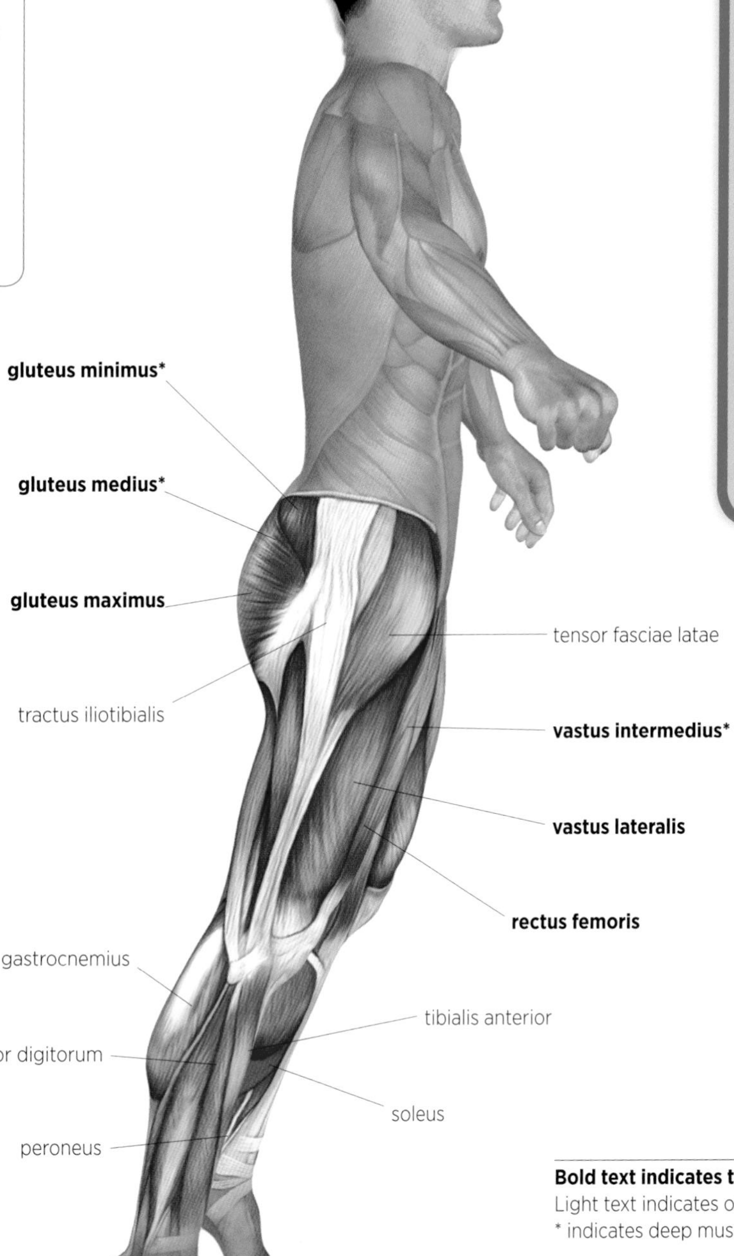

FACT FILE

TARGETS

- Quadriceps
- Hamstrings
- Glutes
- Calves

EQUIPMENT

- Plyo box, aerobics step, or other low platform

BENEFITS

- Strengthens thighs, glutes, and calves
- Produces explosive lower-body power

CAUTIONS

- Hip issues
- Knee issues
- Ankle issues

Annotation Key

Bold text indicates target muscles

Light text indicates other working muscles

* indicates deep muscles

DO IT RIGHT

- Keep a tight core throughout the movement.
- Avoid landing excessively hard.

Speed Skater

The Speed Skater helps you stabilize your knee and hip joints by targeting their supporting muscles, including your iliotibial bands, hip adductors, and hip abductors. Be sure to perform this exercise on a smooth, friction-free surface to bring out your inner skater.

HOW TO DO IT

- Stand in a half-squat position, and place your left leg behind your right.
- Jump to your left as far as possible while swinging your arms toward the left. Land in a half-squat position with your right leg behind your left.
- Immediately jump back toward the right as far as possible, as if you were skating in long strides. Switching back and forth equals one repetition. Repeat for the recommended repetitions.

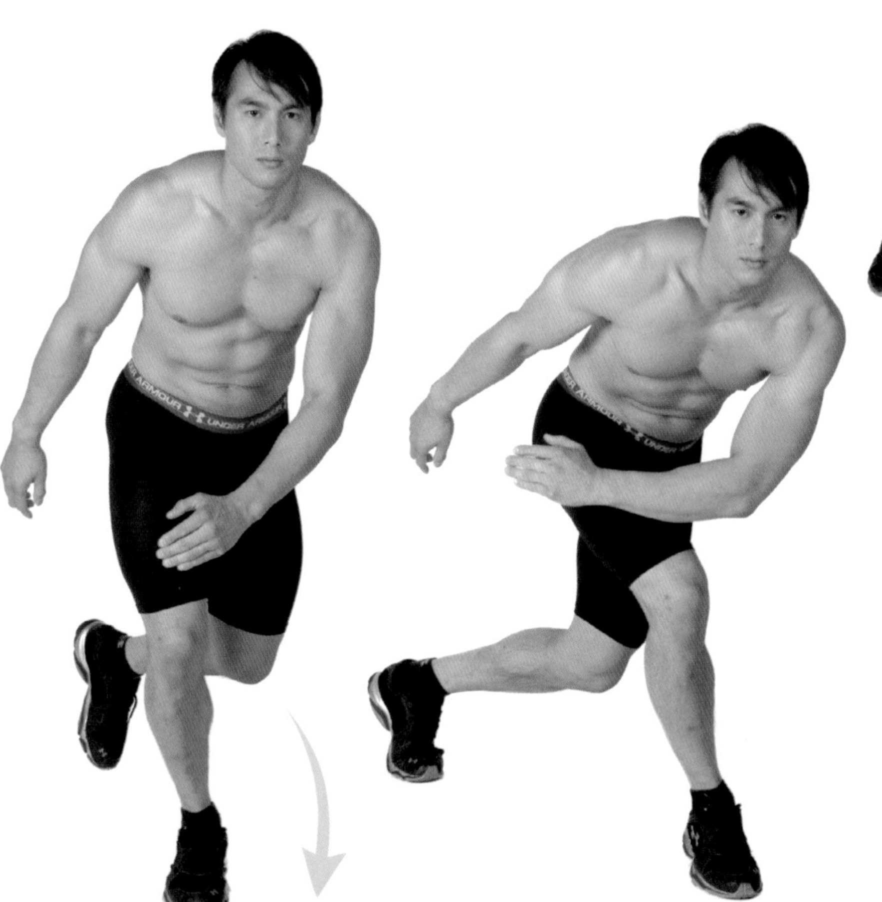

DO IT RIGHT

- Swing your arms together in the direction of the jump.
- Avoid moving your arms in any direction other than the direction of the jump.

FACT FILE

TARGETS
- Inner thighs
- Hips
- Iliotibial band

EQUIPMENT
- None

BENEFITS
- Strengthens hip adductors and abductors
- Keeps iliotibial bands supple

CAUTIONS
- Hip issues
- Knee issues
- Ankle issues

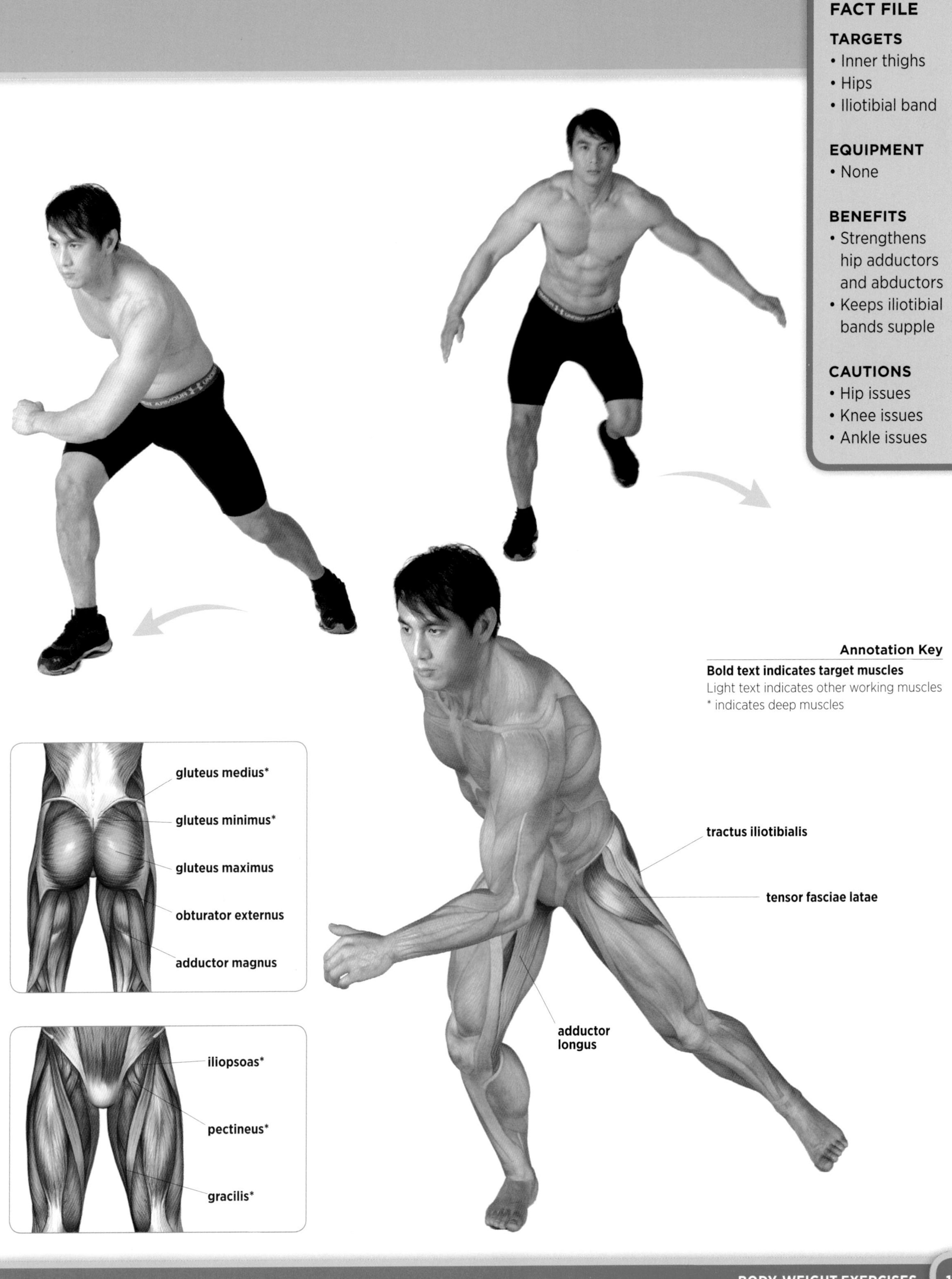

Annotation Key
Bold text indicates target muscles
Light text indicates other working muscles
* indicates deep muscles

Bridge with Leg Lift

Any Bridge exercise is great for toning your glutes and thighs. This version, also known as the Glute Bridge March, allows you to isolate each side of your lower body for an intense workout.

HOW TO DO IT

- Lie faceup with your arms by your sides and lengthened toward your feet. Your legs should be bent, with your feet flat on the floor.
- To assume the bridge position, lift your hips and spine off the floor, creating one long line from your knees to your shoulders. Keep your weight shifted over your feet.
- Keeping your legs bent, bring your left knee toward your chest.
- Keeping your pelvis level, lower your leg until your toe touches the floor.
- Bring your left knee toward your chest again. Repeat for the recommended repetitions, and then repeat on the opposite side.

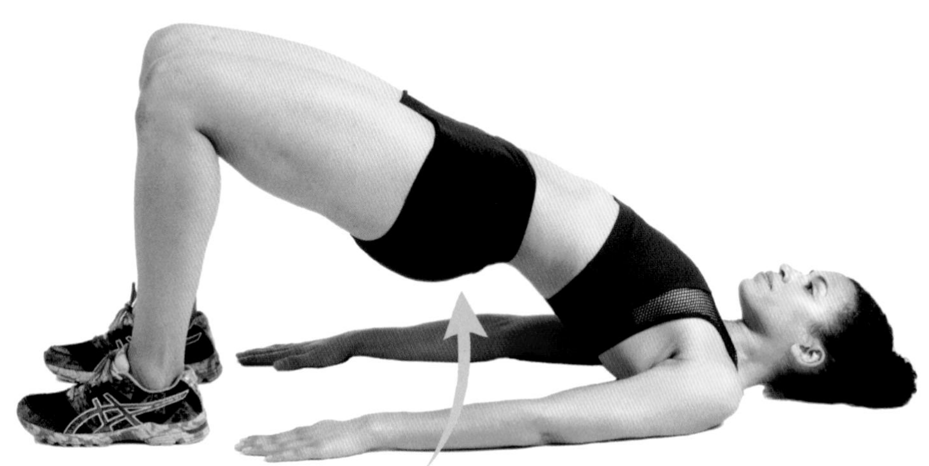

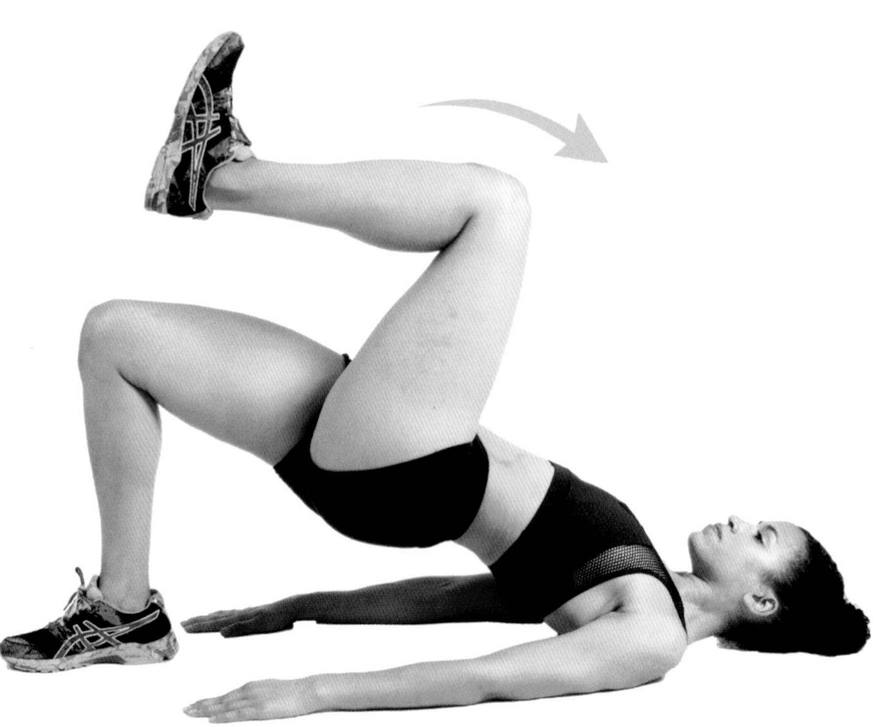

DO IT RIGHT

- Keep your hips and torso stable throughout the exercise. If needed, prop yourself up with your hands beneath your hips once you are in the bridge position.
- Tightly squeeze your glutes as you scoop in your abdominals for stability.
- Avoid allowing your back to do the work by extending out of your hips.
- Avoid lifting your hips so high that your weight shifts onto your neck.

multifidus spinae*
gluteus minimus*
vastus lateraiis
biceps femoris
semitendinosus
semimembranosus

transversus abdominis*
tensor fasciae latae
iliopsoas*
pectineus*
adductor longus

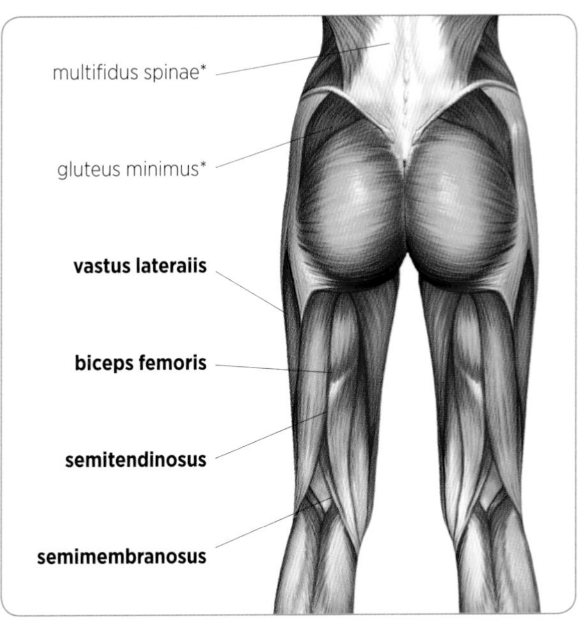

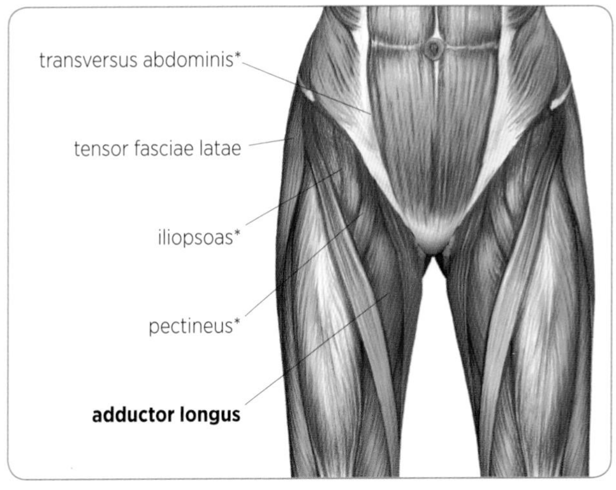

Annotation Key
Bold text indicates target muscles
Light text indicates other working muscles
* indicates deep muscles

FACT FILE

TARGETS
- Hamstrings
- Glutes
- Hip extensors
- Abdominals

EQUIPMENT
- None

BENEFITS
- Increases hip flexor endurance
- Improves pelvic and spinal stability

CAUTIONS
- Neck issues
- Knee injury

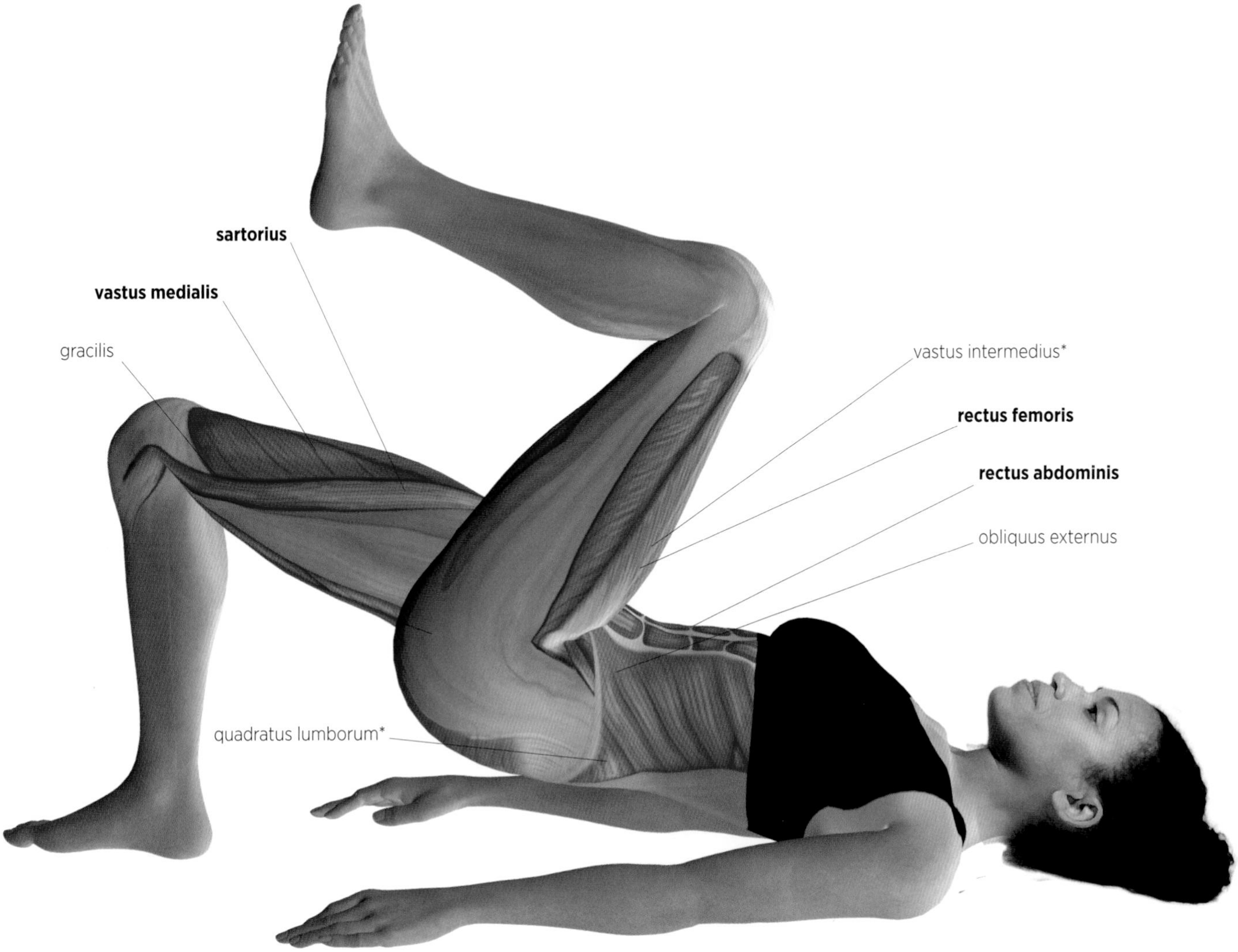

sartorius
vastus medialis
gracilis
vastus intermedius*
rectus femoris
rectus abdominis
obliquus externus
quadratus lumborum*

Plyo Knee Drive

This dynamic exercise uses the form of the standardized lunge combined with the benefits of plyometric training. Focusing on your quadriceps, glutes, calves, and hip flexors, the Plyo Knee Drive will undoubtedly hit nearly every part of your legs.

HOW TO DO IT

- Begin in a staggered stance with your right leg placed forward and your feet approximately hip-width apart.
- Bend both knees to drop the knee of your left leg toward the floor.
- With one explosive motion, extend both legs, launching yourself into the air while drawing your left leg in toward your torso, driving your knee forward.
- Before returning to the floor, return your left leg back behind you, landing in the starting position.
- Repeat on the opposite side. Continue alternating sides for the recommended repetitions.

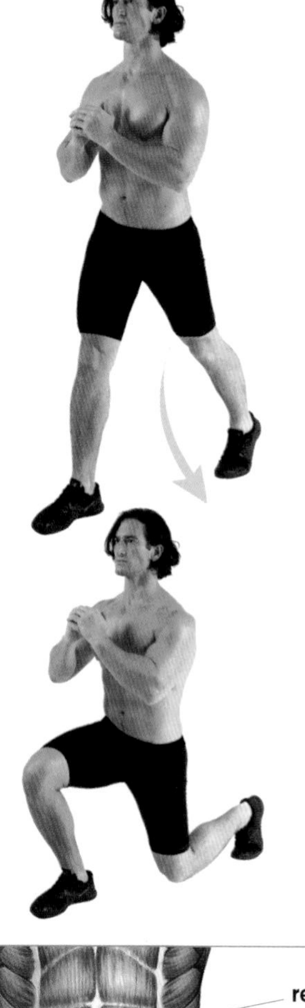

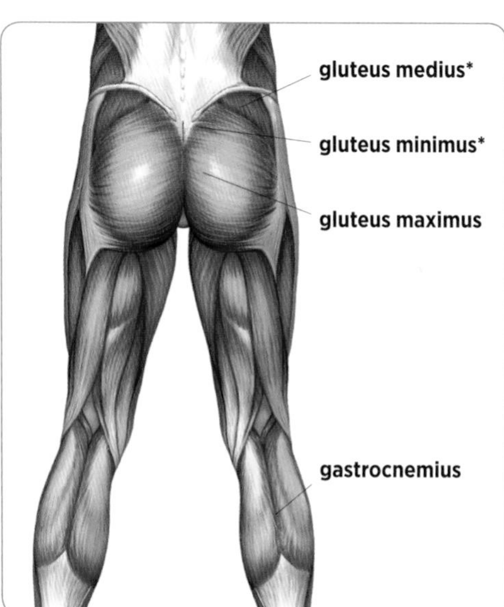

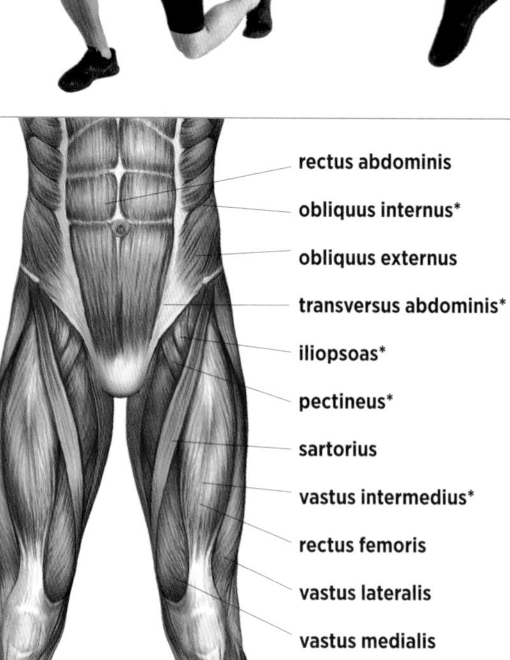

FACT FILE

TARGETS
- Abdominals
- Hip flexors
- Quadriceps
- Glutes

EQUIPMENT
- None

BENEFITS
- Strengthens and tones abdominals and legs
- Increases cardiovascular endurance
- Improves coordination

CAUTIONS
- Lower-back issues

DO IT RIGHT

- Keep your motions quick and powerful.
- Avoid small motions; drive your lifted knee high and outward with exaggerated movements.

Annotation Key

Bold text indicates target muscles
Light text indicates other working muscles
* indicates deep muscles

Pistol

Essentially a single-leg squat, Pistols provide all the lower-body and core benefits of a basic squat, but doubles the intensity. As with any exercise that requires a single-leg stance, they will tax your midline stability, balance, and coordination.

FACT FILE

TARGETS
- Quadriceps
- Glutes
- Back

EQUIPMENT
- None

BENEFITS
- Strengthens and tones back and legs
- Improves balance

CAUTIONS
- Knee issues

HOW TO DO IT

- Stand on your left leg with it centered underneath your center of gravity. Raise your arms straight in front of you at shoulder height, palms facing downward.

- Shift your weight backward, and extend your right leg straight out, flexing at your hip, knee, and ankle as you lower into a squat until the top of your right thigh is parallel with the floor.

- Drive your left foot into the floor, extending your leg and hips to return to the starting position.

- Repeat on the opposite side. Continue alternating sides for the recommended repetitions.

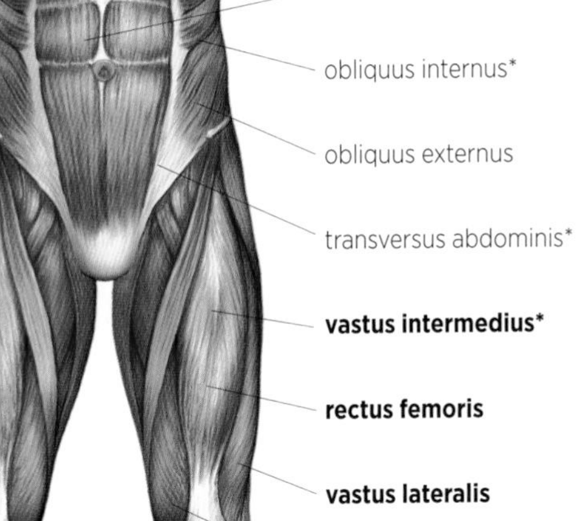

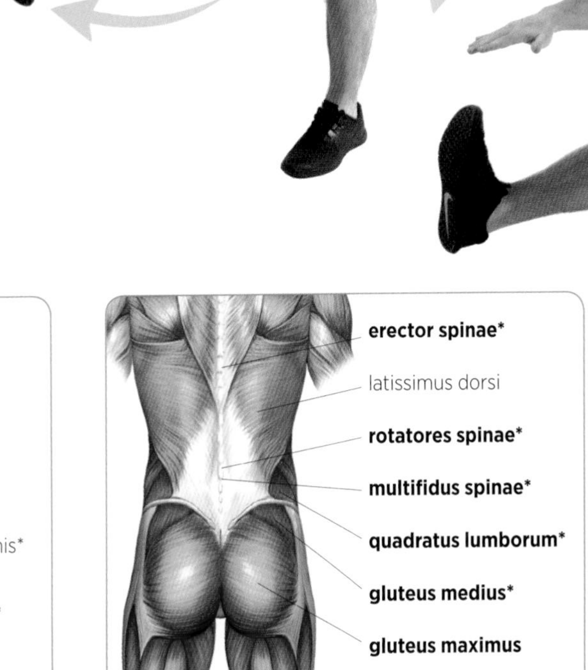

Annotation Key

Bold text indicates target muscles

Light text indicates other working muscles

* indicates deep muscles

DO IT RIGHT

- Keep your back as upright as possible.
- Keep your weight shifted back and through your heel of your supporting foot.

Towel Hamstrings Pull

The Towel Hamstring Pull uses the physical force of friction to your advantage. This exercise works your posterior chain from a bottom-up approach, including your calves, hamstrings, glutes, and, finally, your core.

HOW TO DO IT

- Lie faceup with your legs extended, heels placed on top of towel, and your arms extended down along your sides.
- Engage your hamstrings and glutes by digging your heels into the towel and bridging upward so that your glutes are elevated off the floor, placing your hips in the air.
- Engage your hamstrings to pull your heels toward your trunk while keeping your hips in the air.
- Allow your heels to slide away from you until they return to the floor in the full extended position. Repeat for the recommended repetitions.

DO IT RIGHT

- Keep weight through your heels and on the towel.
- Avoid flaring your knees in or out, keeping them in track and parallel.
- Keep your core engaged to avoid excessive curvature of your spine.
- Perform on a low-friction surface, such as a wood floor.

FACT FILE

TARGETS
- Hamstrings
- Calves
- Glutes
- Abdominals

EQUIPMENT
- Towel

BENEFITS
- Improves coordination
- Strengthens and tones lower calves, hamstrings, and glutes
- Develops core stability

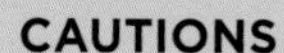

CAUTIONS
- Back issues
- Hip issues

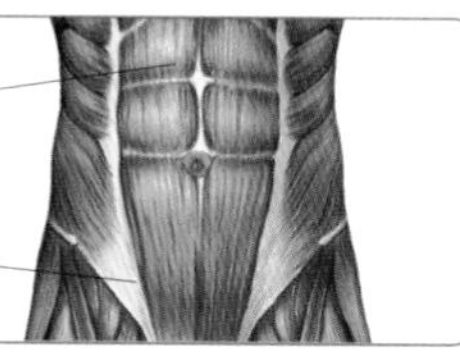

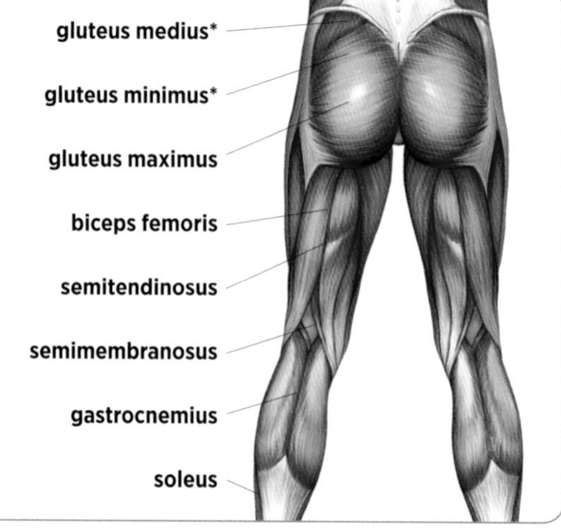

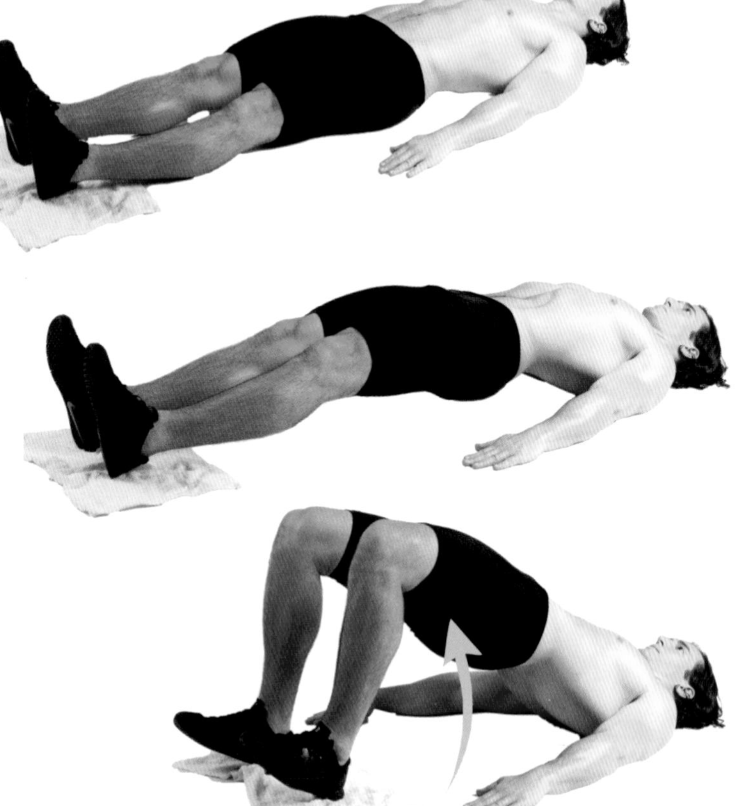

Annotation Key
Bold text indicates target muscles
Light text indicates other working muscles
* indicates deep muscles

Towel Abduction and Adduction

It may resemble cleaning the floor, but this exercise provides its own housekeeping for your inner- and outer-thigh muscles. It is essential to condition these muscles, known as your hip abductors and adductors, if your goal is to have healthier, more powerful legs.

FACT FILE

TARGETS
- Hips
- Abdominals
- Glutes

EQUIPMENT
- Towel

BENEFITS
- Strengthens and tones glutes, abdominals, and legs
- Improves coordination

CAUTIONS
- Hip issues

HOW TO DO IT

- Begin by placing the towel on the floor. Standing on top of the towel, assume a wide stance, spreading your feet approximately twice your hips-width apart.

- While keeping your legs as straight as possible, draw your feet together, pulling the opposite sides of the towel together under your feet.

- Return to the starting position by pressing outward, spreading your legs apart until the towel is taught again under your feet. Repeat for the recommended repetitions.

DO IT RIGHT

- Keep your legs straight.
- Perform on a low-friction surface, such as a wood floor, or use special sliders.
- Perform with smoothly and with control.

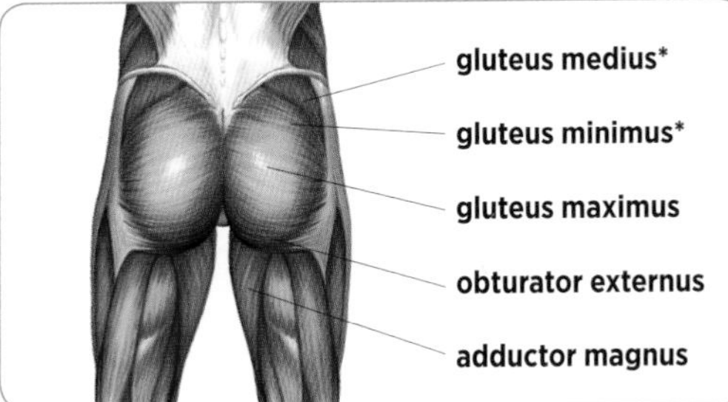

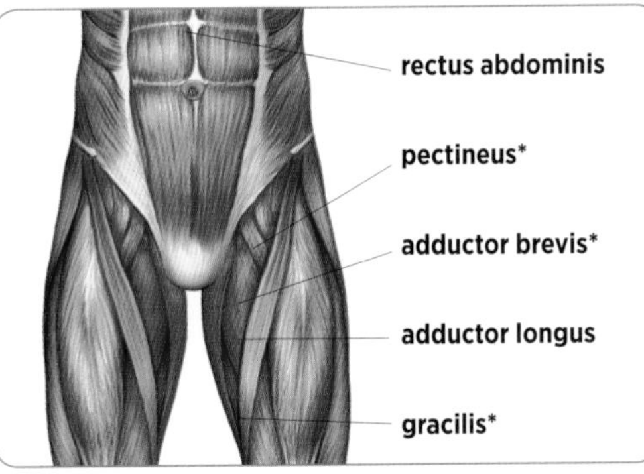

Annotation Key

Bold text indicates target muscles
Light text indicates other working muscles
* indicates deep muscles

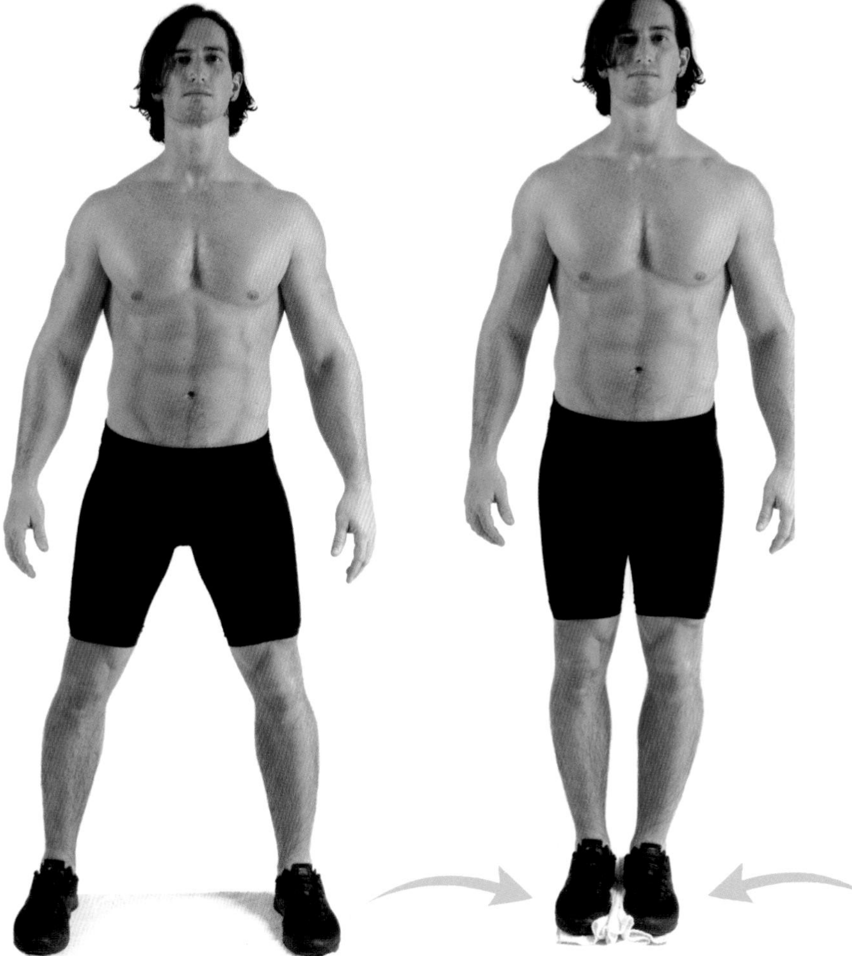

Surrender

"Never quit, never surrender!"—except maybe to this exercise. This beginner body-weight exercise will hit everything from the waist down, including your quadriceps, glutes, calves, and hips.

HOW TO DO IT

- Stand with your feet hip-width apart and your hands clasped behind your head.
- Perform a reverse lunge by flexing at your hips and knees as you step your left leg backward, dropping your knee to the floor.
- Bring your right leg down next to your left leg to come into a kneeling position with both legs.
- Step your left leg in front to again assume the lunge position, this time with your left foot forward.
- Press down into the floor with both feet, performing a lunge to return to the starting position. Continue alternating sides for the recommended repetitions.

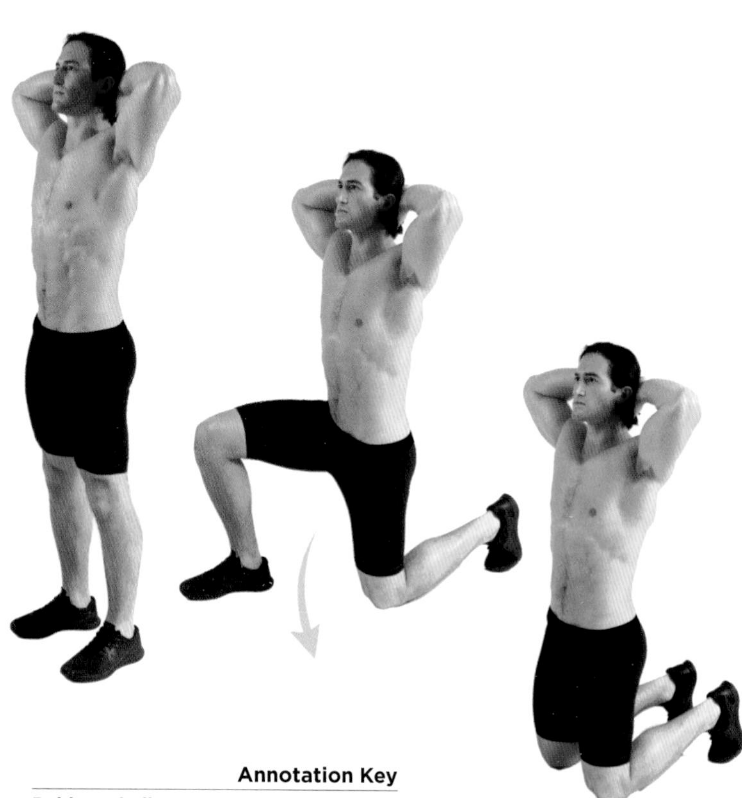

DO IT RIGHT

- Keep your back upright, focusing your gaze slightly higher than the horizon.
- Do use your hands to assist your movements.
- Track your knees over your toes, avoiding any inward or outward deviation of the knee or ankle of your front leg.

Annotation Key
Bold text indicates target muscles
Light text indicates other working muscles
* indicates deep muscles

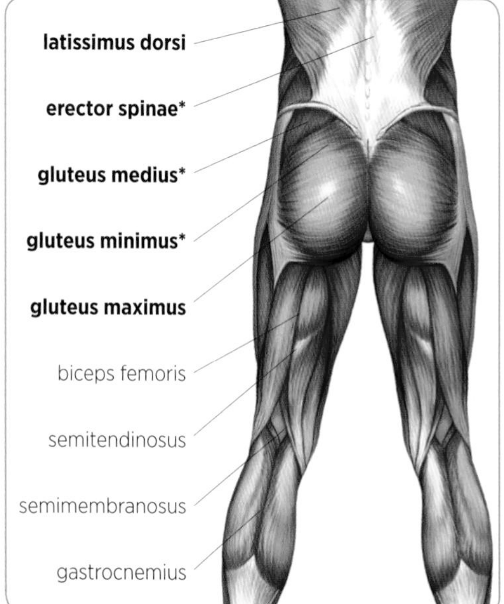

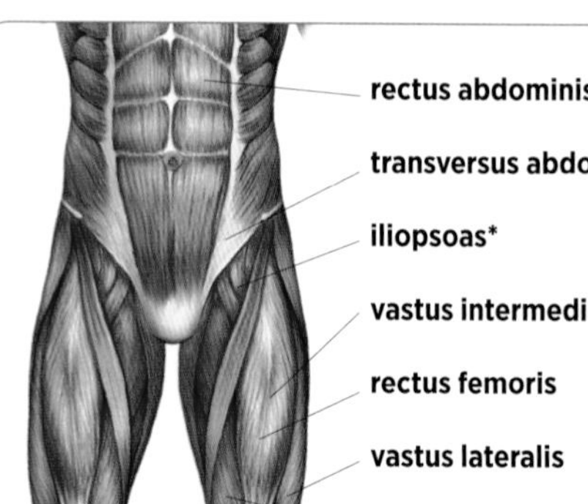

FACT FILE

TARGETS
- Hip flexors
- Quadriceps
- Glutes
- Abdominals
- Back

EQUIPMENT
- None

BENEFITS
- Strengthens and tones core and legs
- Increases lower-extremity muscular endurance
- Improves coordination

CAUTIONS
- Hip issues
- Knee issues

Kneeling Squat Jump

Body-weight leg exercise . . . check. Explosive . . . check. Sweat-inducing . . . check! This advanced, dynamic plyometric exercise targets your quadriceps, glutes, calves, abdominals, and last, but not least, your endurance! A great one to go all out on, this explosive movement demands a lot, but gives even more!

TARGETS
- Hip flexors
- Quadriceps
- Glutes
- Abdominals

EQUIPMENT
- None

BENEFITS
- Strengthens and tones abdominals and legs
- Improves coordination
- Increases cardiovascular endurance
- Increases lower-extremity power

CAUTIONS
- Hip issues
- Knee issues

HOW TO DO IT

- Kneel on the floor with your legs bent and tucked underneath you.
- Drop your hips back, bending at your knees and hips, and swing your arms back and behind you.
- In one explosive motion, swing your arms forward while thrusting your hips forward and extending your legs to power off the floor before pulling your feet underneath you to catch yourself in a squat.
- Come to a standing position by extending your legs and hips.
- Lower yourself back down to the starting position, and then repeat for the recommended repetitions.

Annotation Key
Bold text indicates target muscles
Light text indicates other working muscles
* indicates deep muscles

DO IT RIGHT

- When catching yourself in the squat, make sure to have your feet positioned beneath you, tracking your knees over toes.
- Imagine pressing into the floor as you rise from the squat, creating your body's own resistance in your leg muscles.

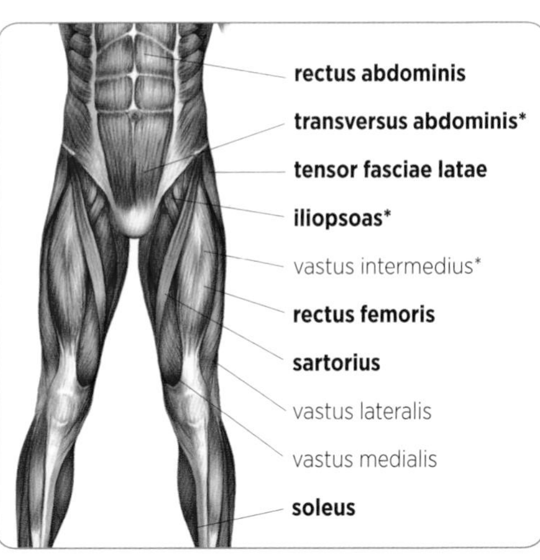

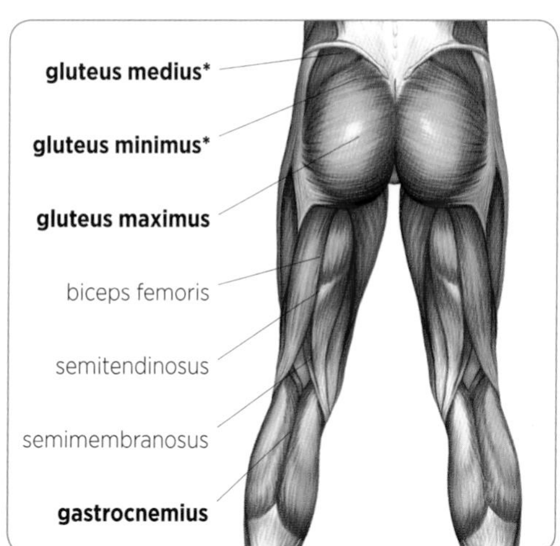

Burpee

The Burpee, a plyometric powerhouse of an exercise, combines the strength-training benefits of a squat or push-up move with high-intensity cardio. Challenge yourself with one of this versatile exercises many variations; for example, you can add different kinds of jumps or perform it on one leg.

HOW TO DO IT

- Stand with your feet together and your arms above your head.
- Drop into a squat, placing your hands on the floor in front of you.
- In one quick, explosive motion, kick your feet back to assume a high plank position.
- Lower your chest to the floor to perform a push-up.
- In another quick motion, jump your feet back into a squat, and then jump into the air.
- Return to the starting position. Continue performing for the desired time or repetitions.

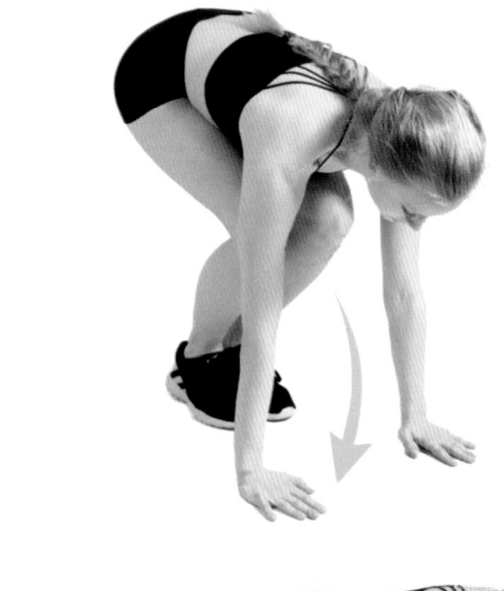

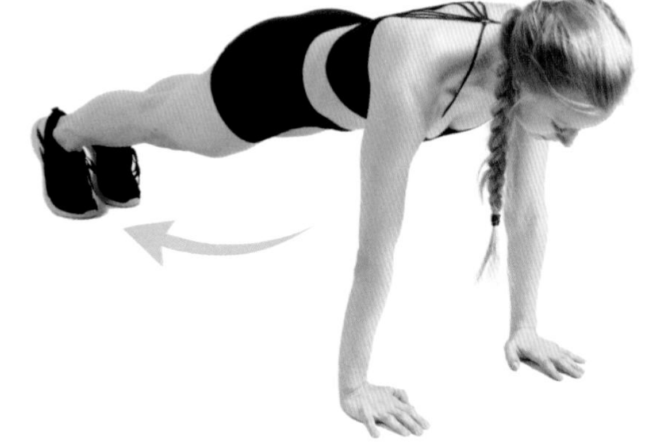

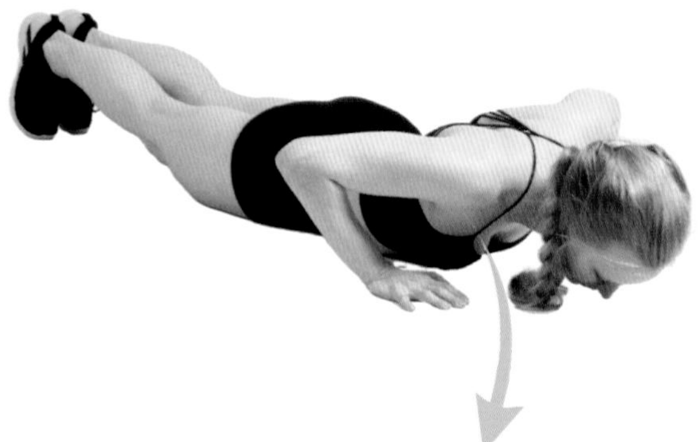

DO IT RIGHT

- Make sure your chest touches the floor during the push-up.
- Jump as high as you can as you rise from the squat.
- Avoid moving with floppy or jerky motions—your movement should be smooth and controlled.

FACT FILE

TARGETS
- Triceps
- Deltoids
- Abdominals
- Back
- Hip flexors
- Quadriceps
- Hamstrings
- Glutes

EQUIPMENT
- None

BENEFITS
- Increases cardiovascular endurance
- Increases agility and speed
- Strengthens entire body

CAUTIONS
- Shortness of breath
- Shoulder issues
- Wrist issues
- Lower-back pain

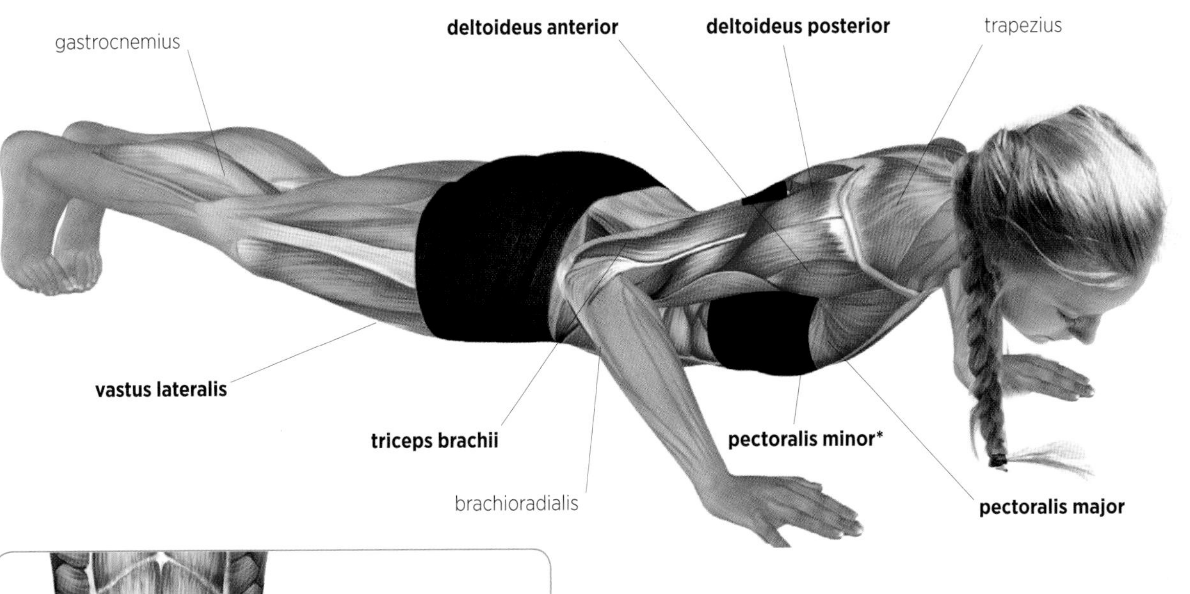

obliquus externus

adductor longus

sartorius

vastus intermedius*

rectus femoris

vastus medialis

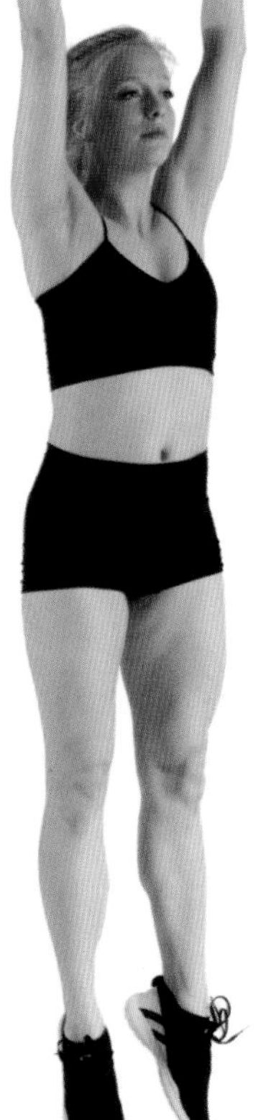

Annotation Key

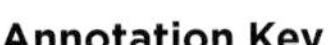

Bold text indicates target muscles

Light text indicates other working muscles

* indicates deep muscles

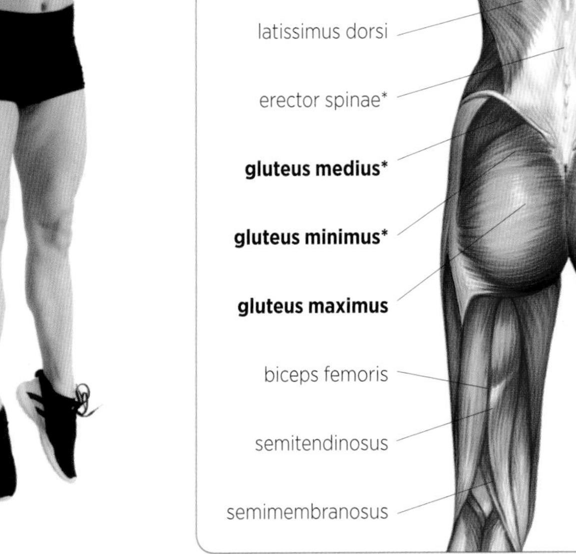

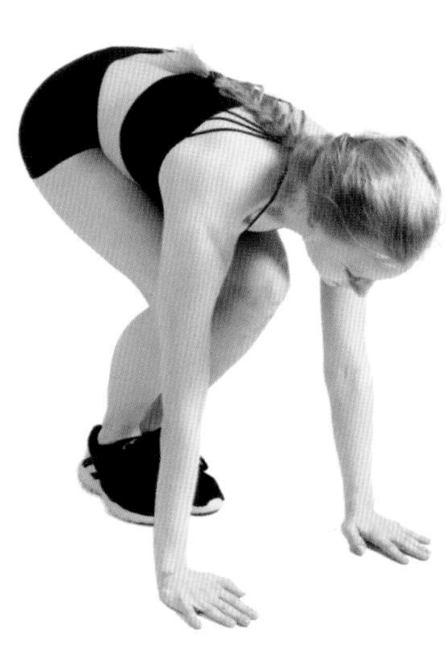

Star Jump

The Star Jump exercise helps develop leg strength and cardio endurance with the Star Jump. It is not easy as it looks—you must be able to jump high enough to simultaneously extend your legs and arms outward.

HOW TO DO IT

- Stand with your feet together, and then squat down, keeping your knees in line with your toes.
- In one explosive movement, jump as high as possible while spreading your arms and legs as wide as you can. Your body will make a star shape in the fully extended point of the jump.
- Bend your knees slightly as you land in the standing position. Sink back to a squat, and repeat. Each jump equals one repetition. Repeat for the recommended repetitions.

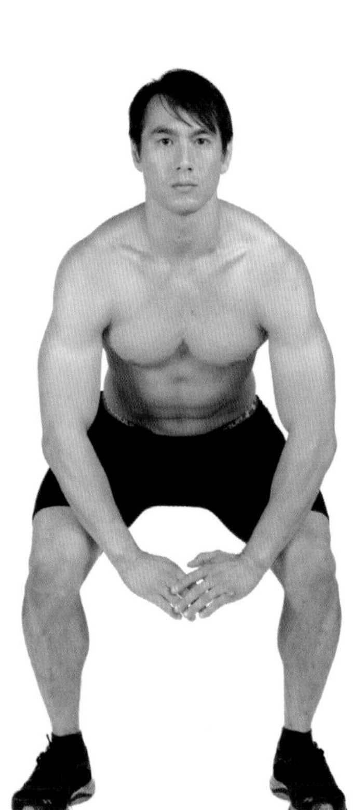

DO IT RIGHT

- Perform these on a soft surface, such as an exercise mat or padded carpeting, to reduce the impact of your landing.
- Flare out your legs as far as possible.
- Avoid twisting in the jump; landing in an awkward position could cause a torque injury.

gluteus medius*
gluteus minimus*
obturator externus
adductor magnus
biceps femoris
semitendinosus
semimembranosus

Annotation Key

Bold text indicates target muscles
Light text indicates other working muscles
* indicates deep muscles

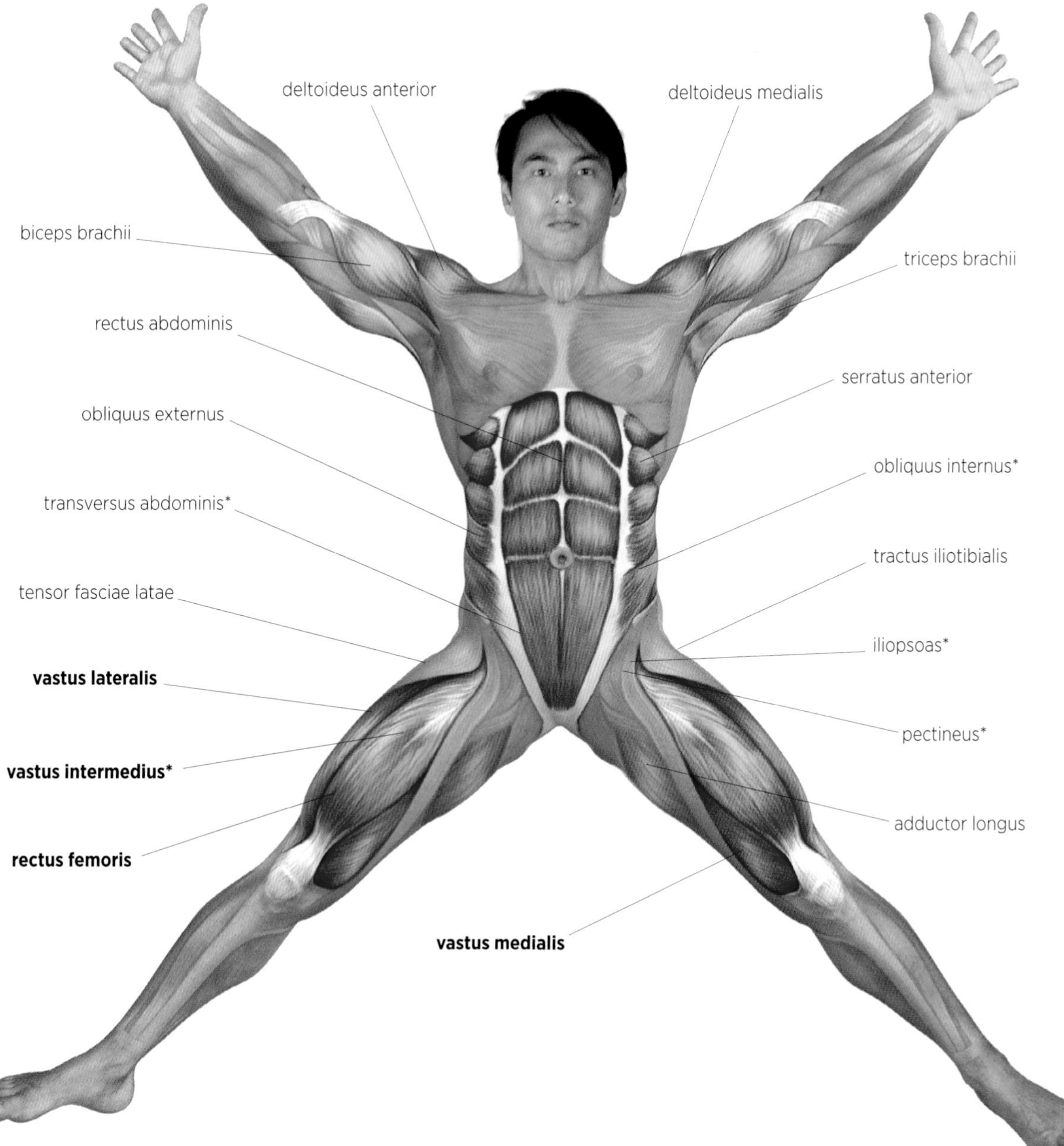

FACT FILE

TARGETS
- Shoulders
- Abdominals
- Quadriceps
- Hamstrings
- Glutes

EQUIPMENT
- None

BENEFITS
- Strengthens upper and lower body
- Increases agility
- Improves coordination
- Increases cardiovascular endurance

CAUTIONS
- Ankle issues

Alligator Crawl

In the fun, but challenging, Alligator Crawl, you imitate an alligator stalking its prey, hovering in a half push-up while steadily moving forward before you slither backward as if in retreat. This move works your chest, shoulders, back, and arms.

HOW TO DO IT

- Begin in a high plank position with your hands shoulder-width apart, your palms on the floor, your feet together, and your back straight.
- Lower into a half push-up position, keeping your back straight. Keeping your body low to the floor, bring your right knee to your right elbow while walking your left hand forward.
- Reverse this movement by walking your right hand forward and bringing your left knee to your left elbow.
- Continue moving forward, reversing your hand and knee positions. Perform for the recommended time, and then reverse your movement to retreat for the recommended time.

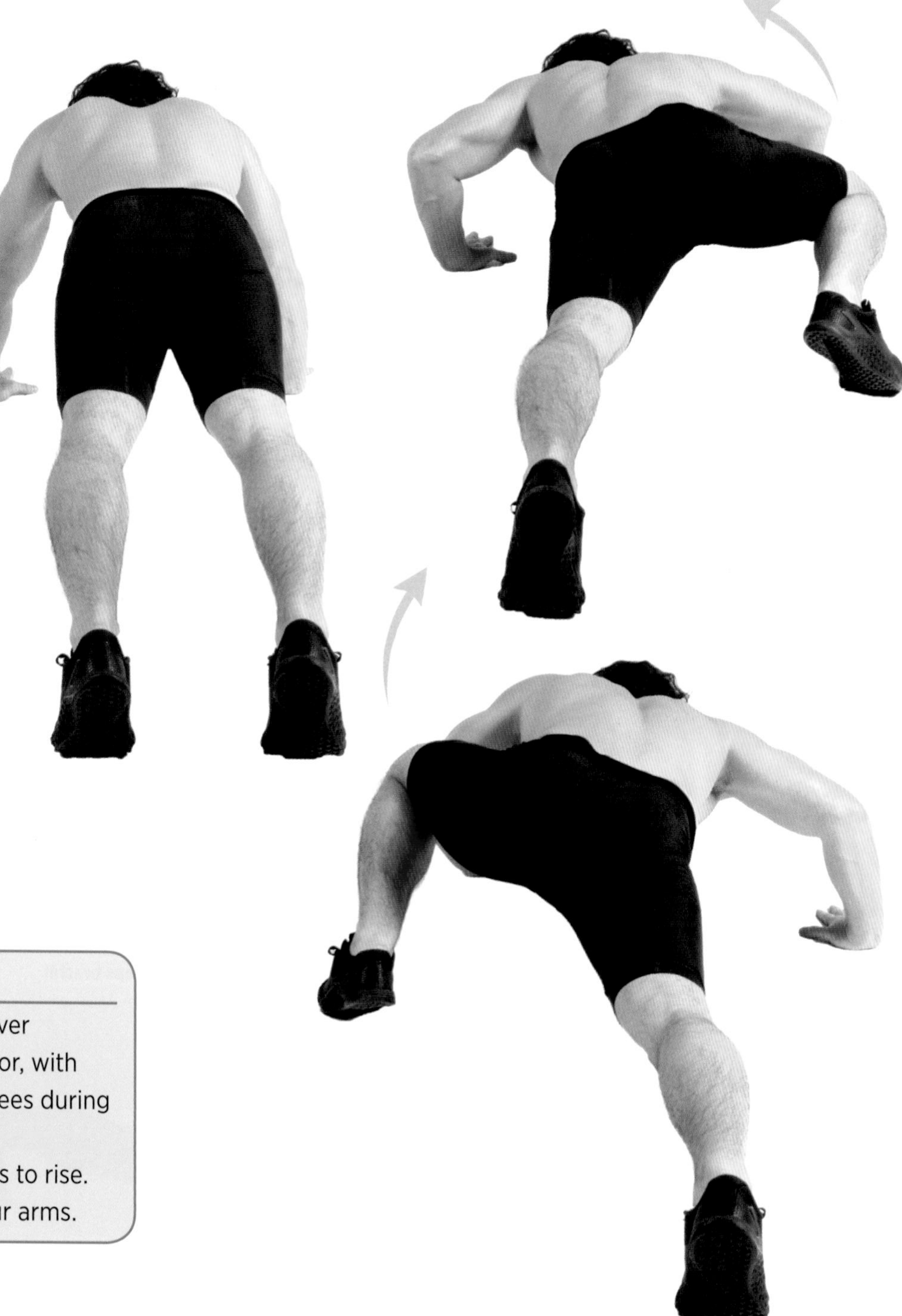

DO IT RIGHT

- Keep your body in a hover position close to the floor, with your elbows at 90 degrees during the entire exercise.
- Avoid allowing your hips to rise.
- Avoid straightening your arms.

Annotation Key

Bold text indicates target muscles

Light text indicates other working muscles

* indicates deep muscles

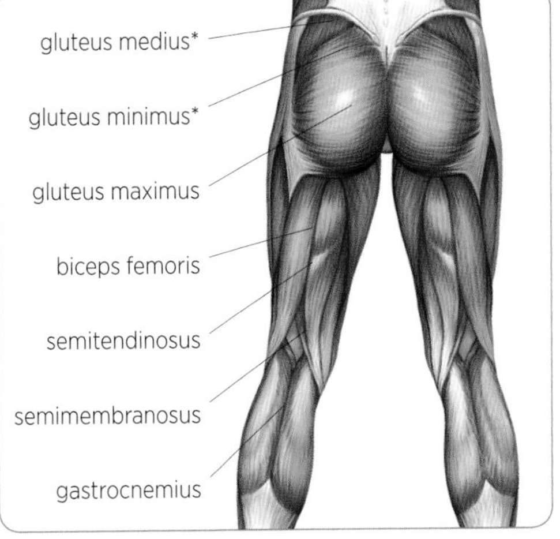

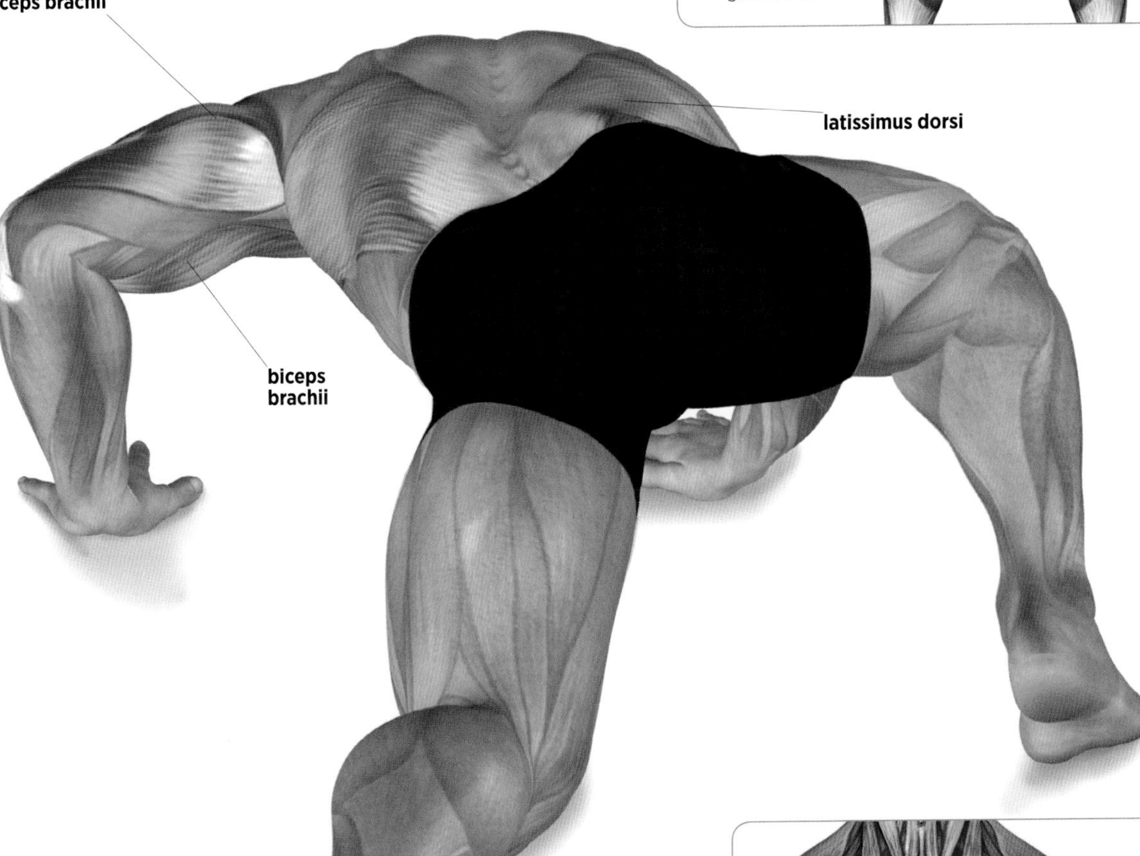

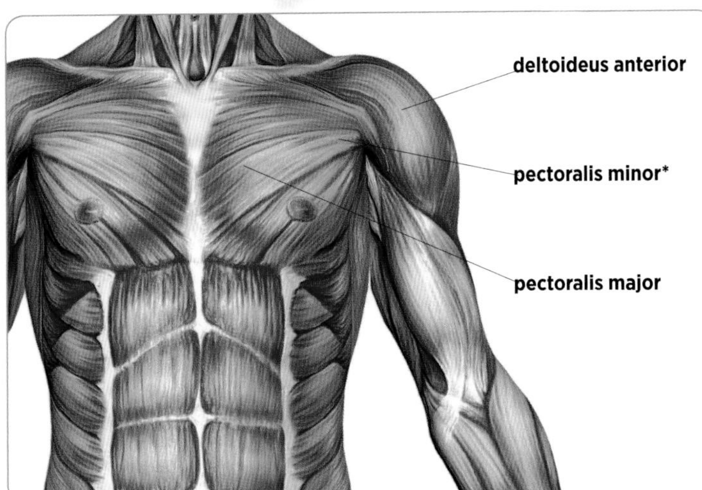

FACT FILE

TARGETS
- Shoulders
- Chest
- Back
- Arms
- Lower body

EQUIPMENT
- None

BENEFITS
- Strengthens upper and lower body
- Increases agility
- Improves coordination

CAUTIONS
- Shoulder issues
- Wrist issues
- Lower-back issues

Slalom Skier

The Slalom Skier is an intense cardio exercise that gets your heart pumping and burns calories. It also strengthen the muscles of your chest, shoulders, arms, and legs.

HOW TO DO IT

- Begin in a high plank position with your feet together.
- Jump both feet to the left so that they land outside your left arm. Tuck your knees toward your chest while you jump.
- Jump your feet back to the leaning rest position, and then jump both feet back across your body to the right, landing with both feet outside your right arm and both knees bent toward your chest.
- Immediately jump back to the left. Both left and right equal one repetition. Continue alternating sides for the recommended repetitions.

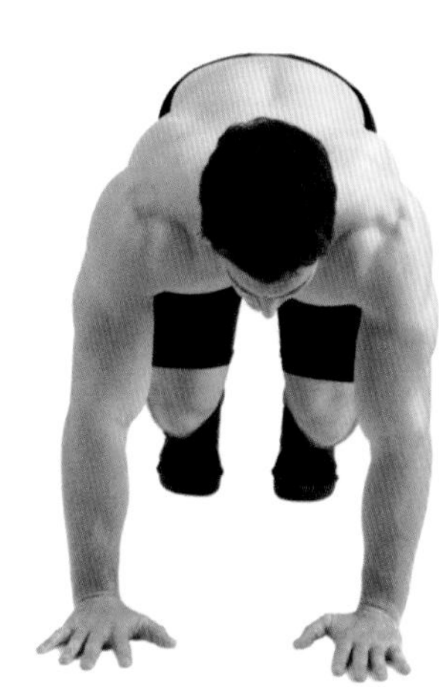

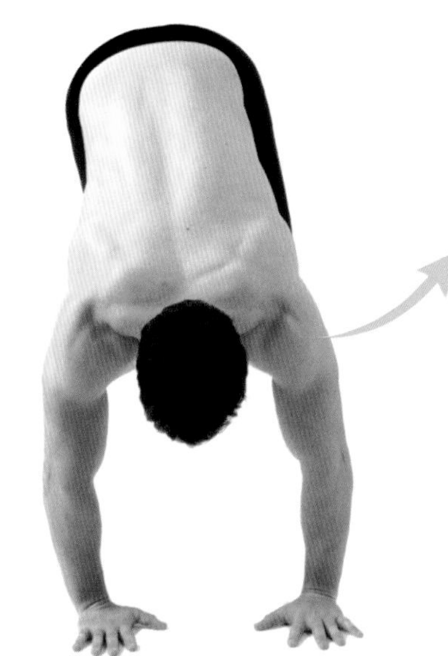

DO IT RIGHT

- When you jump your feet, bend your knees as though they were coming to your chest.
- Avoid jumping your feet too high, which places all of your body weight on your wrists.

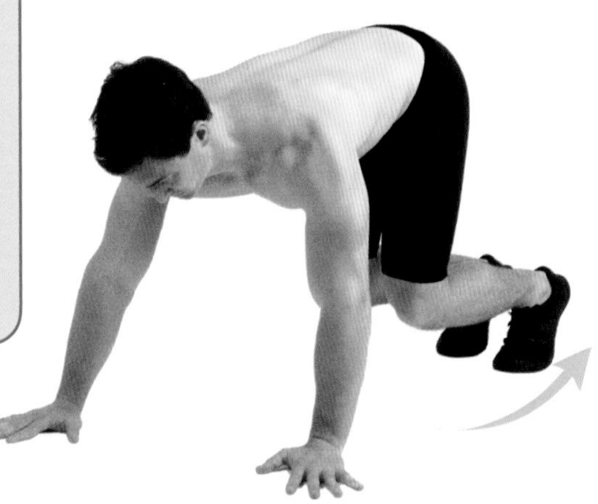

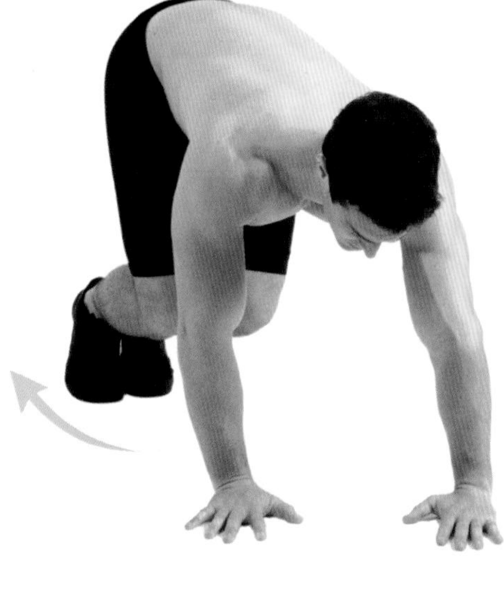

gluteus medius*
gluteus minimus*
adductor magnus
biceps femoris
semitendinosus
semimembranosus

pectoralis major
pectoralis minor*
biceps brachii

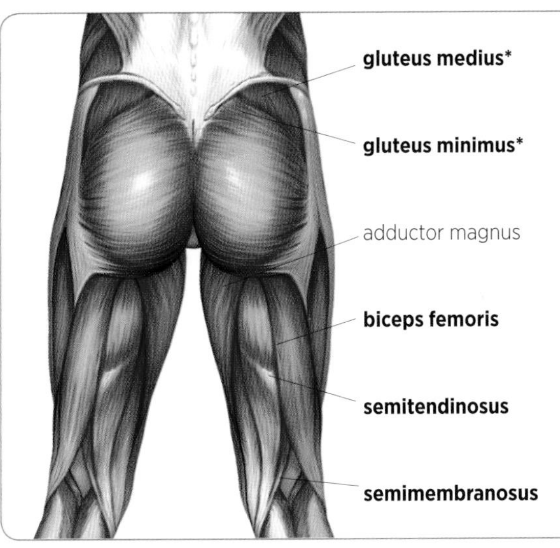

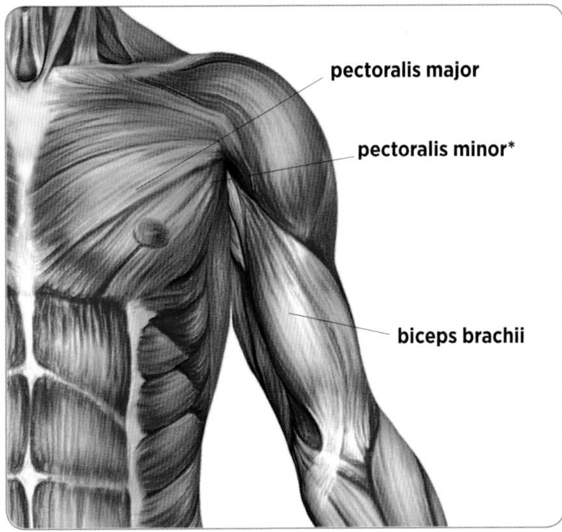

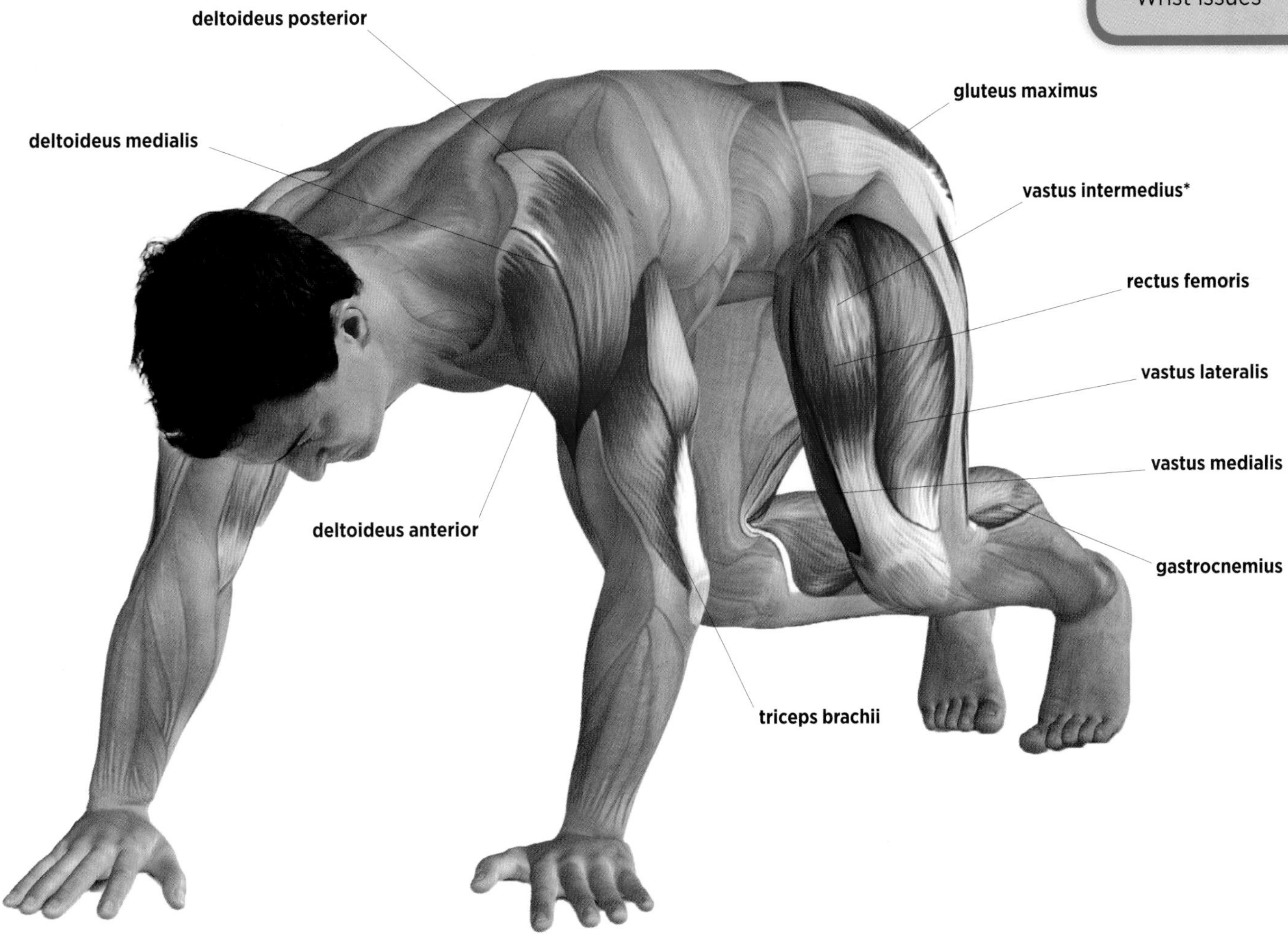

FACT FILE

TARGETS
- Chest
- Shoulders
- Arms
- Glutes
- Thighs
- Calves

EQUIPMENT
- None

BENEFITS
- Strengthens upper body and core
- Increases agility
- Improves coordination
- Increases cardiovascular endurance

CAUTIONS
- Wrist issues

Annotation Key

Bold text indicates target muscles
Light text indicates other working muscles
* indicates deep muscles

deltoideus posterior
deltoideus medialis
deltoideus anterior
gluteus maximus
vastus intermedius*
rectus femoris
vastus lateralis
vastus medialis
gastrocnemius
triceps brachii

Mountain Climber

The explosive Mountain Climber builds upper-body strength while giving your cardiovascular system an intense workout. It also helps hone your balance, coordination, and agility.

HOW TO DO IT

- Begin in a high plank position with your hands shoulder-width apart, your palms on the floor, your feet together, and your back straight.
- Bring your right knee in toward your chest. Rest the ball of your foot on the floor.
- Jump to switch your feet in the air, bringing your left foot in and your right foot back.
- Continue alternating your feet as fast as you can safely go for the recommended repetitions or time.

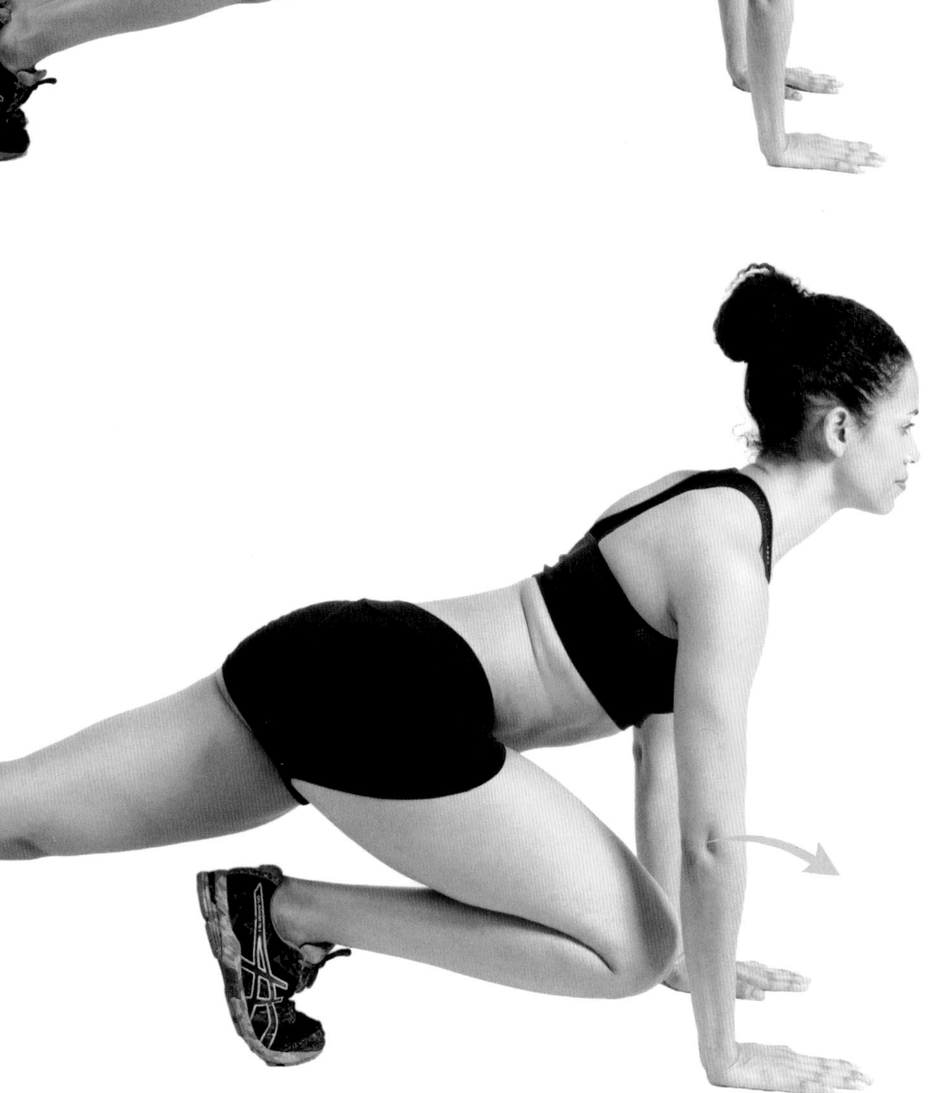

DO IT RIGHT

- Keep your back straight.
- Flare your hands out to ease shoulder stress.
- Avoid small leg movements; attempt to bring each knee to your chest.

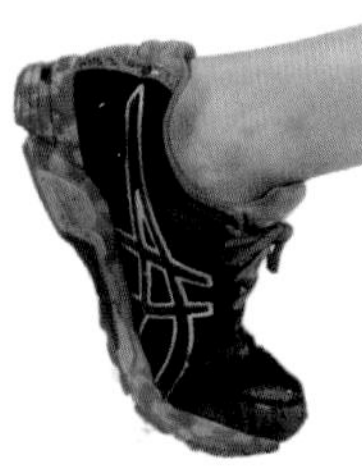

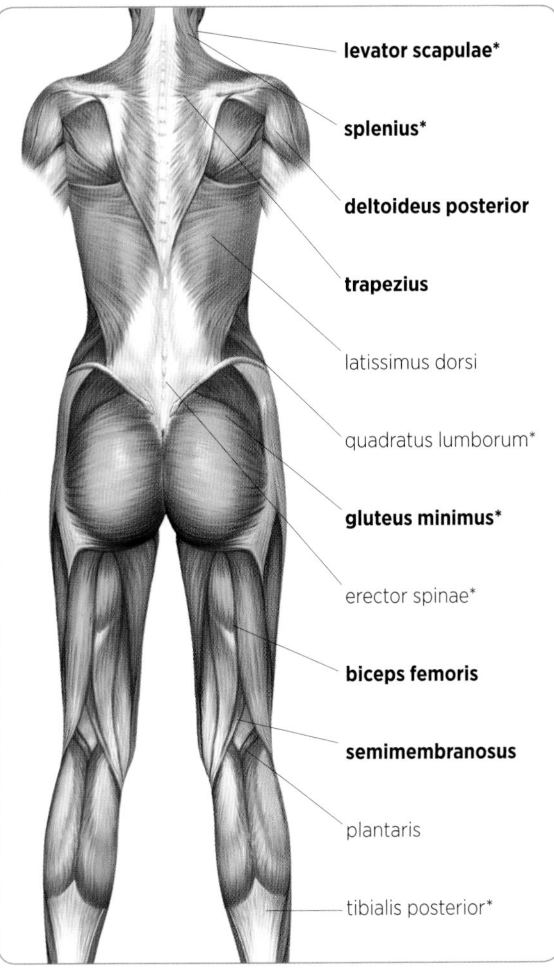

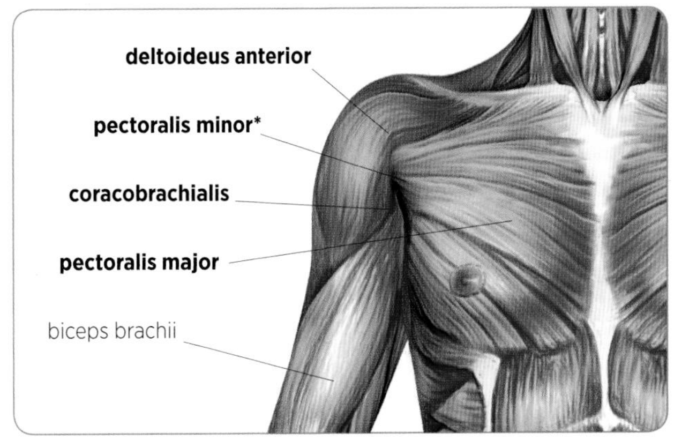

Annotation Key

Bold text indicates target muscles
Light text indicates other working muscles
* indicates deep muscles

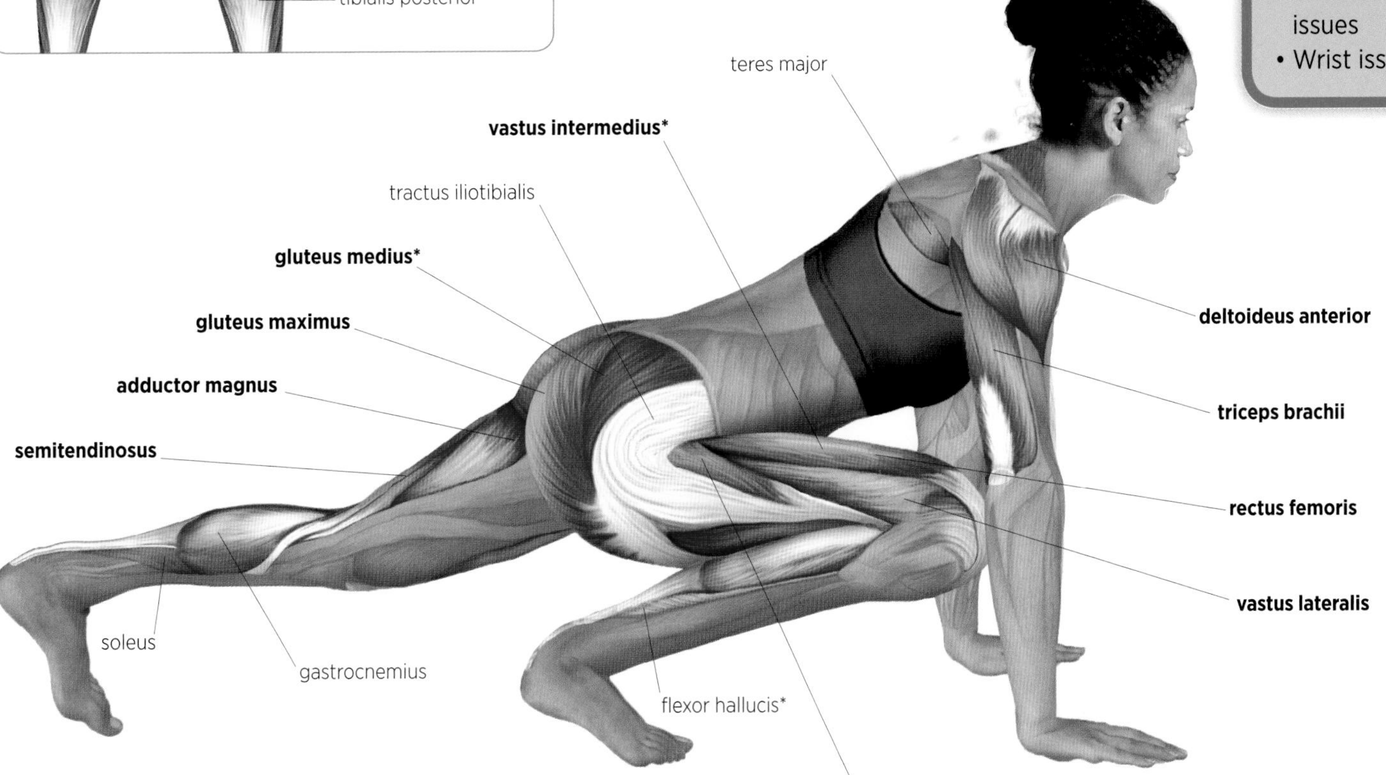

FACT FILE

TARGETS
- Pectorals
- Triceps
- Deltoids
- Abdominals
- Back
- Hip flexors
- Quadriceps
- Hamstrings
- Glutes

EQUIPMENT
- None

BENEFITS
- Warms up muscles
- Improves coordination
- Strengthens and tones abdominals, chest, arms, and legs
- Increases cardiovascular endurance

CAUTIONS
- Shoulder issues
- Wrist issues

Handstand Walk

The Handstand Walk is an advanced exercise that hits your entire body, demanding upper-body strength, as well as midline core and lower-extremity stability. Remember, just one hand after the other!

HOW TO DO IT

- Making sure you have plenty of space on all sides, stand with your feet hip-width apart.
- Raise your hands above your head, and then bend forward to place your hands on the floor in front of you just outside shoulders-width. Stabilize your palms on the floor with your fingers facing away from you.
- When ready, engage your core, and kick up into a handstand by extending one leg toward the ceiling, followed quickly by the other.
- Once in position, shift your body weight toward one side enough to be able to lift one hand and place in front of you.
- Repeat the step above, alternating hands, shifting your body weight over the planting arm. Repeat for the recommended repetitions, or for as long as you can maintain your form and balance.

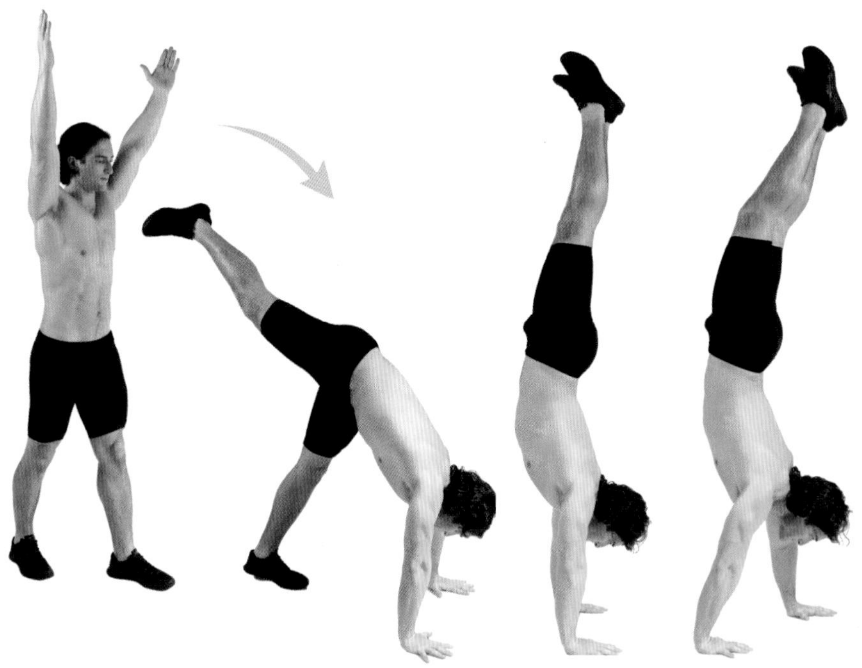

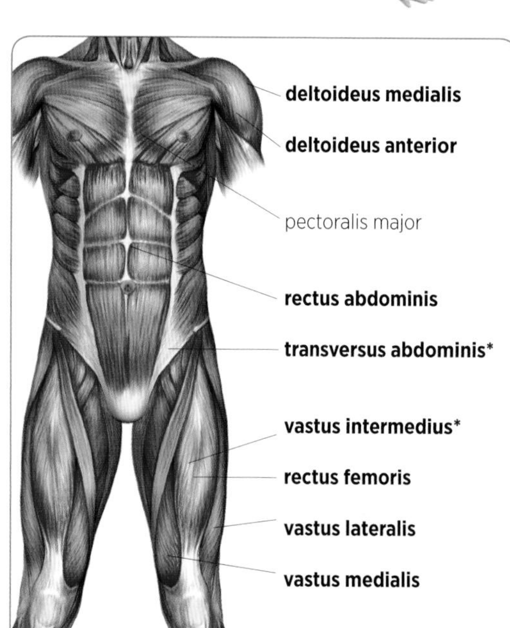

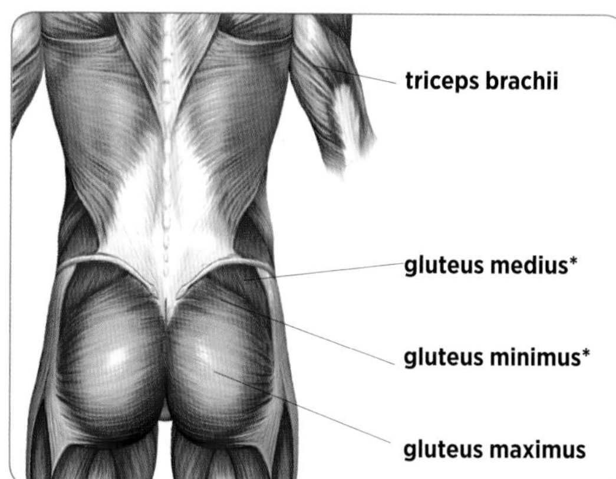

Annotation Key
Bold text indicates target muscles
Light text indicates other working muscles
* indicates deep muscles

FACT FILE

TARGETS
- Quadriceps
- Glutes
- Triceps
- Deltoids
- Abdominals

EQUIPMENT
- None

BENEFITS
- Strengthens and tones arms, chest, and abdominals
- Improves balance and coordination

CAUTIONS
- Shoulder issues
- Wrist issues

DO IT RIGHT
- Keep your core engaged.
- Avoid excessive arching of your spine.
- Keep your shoulders shrugged and activated.
- Perfect the Handstand Push-Up (pages 74–75) before attempting this exercise, and use a spotter for safety.

Muscle-Up

Derived from gymnastics, the Muscle-Up combines the Pull-Up (pages 44–45) and Bar Dip (page 73) to kick your push-and-pull, upper-extremity muscles into full gear. Recruiting help from your core and lower body, this is one elevated exercise.

HOW TO DO IT

- With an overhand grip just outside shoulder-width apart, grasp a pull-up bar.
- Dynamically perform the Pull-Up with enough momentum to pull yourself up and over the bar, resting your chest on the bar, elbows bent and pointing behind you.
- Extend your elbows to push yourself up and away from the bar, pressing down and into the bar, as if performing a Bar Dip.
- Lower yourself until you are hanging underneath the bar once again. Repeat for the recommended repetitions.

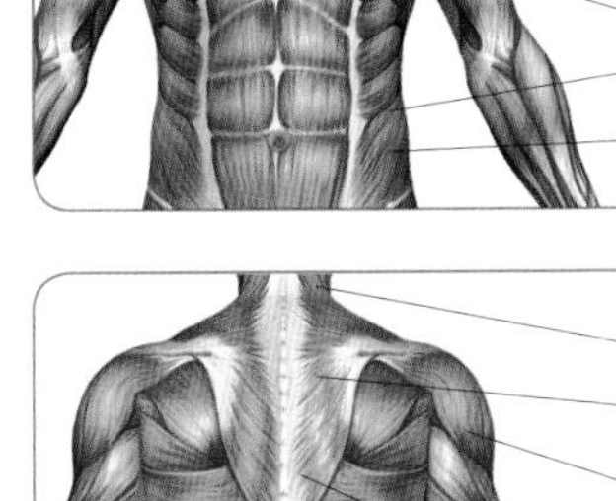

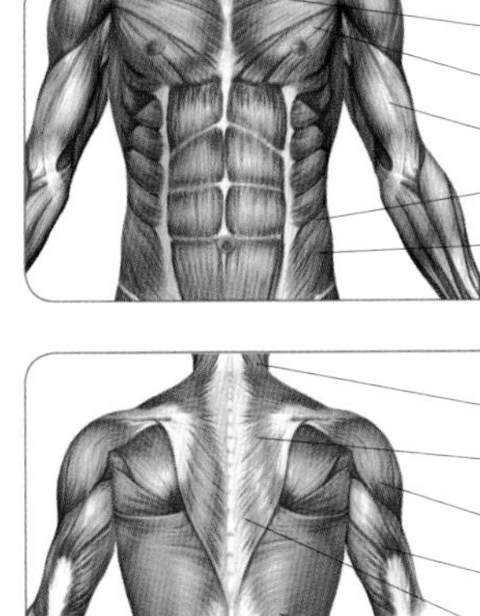

Annotation Key

Bold text indicates target muscles
Light text indicates other working muscles
* indicates deep muscles

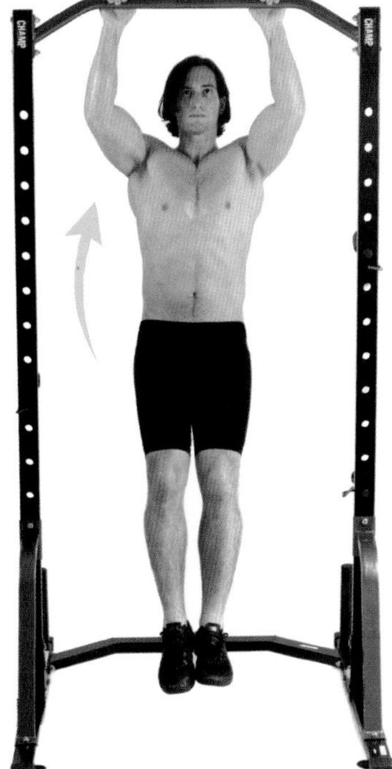

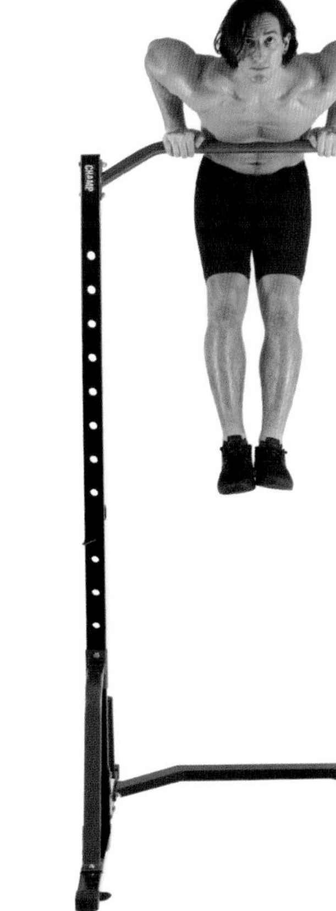

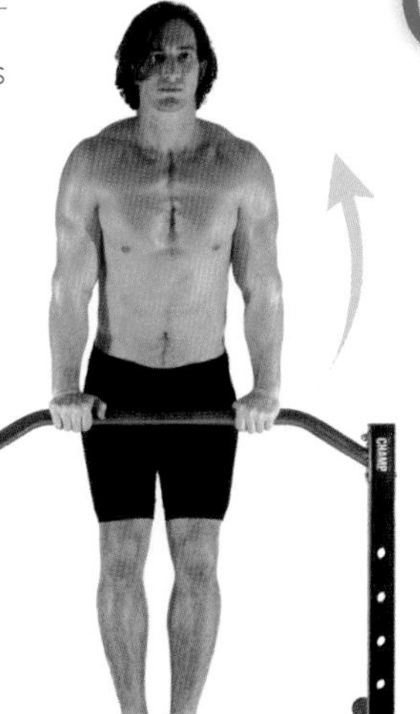

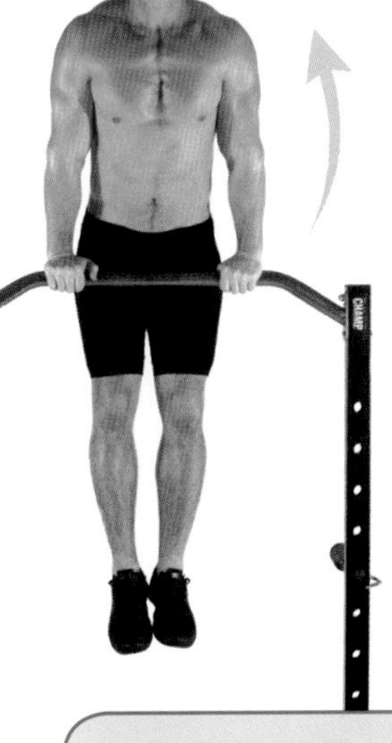

FACT FILE

TARGETS
- Triceps
- Deltoids
- Pectorals
- Abdominals
- Back

EQUIPMENT
- Pull-up bar

BENEFITS
- Strengthens and tones abdominals, back, chest, and arms
- Improves coordination
- Increases cardiovascular endurance

CAUTIONS
- Wrist issues
- Shoulder/ rotator cuff issues

DO IT RIGHT

- Keep your core engaged.
- Keep your movements quick and explosive.
- Simultaneously elevate both shoulders over the bar in order to position yourself on top of it.

Roll-Up

A whole new way to get up in the morning, the Roll-Up is a dynamic full-body exercise that requires core control, lower-extremity power, and balance. This exercise will dynamically challenge your core.

HOW TO DO IT

- Lie faceup with your legs extended and your arms down by your sides.
- Flexing your shoulders, bring your arms above your head.
- With one explosive motion, swing your arms overhead to shoulder height and draw your knees in toward your stomach as you dynamically perform a sit-up. Place your feet on the floor as close to your buttocks as possible.
- Transfer your weight to your feet to come into a low squat. Once you establish balance, press your heels into the floor to rise into a standing position with your legs completely straight.
- Return to the starting position, and then repeat for the recommended repetitions.

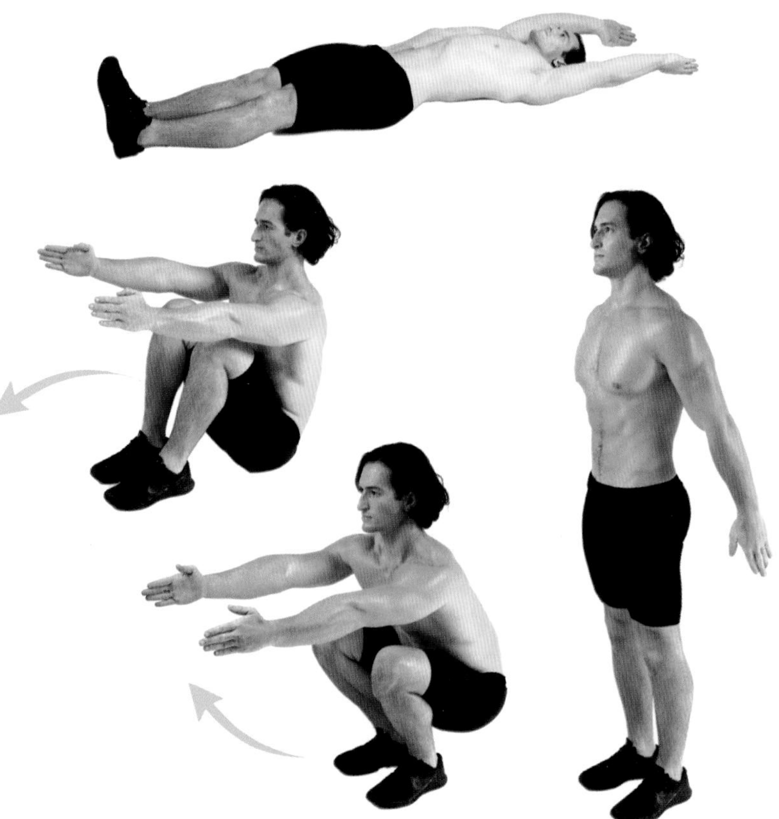

DO IT RIGHT

- Keep your body tight as you roll up.
- Throw your arms forward to transfer your body weight in front of you.
- Keep your back in a neutral position as you come up from the squat.

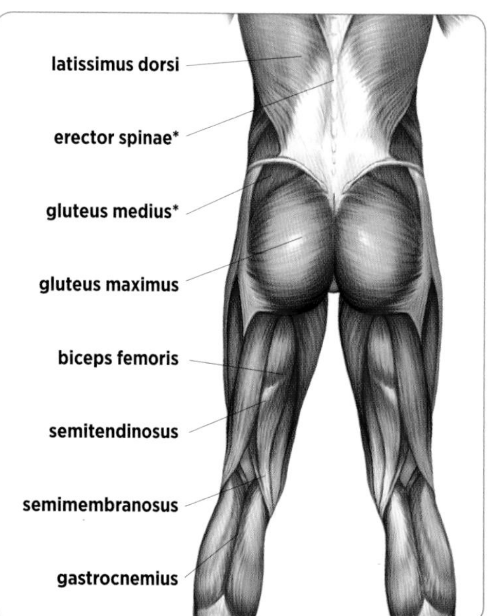

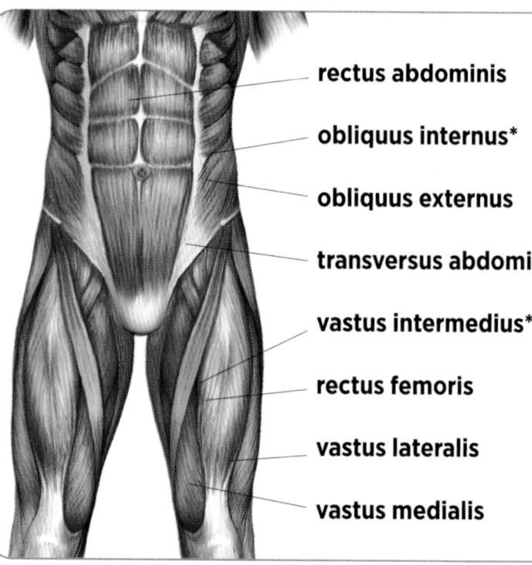

Annotation Key

Bold text indicates target muscles
Light text indicates other working muscles
* indicates deep muscles

FACT FILE

TARGETS
- Abdominals
- Back
- Quadriceps
- Hamstrings
- Glutes

EQUIPMENT
- None

BENEFITS
- Strengthens and tones abdominals, back, and legs
- Improves coordination and balance
- Increases cardiovascular endurance

CAUTIONS
- Lower-back injury

High Plank Kick-Through

The High Plank Kick-Through is a high-intensity exercise that engages your upper body, core, and lower body. A conditioning great exercise, it provides a high-rep sweat maker.

HOW TO DO IT

- Begin in a high plank position with your hands shoulder-width apart, your palms on the floor, your feet together, and your back straight.
- Bring your right leg in toward your body and underneath it while twisting your torso so that your leg crosses your midline toward your left side.
- Without touching the floor with your right leg, draw back underneath your body to return to the high plank position.
- Repeat on the opposite side. Continue alternating sides for the recommended repetitions.

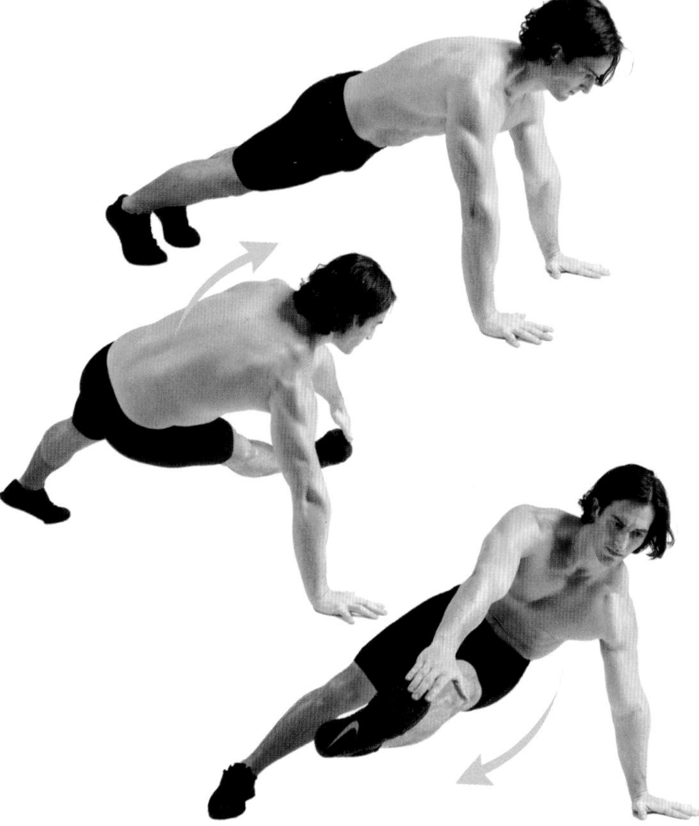

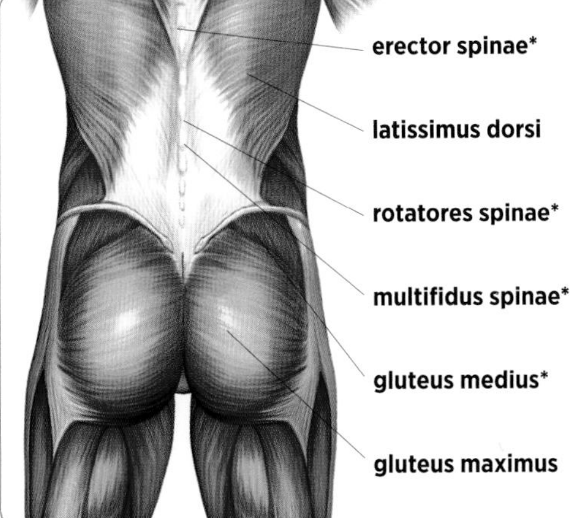

deltoideus medialis
deltoideus anterior
pectoralis minor*
pectoralis major
rectus abdominis
obliquus internus*
obliquus externus
transversus abdominis*
iliopsoas*
pectineus*
sartorius
vastus intermedius*
rectus femoris
vastus lateralis
vastus medialis

Annotation Key

Bold text indicates target muscles

Light text indicates other working muscles

* indicates deep muscles

FACT FILE

TARGETS
- Pectorals
- Triceps
- Deltoids
- Abdominals
- Back
- Hip flexors
- Quadriceps
- Glutes

EQUIPMENT
- None

BENEFITS
- Develops core stability
- Improves coordination
- Strengthens and tones abdominals, chest, arms, and legs

CAUTIONS
- Wrist issues
- Lower-back issues

DO IT RIGHT

- Keep your back straight.
- Bend your elbows when performing the twist.
- Keep your moving leg as straight as possible.

Turkish Get-Up

A simple but powerful exercise, the Turkish Get-Up targets multiple muscles throughout your body, including those in the shoulders, core, thighs, back, glutes, and arms. It also increases hip stability and improves balance and coordination.

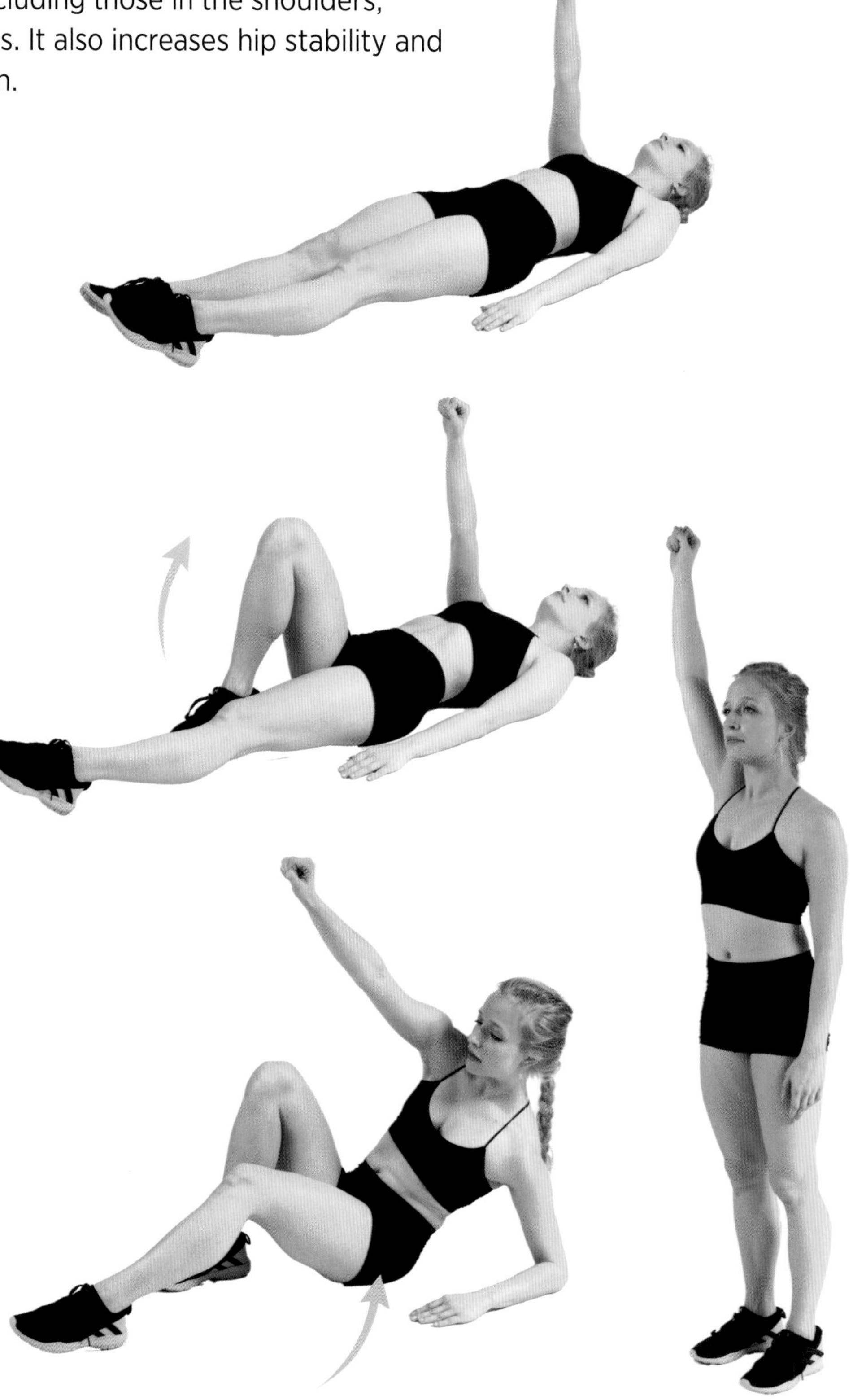

HOW TO DO IT

- Lie faceup with your legs together. Raise your right arm straight up above your chest and extend your left arm along your side.
- Flex your right knee, and place your right foot flat on the floor next to your left knee.
- Rotate your torso slightly to the left, and lift your shoulders off the floor. Plant your left hand on the floor, and lift yourself up to a sitting position.
- Lift your hips upward, and tuck your left leg under your body to support yourself on your left knee.
- Lift your left hand off the floor, and push through your right foot to rise to a standing position, keeping your right arm stretched over your head throughout the exercise.
- Return to the starting position, and then repeat on the other side. Repeat for the recommended repetitions.

DO IT RIGHT

- Keep your abs engaged throughout the movement.
- Avoid performing the exercise at excessive speed.

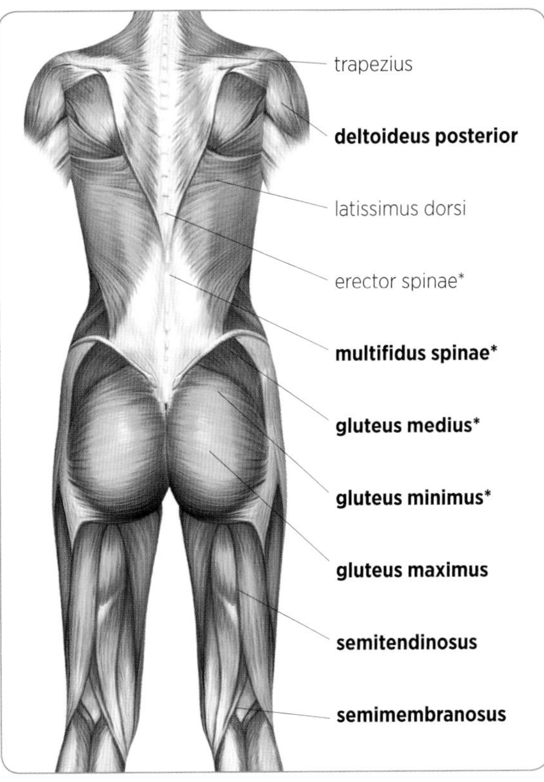

MODIFICATION

HARDER: Perform holding a hand weight or dumbbell in your raised hand.

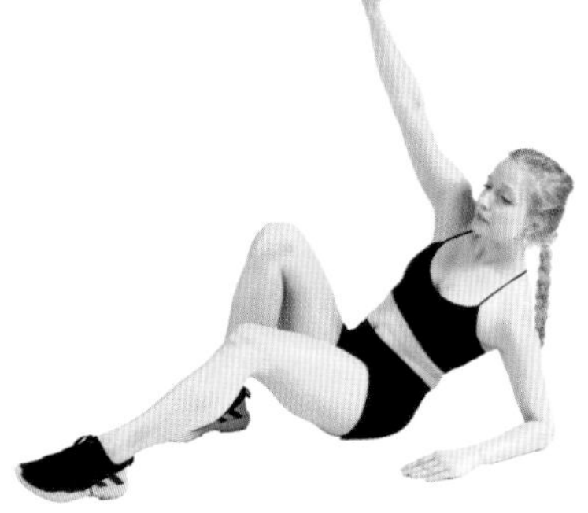

FACT FILE

TARGETS

- Shoulders
- Core
- Thighs
- Glutes
- Upper back
- Triceps

EQUIPMENT

- None

BENEFITS

- Strengthens entire body
- Increases hip stability
- Improves balance and coordination

CAUTIONS

- Back pain

Annotation Key

Bold text indicates target muscles
Light text indicates other working muscles
* indicates deep muscles

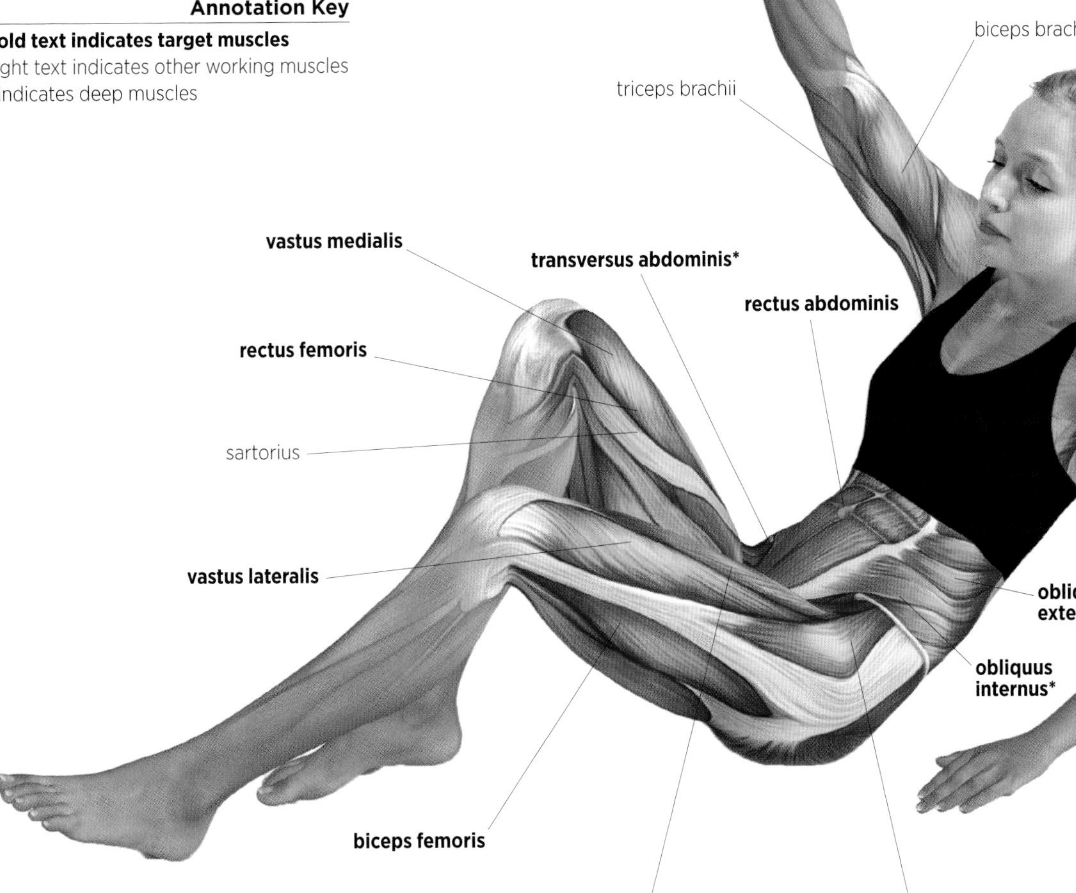

CHAPTER THREE

SEPARABLE FREE-WEIGHT EXERCISES

The following pages provide a compilation of various high-intensity exercises requiring separable free weights, such as dumbbells and kettlebells. These tools are versatile, relatively inexpensive, and easily transportable. The increased use of your core, coordination, and bilateral stabilizers are some of their greatest benefits, taxing your system in positive ways. These tools help turn deficits into strengths. This chapter highlights these tools with a nonexhaustive list that is only limited by your imagination.

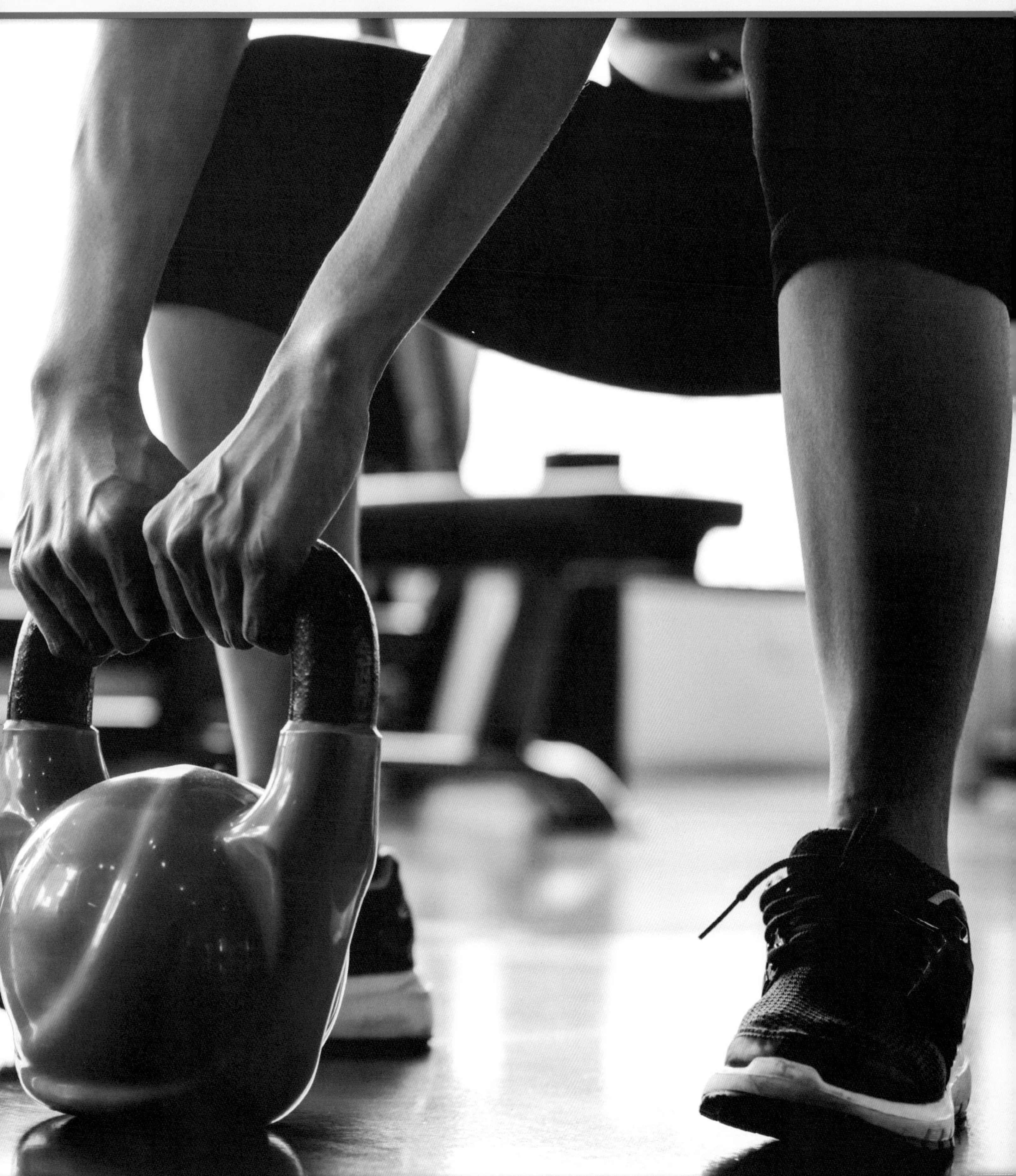

Dumbbell Upright Row

The Dumbbell Upright Row is an essential exercise for upper-body strength. Attacking your "pulling" muscles develops your upper back, as well as your shoulders, arms, and core.

HOW TO DO IT

- Stand with your feet shoulder-width apart, with your arms at your sides and a dumbbell in each hand.
- Leading with your elbows, flex your shoulders and elbows to raise the dumbbells toward your clavicle until they are level with your shoulders.
- Return to the starting position, and then repeat for the recommended repetitions.

trapezius

deltoideus posterior

rhomboideus*

latissimus dorsi

erector spinae*

DO IT RIGHT

- Keep your abdominals engaged.
- Keep your elbows higher than your hands.
- Avoiding leaning back as you lift the weights.

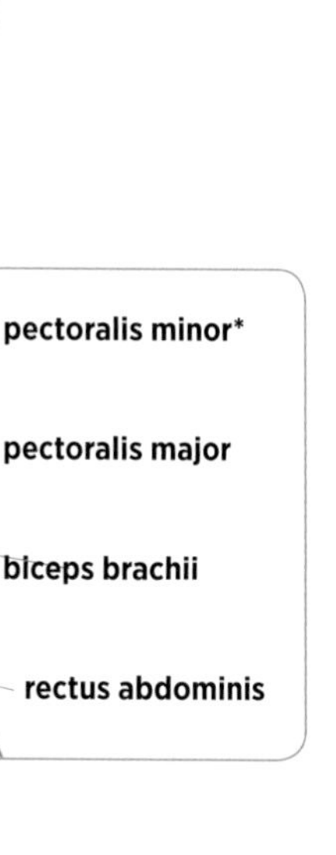

pectoralis minor*

pectoralis major

biceps brachii

rectus abdominis

Annotation Key
Bold text indicates target muscles
Light text indicates other working muscles
* indicates deep muscles

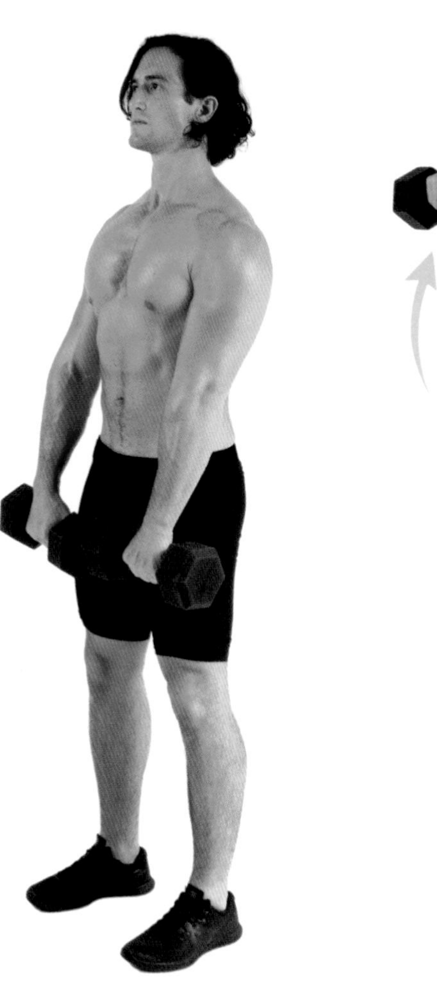

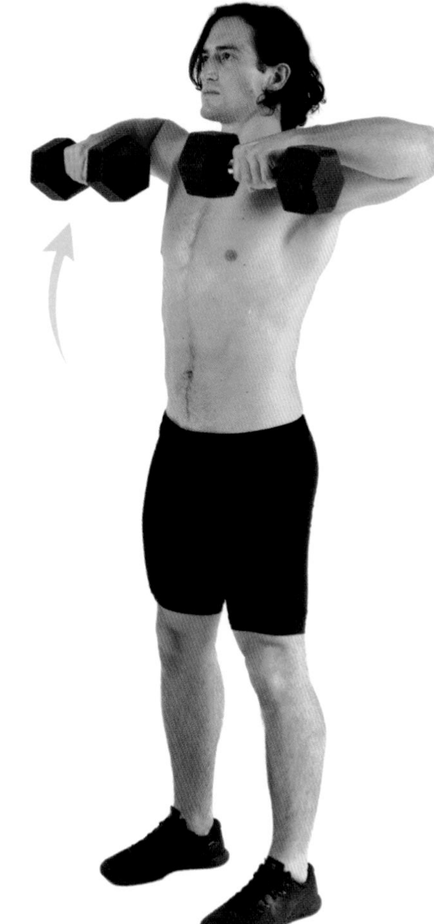

FACT FILE

TARGETS
- Back
- Abdominals
- Deltoids
- Biceps

EQUIPMENT
- Dumbbells

BENEFITS
- Strengthens and tones upper back, shoulders, and biceps
- Increases core stability

CAUTIONS
- Wrist issues
- Shoulder/rotator cuff issues

Kettlebell Bent-Over Row

Use gravity to your advantage by working your entire back with the Kettlebell Bent-Over Row. The dynamic and isometric components to this exercise make it invaluable for a stronger back.

FACT FILE

TARGETS
- Back
- Biceps

EQUIPMENT
- Kettlebell

BENEFITS
- Strengthens and tones back and arms

CAUTIONS
- Shoulder issues

HOW TO DO IT

- Holding a kettlebell straight down beneath your shoulders, stand in a bent-over position with your back in a neutral position and your hips hinged at a 45-degree angle.
- Draw your elbows back, squeezing your shoulder blades together and flexing your elbows to bring the kettlebell in toward your torso.
- Extend your arms to lower the kettlebell back to the starting position. Repeat for the recommended repetitions.

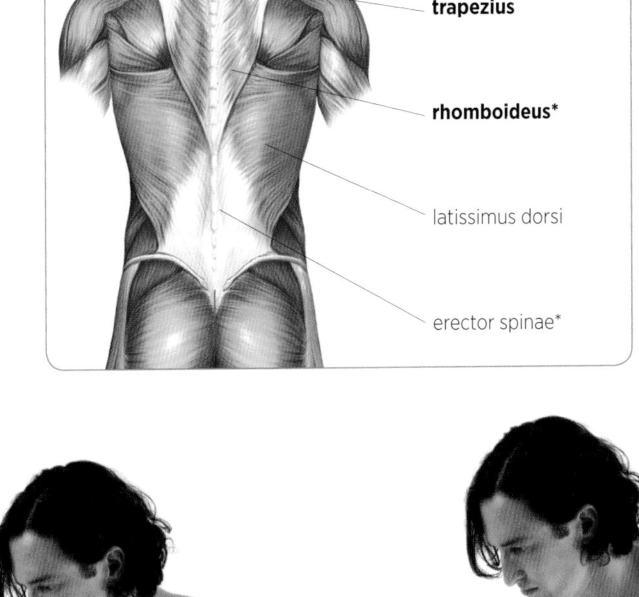
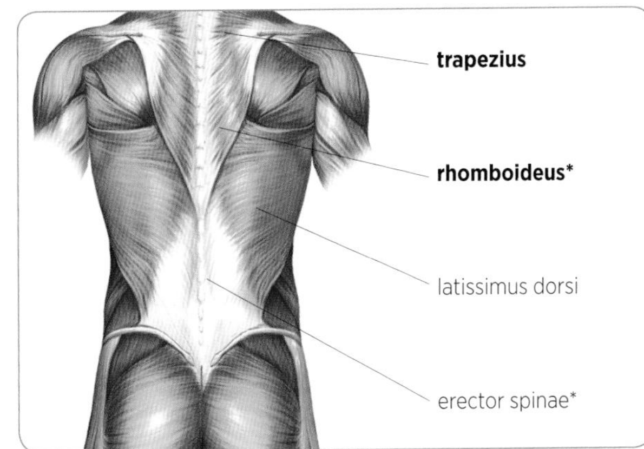

DO IT RIGHT
- Keep your back straight.
- Pinch your shoulder blades together.

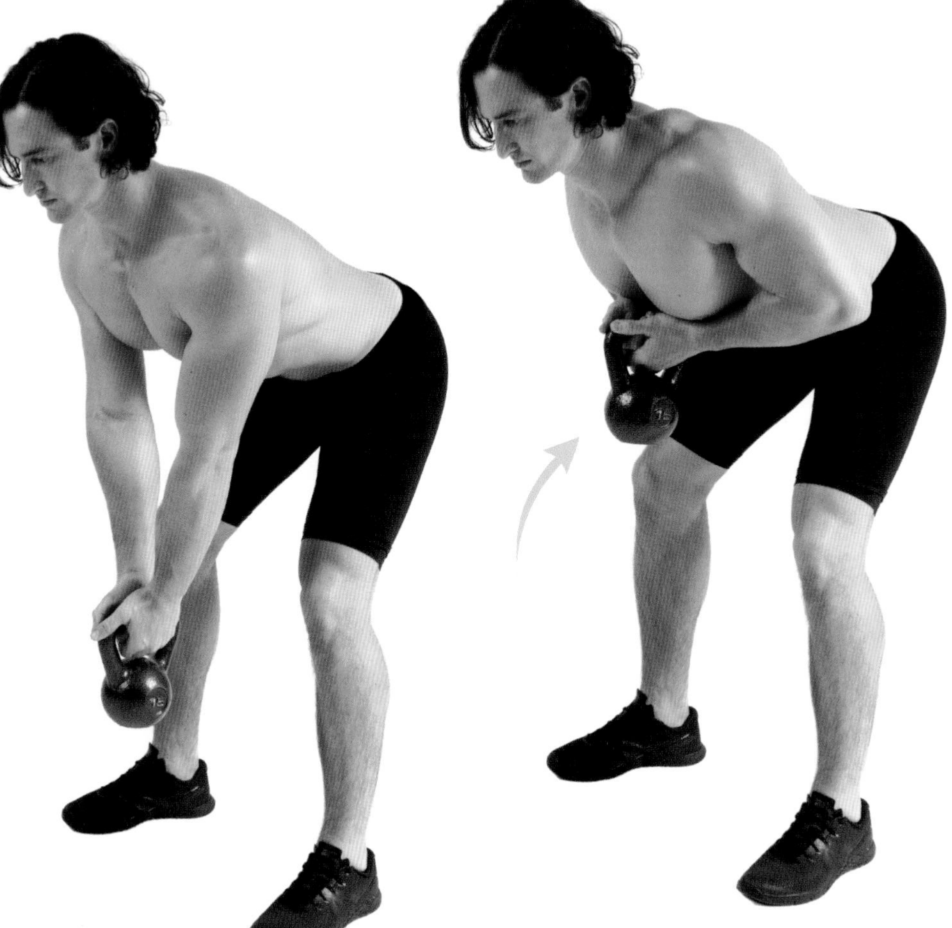

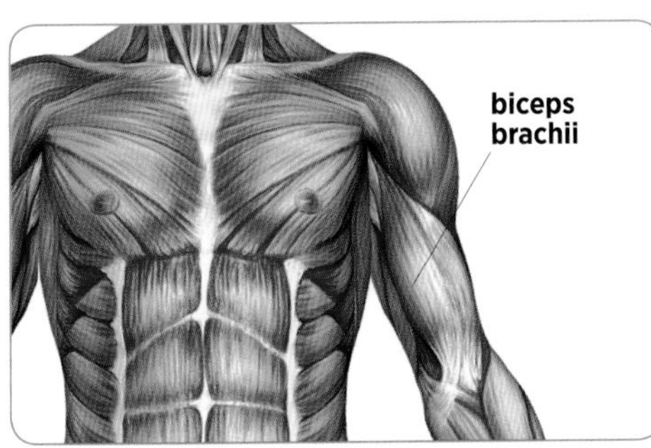

Annotation Key

Bold text indicates target muscles

Light text indicates other working muscles

* indicates deep muscles

Dumbbell Deadlift

A foundational exercise of many strength-training disciplines, the Dumbbell Deadlift is simple exercise. When done correctly, the movement should feel like you are picking up something from the ground.

HOW TO DO IT

- Stand with your feet shoulder-width apart, knees very slightly bent, grasping a dumbbell in each hand, holding them at your side, palms facing each other. Keep your torso upright, and squeeze your shoulder blades together.
- Bend forward from the hips, keeping your knees stationary, and lower the dumbbells toward the tops of your feet. Rotate your palms slightly inward so that they face behind you as you lower the dumbbells until you feel a stretch in your hamstrings.
- Return to the starting position, and then repeat for the recommended repetitions.

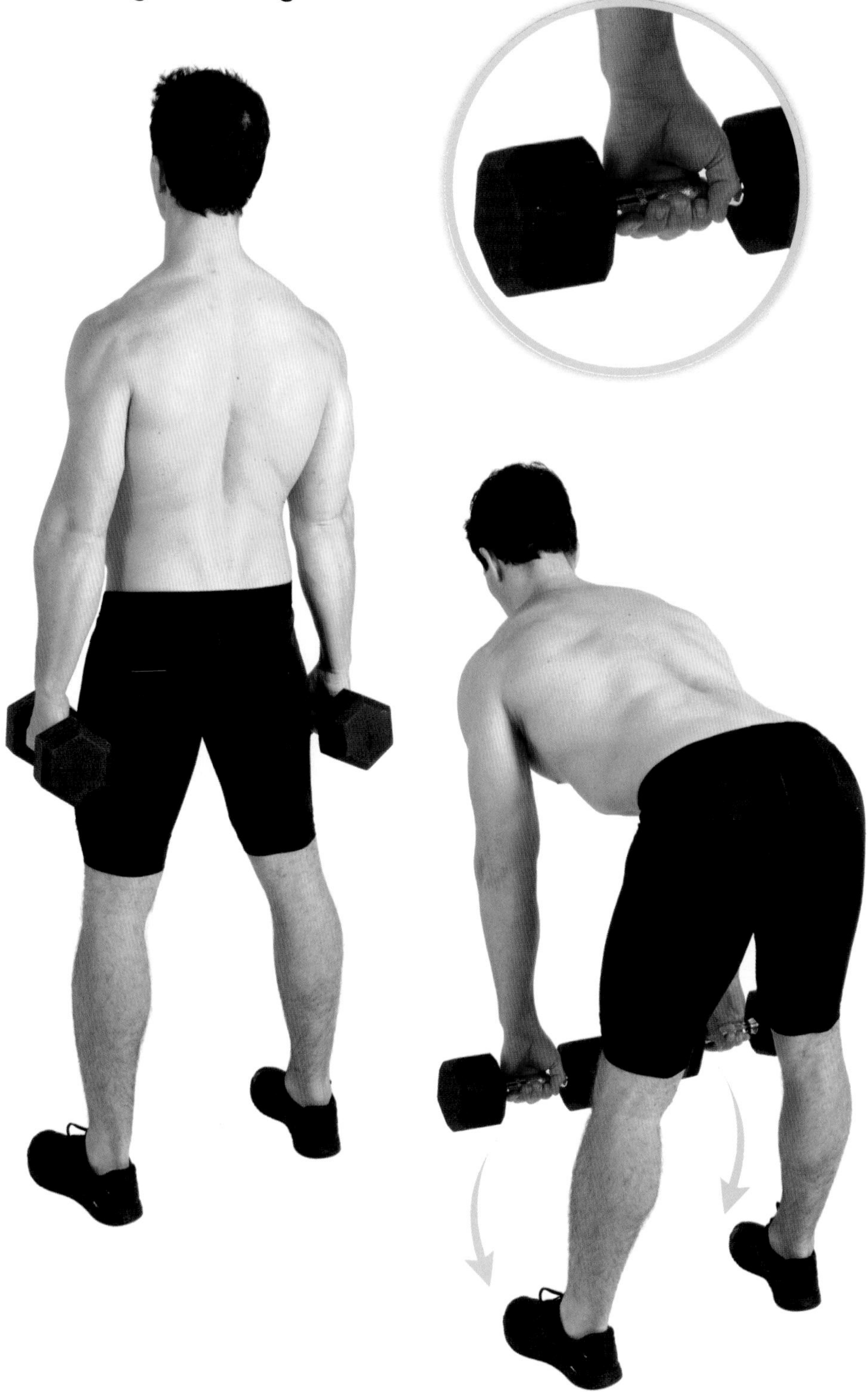

DO IT RIGHT

- Keep your head in line with the rest of your spine; avoid arching your neck to look forward or curling your chin into your chest.
- Exhale as you lower the dumbbells, and inhale as you come up to the starting position.

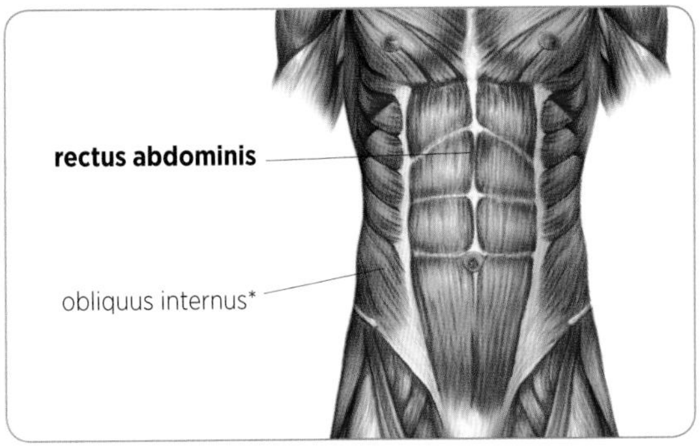

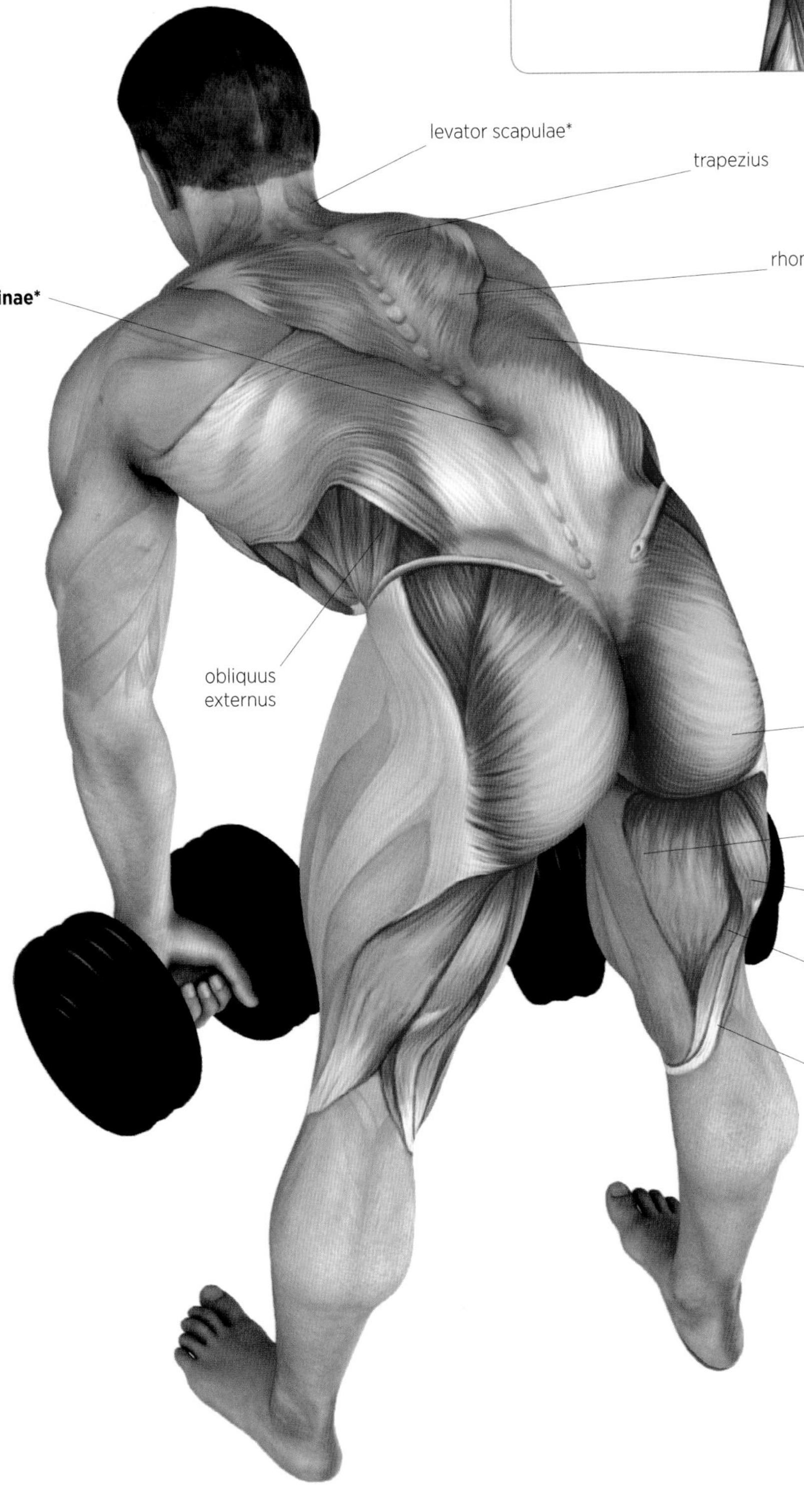

FACT FILE

TARGETS
- Back
- Glutes
- Hamstrings

EQUIPMENT
- Dumbbells

BENEFITS
- Strengthens back and lower body

CAUTIONS
- Shoulder issues
- Wrist issues
- Lower-back pain

Annotation Key

Bold text indicates target muscles

Light text indicates other working muscles

* indicates deep muscles

rectus abdominis

obliquus internus*

levator scapulae*

trapezius

rhomboideus*

erector spinae*

latissimus dorsi

obliquus externus

gluteus maximus

adductor magnus

biceps femoris

semitendinosus

semimembranosus

Single-Arm T-Row

A tough exercise, the Single-Arm T-Row builds strength and stability in your core and upper body. To maintain proper form, use only as much weight as you can carefully and safely control.

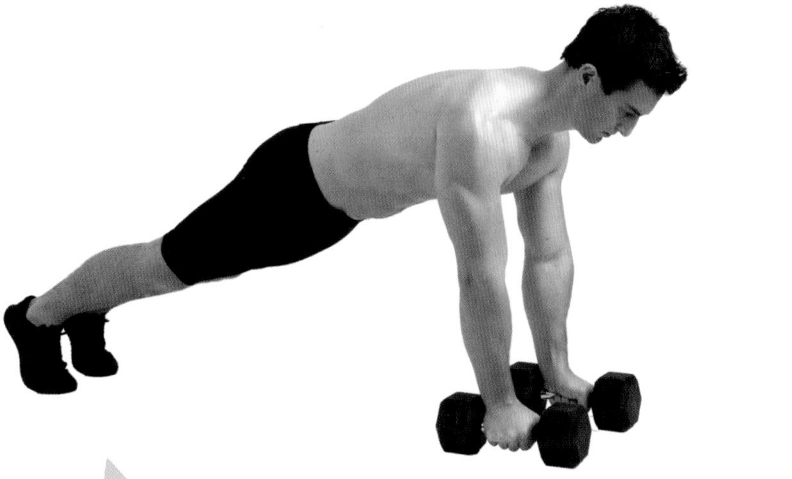

HOW TO DO IT

- Begin in a high plank position, taking a wide stance with your feet planted far apart and holding a dumbbell in each hand.
- Pull the right dumbbell to chest level.
- Lift your right arm straight up, rotating your torso to stack your shoulders, and turn your heels to the left so that your body and arms form a T.
- Slowly lower the weight back to the floor to return to the starting position. Repeat on the opposite side to complete one repetition. Continue alternating sides for the recommended repetitions.

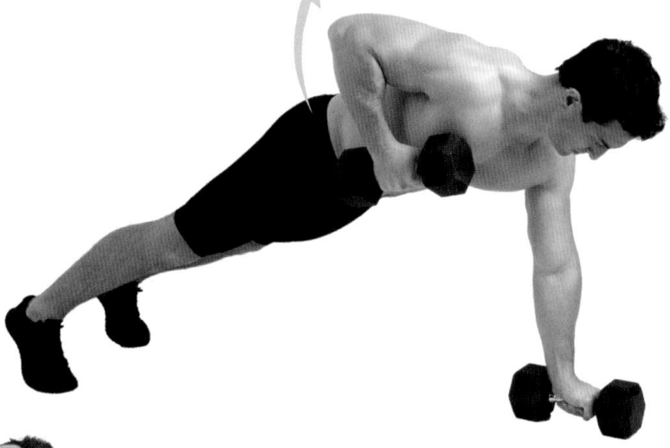

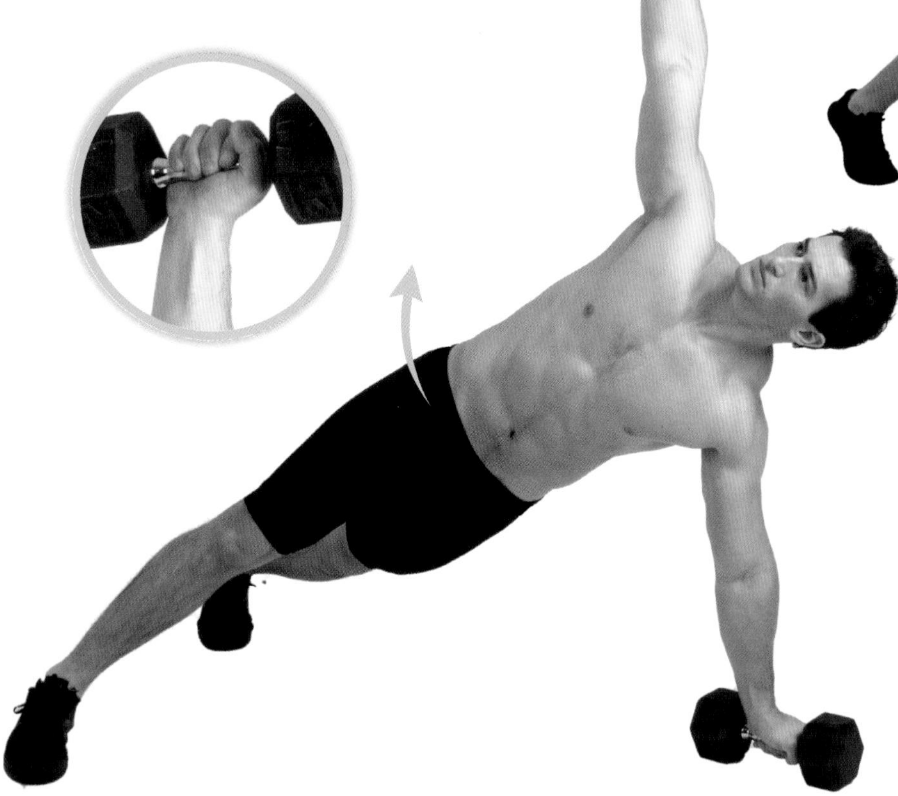

DO IT RIGHT

- Open your stance as wide as possible for stability.
- Move the weight slowly, so as not to knock you off balance.
- Avoid using a weight heavier than you can comfortably lift over your head.

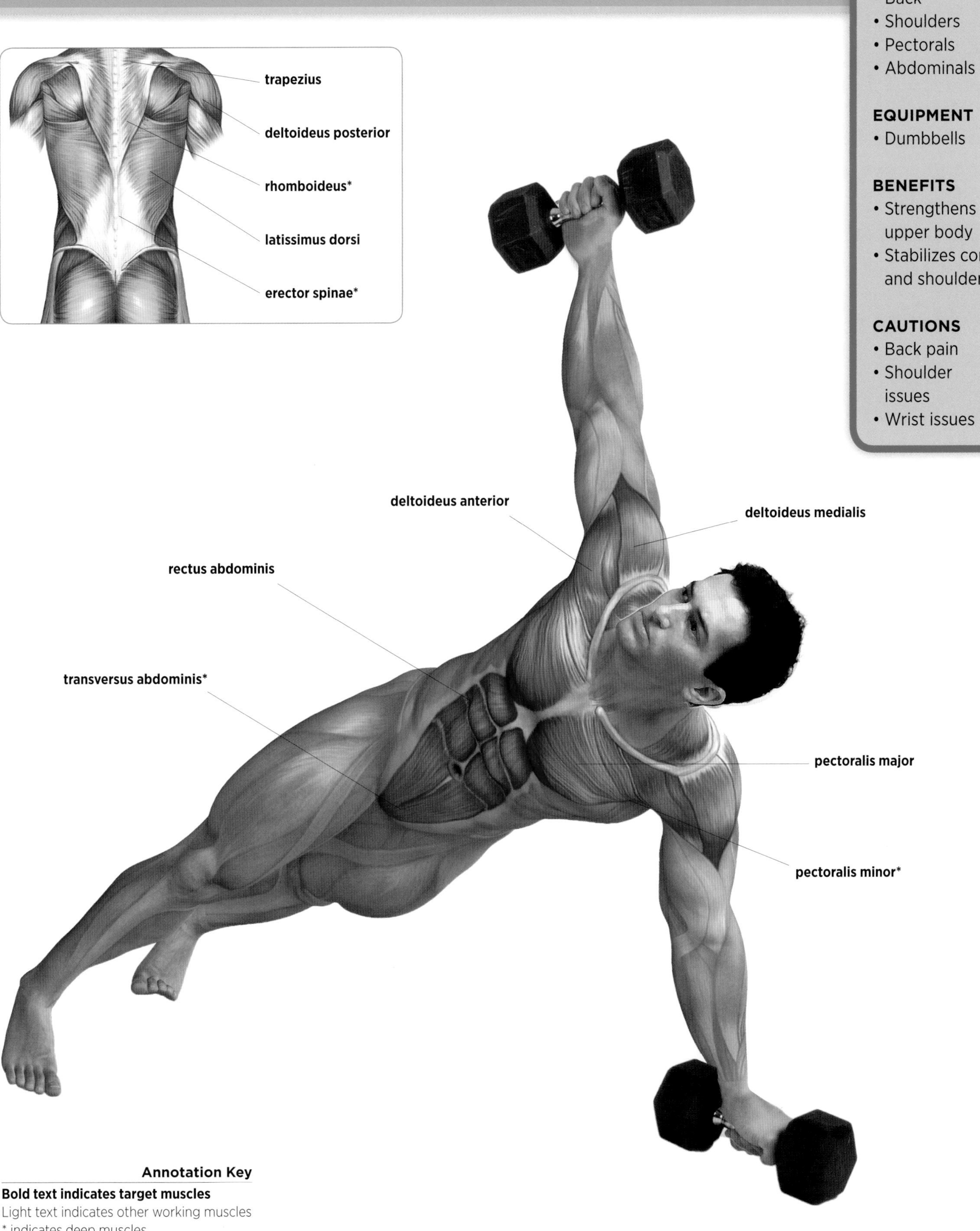

FACT FILE

TARGETS
- Back
- Shoulders
- Pectorals
- Abdominals

EQUIPMENT
- Dumbbells

BENEFITS
- Strengthens upper body
- Stabilizes core and shoulders

CAUTIONS
- Back pain
- Shoulder issues
- Wrist issues

Annotation Key

Bold text indicates target muscles

Light text indicates other working muscles

* indicates deep muscles

Dumbbell Row

A gym staple, the Dumbbell Row is an effective middle-back strengthener. It also targets your arms and shoulders.

HOW TO DO IT

- Holding a dumbbell in your left hand, stand next to an incline bench with your feet placed generously shoulder-width apart.
- Lean forward, and place your right hand on the bench. Your back should be flat and your knees slightly bent. Your left hand should be holding the dumbbell in a hammer-grip position, with your elbow close to your ribs.
- Draw your elbow toward the ceiling.
- Lower the dumbbell to the starting position. Repeat for the recommended repetitions, and then repeat all steps on the opposite side.

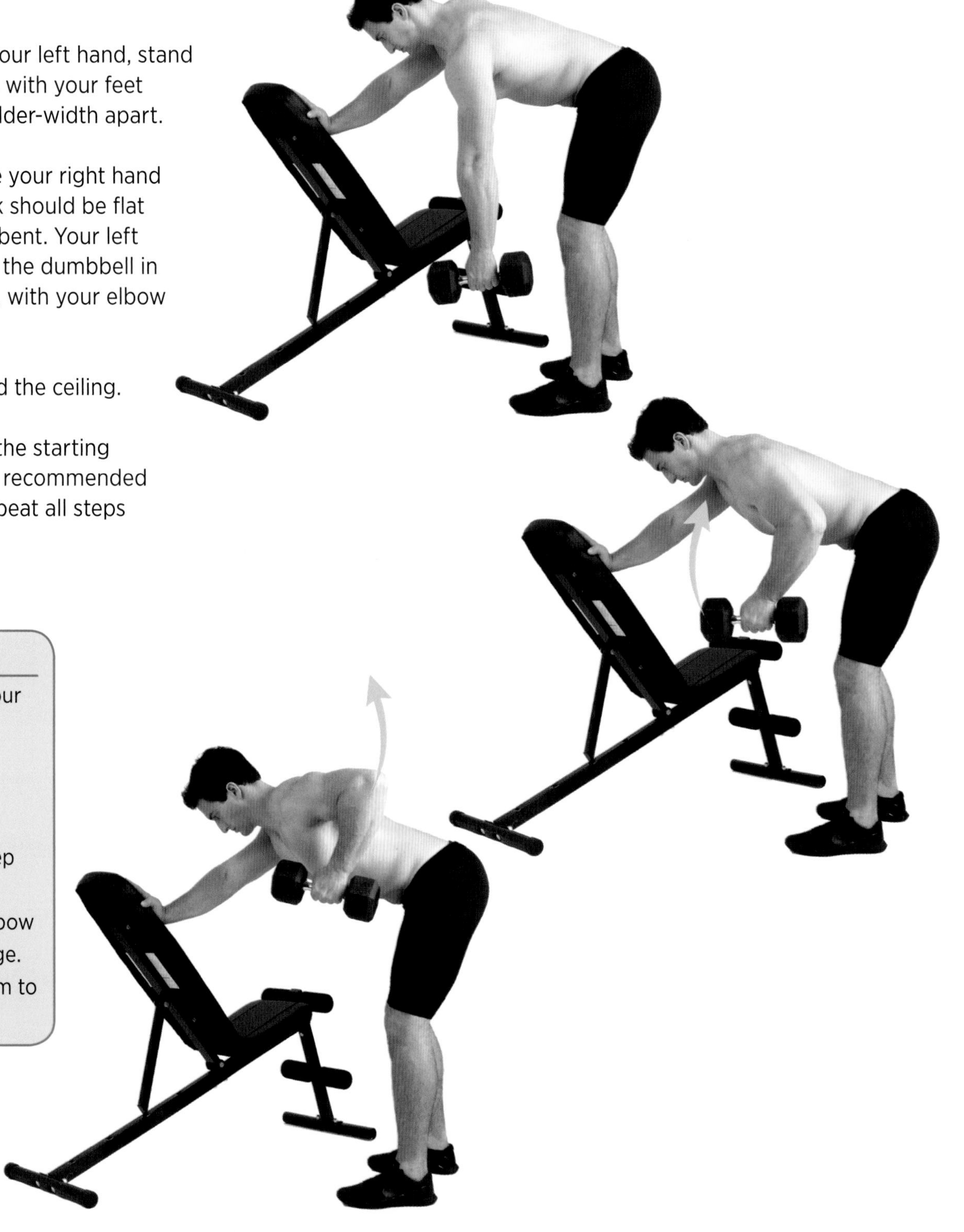

DO IT RIGHT

- Pull the weight with your back, not your biceps.
- Avoid rounding your upper back.
- Keep your chest up.
- Tuck your pelvis to keep your back flat.
- Avoid drawing your elbow away from your rib cage.
- Avoid using momentum to lift the dumbbell.

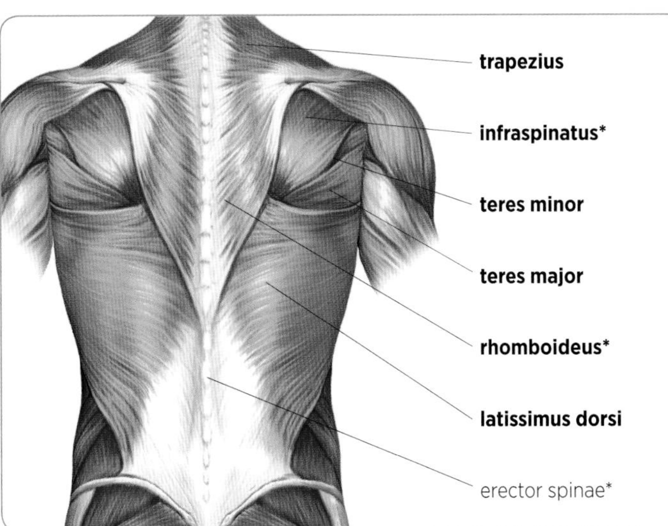

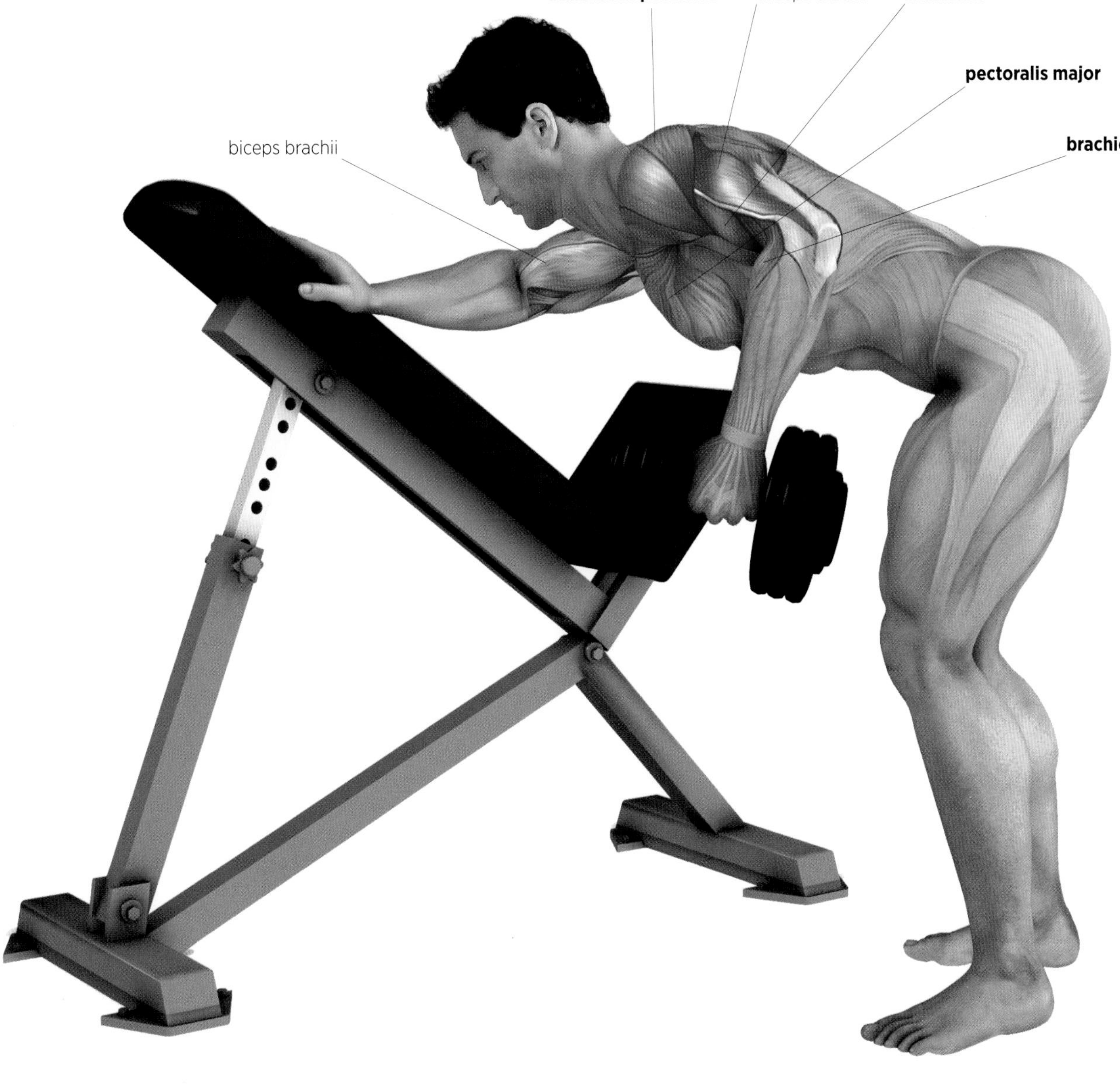

FACT FILE

TARGETS
- Back
- Biceps
- Shoulders

EQUIPMENT
- Dumbbell
- Incline bench

BENEFITS
- Strengthens middle back, biceps, and shoulders

CAUTIONS
- Shoulder issues
- Wrist issues
- Lower-back pain

trapezius
infraspinatus*
teres minor
teres major
rhomboideus*
latissimus dorsi
erector spinae*

Annotation Key

Bold text indicates target muscles

Light text indicates other working muscles

* indicates deep muscles

deltoideus posterior
triceps brachii
brachialis
pectoralis major
biceps brachii
brachioradialis

Alternating Kettlebell Row

Build a strong upper back and core with the Alternating Kettlebell Row. Although the movement is simple, to maintain a steady, even rhythm, choose weights that you can carefully control.

HOW TO DO IT

- Stand with your feet shoulder-width apart and your knees bent. Hold a pair of kettlebells in front of you with an overhand grip. Bend forward slightly at the waist, maintaining a flat back.
- Bend your elbow to pull your left hand up toward your abdomen, and then lower it again.
- Pull your right hand up, and then lower it. Continue alternating sides for the recommended repetitions.

DO IT RIGHT

- Maintain a flat back.
- Keep your knees bent.
- Avoid rotating your torso.

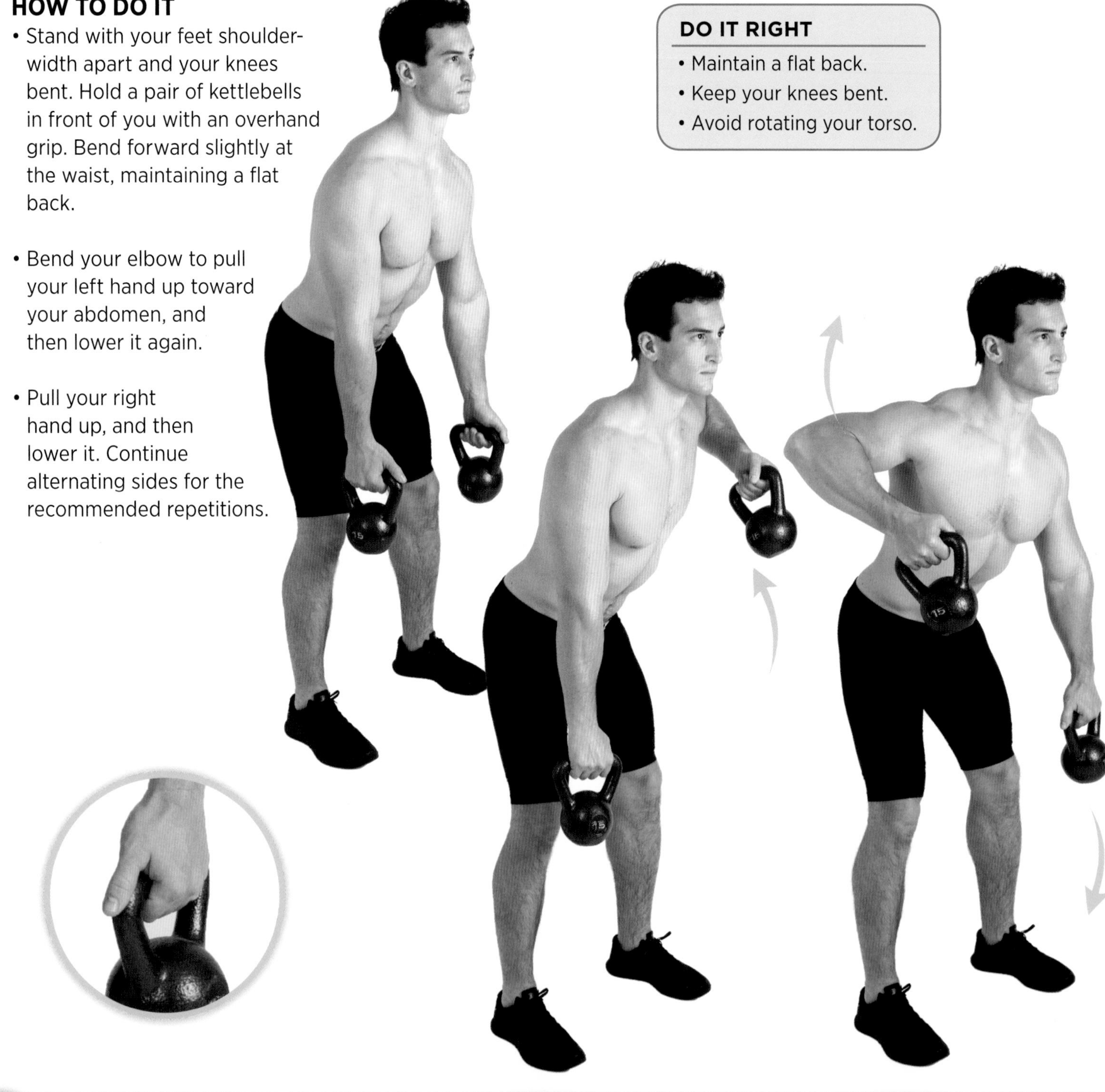

FACT FILE

TARGETS
- Back
- Biceps

EQUIPMENT
- Kettlebells

BENEFITS
- Strengthens back and arms
- Stabilizes lower body

CAUTIONS
- Shoulder issues
- Wrist issues
- Lower-back issues

MODIFICATION
EASIER: Lift with both arms at the same time.

Annotation Key

Bold text indicates target muscles

Light text indicates other working muscles

* indicates deep muscles

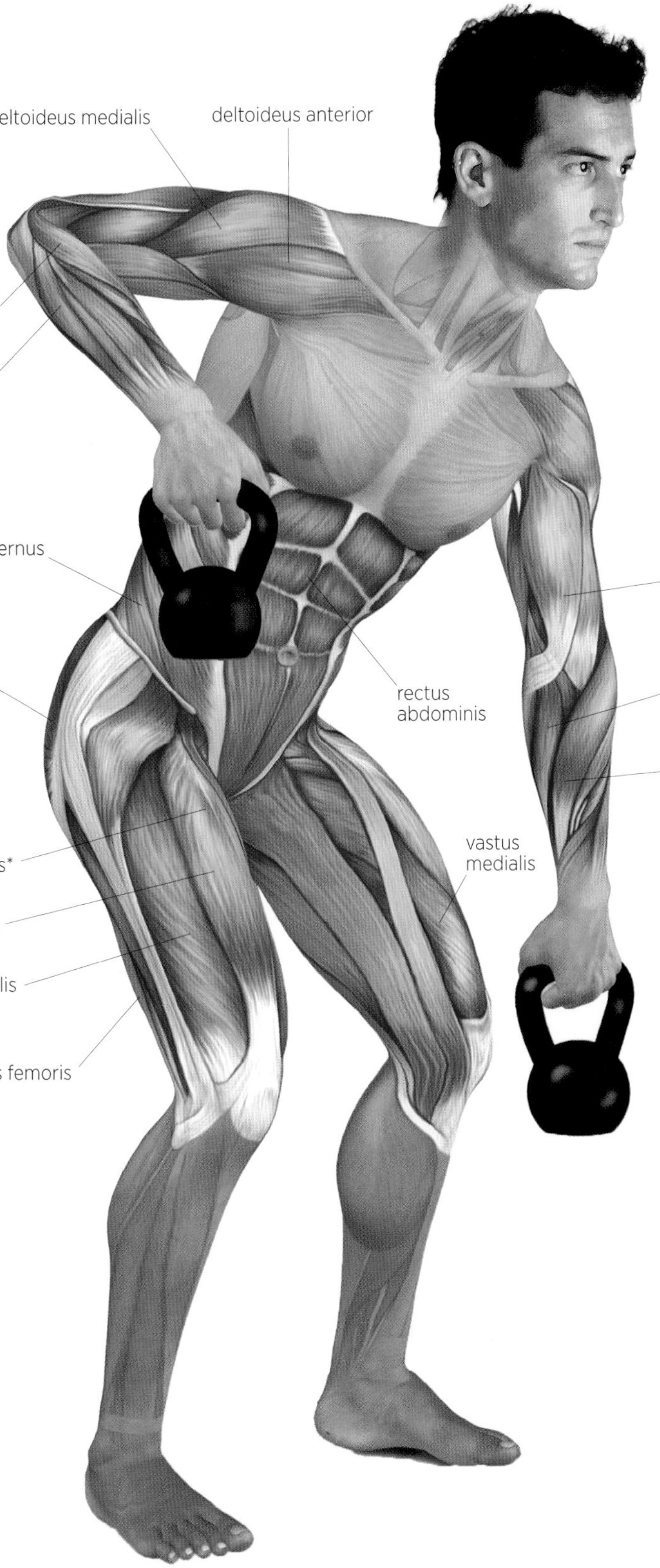

deltoideus medialis
deltoideus anterior
anconeus
extensor digitorum
obliquus externus
biceps brachii
gluteus maximus
palmaris longus
rectus abdominis
flexor digitorum*
vastus intermedius*
vastus medialis
rectus femoris
vastus lateralis
biceps femoris

trapezius
rhomboideus*
triceps brachii
latissimus dorsi
erector spinae*
multifidus spinae*

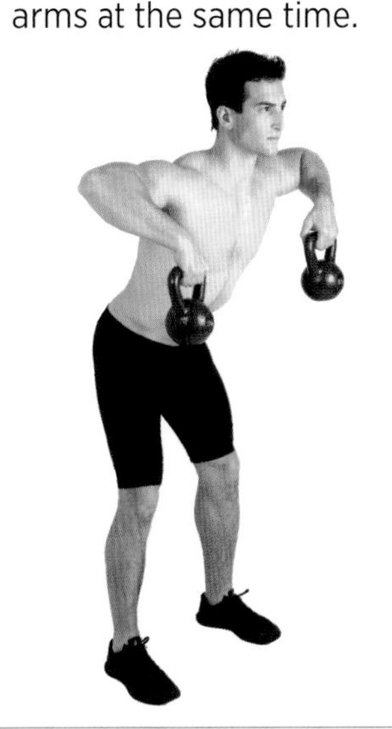

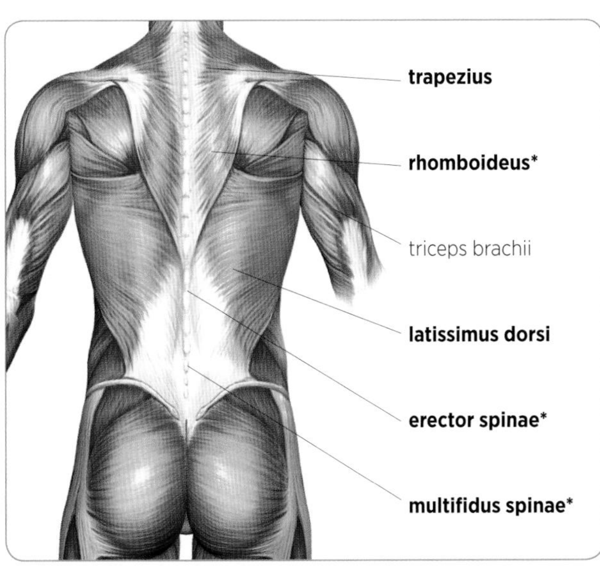

Alternating Renegade Row

The Alternating Renegade Row is a hardworking exercise that combines the benefits of an explosive upper-body move with a powerful core strengthener.

HOW TO DO IT

- With a kettlebell in each hand, assume a high plank position, balancing your feet on your toes.
- While staying on your toes and keeping your core stable and parallel to the floor, pull the kettlebell in your right hand up toward your chest while straightening your left arm and pushing that kettlebell into the floor.
- Lower your right arm, and then repeat the movement with the left. Continue alternating sides for the recommended repetitions.

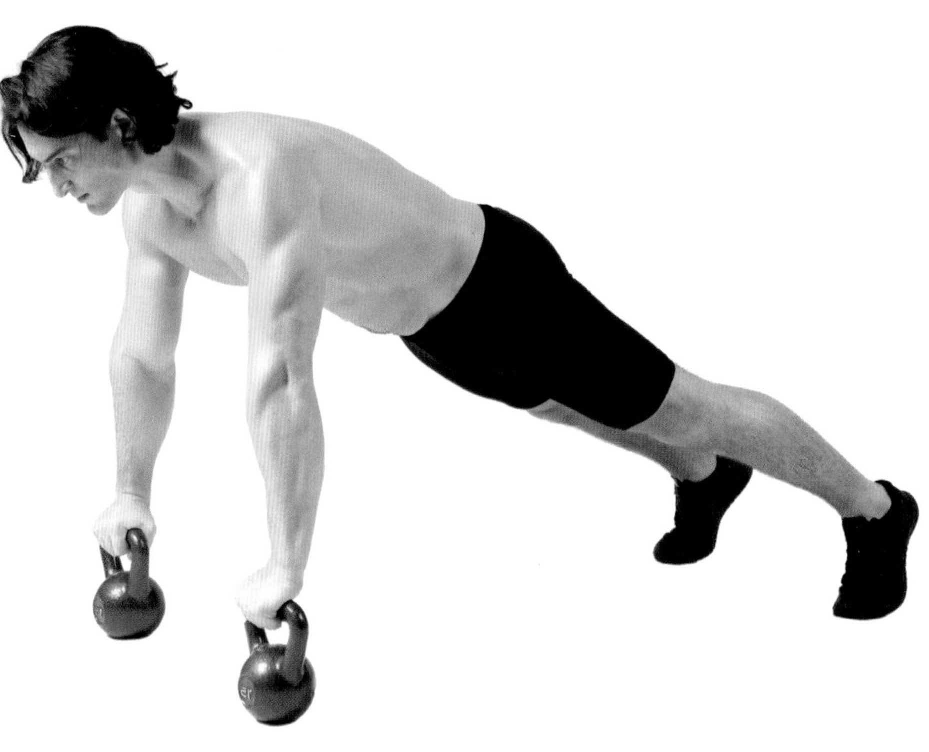

DO IT RIGHT

- Make sure the kettlebells have a flat surface on the bottom for stability.
- Keep your wrists strong to ensure the kettlebell doesn't flip.
- Keep your hips level and square to the floor.
- Keep your core stable and straight on.
- Avoid allowing your hips to sag.
- Avoid dropping or slamming the weight into the floor.

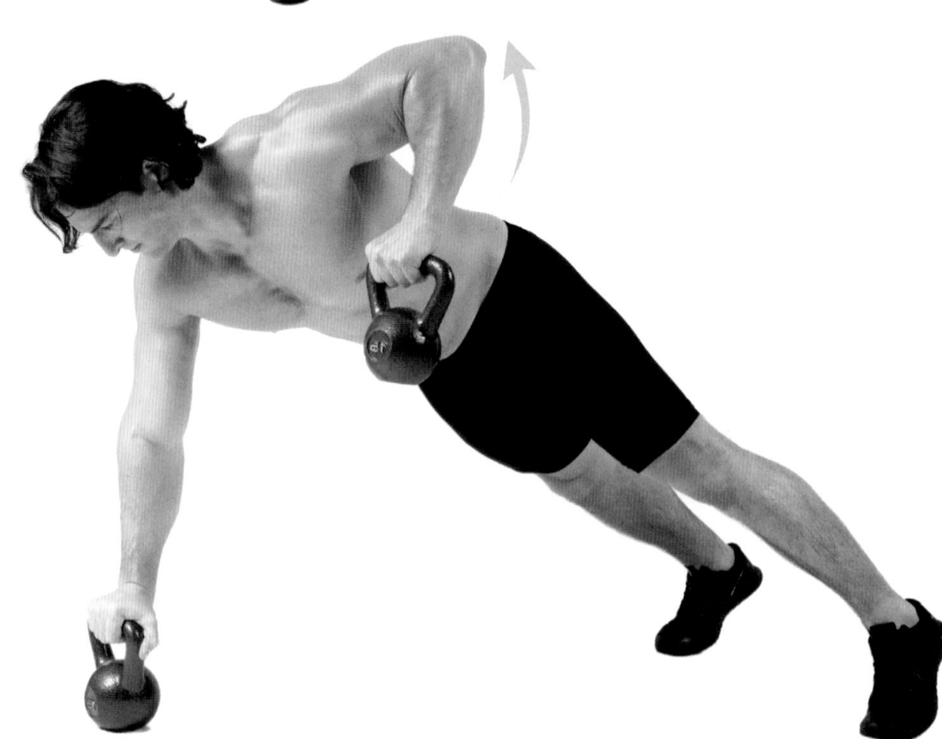

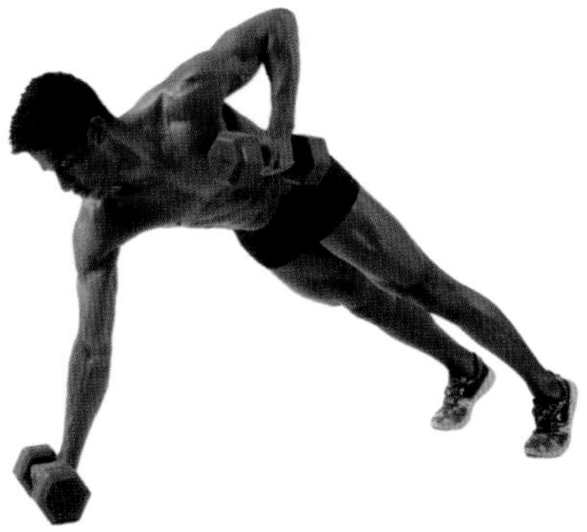

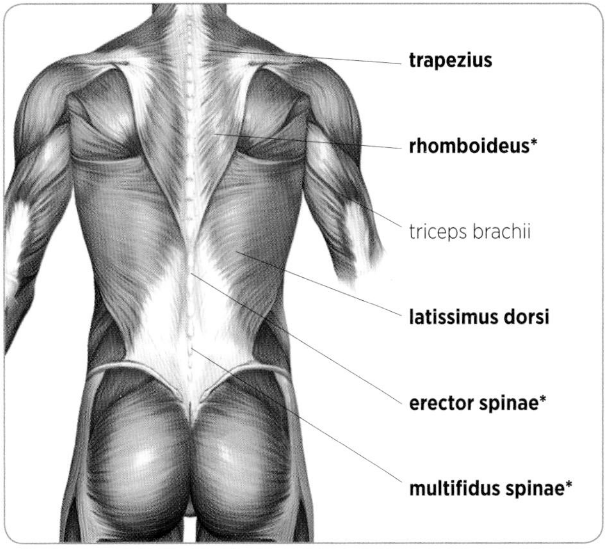

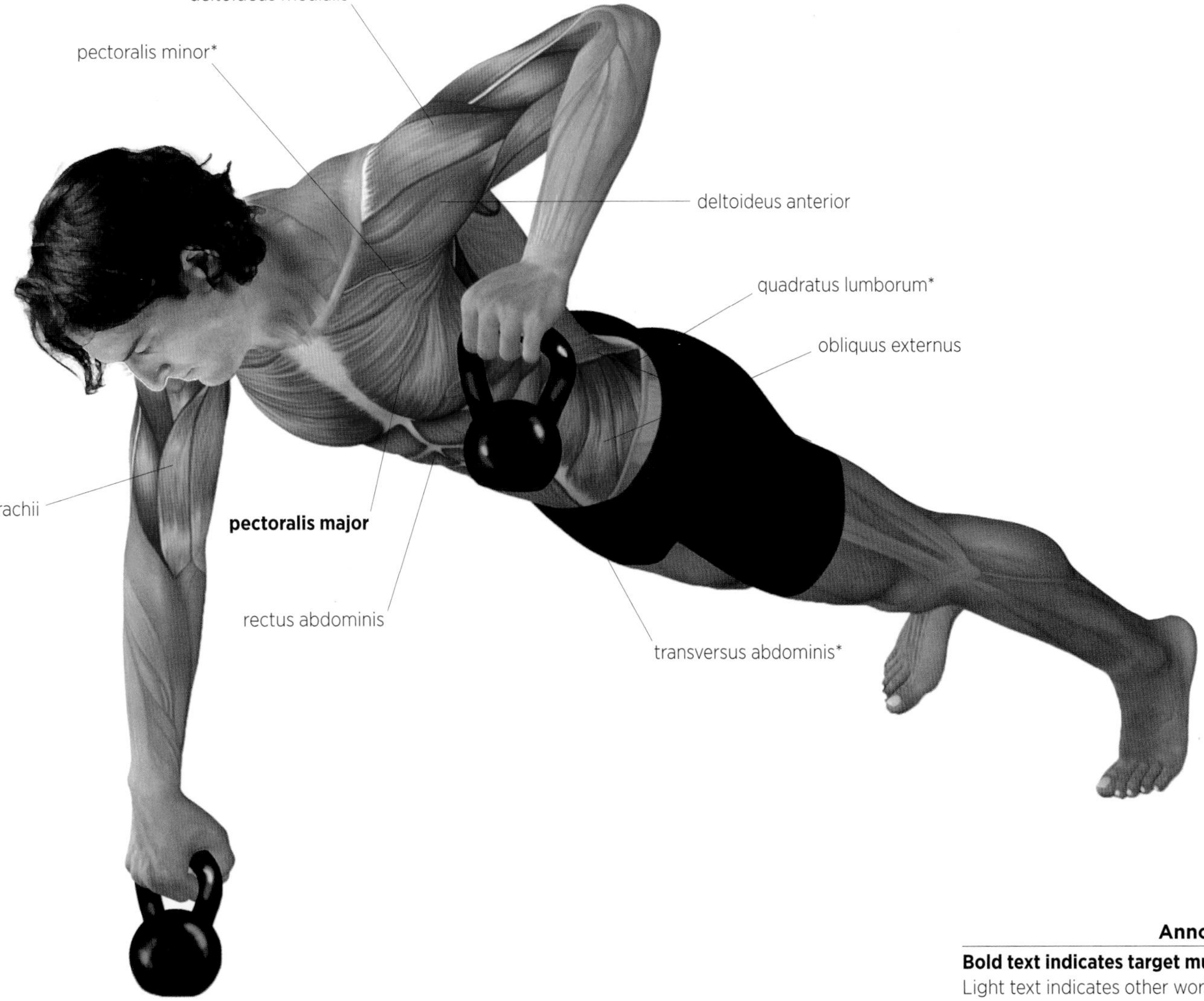

FACT FILE

TARGETS
- Middle back
- Abdominals
- Biceps
- Chest

EQUIPMENT
- Kettlebells

BENEFITS
- Strengthens back, arms, chest, and abdominals

CAUTIONS
- Shoulder issues
- Wrist issues
- Lower-back pain

MODIFICATION

EASIER: Use hexagonal dumbbells in place of the kettlebells.

trapezius
rhomboideus*
triceps brachii
latissimus dorsi
erector spinae*
multifidus spinae*

deltoideus medialis
pectoralis minor*
deltoideus anterior
quadratus lumborum*
obliquus externus
biceps brachii
pectoralis major
rectus abdominis
transversus abdominis*

Annotation Key

Bold text indicates target muscles

Light text indicates other working muscles

* indicates deep muscles

Rear Lateral Raise

The Rear Lateral Raise targets your upper back and shoulders, building the strength and size of your deltoid muscles. Focusing on these muscles improves general back and shoulder health, and promotes good posture.

HOW TO DO IT

- Lie facedown on a Swiss ball holding a pair of dumbbells at your sides, your palms facing inward, and your legs spaced slightly apart for stability.
- Raise your arms directly out to the sides in a reverse hugging motion, bending your arms slightly.
- Lower your arms back to the starting position, and then repeat for the recommended repetitions.

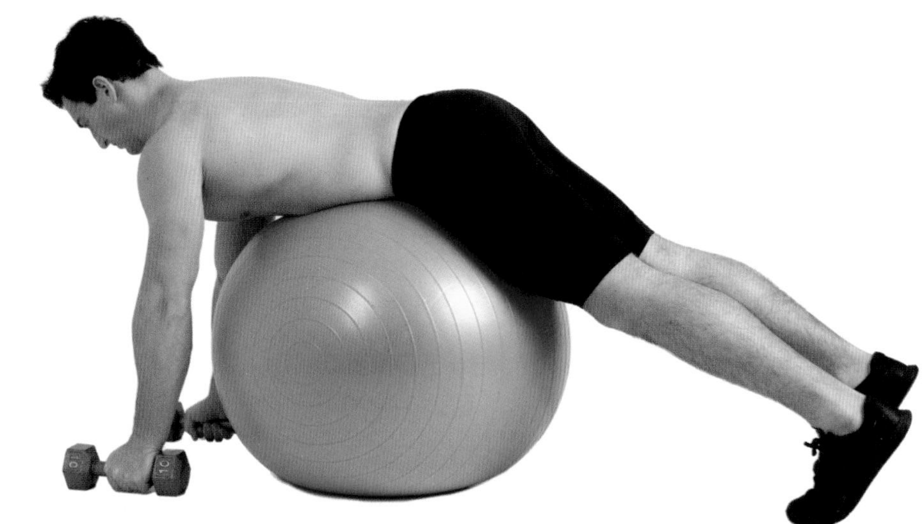

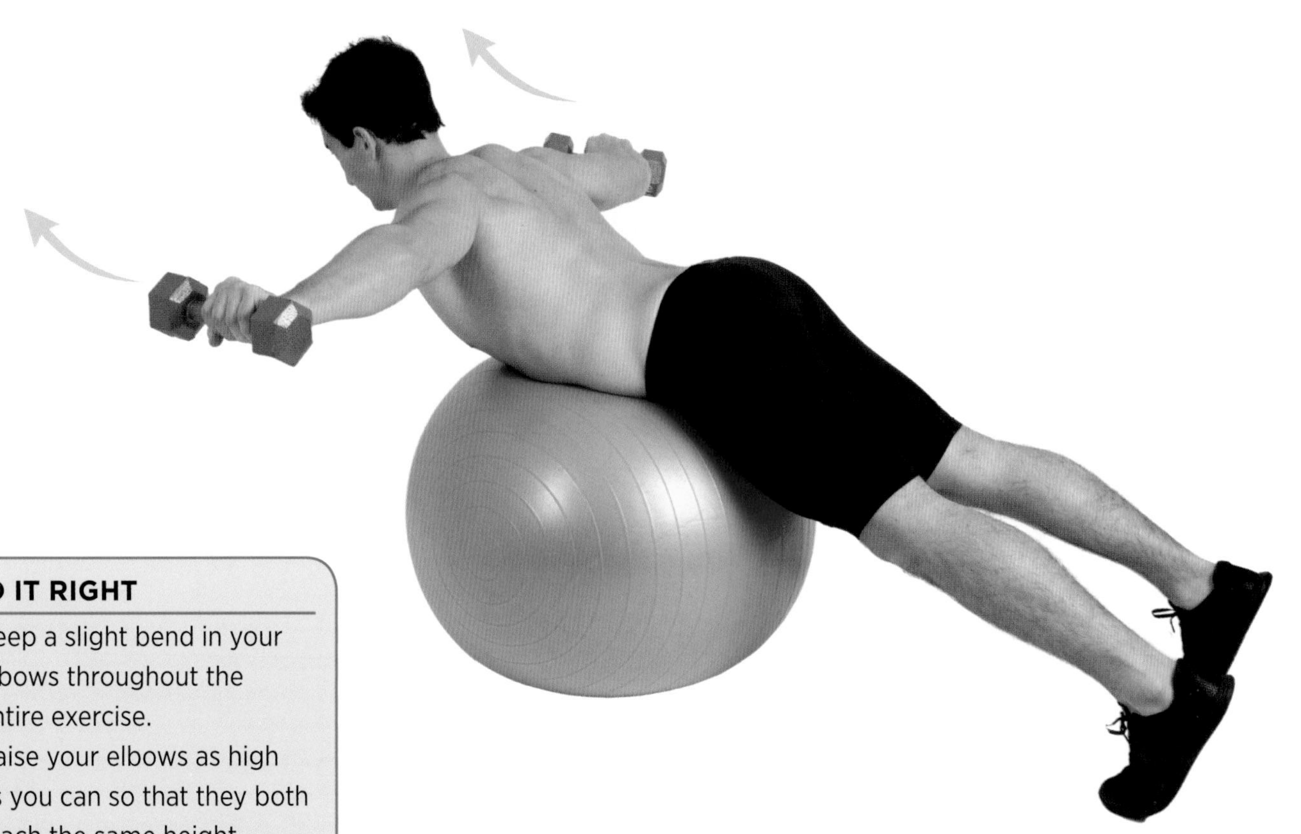

DO IT RIGHT

- Keep a slight bend in your elbows throughout the entire exercise.
- Raise your elbows as high as you can so that they both reach the same height.

scalenus*
pectoralis major
obliquus externus
obliquus internus*
extensor carpi radialis
flexor carpi radialis

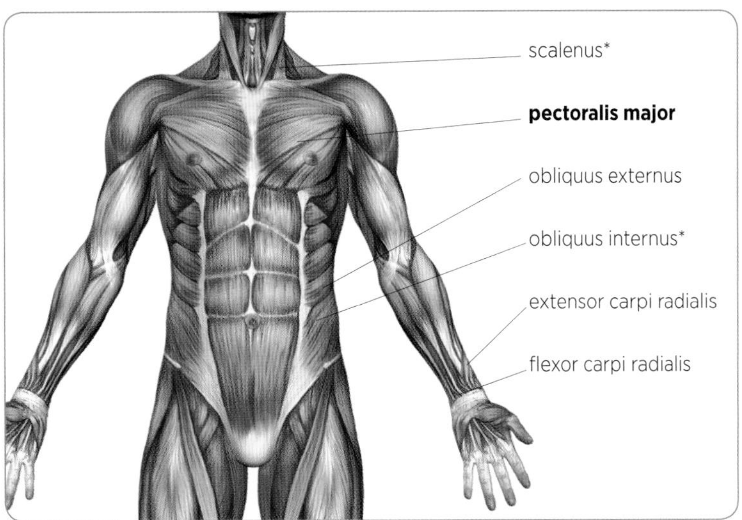

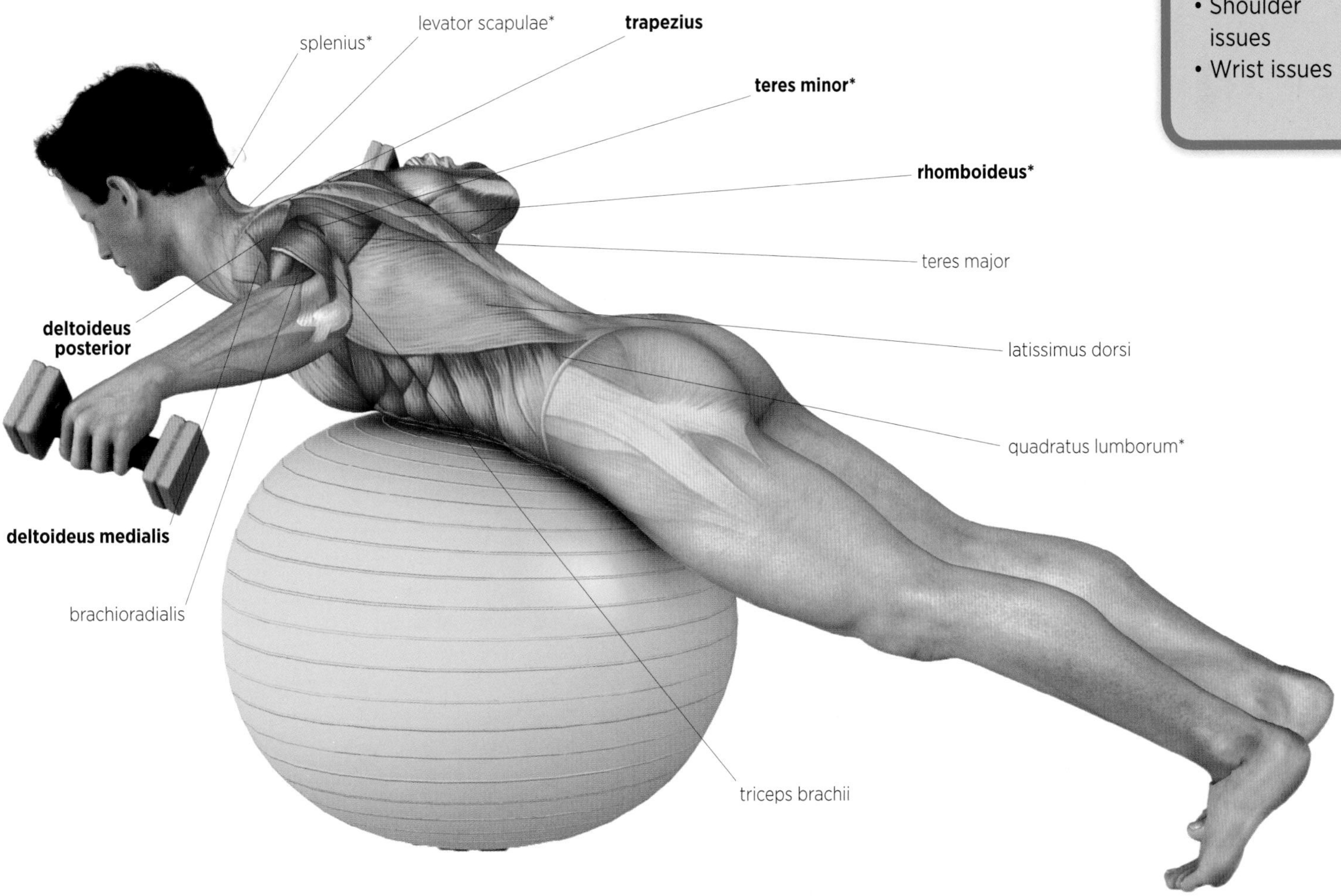

splenius*
levator scapulae*
trapezius
teres minor*
rhomboideus*
teres major
latissimus dorsi
quadratus lumborum*
deltoideus posterior
deltoideus medialis
brachioradialis
triceps brachii

FACT FILE

TARGETS
- Shoulders
- Upper back
- Chest

EQUIPMENT
- Dumbbells
- Swiss ball

BENEFITS
- Strengthens shoulders and upper back
- Improves posture
- Stretches and tones chest

CAUTIONS
- Neck issues
- Lower-back pain
- Shoulder issues
- Wrist issues

Annotation Key

Bold text indicates target muscles
Light text indicates other working muscles
* indicates deep muscles

Dumbbell Pullover

This exercise should be done with extreme caution. Have a spotter assist you with this exercise if you are new to it.

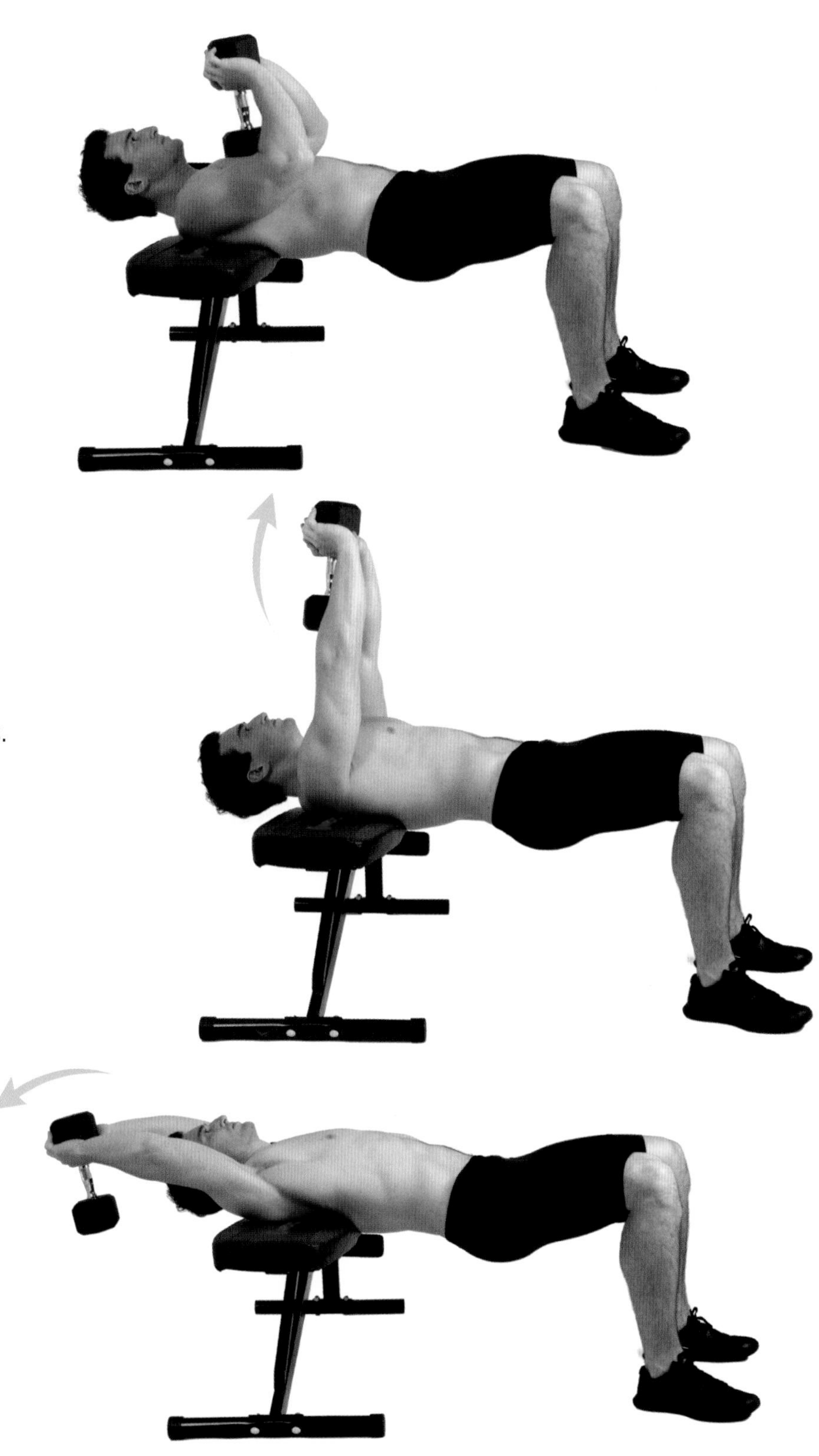

HOW TO DO IT

- Place a dumbbell on a flat bench, and lower your upper body onto the bench.
- Pick up the dumbbell, placing the palms of your hands underneath the top part of the weight. Lift the dumbbell onto your chest, and slightly lower your body on the bench so that your head, neck, and upper back are on and supported by the bench.
- Raise the dumbbell above your chest to assume the starting position.
- With your elbows slightly bent, lower the dumbbell over and behind you. Do not lower the dumbbell lower than your head.
- Carefully return to the starting position, and then repeat for the recommended repetitions.

DO IT RIGHT

- Keep your back, glutes, and hamstrings in a straight line while executing the full range of movement.
- Avoid locking your elbows.
- Avoid lowering the weight too far behind your head; dropping too low can cause strain on the neck, back, and arms.
- Make sure the dumbbell is always secure.

FACT FILE

TARGETS
- Back
- Chest

EQUIPMENT
- Dumbbell
- Flat bench

BENEFITS
- Strengthens back and chest

CAUTIONS
- Shoulder issues
- Wrist issues
- Lower-back issues

Annotation Key

Bold text indicates target muscles

Light text indicates other working muscles

* indicates deep muscles

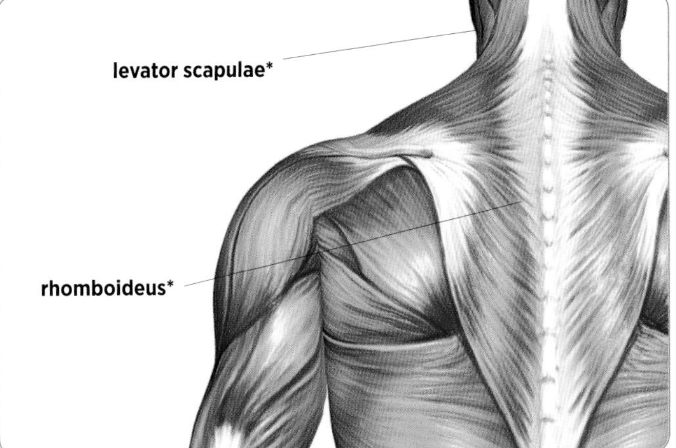

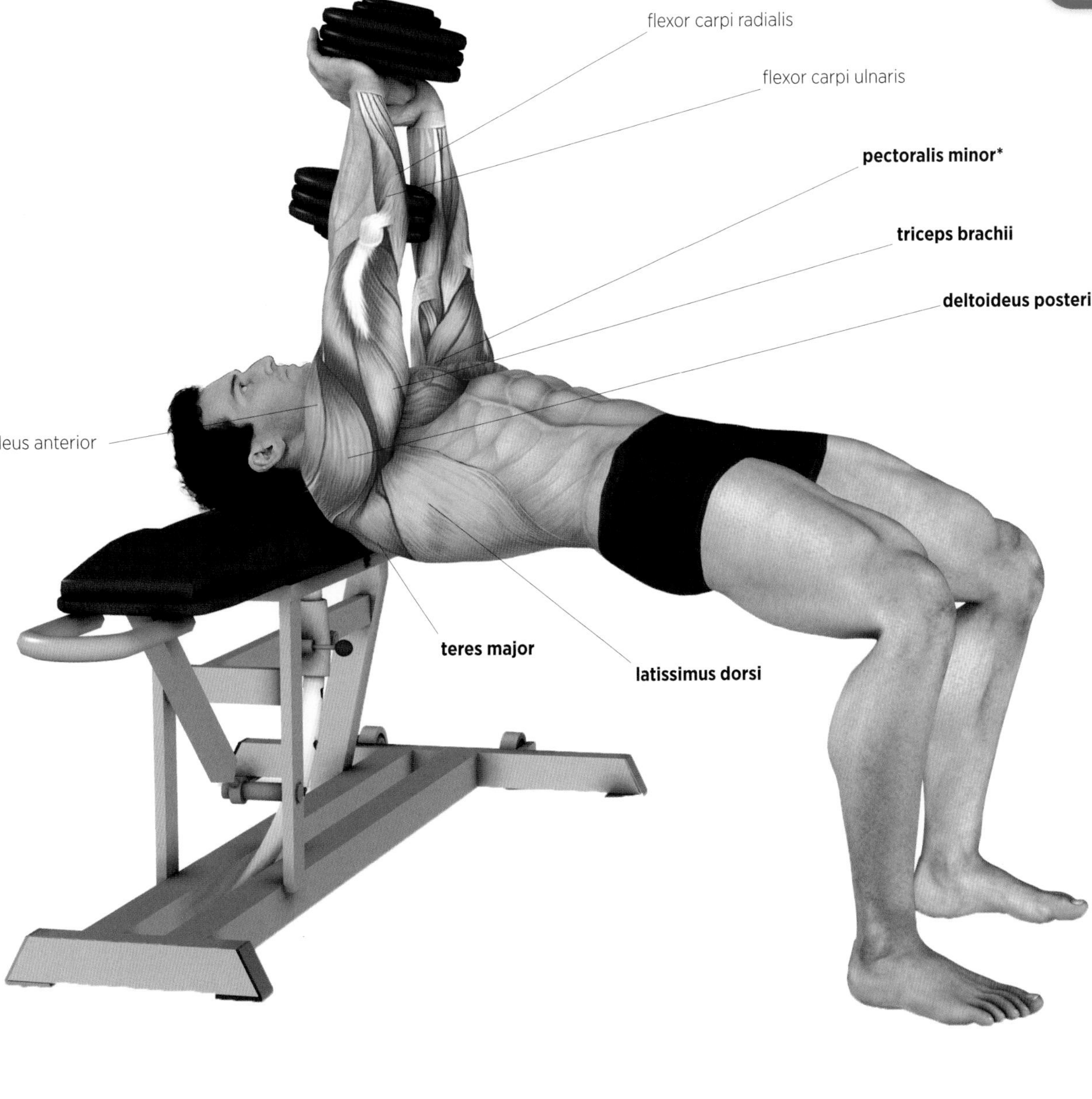

Alternating Hammer Curl

The Alternating Hammer Curl targets your biceps. It takes its name from the position of your hands. For this exercise, you hold the dumbbells with your palms facing inward, similar to how you would hold a hammer to drive a nail into a wall.

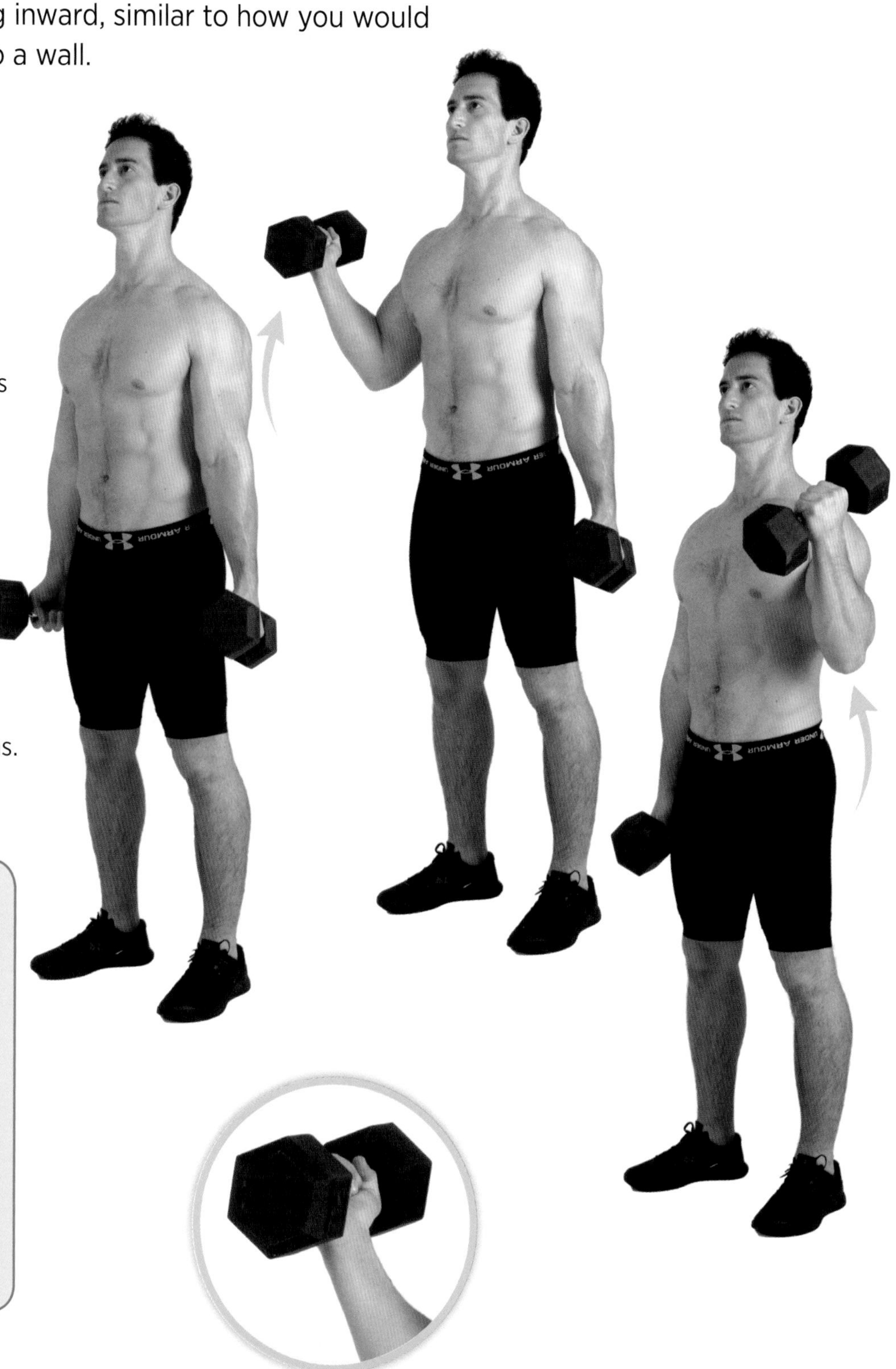

HOW TO DO IT

- Stand with your feet parallel and shoulder-width apart, your knees slightly bent an your pelvis slightly tucked in.
- Grasp a dumbbell in each hand using hammer-grip position with your palms facing your thighs. Keep your elbows close to your torso.
- Keeping your upper arms stationary, curl the right dumbbell toward your upper chest.
- Slowly lower the weight back to the starting position, and then repeat on the other side. Continue alternating sides for the recommended repetitions.

DO IT RIGHT

- Fully contract your biceps at the top range of the movement.
- Avoid using momentum to lift the weight—keep your torso upright and concentrate on isolating and engaging your biceps.
- Avoid bending at the wrists; keep them aligned with your forearms.
- Exhale as you lift the dumbbell up, and inhale as you lower it back to the starting position.

FACT FILE

TARGETS
- Biceps

EQUIPMENT
- Dumbbells

BENEFITS
- Strengthens biceps, shoulders, and upper back

CAUTIONS
- Shoulder issues
- Wrist issues

Annotation Key

Bold text indicates target muscles
Light text indicates other working muscles
* indicates deep muscles

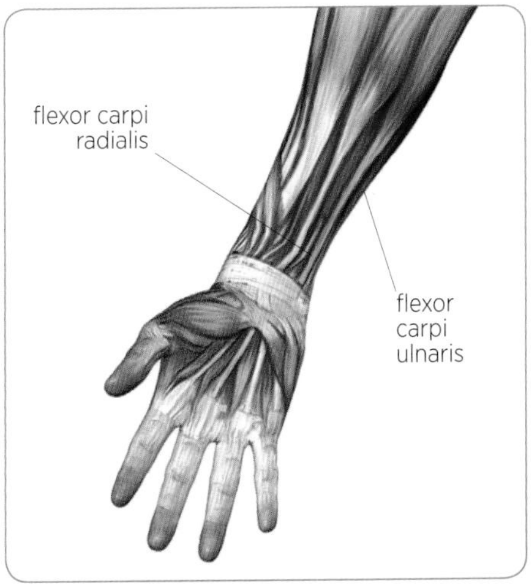

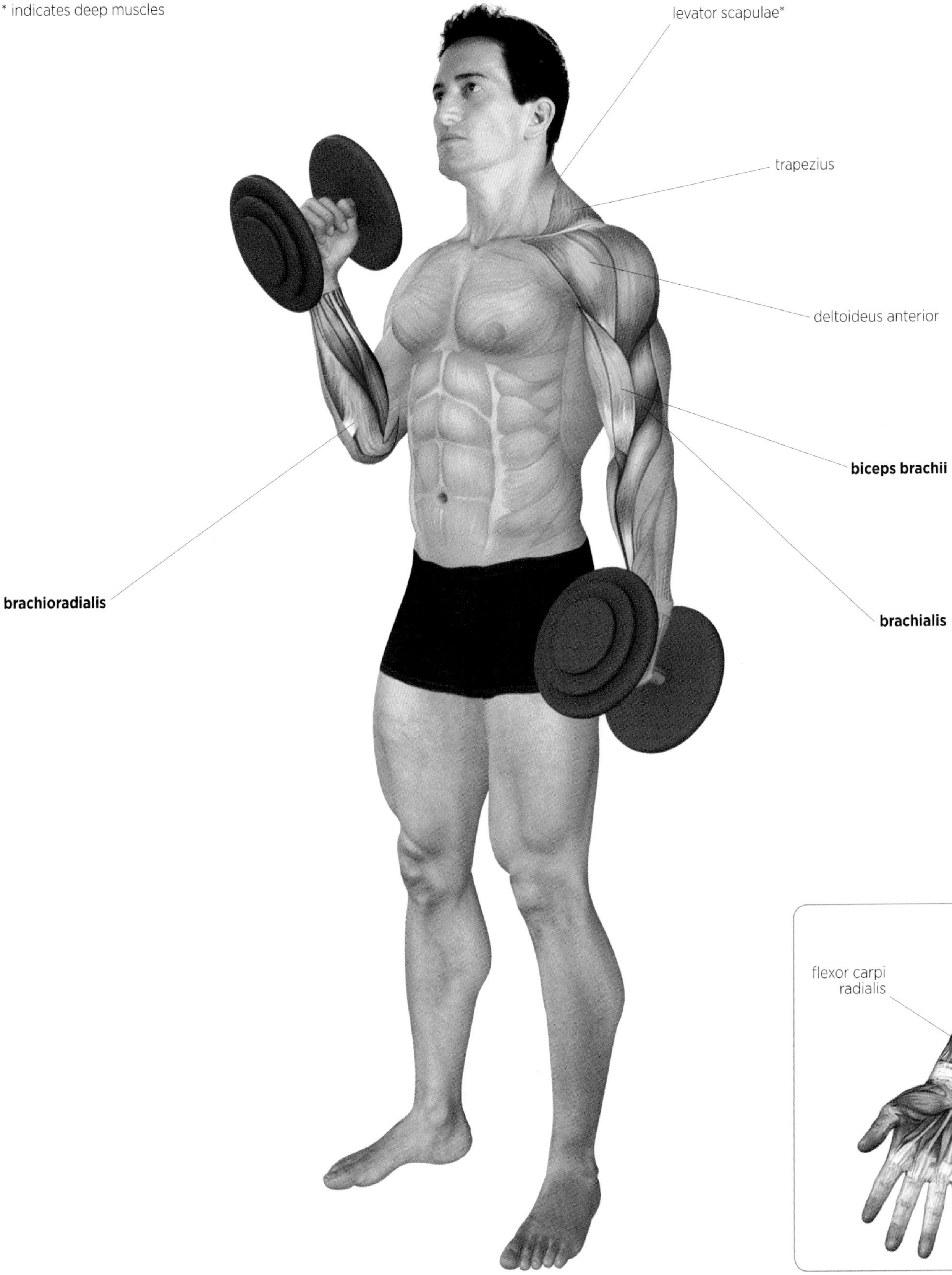

Alternating Dumbbell Biceps Curl

The Alternating Dumbbell Biceps Curl is a standard exercise that should be in every exerciser's toolbox. This movement will condition and sculpt your arms, while demanding core stability. It uses a supinated grip, meaning you hold the dumbbell with your palms facing forward.

FACT FILE

TARGETS
- Biceps

EQUIPMENT
- Dumbbells

BENEFITS
- Strengthens and tones arms and core
- Increases cardiovascular endurance

CAUTIONS
- Wrist issues

HOW TO DO IT

- Stand with your feet hip-width apart holding a dumbbell in each hand, palms facing forward.
- Flex your elbow to bring the right dumbbell up toward your shoulder so that your palm faces upward.
- Lower the dumbbell back down to your side to return to the starting position, and then repeat on the opposite side. Continue alternating sides for the recommended repetitions.

DO IT RIGHT
- Keep your back straight and shoulders retracted.
- Keep your palms facing up.
- Avoid excessive trunk movement.

Annotation Key
Bold text indicates target muscles
Light text indicates other working muscles
* indicates deep muscles

biceps brachii

Arnold Press

Named after the one and only Arnold Schwarzenegger, you know the Arnold Press will blast your shoulders. It strengthens and conditions all three of your main shoulder muscles, making it an essential part of your HIIT routine.

FACT FILE

TARGETS
- Deltoids

EQUIPMENT
- Dumbbells

BENEFITS
- Strengthens shoulders
- Warms up muscles
- Improves coordination
- Increases cardiovascular endurance

CAUTIONS
- Wrist issues
- Shoulder pain

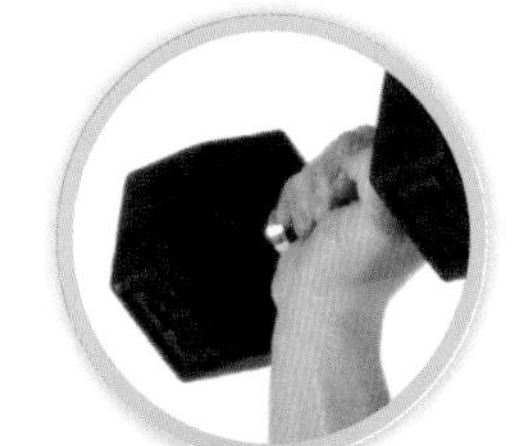

HOW TO DO IT

- Stand with your feet hip-width apart holding a dumbbell in each hand positioned at the level of your shoulders, palms facing inward.
- Spread your arms to each side laterally so that your shoulders are abducted to 90 degrees, and then press your arms up and twist your hands so that your palms face forward.

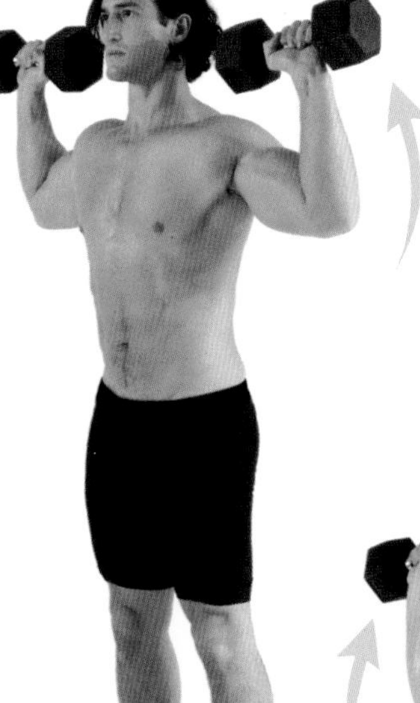

- Extend your arms straight upward to press the dumbbells overhead.
- Bring your arms back down to 90 degrees.
- To return the starting position, draw your elbows in front of your body, lowering the dumbbells to shoulder level with your palms facing inward. Repeat for the recommended repetitions.

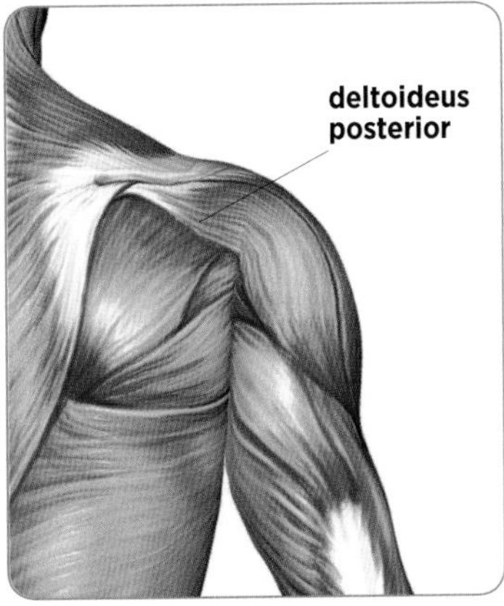

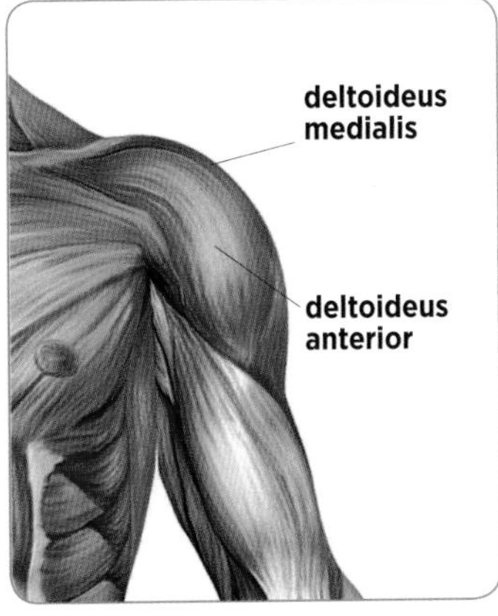

DO IT RIGHT
- Keep your back straight.
- Avoid excessive trunk movement.

Annotation Key
Bold text indicates target muscles
Light text indicates other working muscles
* indicates deep muscles

Curling Step and Raise

Combining a classic biceps exercise with a lower-body move, the Curling Step and Raise is an exercise for multitaskers. Also known as the Dumbbell Step-Up Single-Leg Balance, it works your muscles while honing your balance and coordination.

DO IT RIGHT

- Keep your upper arms stationary.
- Keep your torso facing forward.
- Pull your abdominal muscles inward.
- Press your shoulders away from your ears.
- Avoid twisting your neck.
- Avoid arching your back or hunching forward.
- Avoid rushing through the movement; keep your movements smooth and controlled.

HOW TO DO IT

- Stand with your feet hip-width apart, your arms at your sides, and a dumbbell in each hand. Position a step beside your left foot.
- Place your left foot on the step.
- Shift your weight onto your left foot. Bend your elbows, curling the dumbbells toward your chest. At the same time, raise your right knee as the foot comes off the floor. Continue raising and curling until your right leg forms a 90-degree angle and the dumbbells are nearly at shoulder height.
- Lowering the dumbbells, cross your right leg over your left leg, which should bend slightly as you lower your right leg to the floor, left of the platform. Simultaneously, bend your left leg slightly.
- Step your left leg onto the floor so that you are in starting position on the other side of the step. Repeat on the opposite side. Continue alternating sides for the recommended repetitions.

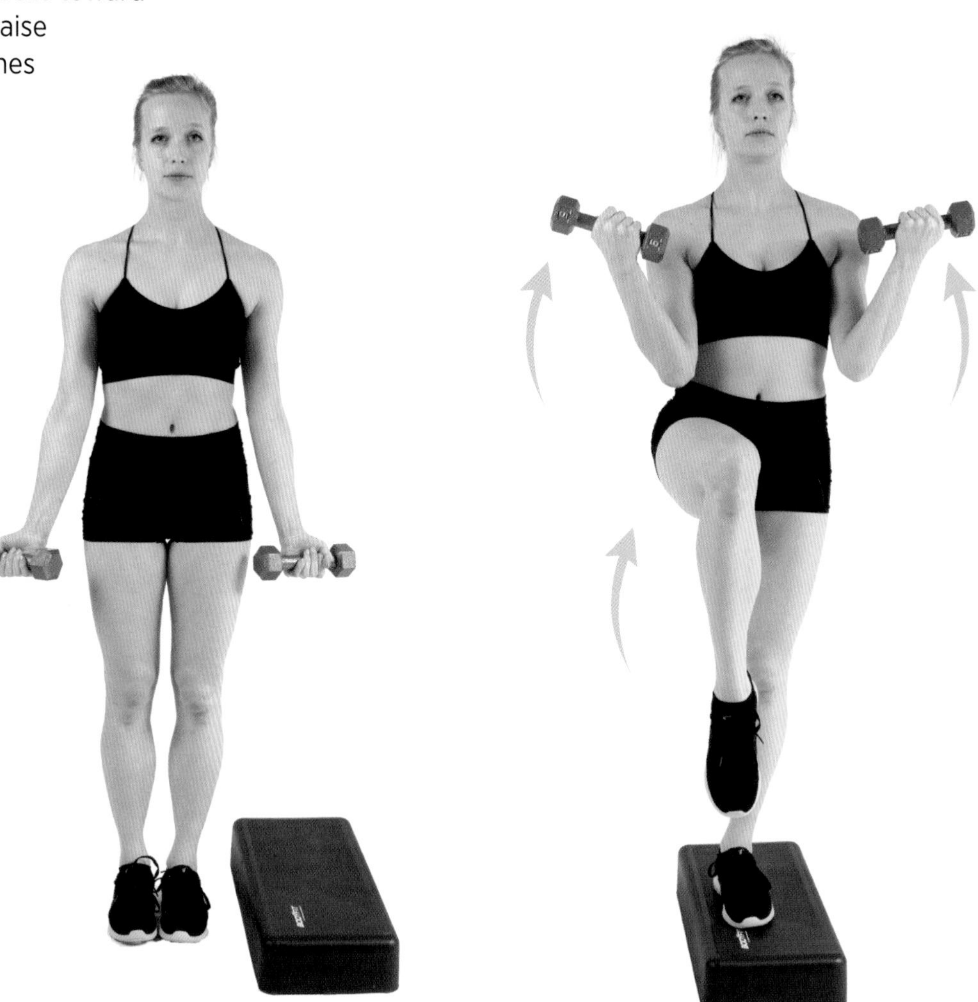

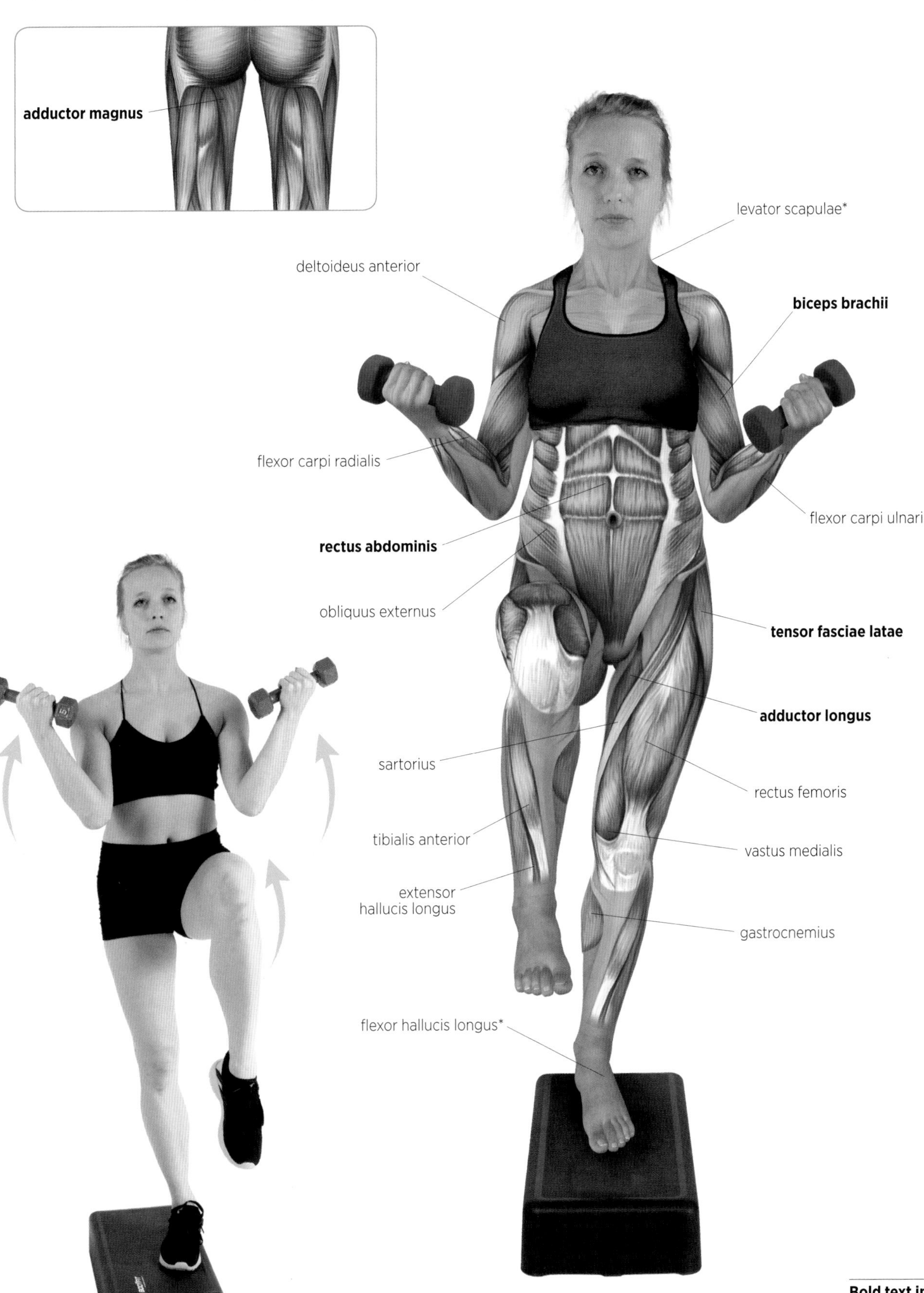

FACT FILE

TARGETS
- Biceps
- Abdominals
- Hip adductors

EQUIPMENT
- Dumbbells
- Plyo box, aerobics step, or other low platform

BENEFITS
- Strengthens and tones abdominals, hips, and biceps
- Improves balance and coordination

CAUTIONS
- Shoulder issues
- Wrist issues
- Knee issues

Annotation Key

Bold text indicates target muscles

Light text indicates other working muscles

* indicates deep muscles

Shoulder Raise and Pull

The Shoulder Raise and Pull offers the benefits of two effective arm exercises. The raise portion works your deltoids, especially the anterior delts. The pulling portion works the muscles of your upper back.

HOW TO DO IT

- Holding a dumbbell in each hand, stand with your legs and feet parallel and shoulder-width apart. Bend your knees very slightly, and tuck your pelvis slightly forward as you lift your chest and press your shoulders downward and back.
- Lift the dumbbells straight up to shoulder height.
- Pull the dumbbells to the front of your shoulders with your elbows leading out to sides.
- Lower back to the starting position, and then repeat for the recommended repetitions.

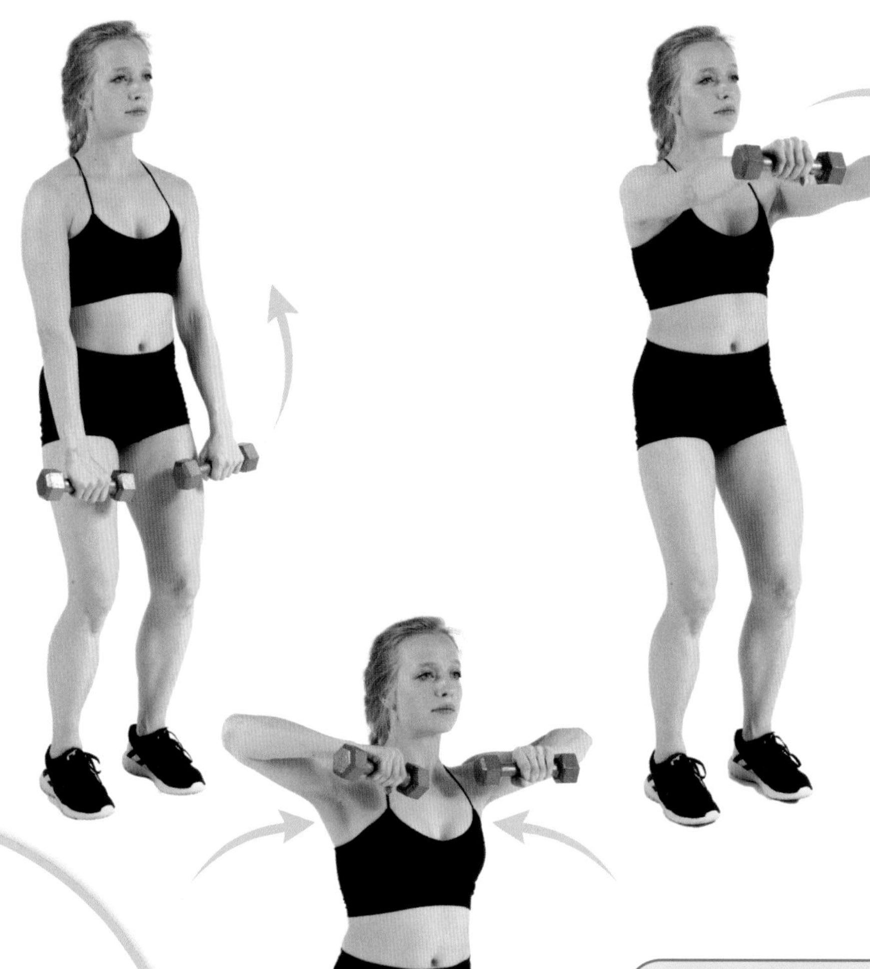

DO IT RIGHT

- Keep a slight bend in your elbow as you lift upward to avoid stress on the joints.
- Avoid raising your elbows or the weights higher than your shoulders.

FACT FILE

TARGETS
- Shoulders
- Chest

EQUIPMENT
- Dumbbells

BENEFITS
- Strengthens shoulders and chest

CAUTIONS
- Shoulder issues
- Rotator cuff injury
- Wrist issues

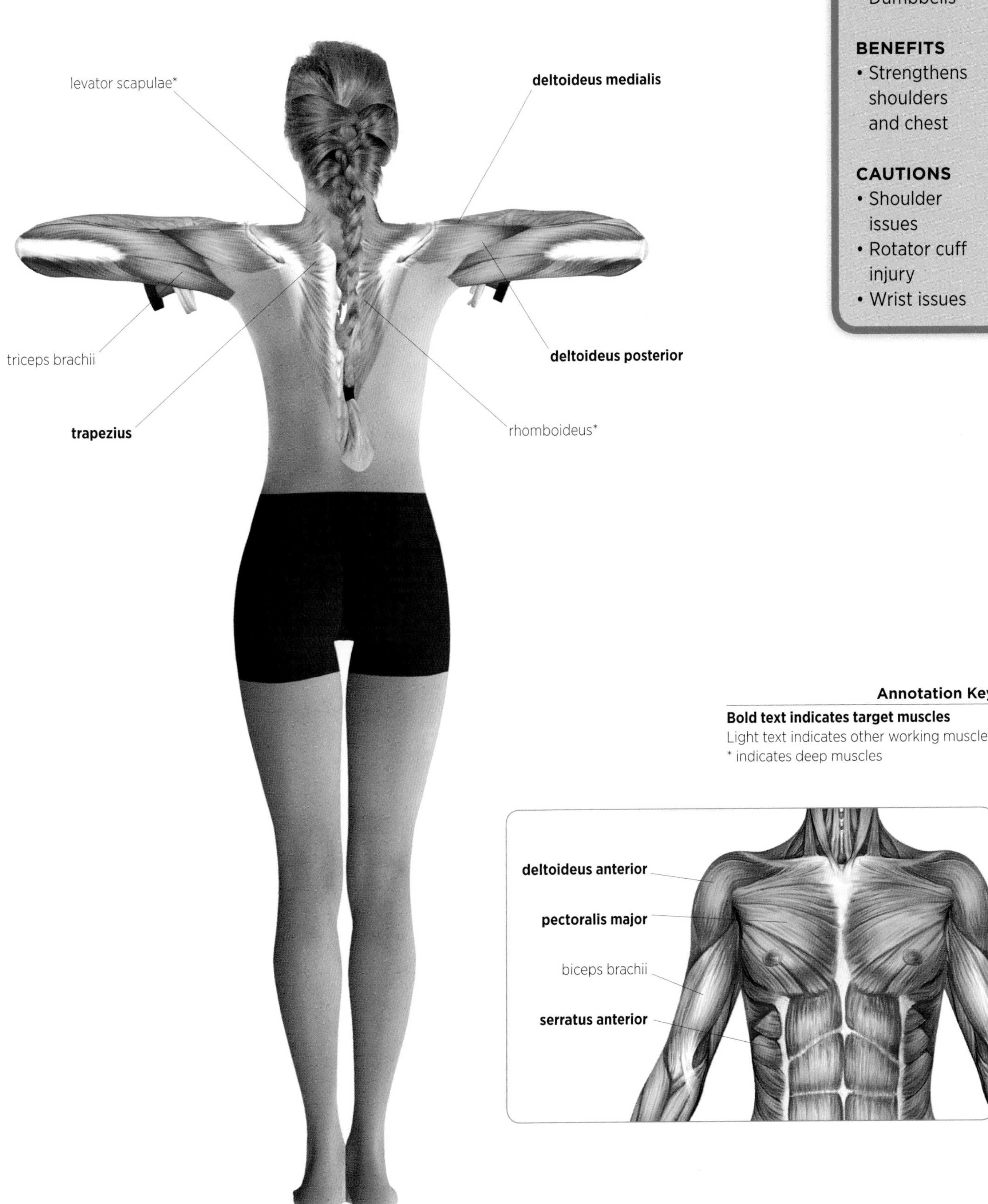

Annotation Key

Bold text indicates target muscles
Light text indicates other working muscles
* indicates deep muscles

Alternating Kettlebell Press

The Alternating Kettlebell Press targets your deltoids and your triceps. It is a simple, but effective, way to build shoulder strength.

HOW TO DO IT

- Stand with your feet shoulder-width apart and a pair of dumbbells at your feet. Bend forward to grasp the handles, and raise the kettlebells to your shoulders in one smooth motion to prepare for the overhead lift.

- Raise the right kettlebell directly overhead until your arm locks out. Keep the other kettlebell as still as possible.

- Lower your right arm to the starting position, and then repeat on the opposite side. Continue alternating sides for the recommended repetitions.

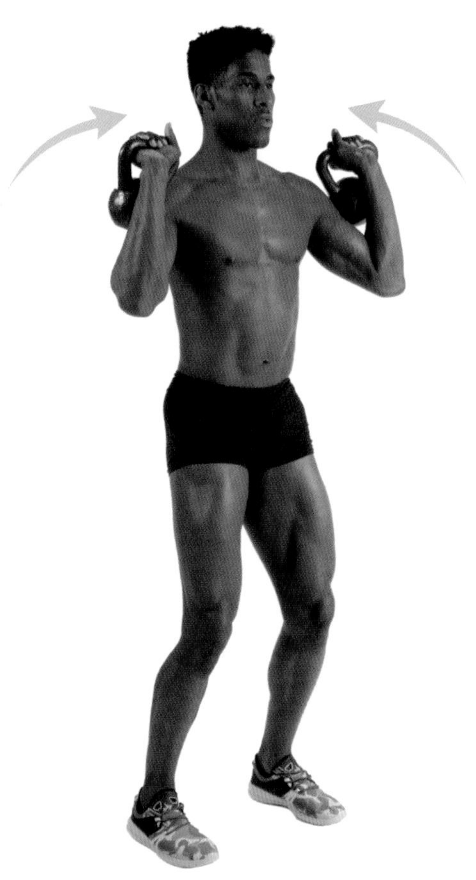

DO IT RIGHT

- Keep your core engaged.
- Avoid twisting your torso.
- Avoid leaning back when executing the movement.

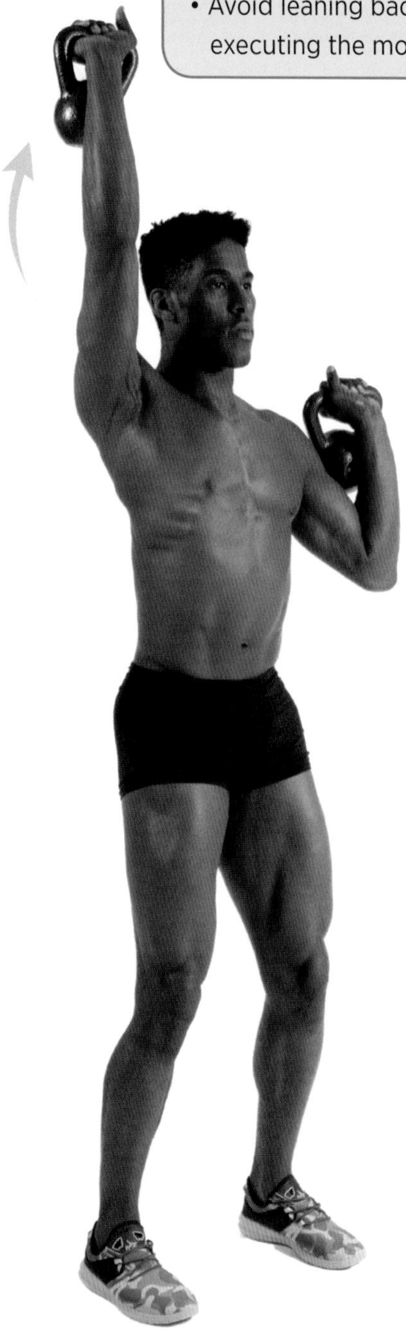

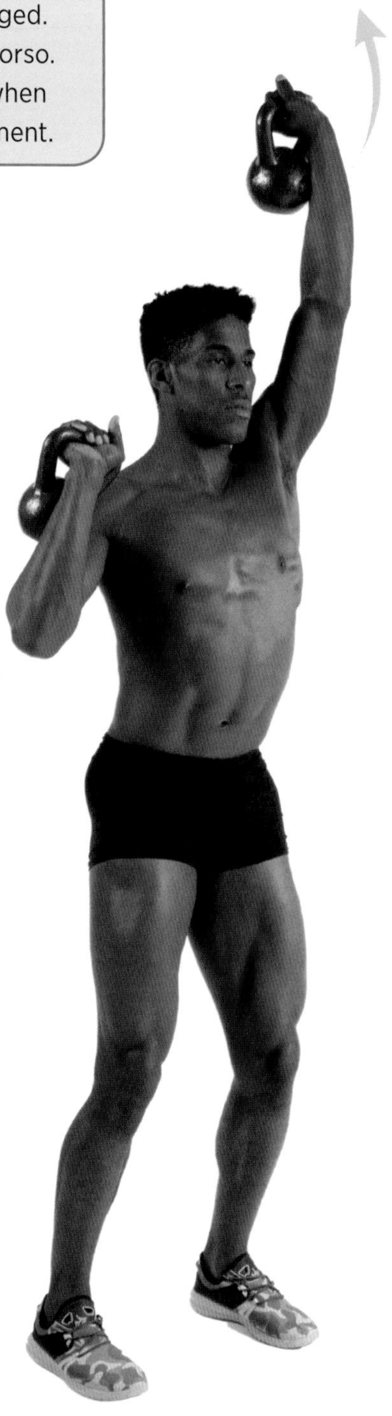

FACT FILE

TARGETS
- Deltoids
- Triceps

EQUIPMENT
- Kettlebells

BENEFITS
- Strengthens shoulders and upper arms

CAUTIONS
- Hip issues
- Knee issues

MODIFICATION

EASIER: Press upward with both arms at the same time.

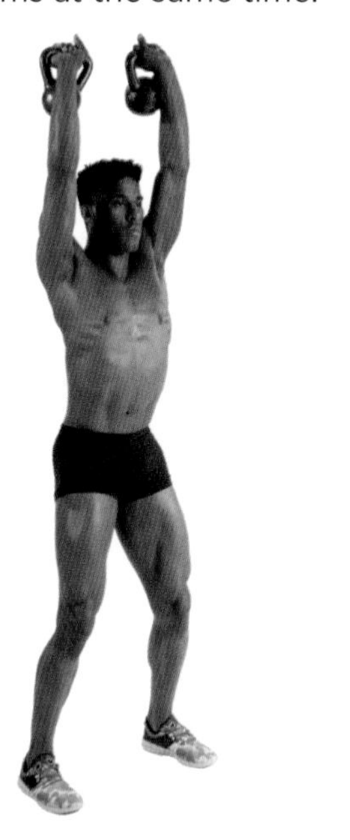

flexor carpi radialis

pronator teres

deltoideus anterior

pectoralis minor*

pectoralis major

obliquus externus

obliquus internus*

deltoideus medialis

deltoideus posterior

triceps brachii

quadratus lumborum*

Annotation Key

Bold text indicates target muscles

Light text indicates other working muscles

* indicates deep muscles

4-Count Overhead

The 4-Count Overhead draws its inspiration from military endurance and stamina exercises. Performed to a steady four-count beat, it simulates this kind of training while it works the muscles of your shoulders.

HOW TO DO IT

- Stand with your feet hip-width apart. With both hands, grasp a dumbbell of any weight you can press overhead, and bring it to your right shoulder.
- Press the weight overhead with your arms straight for count 1.
- Lower the weight to your left shoulder for count 2.
- Press the weight overhead with your arms straight for 3.
- Lower the weight to your right shoulder for count 4. Each time the weight touches your right shoulder equals one rep. Repeat for the recommended repetitions.

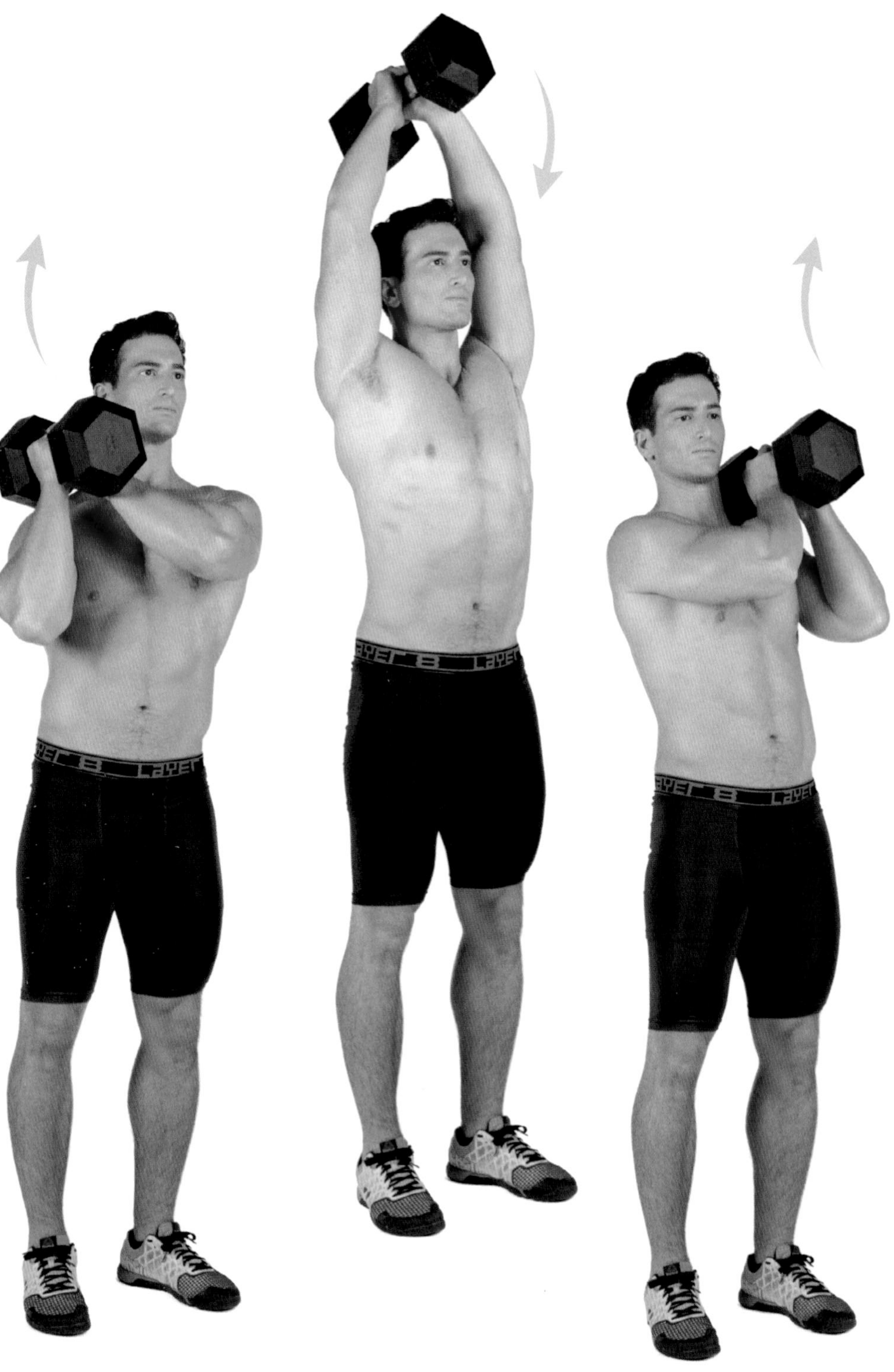

DO IT RIGHT

- Maintain a steady beat, moving quickly but with control.
- Move the weight around your head—not your head around the weight.
- Avoid arching your lower back.

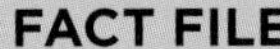

FACT FILE

TARGETS
- Deltoids

EQUIPMENT
- Dumbbell

BENEFITS
- Strengthens shoulders

CAUTIONS
- Shoulder issues
- Lower-back pain
- Wrist issues
- Elbow issues

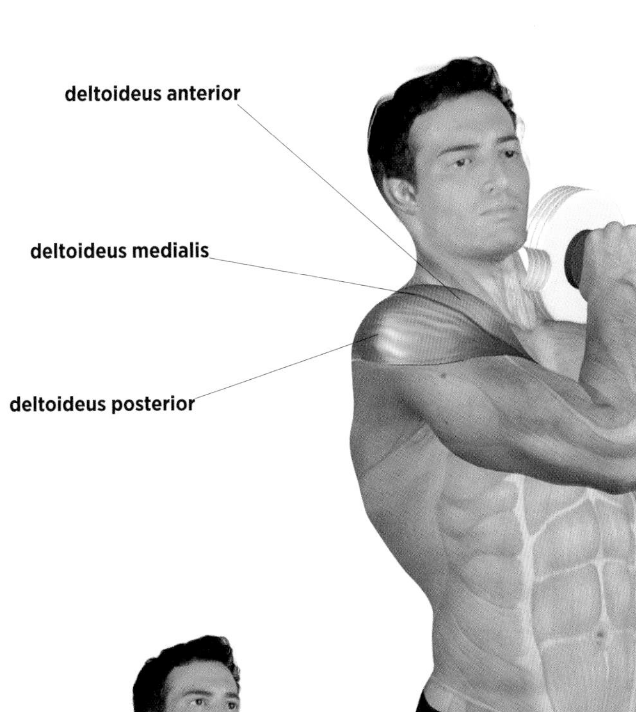

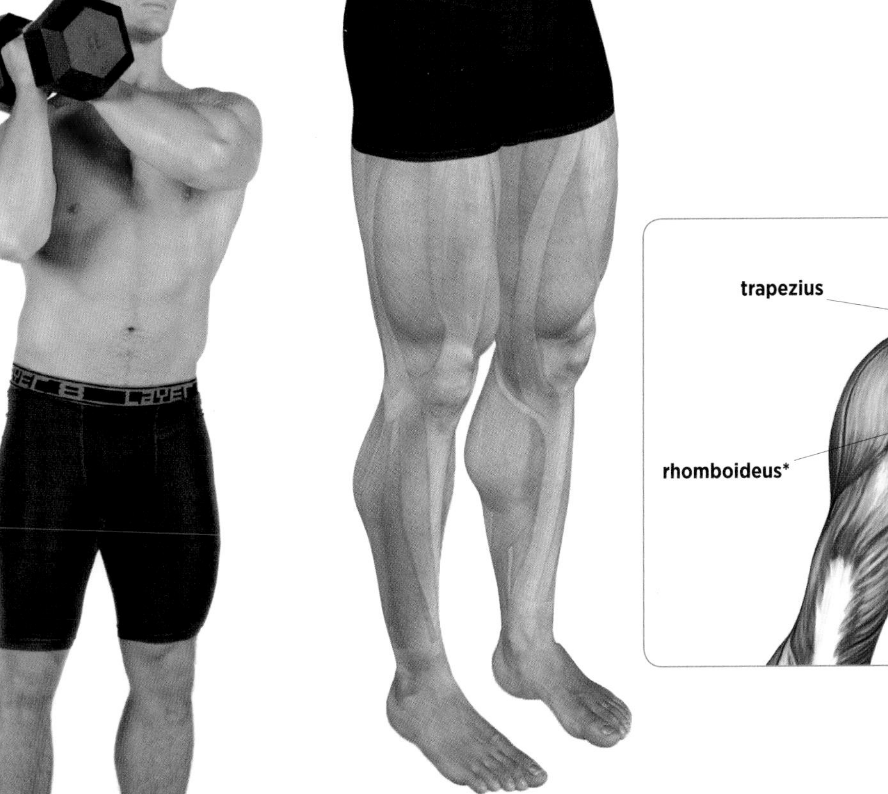

Annotation Key

Bold text indicates target muscles

Light text indicates other working muscles

* indicates deep muscles

Shoulder Crusher

The Shoulder Crusher homes in on your deltoids to give your shoulders an intense workout. It calls for you to perform a series of positions in rapid succession to an eight-count beat.

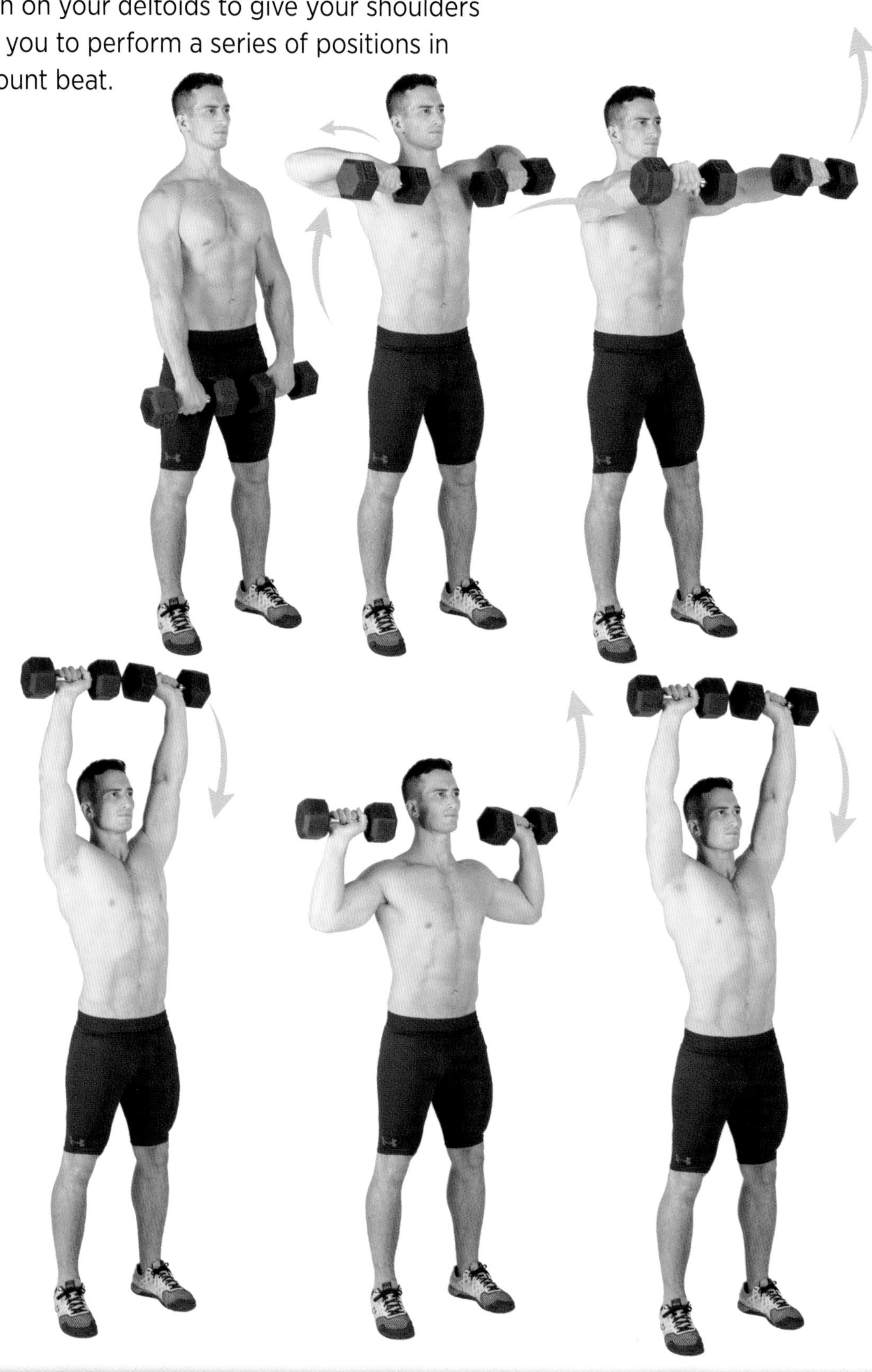

HOW TO DO IT

- Stand with your feet hip-width apart with a dumbbell in each hand resting at the front of your thighs, your palms facing inward.
- Bring your hands to your chest for count 1.
- Move your arms straight out in front of your body at chest level for count 2.
- Keeping your arms straight, bring your hands overhead, and hold for count 3.
- Lower the weight to your shoulders, and hold for count 4.
- Press your arms overhead, and hold for count 5.
- Keeping your arms straight, bring them back in front of your chest for count 6.
- Pull your hands into the chest for count 7.
- Drop your arms to the front of each thigh for count 8. Each time your hands hit your thighs equals one rep. Repeat for the recommended repetitions.

FACT FILE

TARGETS
- Deltoids

EQUIPMENT
- Dumbbells

BENEFITS
- Strengthens shoulders

CAUTIONS
- Shoulder issues
- Lower-back pain
- Wrist issues
- Elbow issues

DO IT RIGHT

- Maintain a steady beat, moving quickly but with control.
- When bringing the dumbbells overhead, make sure that your hands are directly above you, and not in front of your center of gravity.
- Be sure to work with weights that are not too heavy for your strength level.
- Avoid arching your lower back.

Annotation Key
Bold text indicates target muscles
Light text indicates other working muscles
* indicates deep muscles

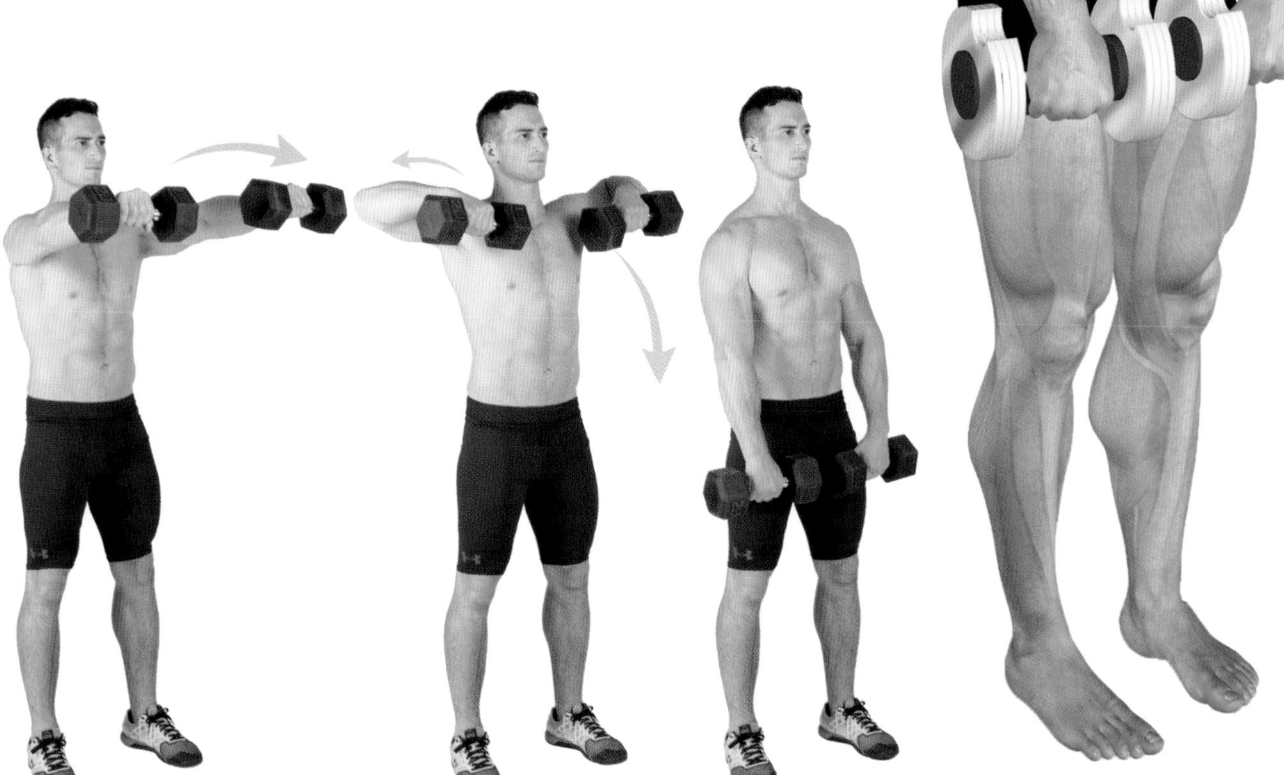

Da Vinci

Inspired by the Vitruvian Man, Leonardo da Vinci's famous anatomical diagram, this exercise will expose your muscles to their own renaissance! Using full range of motion, it engages your shoulders, biceps, forearms, upper back, and triceps to give you a complete arm workout.

HOW TO DO IT

- Stand with your feet hip-width apart with a dumbbell in each hand resting at the front of your thighs and your palms facing outward.
- Leading with your thumbs, bring the dumbbells overhead in a large arc to touch the dumbbells together.
- Lower the dumbbells in the same arc until the weights are once more down by your sides to return to the starting position. Repeat for the recommended repetitions.

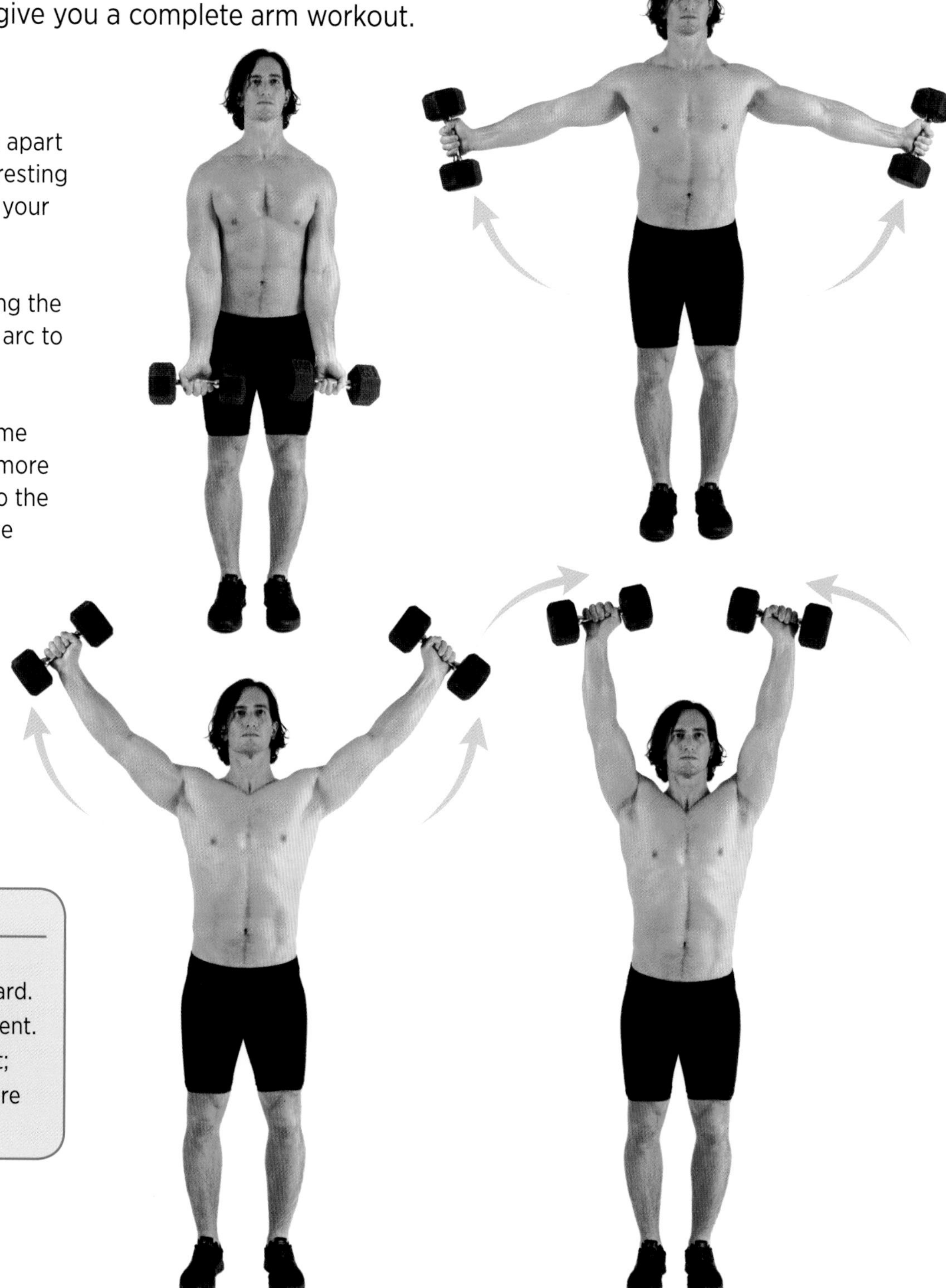

DO IT RIGHT

- Keep your core engaged.
- Keep your palms facing outward.
- Avoid excessive trunk movement.
- Choose an appropriate weight; this movement does not require high resistance.

FACT FILE

TARGETS
- Arms
- Shoulders
- Back
- Abdominals

EQUIPMENT
- Dumbbells

BENEFITS
- Encourages full range of motion
- Strengthens and tones arms, back, and core

CAUTIONS
- Shoulder/ rotator cuff issues
- Wrist issues
- Elbow issues

palmaris longus
flexor carpi radialis
flexor carpi ulnaris
extensor carpi radialis
extensor carpi ulnaris
scalenus*
biceps brachii
rectus abdominis
serratus anterior
obliquus internus*
obliquus externus*
transversus abdominis*

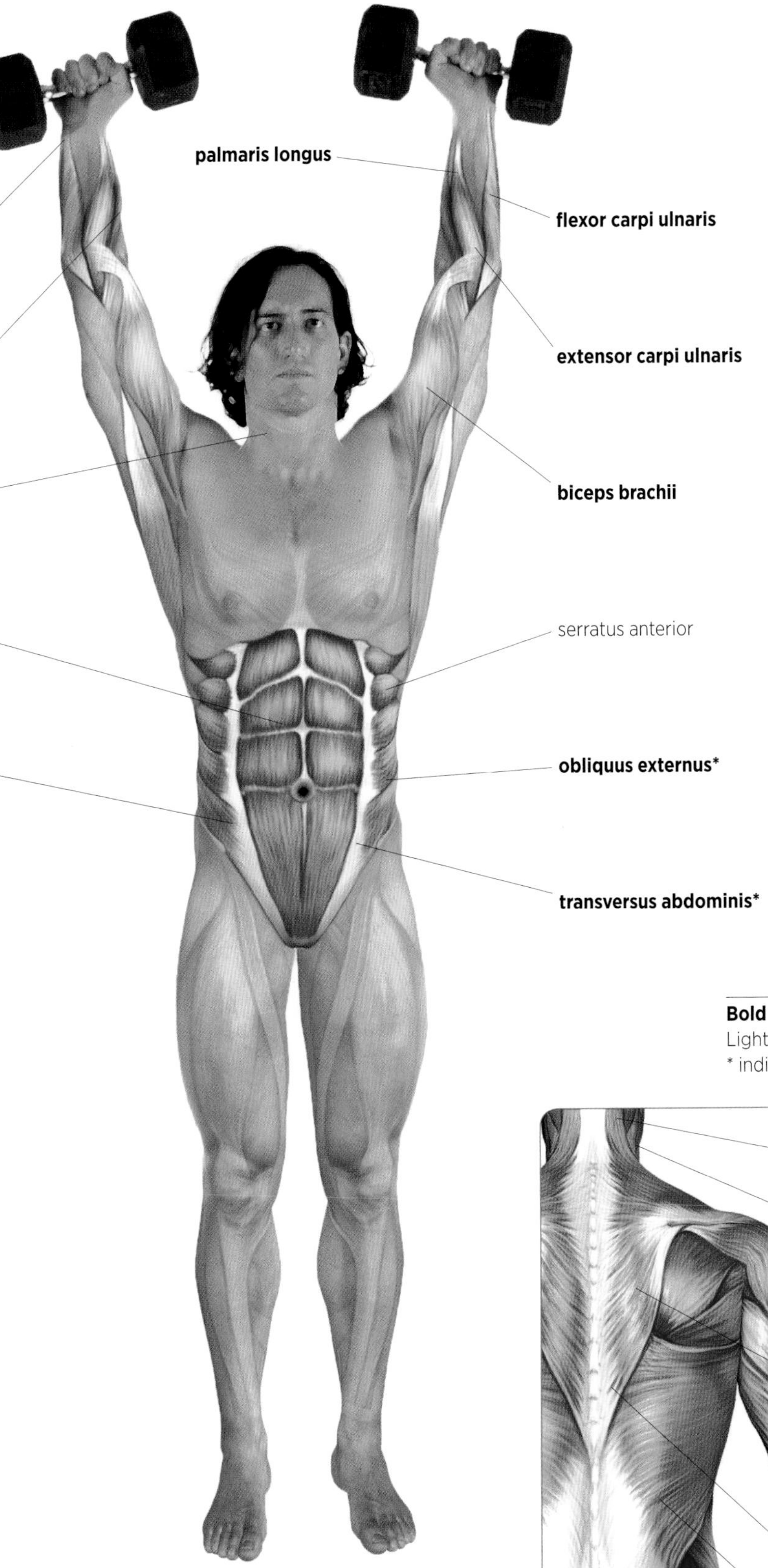

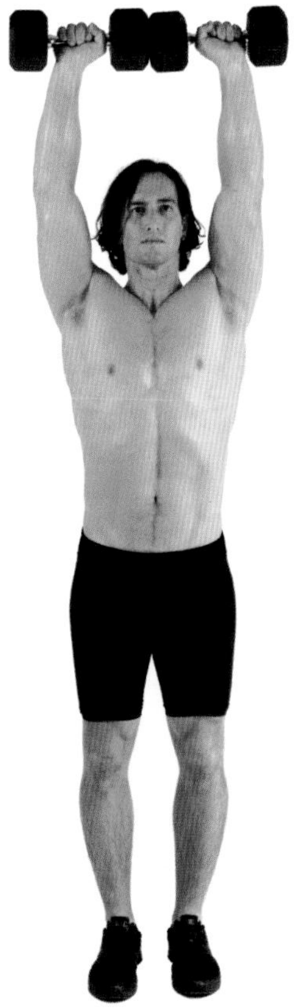

Annotation Key

Bold text indicates target muscles

Light text indicates other working muscles

* indicates deep muscles

splenius*
levator scapulae*
deltoideus medialis
deltoideus posterior
trapezius
triceps brachii
rhomboideus*
latissimus dorsi

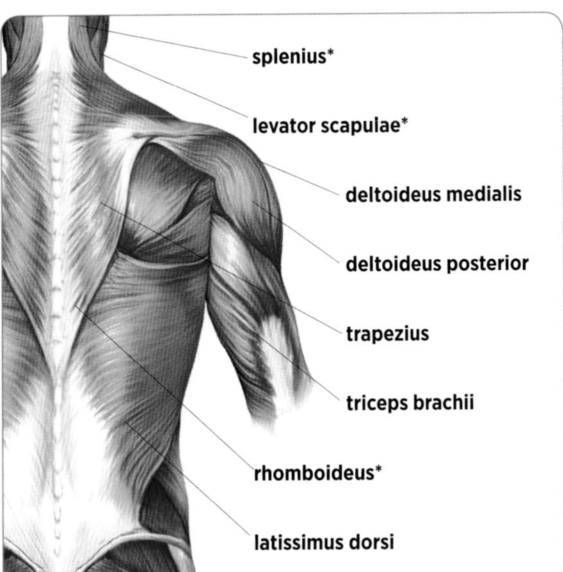

Double-Arm Triceps Kickback

A fundamental exercise for the triceps brachii, the Triceps Kickback is based on the theory of active insufficiency. This means you utilize a muscle that is activated already to its advantage to put your posterior arms under tension and give them a great workout. In this version, you move both arms at the same time.

FACT FILE

TARGETS
- Triceps
- Upper back

EQUIPMENT
- Dumbbells

BENEFITS
- Strengthens triceps
- Develops upper-body control

CAUTIONS
- Elbow injury
- Lower-back issues

HOW TO DO IT

- Begin in a staggered stance with one leg in front of the other and with your hips bent at 45 degrees, your back in a neutral position, and your arms drawn back so that your upper arm is parallel with the floor.
- Extend your elbows, pushing the dumbbells back behind you until your arms are straight. Keep your wrists neutral, with your palms facing each other.
- To return to the starting position, bend your elbows to 90 degrees to lower the weights so that they hang toward to floor. Repeat for the recommended repetitions.

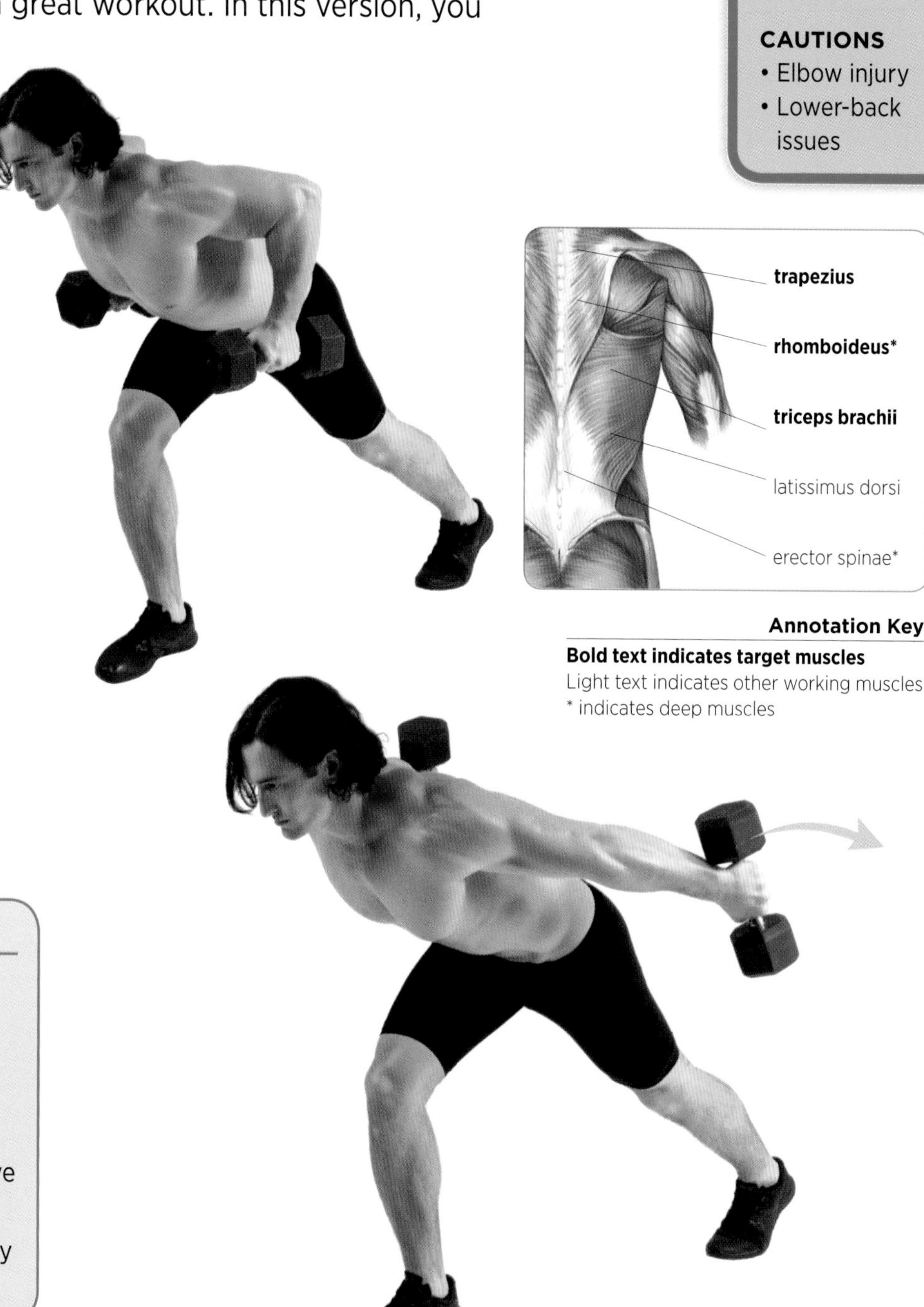

Annotation Key
Bold text indicates target muscles
Light text indicates other working muscles
* indicates deep muscles

DO IT RIGHT

- Keep your back straight.
- Keep your core engaged.
- Avoid excessive trunk motion.
- Hold the weights directly under your shoulder.
- Avoid swinging your arm to move from one position to the next.
- Avoid overextending your arm by locking your elbows.

Single-Arm Triceps Kickback

The Single-Arm Triceps Kickback version of this upper-arm move is an excellent, and relatively simple, exercise that tones the hard-to-activate triceps brachii. Balancing on three limbs will also engage your core.

HOW TO DO IT

- WIth a dumbbell near your right hand, kneel on all fours, with your wrists directly under your shoulders, your fingers facing forward, and your knees directly under your hips. Press your navel toward your spine.
- Flex your right elbow tightly into your side. Keep pressing your shoulder blades down your back, and then extend your right arm straight behind you.
- Flex your elbow forward again, controlling the movement all the way. Repeat for the recommended repetitions, and then repeat on the opposite side.

DO IT RIGHT

- Keep your pelvis and spine in a neutral position.
- Keep your core engaged.
- Gaze toward the floor.
- Hold the weight directly under your shoulder.
- Avoid swinging your arm.
- Avoid locking your elbow.

deltoideus anterior

triceps brachii

rhomboideus*

serratus anterior

rectus abdominis

transversus abdominis*

Annotation Key

Bold text indicates target muscles

Light text indicates other working muscles

* indicates deep muscles

FACT FILE

TARGETS

- Triceps
- Upper back
- Core

EQUIPMENT

- Dumbbells

BENEFITS

- Strengthens triceps
- Develops upper-body control
- Strengthens core

CAUTIONS

- Elbow injury
- Lower-back issues

Single-Arm Dumbbell Press

The Single-Arm Dumbbell Press is a fantastic resistance exercise to develop your pectorals. By using separable weights in an alternating pattern, it ensures that each side receives a great chest workout.

FACT FILE

TARGETS
- Pectorals
- Triceps
- Abdominals

EQUIPMENT
- Dumbbells
- Flat bench

BENEFITS
- Strengthens and tones chest, arms, and core
- Improves coordination

CAUTIONS
- Wrist issues

HOW TO DO IT

- Lie faceup on a flat bench with a dumbbell in each hand, your elbows flared out, and your feet planted on the floor.
- Press the right dumbbell directly above you with your right arm, until your arm is fully extended.
- Bend your elbow to lower the weight back to the starting position. Repeat on the opposite side, and then continue alternating sides for the recommended repetitions.

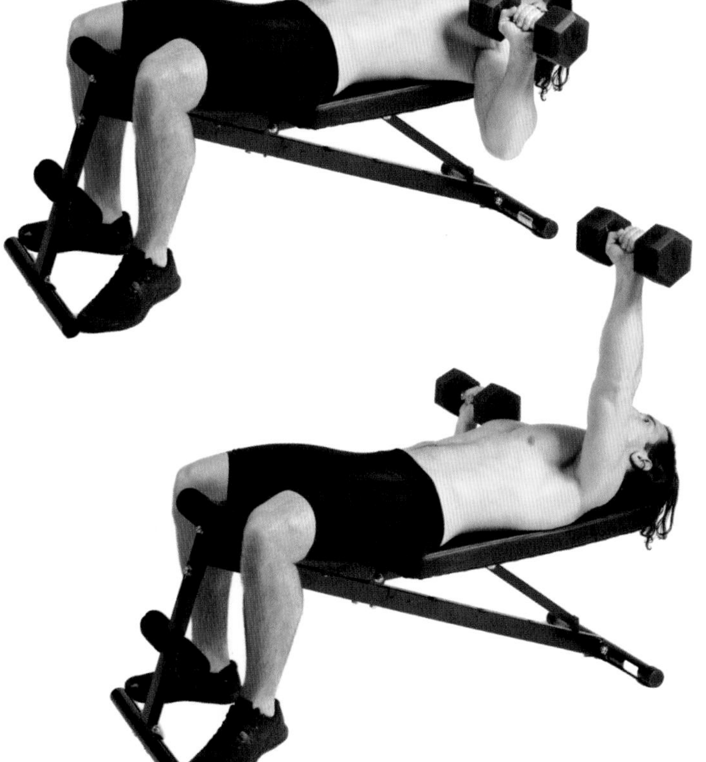

DO IT RIGHT

- Keep your core engaged.
- Avoid arching your back.
- Keep your elbows slightly below the level of your shoulders to ease shoulder stress.

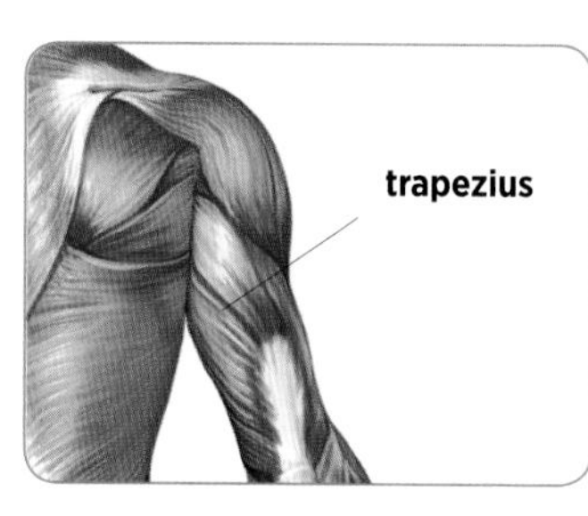

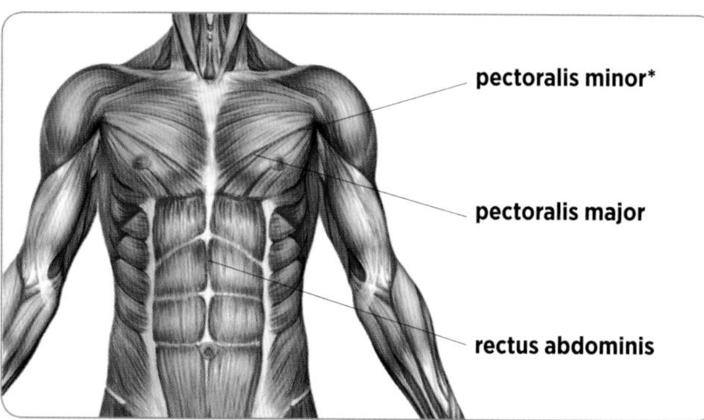

Annotation Key
Bold text indicates target muscles
Light text indicates other working muscles
* indicates deep muscles

Swiss Ball Incline Dumbbell Press

To build and strengthen the often-neglected upper portion of your chest, try the Swiss Ball Incline Dumbbell Press. Performed on the unstable surface of a ball, it also recruits your core muscles to help with balance.

FACT FILE

TARGETS
- Chest
- Core

EQUIPMENT
- Dumbbells
- Swiss ball

BENEFITS
- Strengthens pectorals
- Strengthens and stabilizes core

CAUTIONS
- Shoulder issues
- Wrist issues
- Lower-back issues

HOW TO DO IT

- Lie faceup on a Swiss ball, with your upper back, neck, and head supported. Keep your torso elongated, and bend your knees at a right angle. Plant your feet on the floor a little wider than shoulder-width apart. Drop your buttocks slightly so that your torso takes on an incline position.

- Grasp a hand weight or dumbbell in each hand, and bend your elbows so that the weights are in line with your shoulders.

- Press your arms upward and slightly inward until the dumbbells are nearly touching at the top.

- Bend your elbows as you lower the weights toward your shoulders back to the starting position. Repeat for the recommended repetitions.

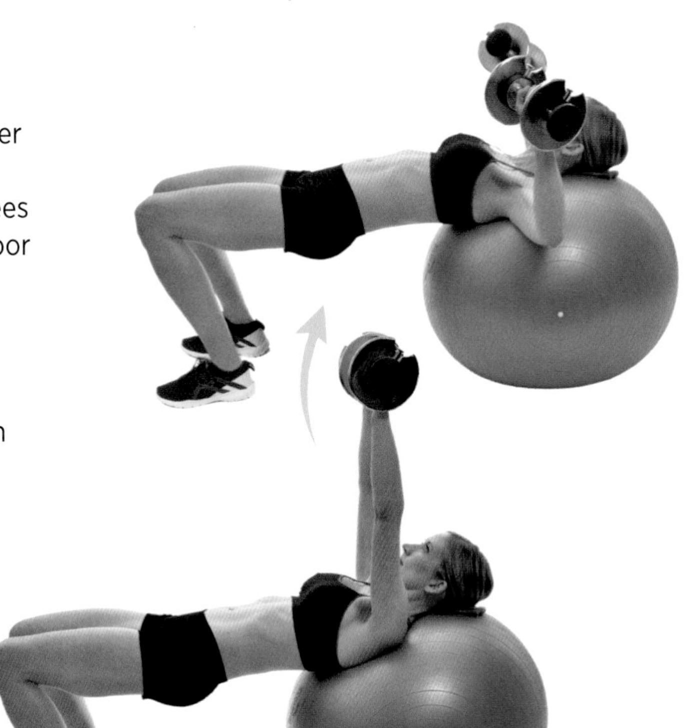

DO IT RIGHT
- Avoid excessive speed; lower the weight smoothly and with control.
- Keep your heels firmly pressed into the floor.
- Avoid bouncing the dumbbells off your chest.
- Avoid arching your back.

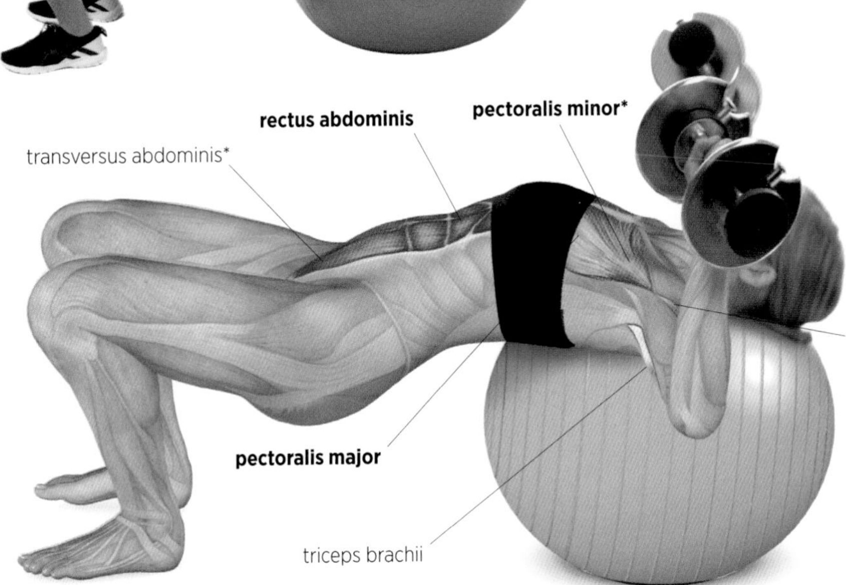

Annotation Key
Bold text indicates target muscles
Light text indicates other working muscles
* indicates deep muscles

Swiss Ball Flat Dumbbell Press

The Swiss Ball Flat Chest Press targets the mid to lower sections of your chest. Performing it on the Swiss ball calls for you to also engage your core to keep yourself steady and stable.

HOW TO DO IT

- Lie faceup on a Swiss ball with a dumbbell in each hand, your elbows flared out and your feet planted on the floor. Move forward until your back is flat against the ball, as well as your head and neck. Keep your glutes raised and your back flat.

- Raise the dumbbells directly above you until your arms are fully extended.

- Bend your elbows to lower the weights back to the starting position. Repeat for the recommended repetitions.

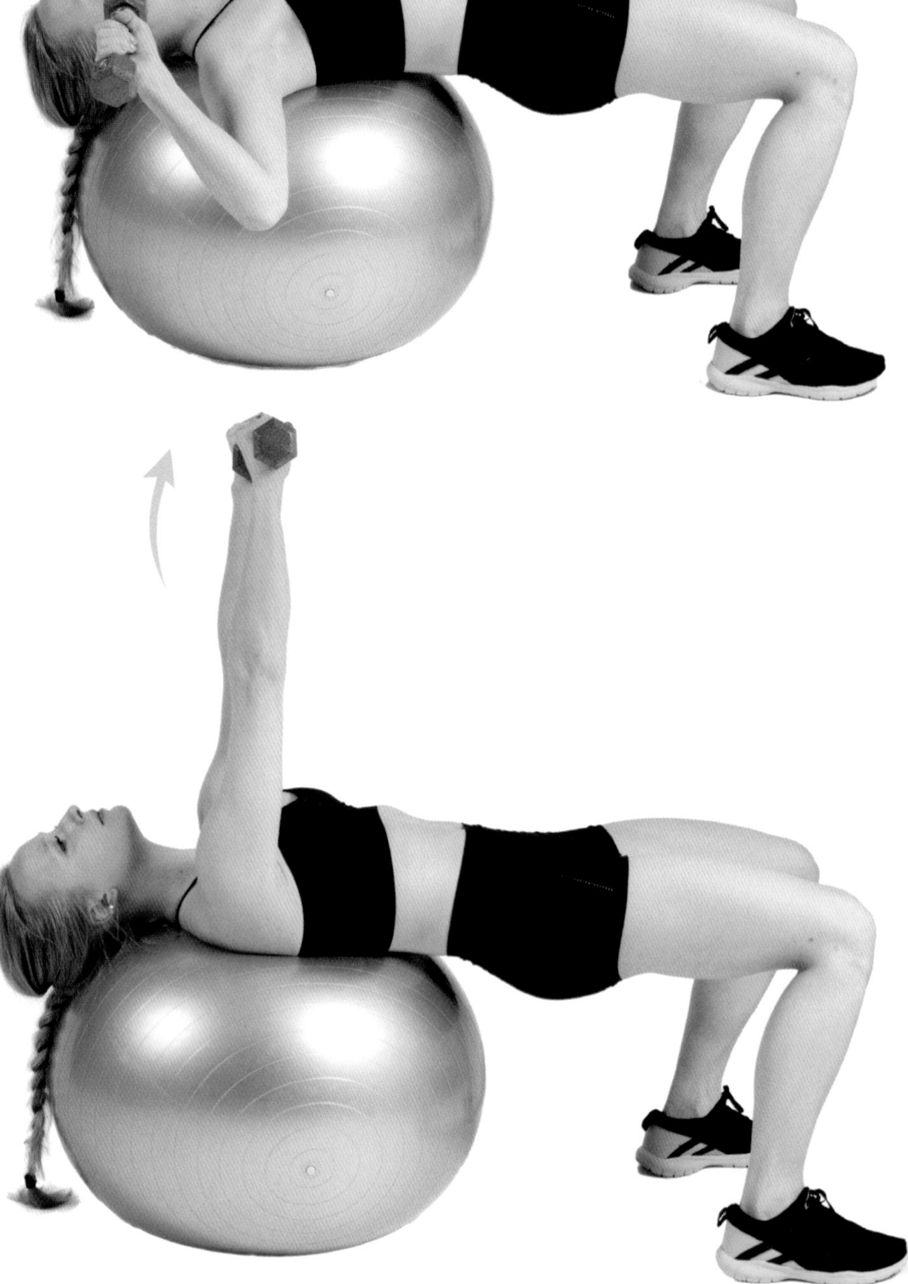

DO IT RIGHT

- Keep your heels firmly pressed into the floor.
- Keep your wrists in line with your shoulders.
- Avoid excessive speed; lower the weight smoothly and with control.
- Avoid bouncing the dumbbells off your chest.
- Avoid arching your back.

trapezius
infraspinatus*
supraspinatus*
teres minor
subscapularis*
rhomboideus*

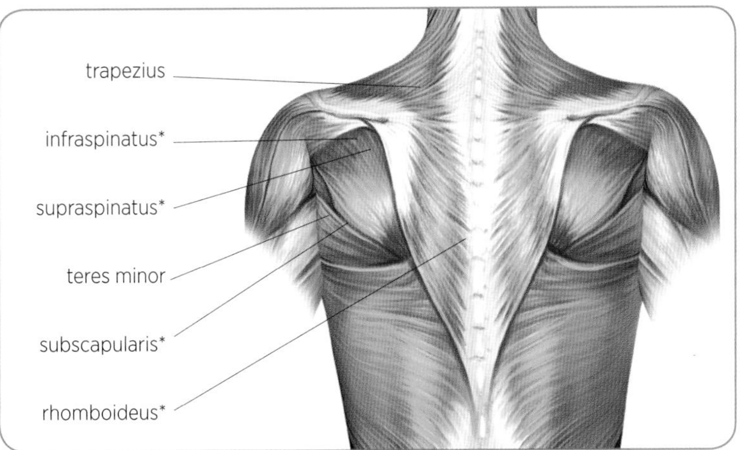

Annotation Key

Bold text indicates target muscles

Light text indicates other working muscles

* indicates deep muscles

FACT FILE

TARGETS
- Pectorals
- Deltoids
- Triceps
- Abdominals

EQUIPMENT
- Dumbbells
- Swiss ball

BENEFITS
- Strengthens and tones chest, shoulder, arms, and core
- Improves coordination

CAUTIONS
- Shoulder issues
- Lower-back pain
- Wrist issues

pectoralis minor*
pectoralis major
serratus anterior
triceps brachii
latissimus dorsi
teres major
levator scapulae*
deltoideus posterior

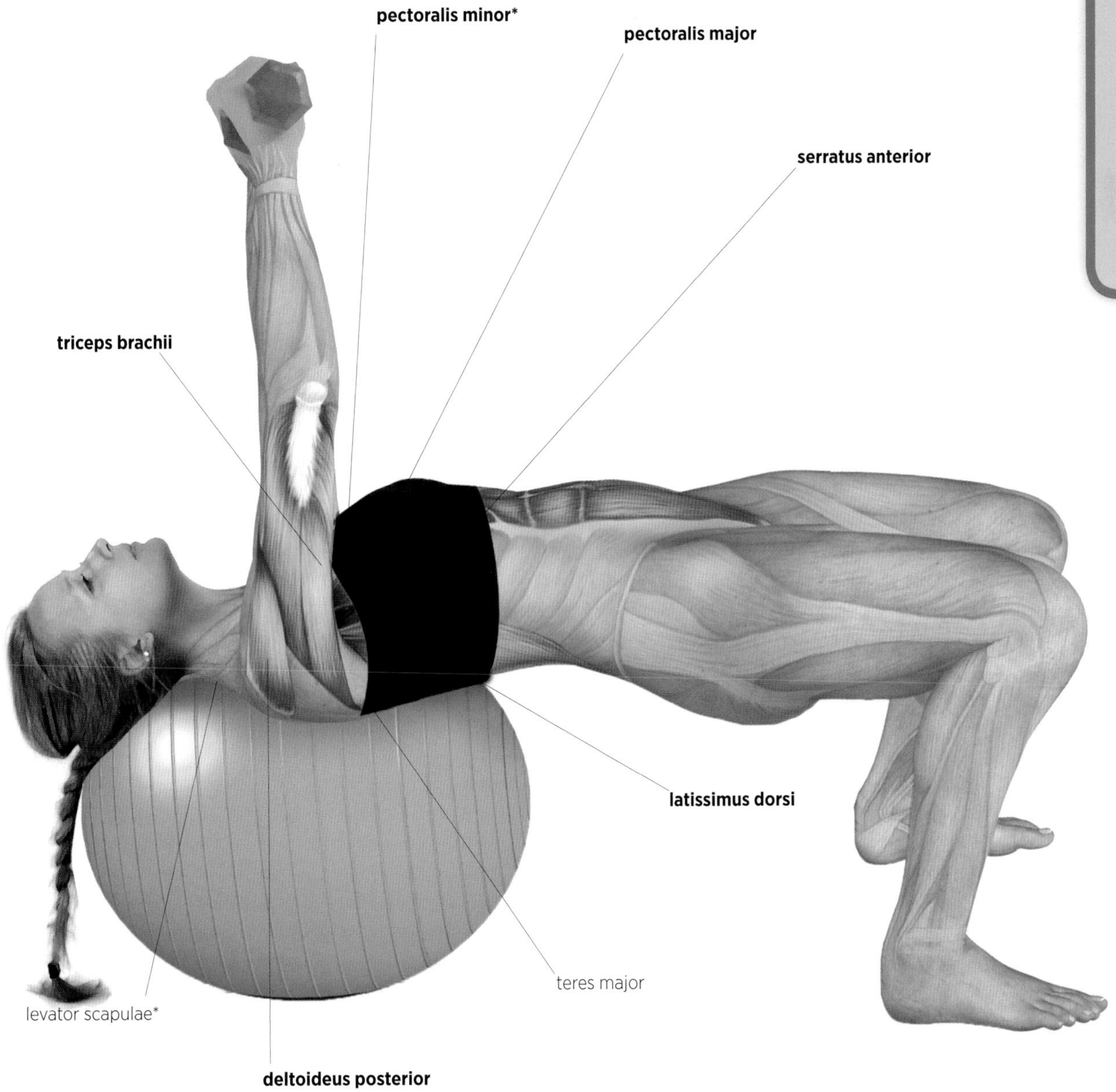

Hammer-Grip Press

The Hammer Grip Press, performed on an incline bench, targets your chest, arms, and shoulders. Be sure to use a weight that you can carefully and safely control.

HOW TO DO IT

- Sit on an incline bench, grasping a dumbbell in each hand and resting them on your thighs.
- Kick up while leaning back on the bench, so that you can start the movement with your elbows near your ribs and the dumbbells to the sides of your chest. Your palms should be facing each other in a hammer-grip position.
- Raise the dumbbells toward the ceiling until they are directly above your shoulders. Hold this top position for a moment.
- Slowly lower the dumbbells to your shoulders, and then bring the dumbbells back to the starting position. Repeat for the recommended repetitions.

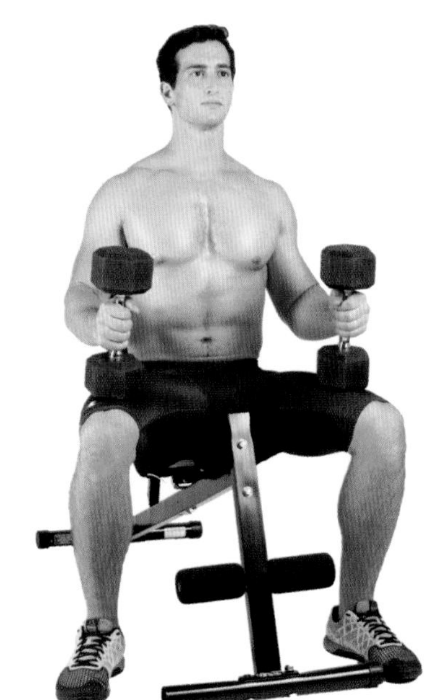

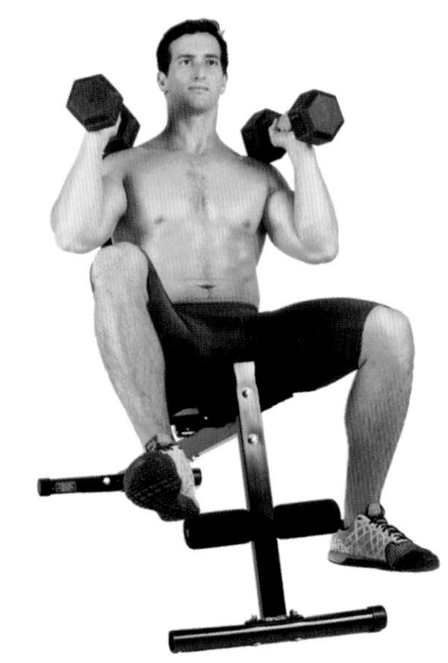

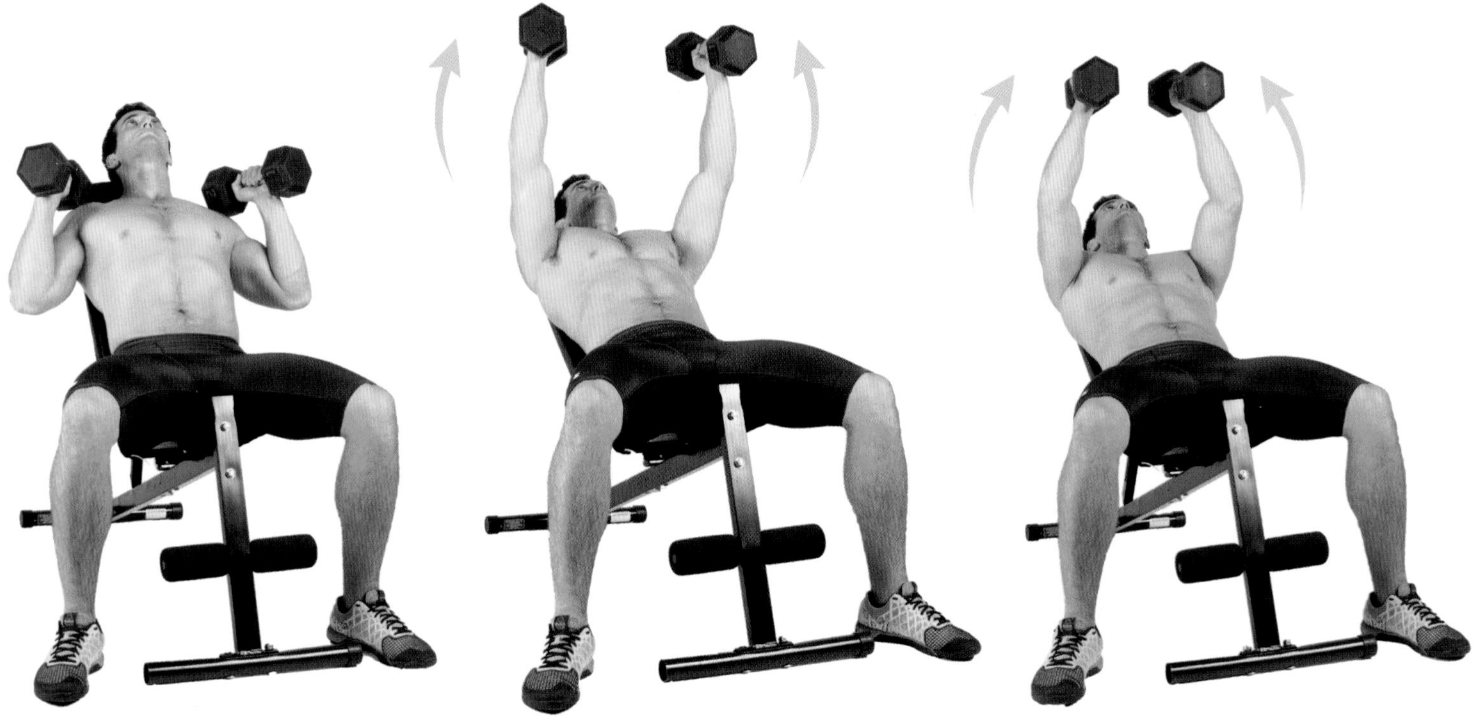

FACT FILE

TARGETS
- Pectorals
- Deltoids
- Triceps

EQUIPMENT
- Dumbbells
- Incline bench

BENEFITS
- Strengthens upper chest, arms, and shoulders

CAUTIONS
- Shoulder issues
- Lower-back pain
- Wrist issues

pectoralis minor*

triceps brachii

deltoideus anterior

pectoralis major

DO IT RIGHT
- Keep your chest muscles engaged.
- Be sure the dumbbells face each other as you execute the movement.
- Avoid lifting your feet off the floor.
- Avoid lifting your glutes and back while executing the exercise.
- Avoid hyperextending your arms at the top range of the movement.

Annotation Key

Bold text indicates target muscles

Light text indicates other working muscles

* indicates deep muscles

Dumbbell Fly

The Dumbbell Fly gives your chest and shoulders a thorough workout. When done right, this move feels as if you are hugging a large tree.

HOW TO DO IT

- Sit on an incline bench, grasping a dumbbell in each hand and resting them on your thighs.
- Kick up while leaning back on the bench, so that you can start the movement with your elbows near your ribs and the dumbbells to the sides of your chest. Your palms should be facing each other in a hammer-grip position.
- Keeping your spine in a neutral position, place your feet flat on the floor. Raise the dumbbells above your chest until your elbows are only very slightly bent.
- With a slight bend in your elbow, open up your chest and slowly lower the dumbbells to the sides.
- To return to the starting position, bring the dumbbells back along the same path as the descent, exhaling as you do so. Repeat for the recommended repetitions.

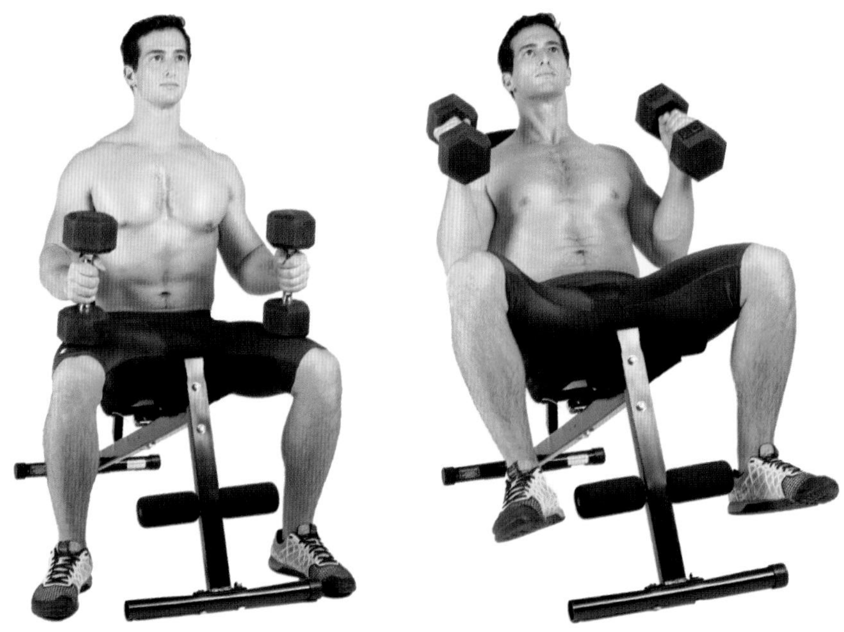

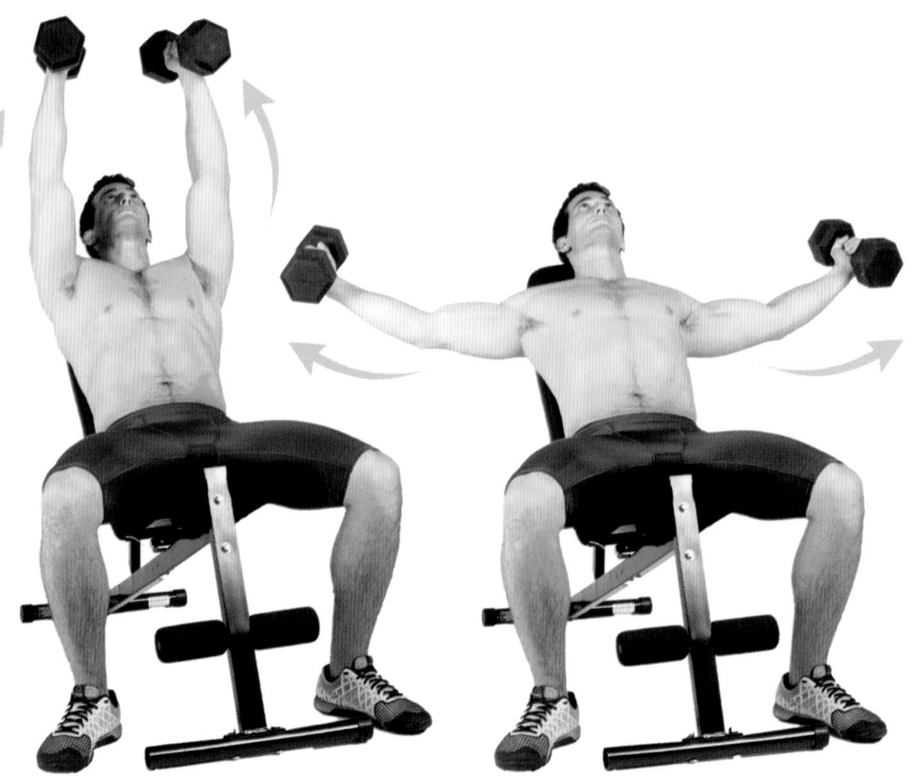

DO IT RIGHT

- Look for your chest and rib cage to rise as the dumbbells descend.
- Keep your spine and shoulders in the same position as you return to the starting position.
- Avoid moving your head or chin forward or off the bench.
- Avoid elevating your shoulders.
- Avoid bending your elbows excessively as the dumbbells descend, or flattening them as the dumbbell ascend.

FACT FILE

TARGETS
- Pectoral
- Shoulders
- Arms

EQUIPMENT
- Dumbbell
- Incline bench

BENEFITS
- Strengthens chest and shoulders

CAUTIONS
- Shoulder issues
- Lower-back pain
- Wrist issues

deltoideus medialis
deltoideus posterior
subscapularis*

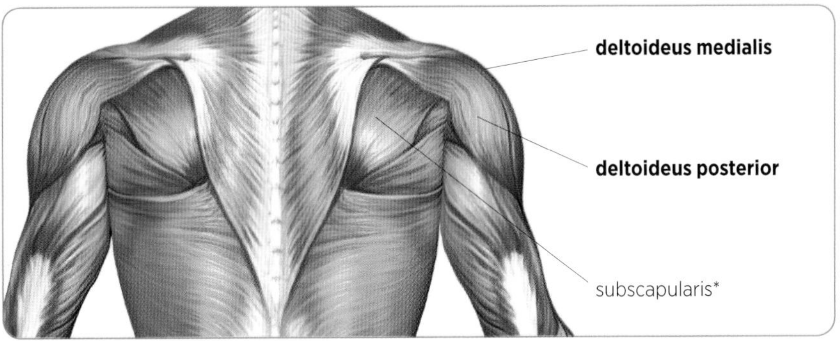

Annotation Key
Bold text indicates target muscles
Light text indicates other working muscles
* indicates deep muscles

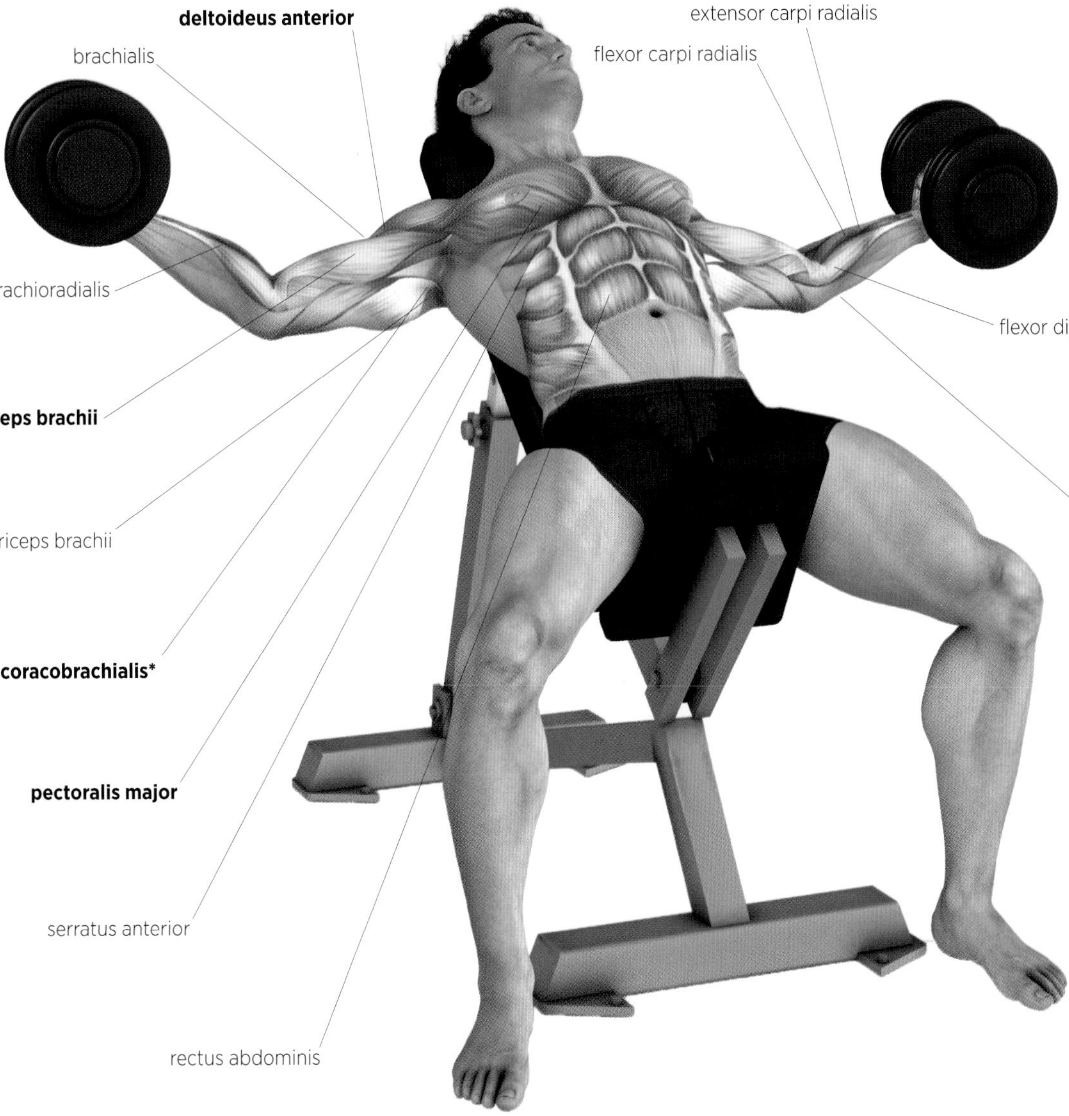

deltoideus anterior
brachialis
extensor carpi radialis
flexor carpi radialis
brachioradialis
flexor digitorum*
biceps brachii
extensor digitorum
triceps brachii
coracobrachialis*
pectoralis major
serratus anterior
rectus abdominis

Plyo Power Stand Push-Up

Also known as the Plyometric Push-up, this advanced version of a basic push-up demands strength, agility, and coordination. Performed with a push-up stand, this exercise will truly challenge your pectoral strength and your core stability.

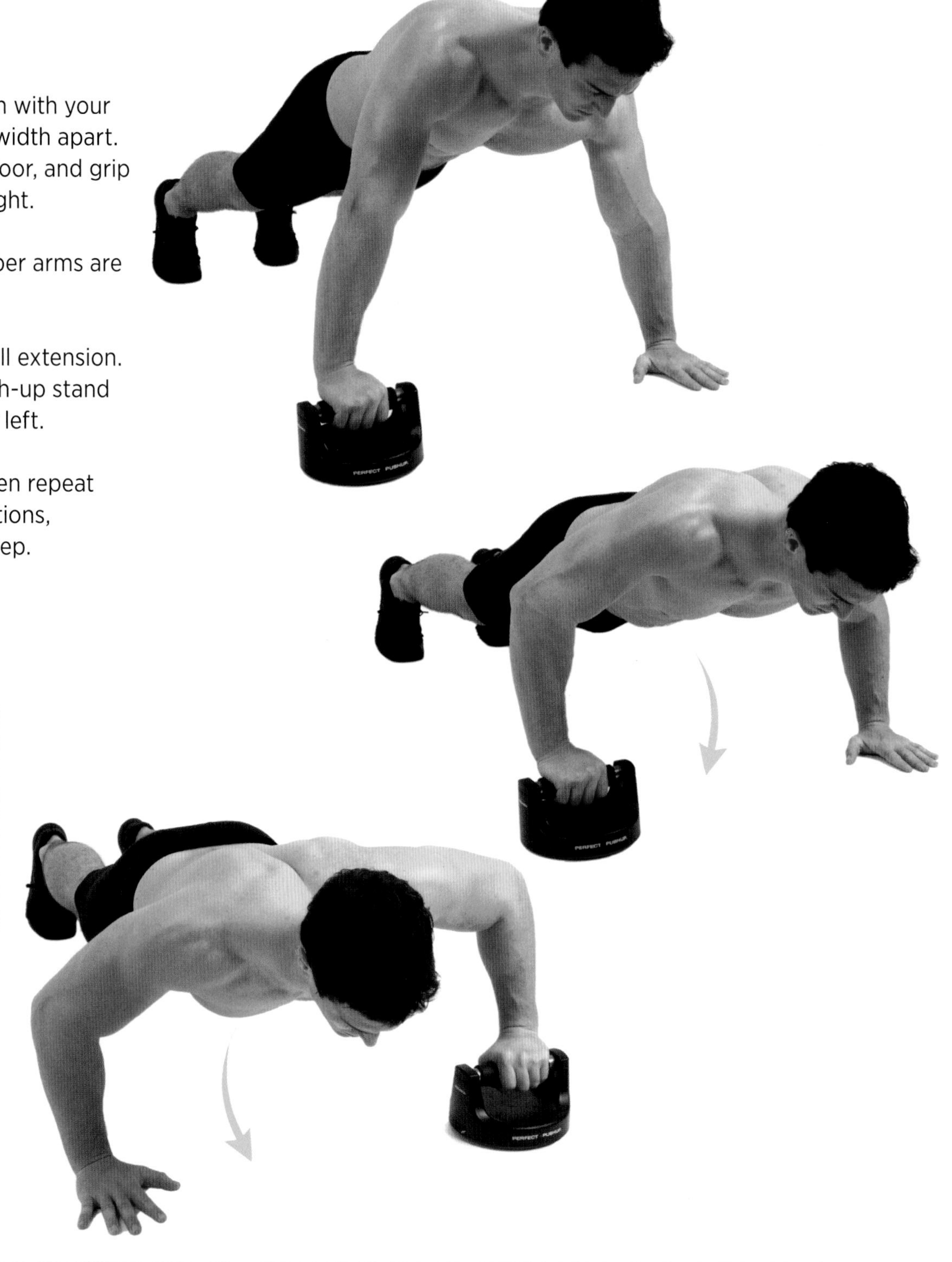

HOW TO DO IT

- Begin in a high plank position with your feet spread wider than hips-width apart. Plant your left hand on the floor, and grip a push-up stand with your right.
- Lower yourself until your upper arms are parallel to the floor.
- Quickly push your arms to full extension. As you do so, switch the push-up stand from your right hand to your left.
- Lower yourself again, and then repeat for the recommended repetitions, alternating arms with every rep.

DO IT RIGHT

- Keep your back flat.
- Avoid excessive bouncing.
- Avoid using momentum to drive the movement.

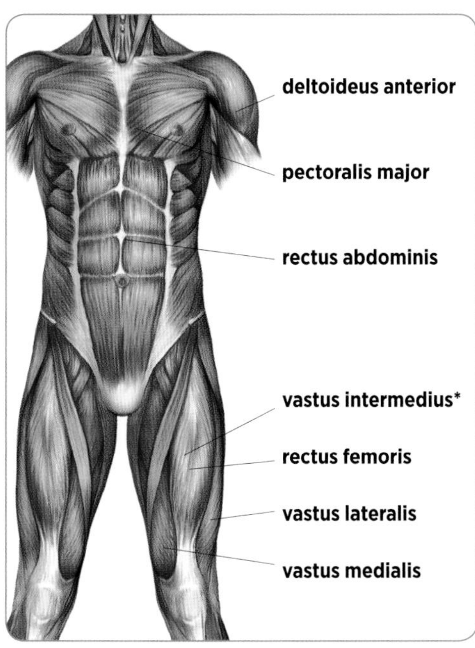

MODIFICATION

HARDER: Perform the push-ups with both hands gripping flat-bottomed kettlebells. Be very careful to ensure that the kettlebells don't flip over!

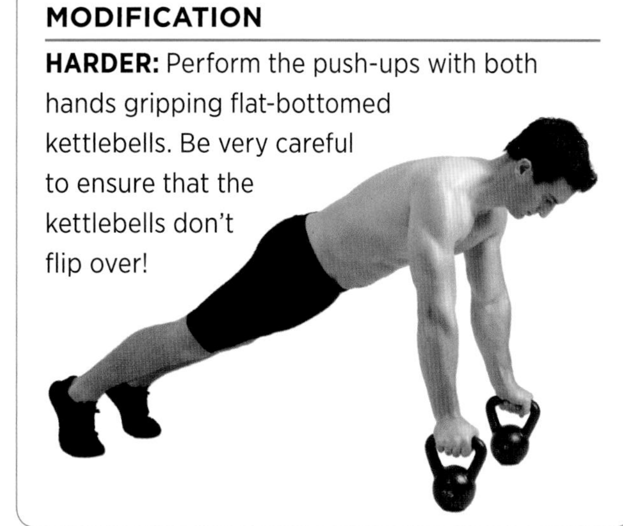

FACT FILE

TARGETS
- Pectorals
- Deltoids
- Abdominals
- Quadriceps

EQUIPMENT
- Push-up stand

BENEFITS
- Improves balance
- Improves coordination
- Strengthens and tones chest, arms, abdominals, and legs

CAUTIONS
- Knee issues

Annotation Key
Bold text indicates target muscles
Light text indicates other working muscles
* indicates deep muscles

triceps brachii
deltoideus medialis
deltoideus posterior
biceps brachii
extensor digitorum
palmaris longus
deltoideus anterior
pectoralis major

Single Dumbbell Push-Up

The Single Dumbbell Push-Up uses the weight to focus gravitational stresses that engage your chest muscles in a concentrated way. This exercise will recruit your pectorals to establish a full contraction and give you a great chest workout.

FACT FILE

TARGETS
- Pectorals
- Triceps
- Deltoids
- Abdominals

EQUIPMENT
- Hexagonal dumbbells

BENEFITS
- Strengthens and tones chest, arms, and abdominals
- Improves balance

CAUTIONS
- Wrist issues

HOW TO DO IT

- Begin in a high plank position with your feet splayed wider than hip-width apart and with both hands holding onto a dumbbell.

- Keeping your core engaged, bend your elbows to lower your body to the dumbbell.

- Press down into the dumbbell, extending your arms until you have returned to the starting position. Repeat for the recommended repetitions.

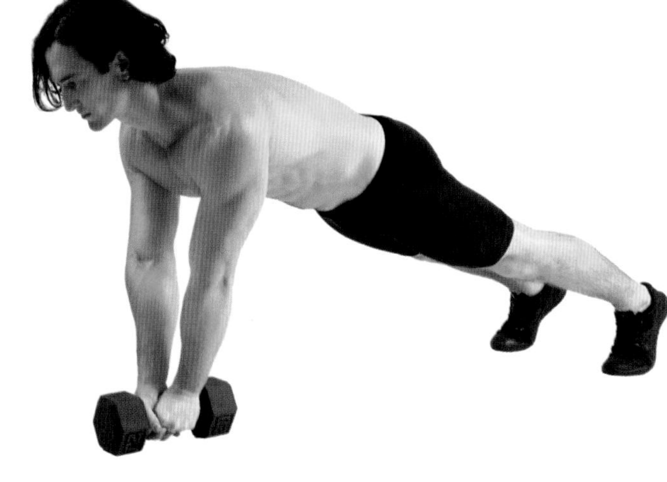

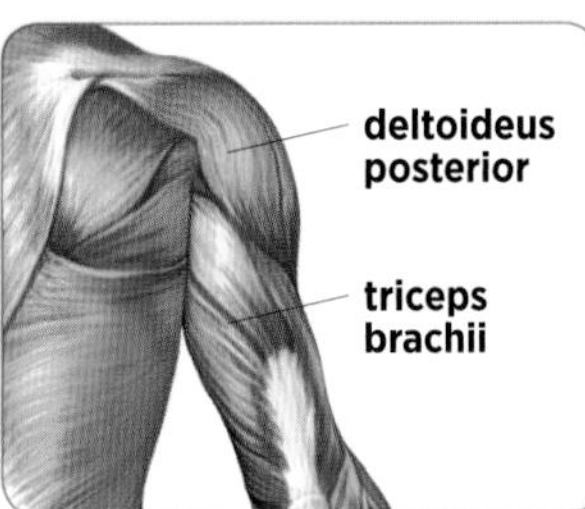

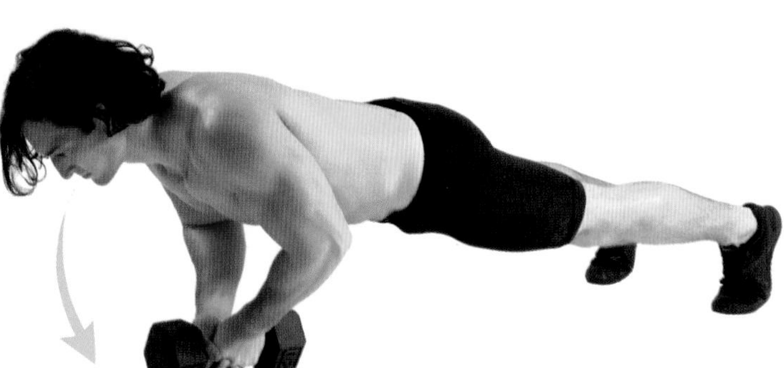

DO IT RIGHT

- Make sure the dumbbell is stable on the floor, with the flat side fixed on the floor.
- Avoid arching your back.
- Avoid flaring out your elbows; keep your arms close to your torso.

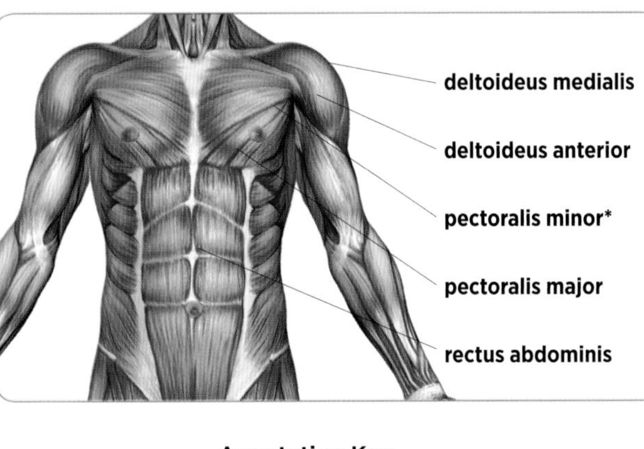

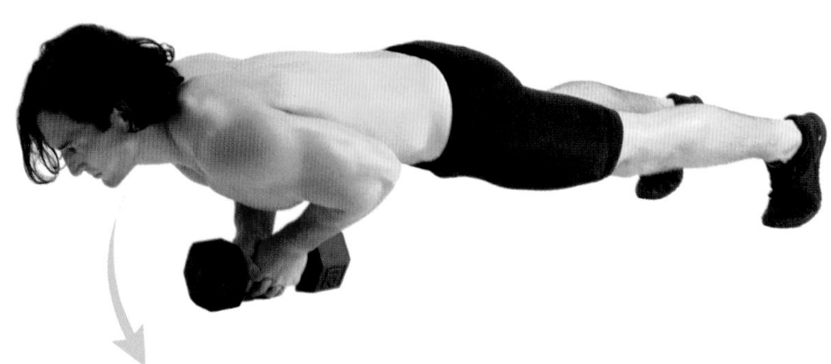

Annotation Key

Bold text indicates target muscles
Light text indicates other working muscles
* indicates deep muscles

Rolling Dumbbell Fly

The Rolling Dumbbell Fly is another exercise that uses gravity as resistance to engage your pectorals, deltoids, core, and more. Requiring full range of motion, this exercise will get the best out of your chest.

HOW TO DO IT

- Begin in a high plank position, balancing your feet on your toes. With your hands directly beneath your shoulders, grasp the parallel-positioned handles of two dumbbells. Keep your back straight and your feet together.

- Roll the dumbbells away from each other, keeping your arms as straight as possible, allowing gravity to drop your body toward the floor. The movement ends when you reach the floor or you can no longer control your descent.

- Draw your arms together, keeping them as straight as possible, rolling the dumbbells in toward each other to return to the starting position. Repeat for the recommended repetitions.

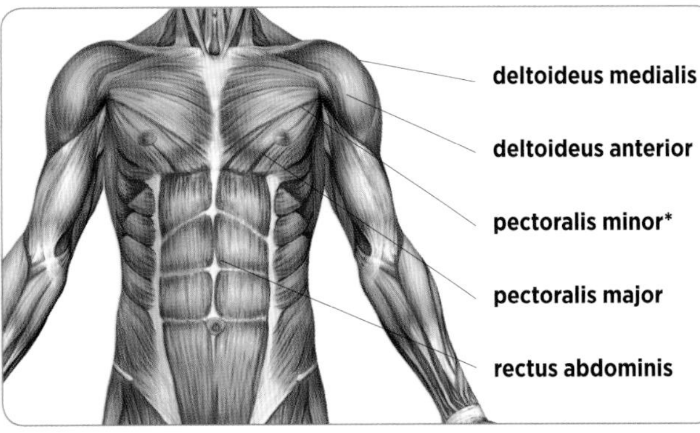

Annotation Key

Bold text indicates target muscles

Light text indicates other working muscles

* indicates deep muscles

FACT FILE

TARGETS
- Pectorals
- Deltoids
- Abdominals

EQUIPMENT
- Dumbbells

BENEFITS
- Strengthens and tones chest, arms, and abdominals
- Increases eccentric and concentric strength

CAUTIONS
- Wrist issues

DO IT RIGHT

- Keep your back straight.
- Keep your arms as straight as possible.
- Avoid extra movement at your wrists.

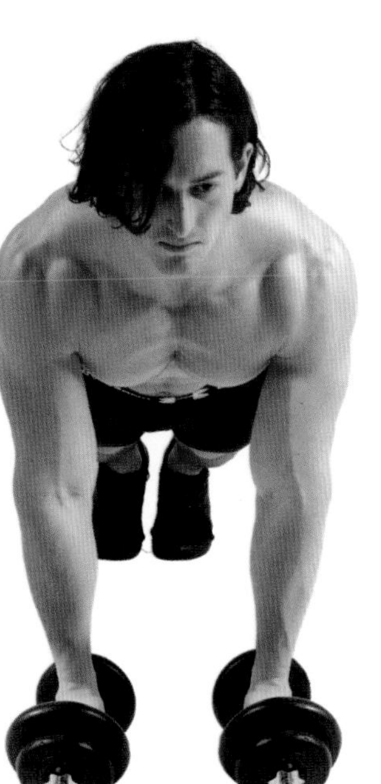

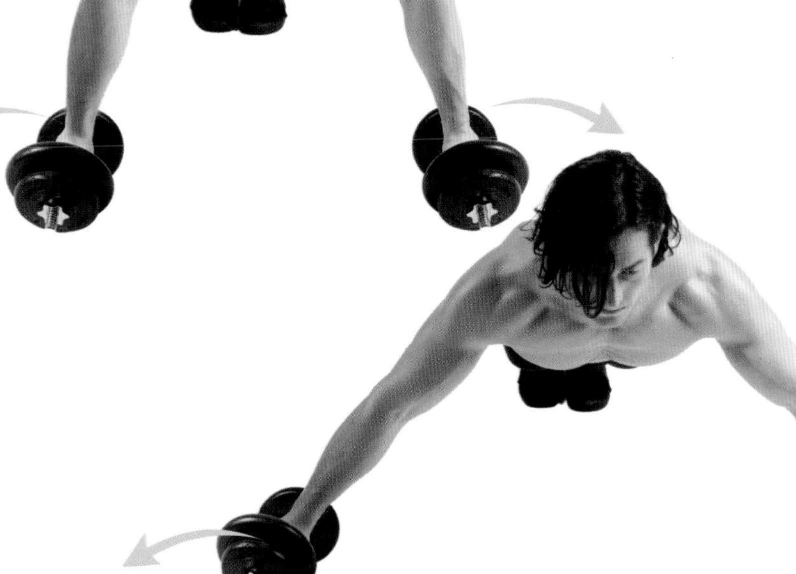

Scissors over Dumbbells

If you were told to never run with scissors, this may be your chance. This exercise uses dumbbells, rather than resistance, to target your hip flexors, core, and legs. It requires coordination, balance, and core stability.

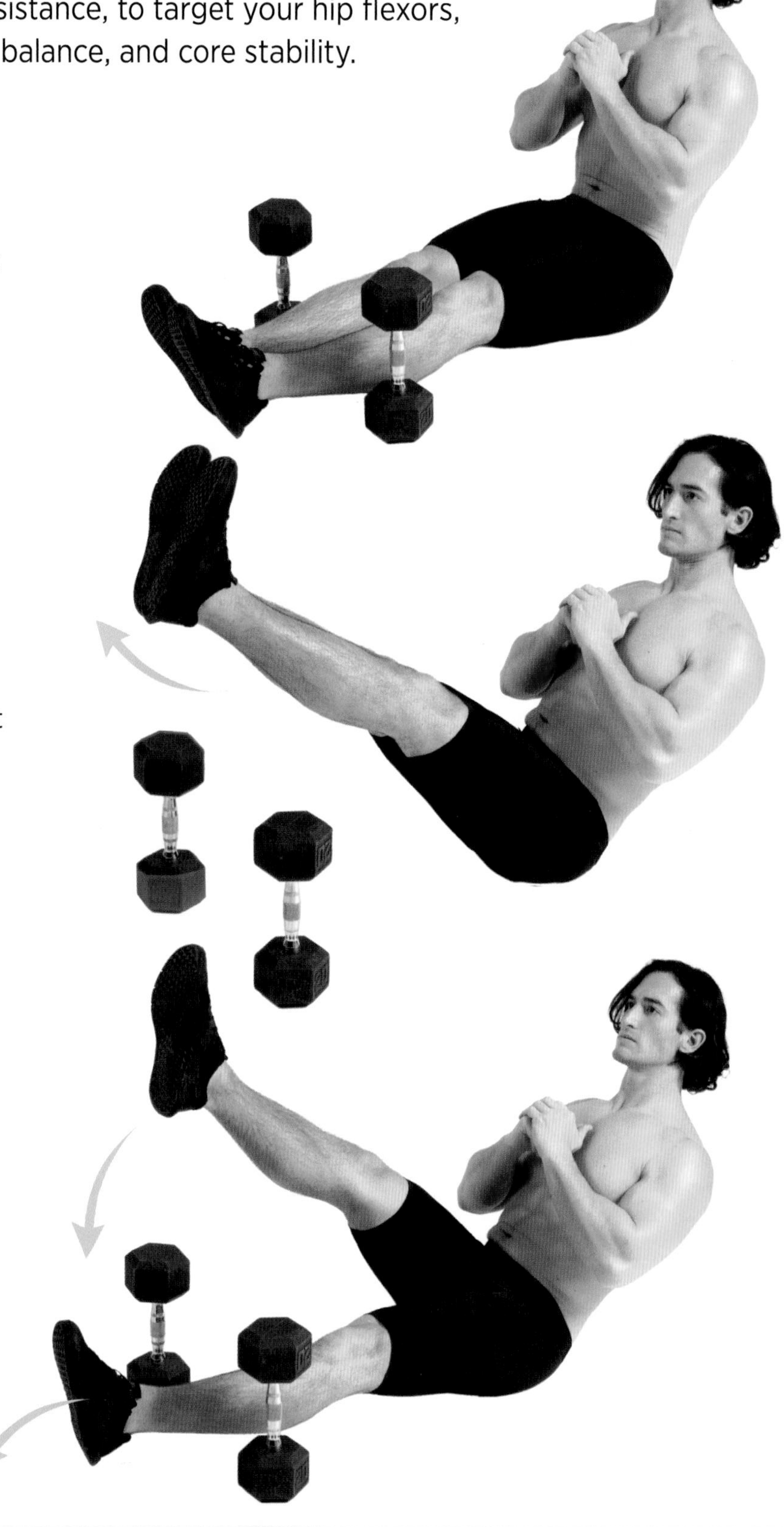

HOW TO DO IT

- Place two dumbbells upright on the floor approximately 1 foot apart from each other. Sit with your legs outstretched and your feet between the dumbbells.
- Bring your legs up and away from the floor, and roll backwards to counterbalance your lower extremities. Keep your core engaged and your spine in a neutral position.
- To scissor your legs, drop your left leg towards the floor, but not touching it, between the dumbbells.
- Drop your right leg between the dumbbells while you draw the left one up, and elevate it in the air.
- Repeat the scissoring motion, alternating which leg elevates and drops, until both legs are positioned on the left side of the dumbbells.
- Return to the starting position by reversing the steps above, performing the scissor motion toward the right and leading with the right leg. Continue alternating sides for the recommended repetitions.

DO IT RIGHT

- Keep your back straight.
- Keep your core engaged.

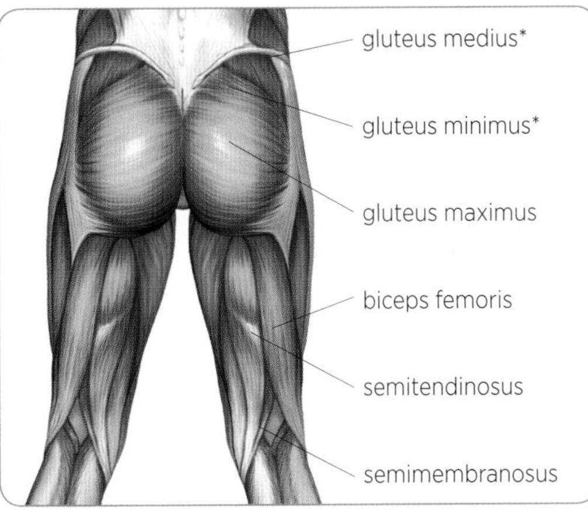

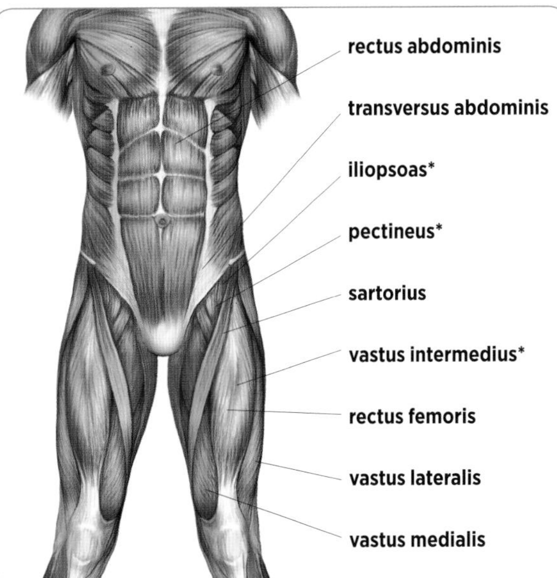

Annotation Key

Bold text indicates target muscles
Light text indicates other working muscles
* indicates deep muscles

FACT FILE

TARGETS
- Abdominals
- Hip flexors
- Quadriceps

EQUIPMENT
- Dumbbells

BENEFITS
- Strengthens and tones abdominals and legs
- Improves sitting balance
- Improves coordination

CAUTIONS
- Back issues

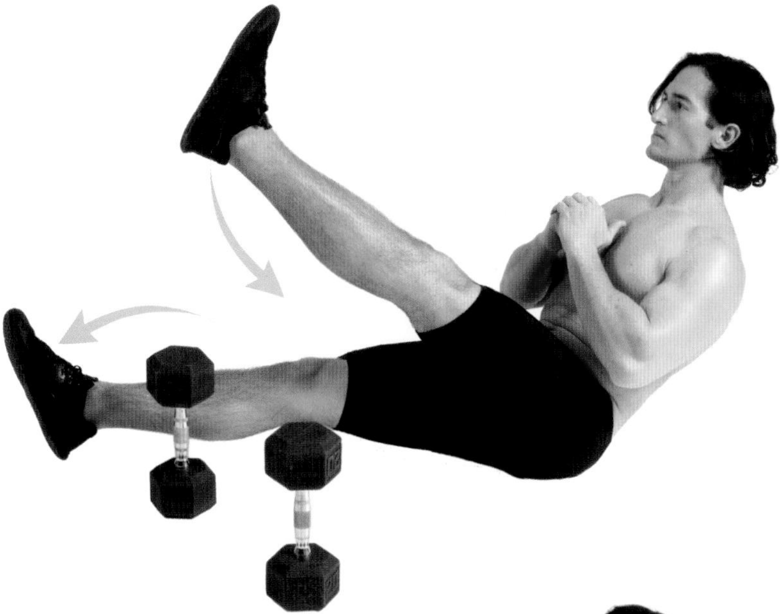

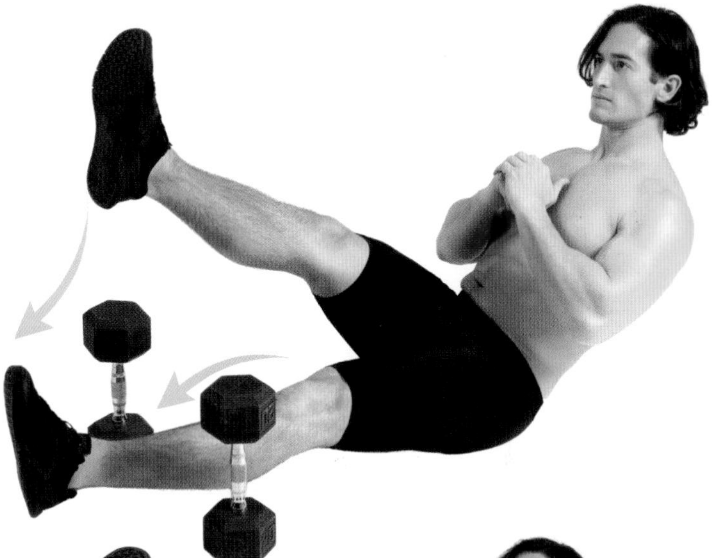

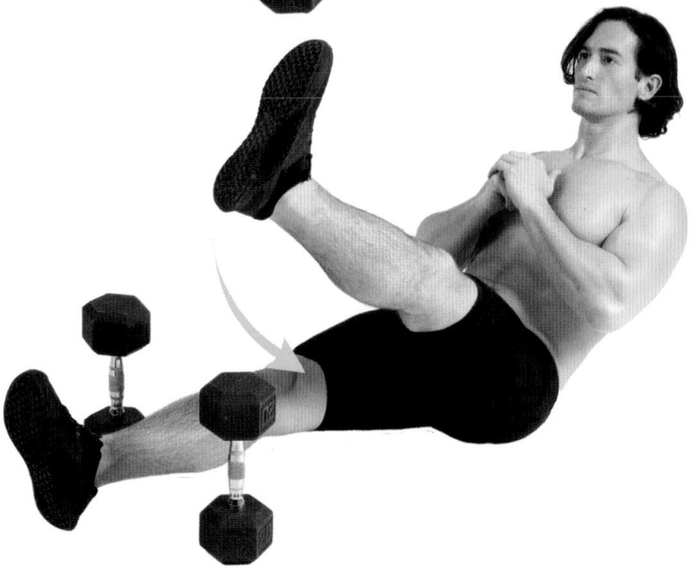

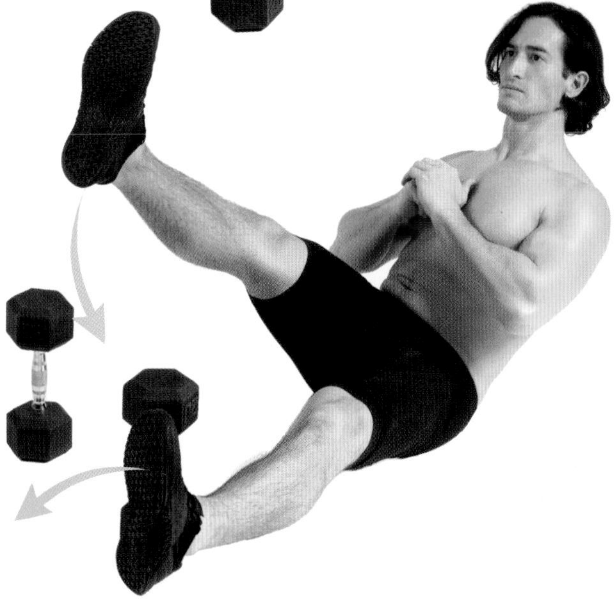

Dumbbell Sit-Up

Sit-ups train your core muscles to increase your flexibility and hone your balance. They also improve overall body strength, helping you build the muscles in your abdominals, lower back, and hip flexors. Adding dumbbells increases the intensity of the move.

FACT FILE

TARGETS
- Abdominals
- Back
- Chest
- Hip flexors

EQUIPMENT
- Dumbbells

BENEFITS
- Strengthens core, back, chest, and hips

CAUTIONS
- Lower-back issues
- Wrist issues

HOW TO DO IT

- Lie faceup with your knees slightly bent holding a dumbbell in each hand.
- Contract your abdominals as you raise your torso into a sit-up position, keeping the dumbbells at shoulder level.
- Lower yourself slowly back to the starting position. Repeat for the recommended repetitions.

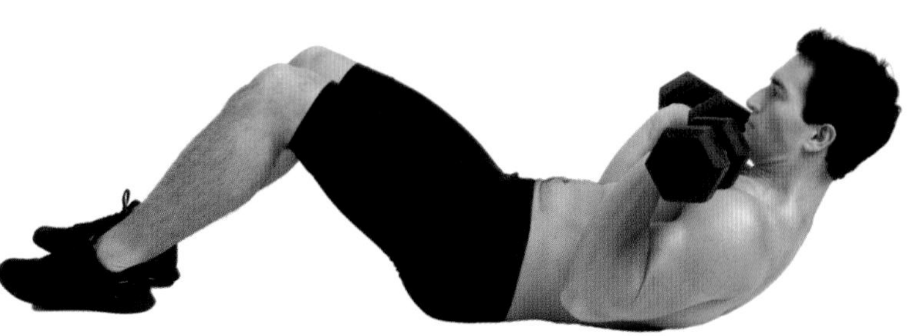

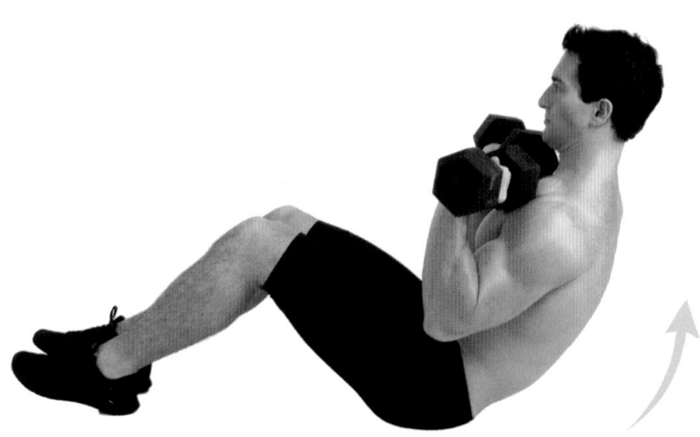

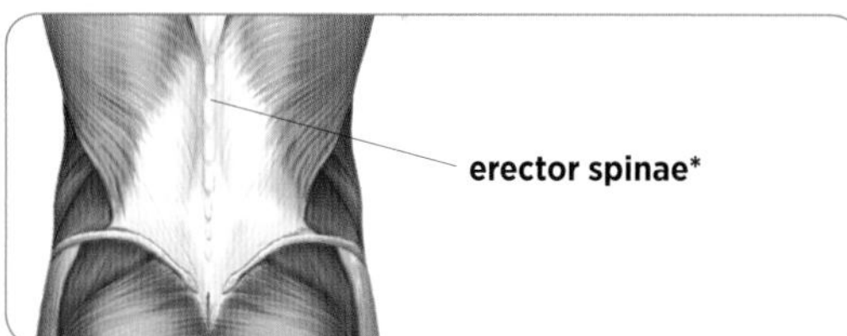

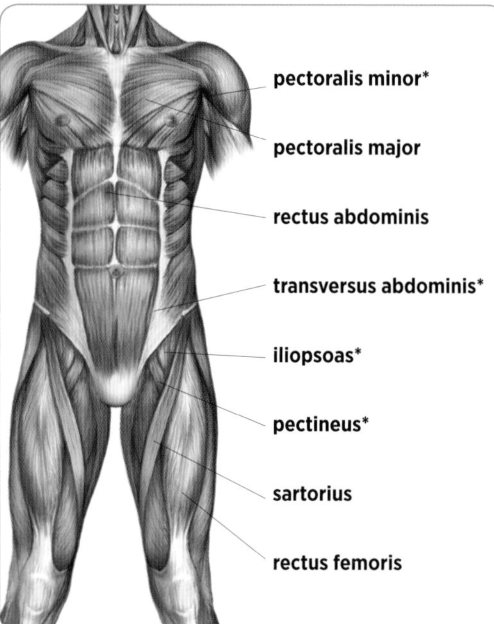

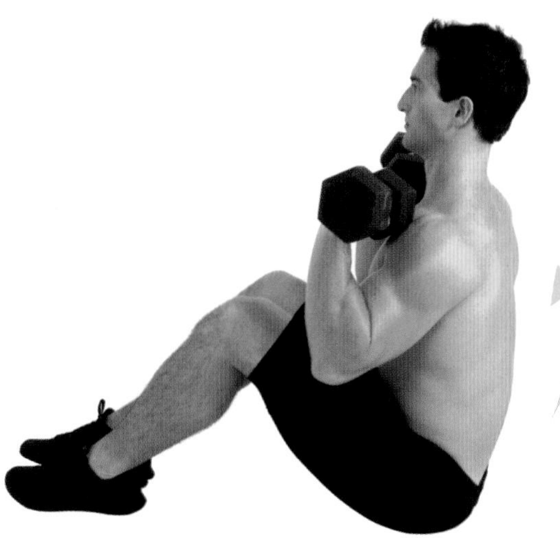

Annotation Key
Bold text indicates target muscles
Light text indicates other working muscles
* indicates deep muscles

DO IT RIGHT

- Maintain a smooth range of motion.
- Keep the dumbbells at shoulder level.
- Avoid moving too quickly—the slower the movement, the more effective the exercise.
- Avoid placing too much stress on your lower back.

V-Sit Kettlebell Hold with Leg Lift

The V-Sit Kettlebell Hold with Leg Lift combines the best benefits of an isometric resistance hold with the dynamic stress of a leg lift. In this way, it will challenge your sitting balance, hip flexors, and core stability.

FACT FILE

TARGETS
- Abdominals
- Hip flexors
- Quadriceps
- Deltoids

EQUIPMENT
- Kettlebell

BENEFITS
- Improves sitting balance
- Improves coordination
- Strengthens and tones abdominals, shoulders, and legs

CAUTIONS
- Lower-back issues

HOW TO DO IT

- Sit with your legs outstretched, grasping a kettlebell in front of your chest with both hands.
- Keeping your feet together, lift both legs off the floor, shifting your weight back and using the kettlebell as a counterbalance.
- Lower your legs to just a few inches off the floor.
- Repeat for the recommended repetitions, never letting your feet touch the floor.

DO IT RIGHT

- Keep your back in a neutral position.
- Hold the kettlebell with your elbows bent softly.
- Avoid letting with your feet touch the floor.

deltoideus posterior
erector spinae*
latissimus dorsi
multifidus spinae*

deltoideus anterior
pectoralis minor*
pectoralis major
rectus abdominis
iliopsoas*
pectineus*
sartorius
vastus intermedius*
rectus femoris
vastus lateralis
vastus medialis

Annotation Key
Bold text indicates target muscles
Light text indicates other working muscles
* indicates deep muscles

Seated Dumbbell Russian Twist

The Russian Twist is classic exercise that targets your obliques. In the Seated Dumbbell Russian Twist version, the added weight of the dumbbell increases the challenge.

HOW TO DO IT

- Holding a dumbbell in both hands, sit with your legs extended in front of you, your knees bent and your feet about hip-width apart. Lean back slightly.
- Engage your core muscles and rotate your torso to bring the dumbbell to your right.
- Bring the dumbbell back to the starting position, and then repeat on the other side. Continue alternating sides for the recommended repetitions.

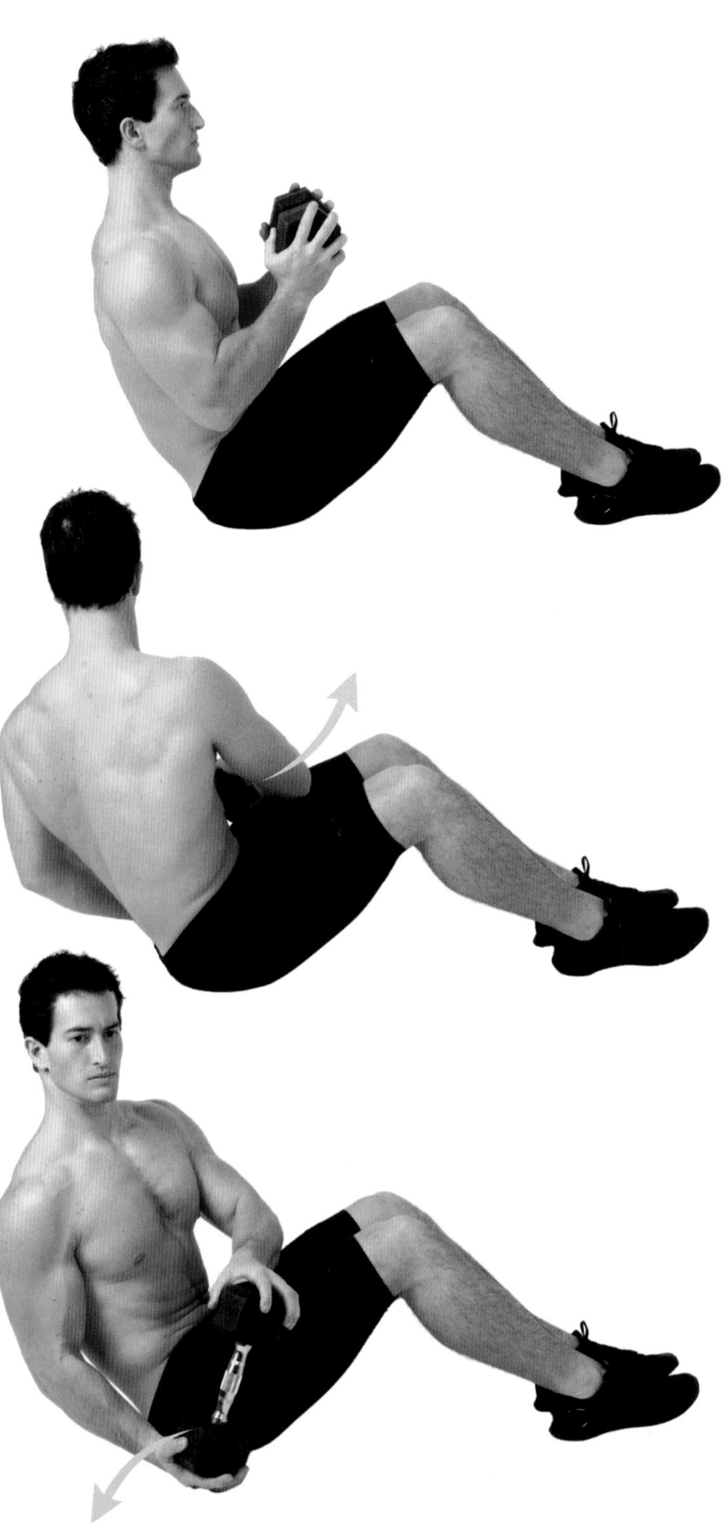

DO IT RIGHT

- Keep your core engaged.
- Anchor your heels to the floor.
- Move smoothly and with control.
- Avoid arching or rounding your back.
- Avoid hunching your shoulders.
- Avoid swinging your arms or moving in a jerky manner.
- Avoid tensing your neck as you twist.

obliquus internus*
transversus abdominis*
iliopsoas*
vastus intermedius*
rectus femoris
vastus medialis

triceps brachii
erector spinae*
latissimus dorsi

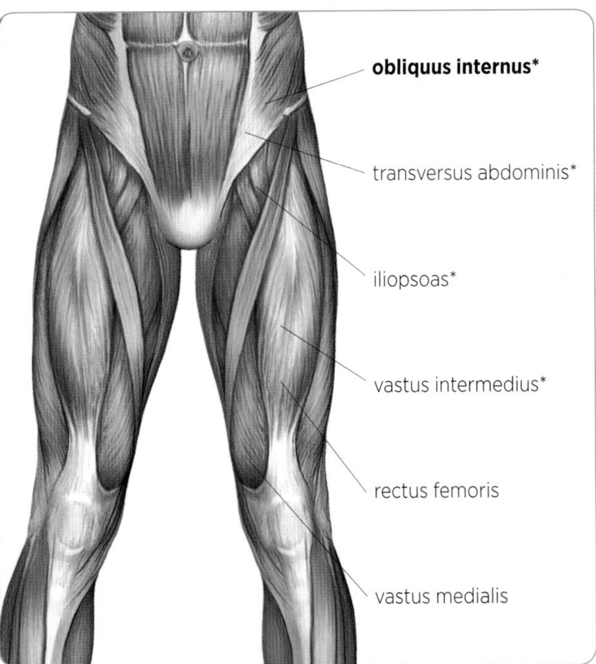

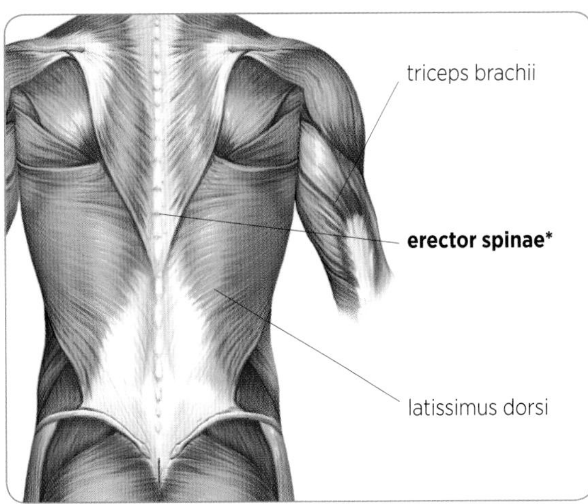

Annotation Key

Bold text indicates target muscles
Light text indicates other working muscles
* indicates deep muscles

FACT FILE

TARGETS
- Abdominals
- Obliques
- Spine

EQUIPMENT
- Dumbbells

BENEFITS
- Strengthens obliques, lower-back extensors, abdominals, and deep core stabilizers

CAUTIONS
- Back injury
- Wrist injury

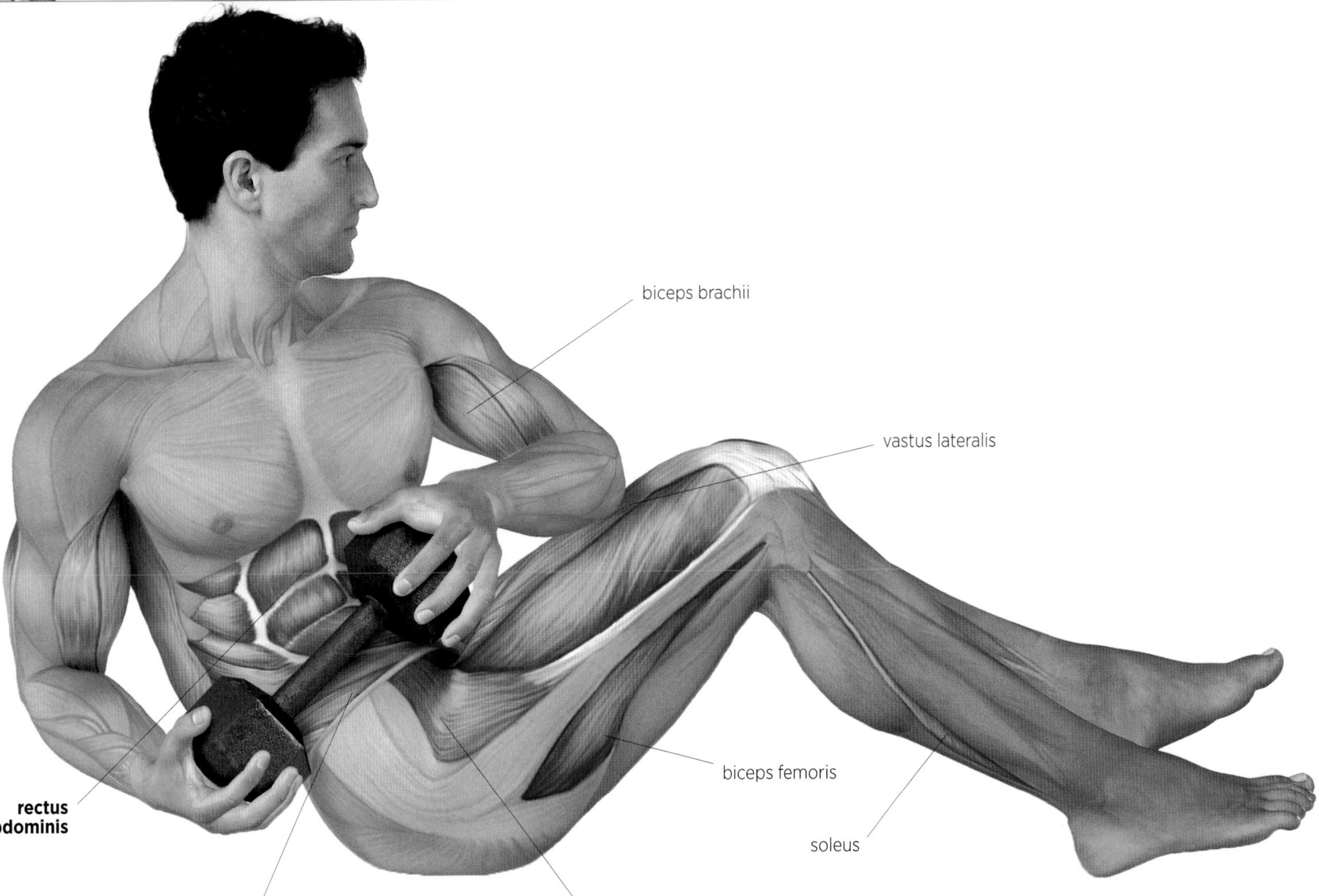

biceps brachii
vastus lateralis
biceps femoris
soleus
tensor fasciae latae
rectus abdominis
obliquus externus

Kettlebell Windmill

The Kettlebell Windmill is more than a core exercise. Along with strengthening your obliques and abdominals, it also works your deep shoulder muscles, improves overall joint mobility, and increases hip and hamstring flexibility.

HOW TO DO IT

- With your right arm by your side and your feet shoulder-width apart, stand with a kettlebell in your left hand, raised overhead.
- Push your left hip out to the left, and slightly bend your knees while lowering your torso to the right as far as possible. Pause, and then return to the starting position. Repeat for the recommended repetitions.
- Switch hands, and then repeat on the opposite side.

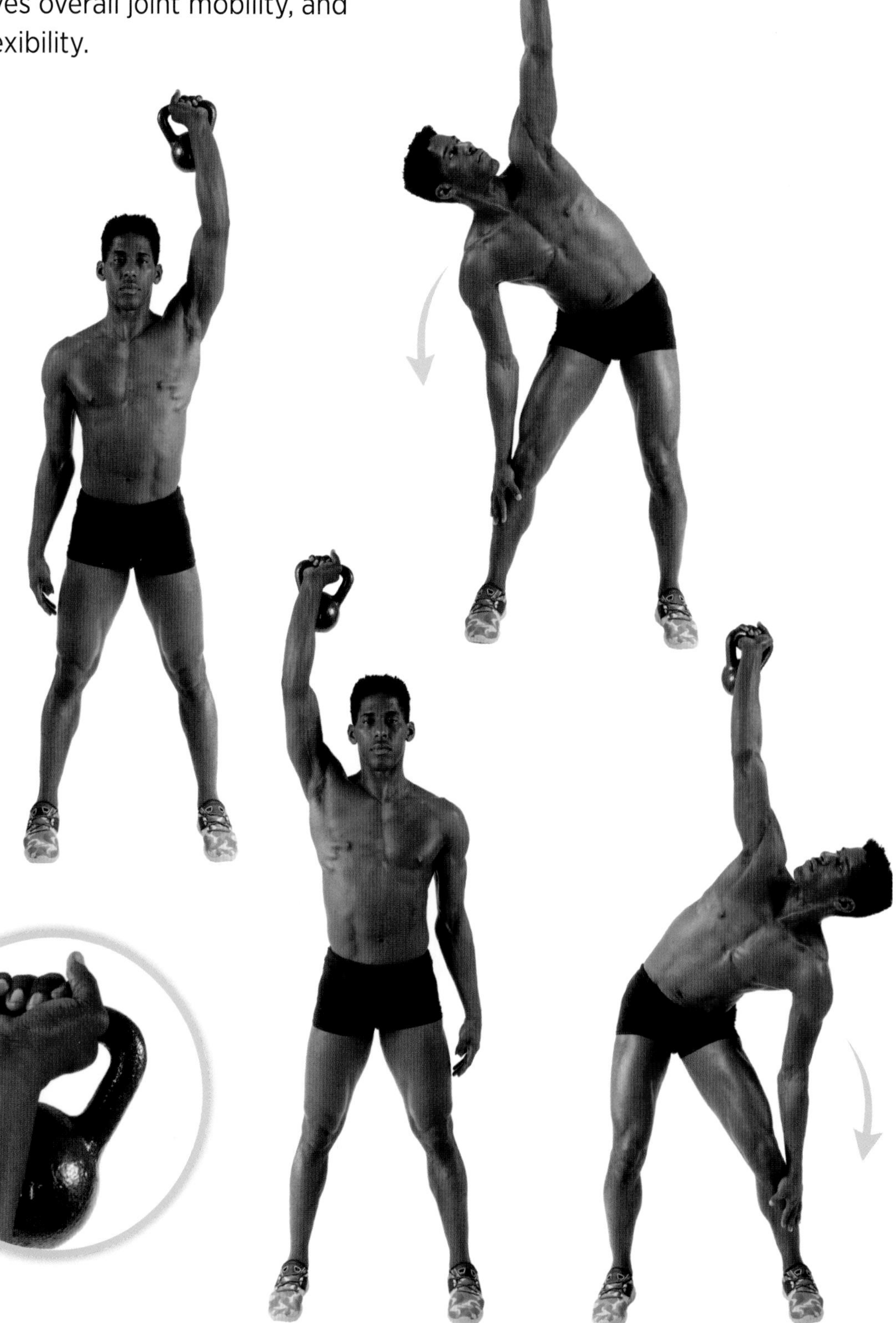

DO IT RIGHT

- Keep your back flat.
- Avoid bouncing excessively or using momentum to drive the movement.

Annotation Key

Bold text indicates target muscles
Light text indicates other working muscles
* indicates deep muscles

palmaris longus
pronator teres
triceps brachii
deltoideus anterior
serratus anterior
rectus abdominis
obliquus internus*
transversus abdominis*
tensor fasciae latae
deltoideus medialis
biceps brachii
obliquus externus
flexor carpi ulnaris
vastus intermedius*
rectus femoris
vastus medialis
vastus lateralis

gluteus medius*
gluteus minimus*
gluteus maximus
biceps femoris
semitendinosus
semimembranosus

FACT FILE

TARGETS
- Abdominals
- Obliques
- Shoulders
- Hips
- Hamstrings

EQUIPMENT
- Kettlebell

BENEFITS
- Strengthens core, upper body, and lower body
- Builds cardio and muscle endurance

CAUTIONS
- Shoulder issues
- Wrist issues
- Lower-back issues

MODIFICATION

EASIER: Perform the exercise without holding a kettlebell.

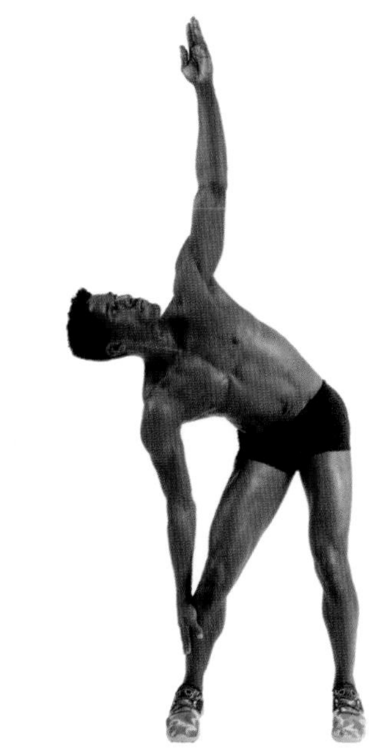

Farmer's Walk

The Farmer's Walk is fairly simple, but it is one of the best ways to increase strength, stamina and endurance. It involves walking carrying a weight in each hand for a set distance (for example, the length of the gym) or time (say, 20 to 30 seconds).

HOW TO DO IT

- Stand with your feet shoulder-width apart holding a pair of kettlebells at your sides.
- Walk rapidly for a predetermined distance or time. Lower the weights, rest, and then repeat for the recommended sets.

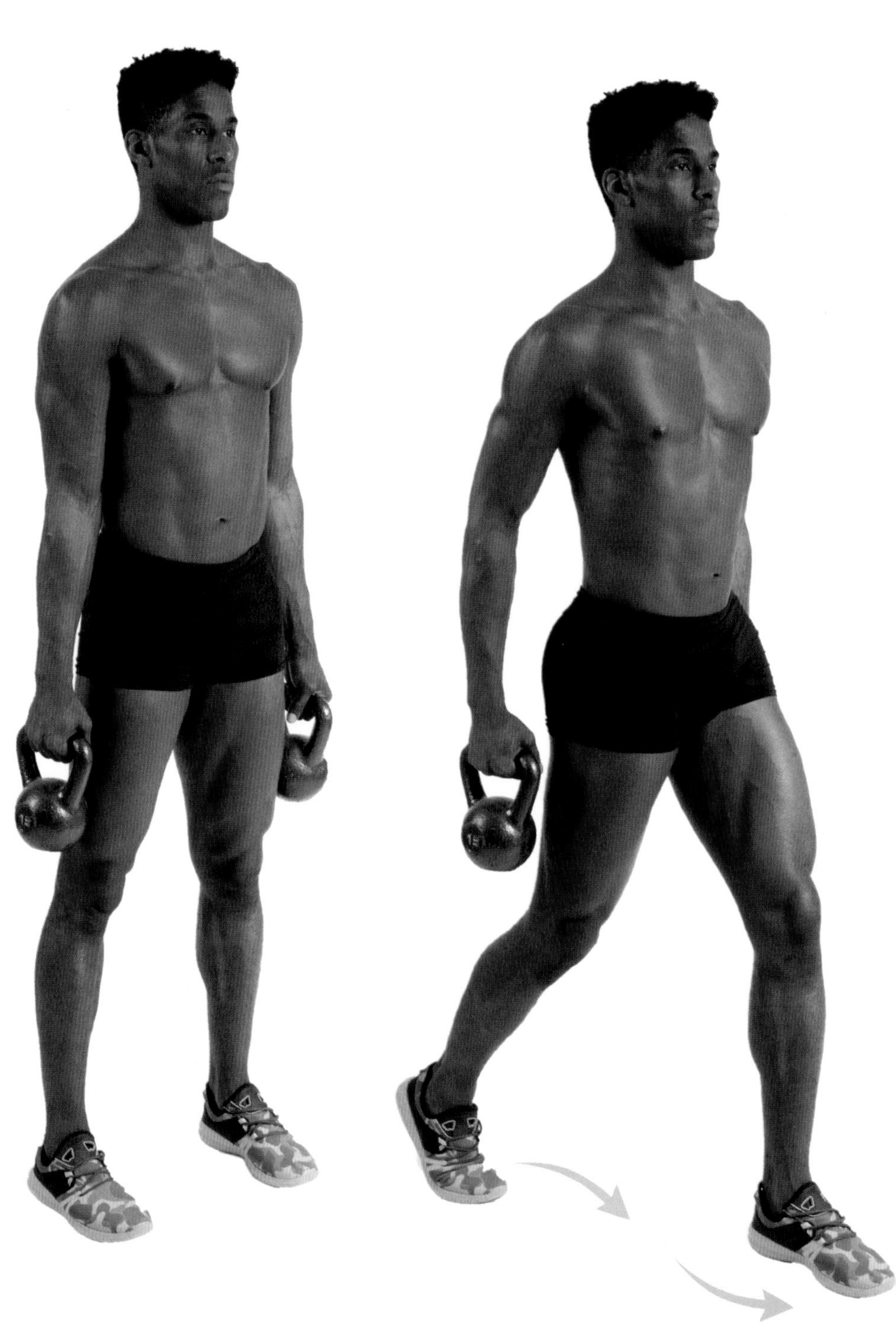

DO IT RIGHT

- Keep your core engaged.
- Keep your lower back and pelvis aligned.
- Keep your shoulders as tight as possible to improve joint stability.
- Breathe in through your nose and then forcefully out through your mouth; this will push your ribs down.
- Keep your ears directly over your shoulders and hips.
- Avoid using heavier weights than you can safely handle.

FACT FILE

TARGETS
- Abdominals
- Spine
- Forearms
- Biceps

EQUIPMENT
- Kettlebells

BENEFITS
- Strengthens and stabilizes core
- Develops grip strength in forearms

CAUTIONS
- Wrist issues

trapezius
deltoideus medialis
latissimus dorsi
triceps brachii
brachialis
biceps brachii
palmaris longus
extensor digitorum
flexor carpi ulnaris
deltoideus anterior
rectus abdominis
obliquus externus
obliquus internus*
transversus abdominis*

deltoideus posterior
teres major
trapezius
erector spinae*
latissimus dorsi
multifidus spinae*

deltoideus anterior
biceps brachii
palmaris longus
flexor digitorum*
pronator teres

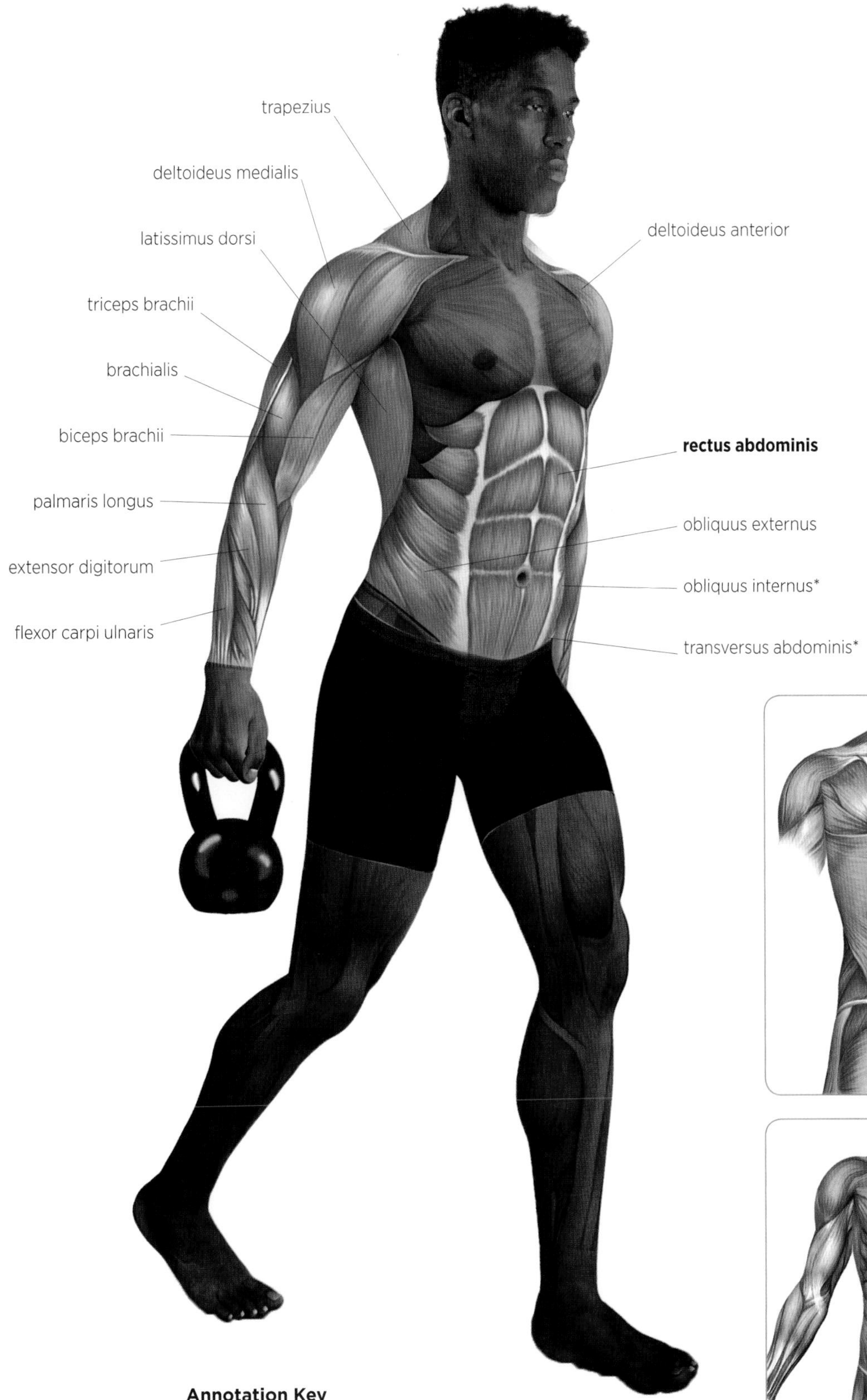

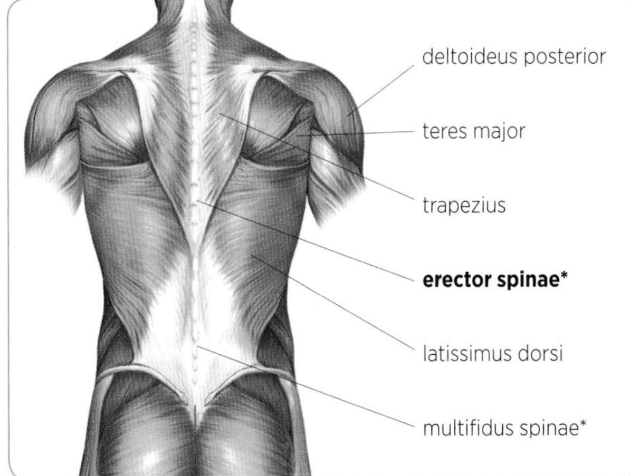

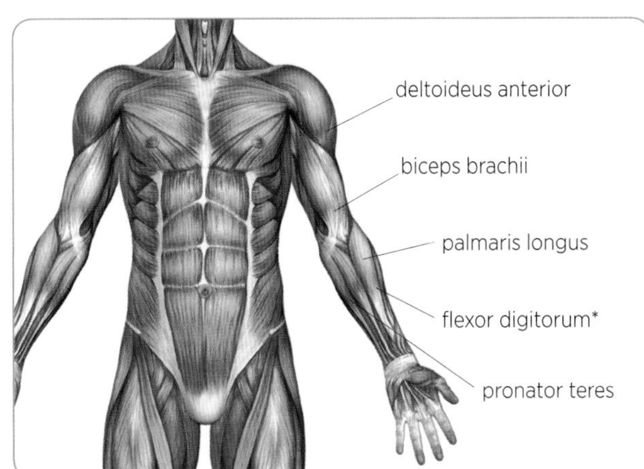

Annotation Key
Bold text indicates target muscles
Light text indicates other working muscles
* indicates deep muscles

Single-Arm Kettlebell Press-Up

The Single-Arm Kettlebell Press-up uses resistance to make an already effective exercise that much more difficult and beneficial. Requiring midline stability, core strength, and upper-extremity strength, this exercise will condition everything from the waist up.

FACT FILE

TARGETS
- Abdominals
- Deltoids
- Triceps
- Pectorals
- Hip flexors

EQUIPMENT
- Kettlebell

BENEFITS
- Strengthens and tones abdominals, chest, and arms
- Improves midline stability

CAUTIONS
- Lower-back issues
- Wrist issues

HOW TO DO IT
- Holding a kettlebell in your right hand, lie faceup with your legs extended.
- Contracting your core, perform a sit-up while pressing the kettlebell up toward the ceiling.
- With a controlled descent, lower both your torso and your arm to return to the starting position. Repeat for the recommended repetitions.
- Switch hands, and then repeat on the opposite side.

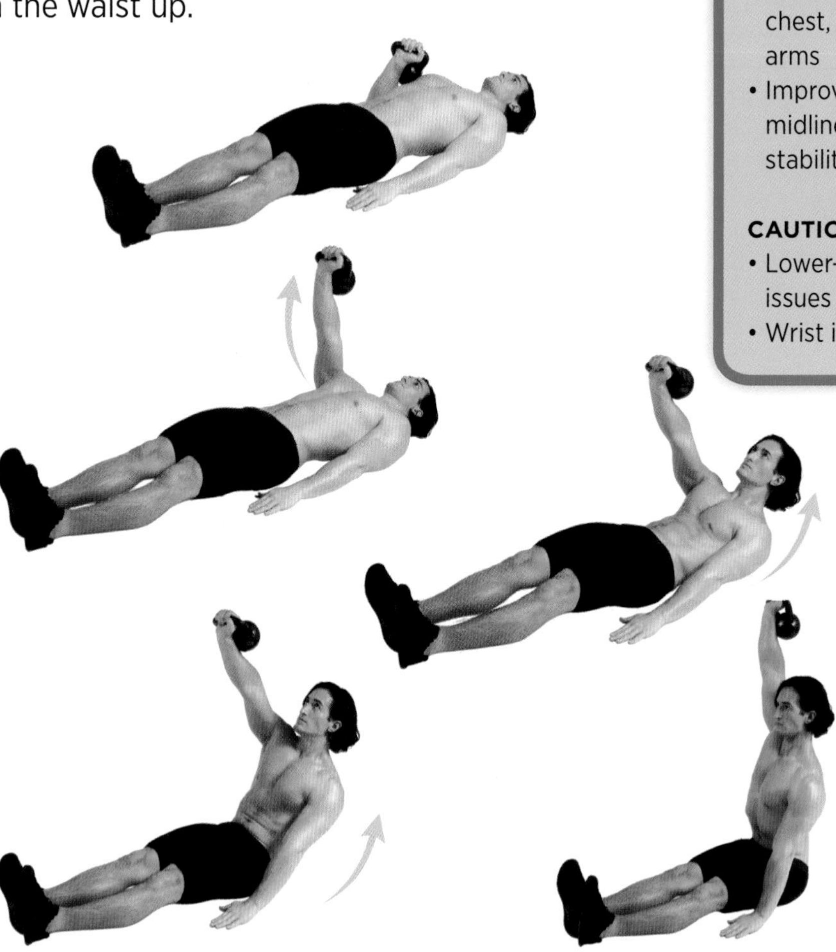

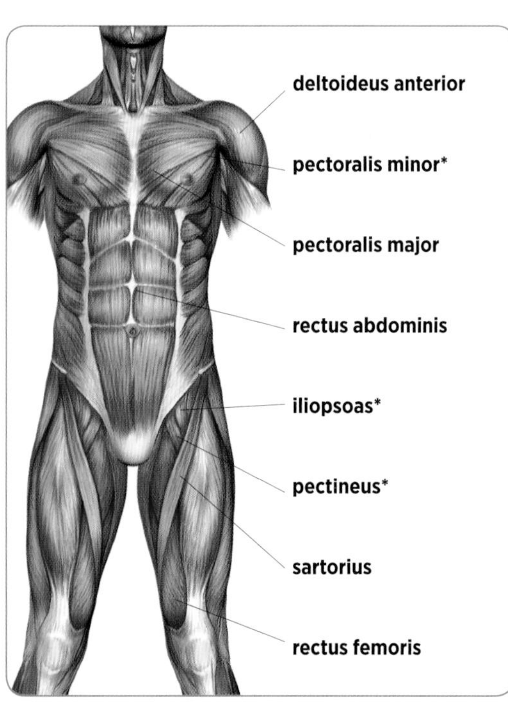

triceps brachii

DO IT RIGHT
- Keep your core engaged.
- Avoid swaying your trunk away from your midline.

Annotation Key

Bold text indicates target muscles
Light text indicates other working muscles
* indicates deep muscles

Kettlebell Toe Toucher

The Kettlebell Toe Toucher engages the full length of your abdominal muscles, requiring full contraction against resistance and gravity, sitting balance, and coordination. This is an excellent core exercise to add to your program.

FACT FILE

TARGETS
- Abdominals
- Back
- Shoulders
- Hip flexors

EQUIPMENT
- Kettlebell

BENEFITS
- Strengthens and tones abdominals, arms, and legs
- Improves sitting balance
- Improves coordination

CAUTIONS
- Lower-back issues

HOW TO DO IT

- Lie faceup with your legs extended holding a kettlebell in both hands with your arms extended above your head.
- Contracting your core, draw the kettlebell forward over your chest as you sit up. Simultaneously perform a leg lift, so that your body forms a V, reaching the kettlebell toward your feet to touch your toes.
- Lower your torso and legs to the floor, allowing the kettlebell to travel overhead and toward the floor to return to the starting position. Repeat for the recommended repetitions.

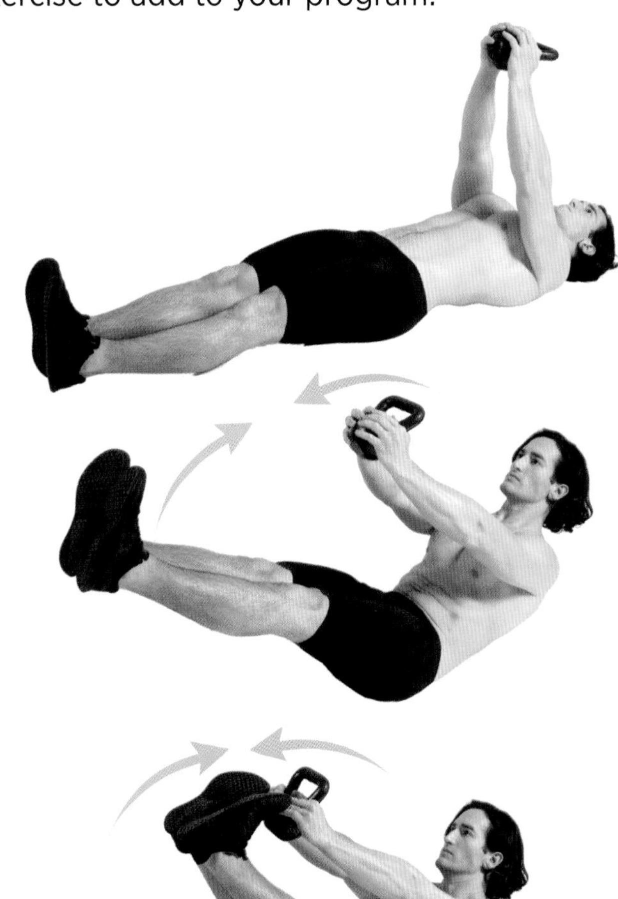

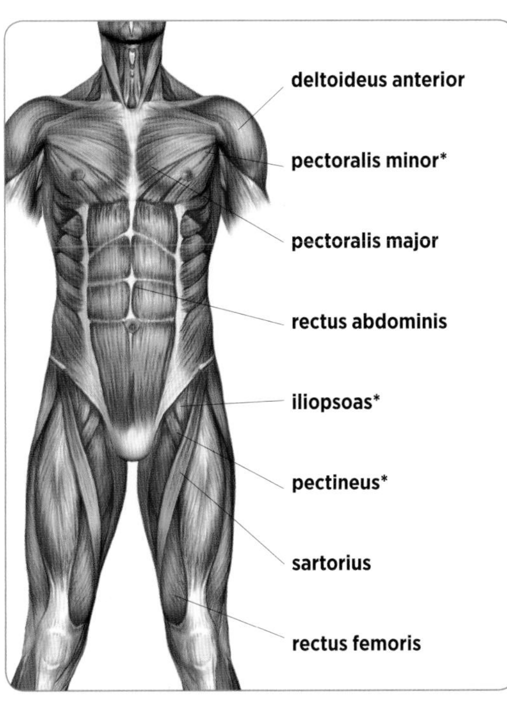

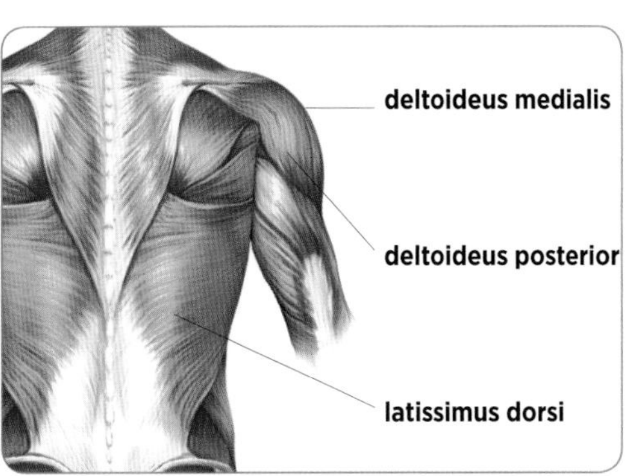

DO IT RIGHT
- Keep your core engaged.
- Avoid excessively arching in your lower back.

Annotation Key

Bold text indicates target muscles
Light text indicates other working muscles
* indicates deep muscles

Flat Bench Dumbbell Squat

The Flat Bench Dumbbell Squat takes squat exercises to another level. Descending to the bench ensures that you execute a deep squat, and the added weight of the dumbbells increases the exercise's intensity.

HOW TO DO IT

- Stand about 1 to 2 feet in front of a flat bench with your feet parallel and placed generously outside of shoulder width. Grasp a dumbbell in each hand using hammer grip with your palms facing each other.
- Squat down toward the bench, lightly touching the bench with your glutes.
- Slowly raise back to the starting position. Repeat for the recommended repetitions.

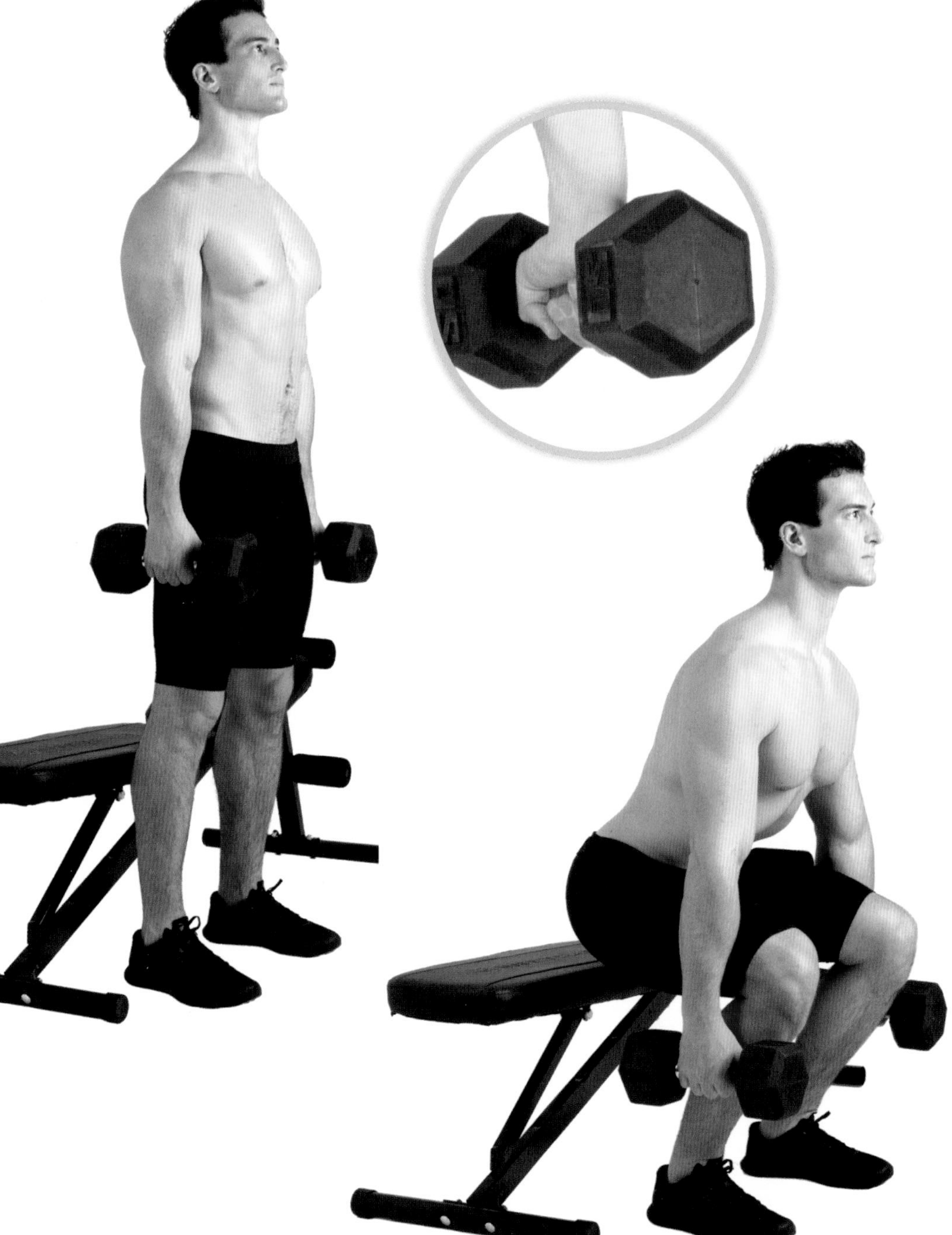

DO IT RIGHT

- Keep your torso upright.
- Align your head with your spine, and keep your chin slightly up.
- Avoid rolling your shoulders and upper back forward.

FACT FILE

TARGETS
- Quadriceps
- Glutes

EQUIPMENT
- Dumbbells
- Flat bench

BENEFITS
- Strengthens thighs and glutes

CAUTIONS
- Shoulder issues
- Wrist issues
- Knee issues

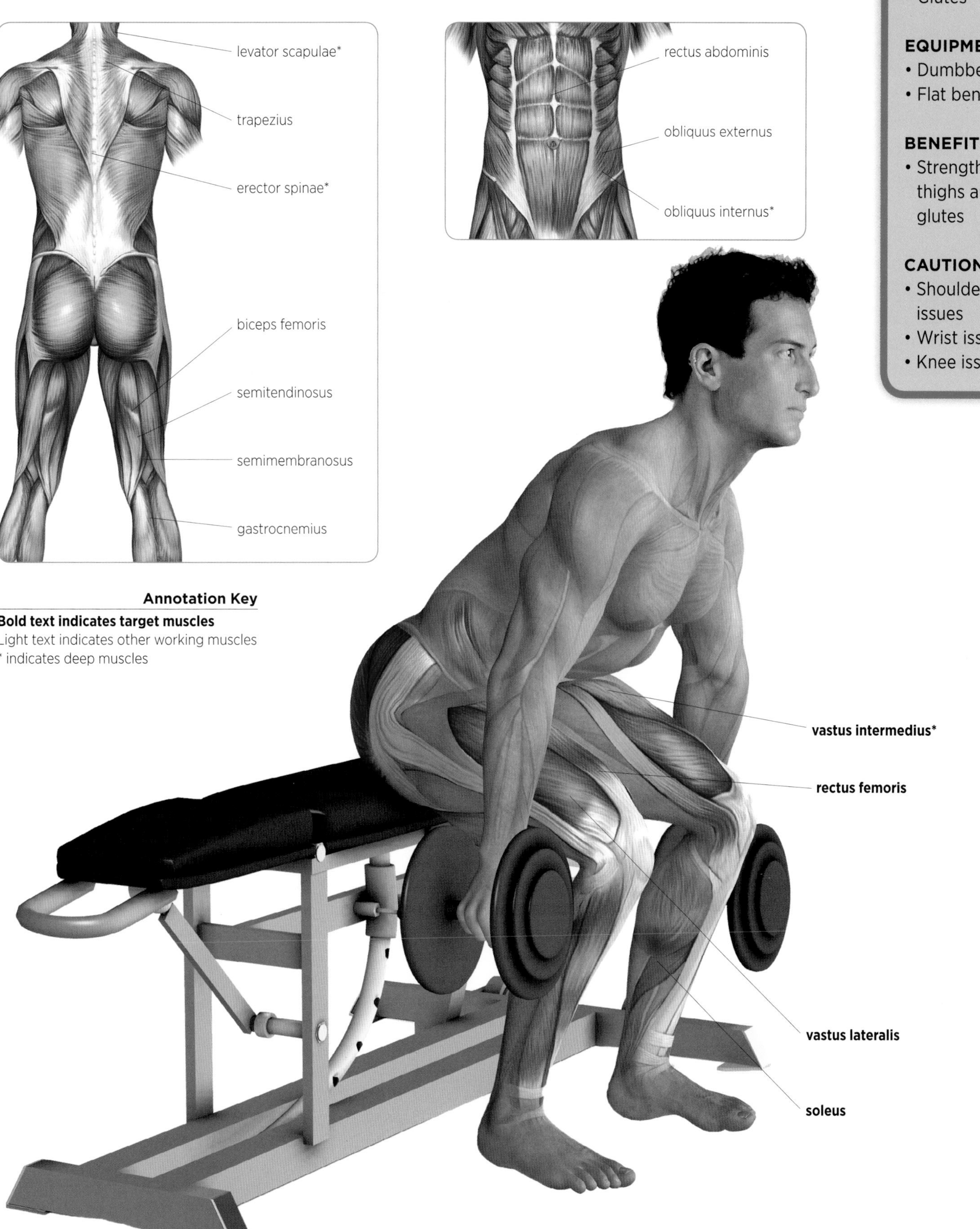

Annotation Key

Bold text indicates target muscles

Light text indicates other working muscles

* indicates deep muscles

Flat Bench Step-Up

The demanding Flat Bench Step-Up challenges your strength, balance, and coordination in an stepping-upward action that targets your glutes and hamstrings. If you don't have a flat bench, try it with a sturdy chair or solid coffee table.

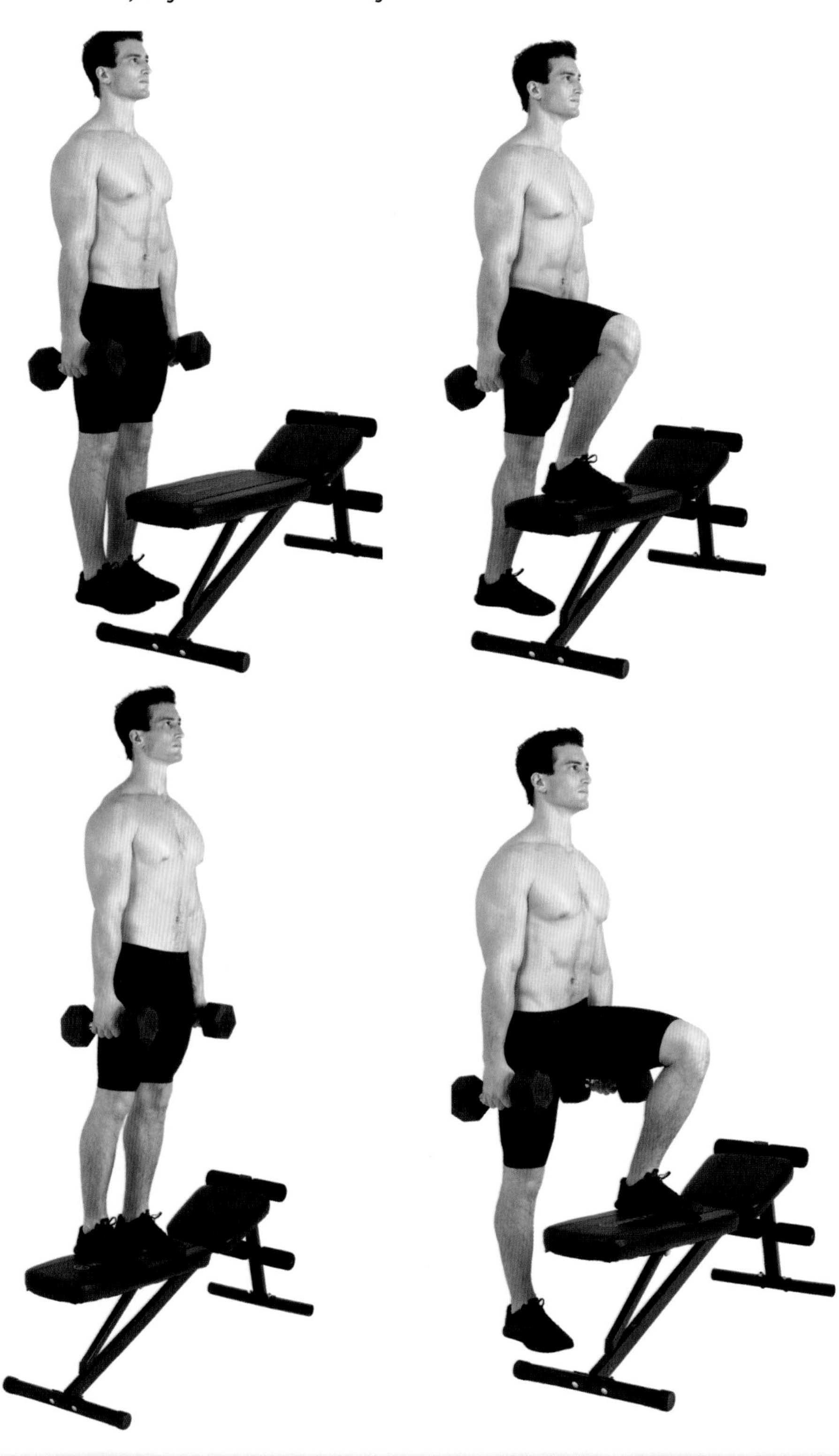

HOW TO DO IT

- Stand about 1 foot behind a flat bench with your feet parallel and close together. Grip a dumbbell in each hand.
- Step your right leg onto the bench.
- Bring your left leg up beside your right leg.
- Step down with your right leg, and then step down with your left to return to the starting position.
- Continue leading with the right foot up and off the bench for the recommended repetitions. Switch legs, and then repeat on the opposite side.

DO IT RIGHT

- Keep your torso upright.
- Maintain a slow, even, and steady pace with both the step-ups and the step-downs.
- Avoid rolling your shoulders and upper back forward.
- Avoid using the leg on the floor to help lift yourself onto the bench.
- Avoiding letting the knee of the stepping leg cave inward.

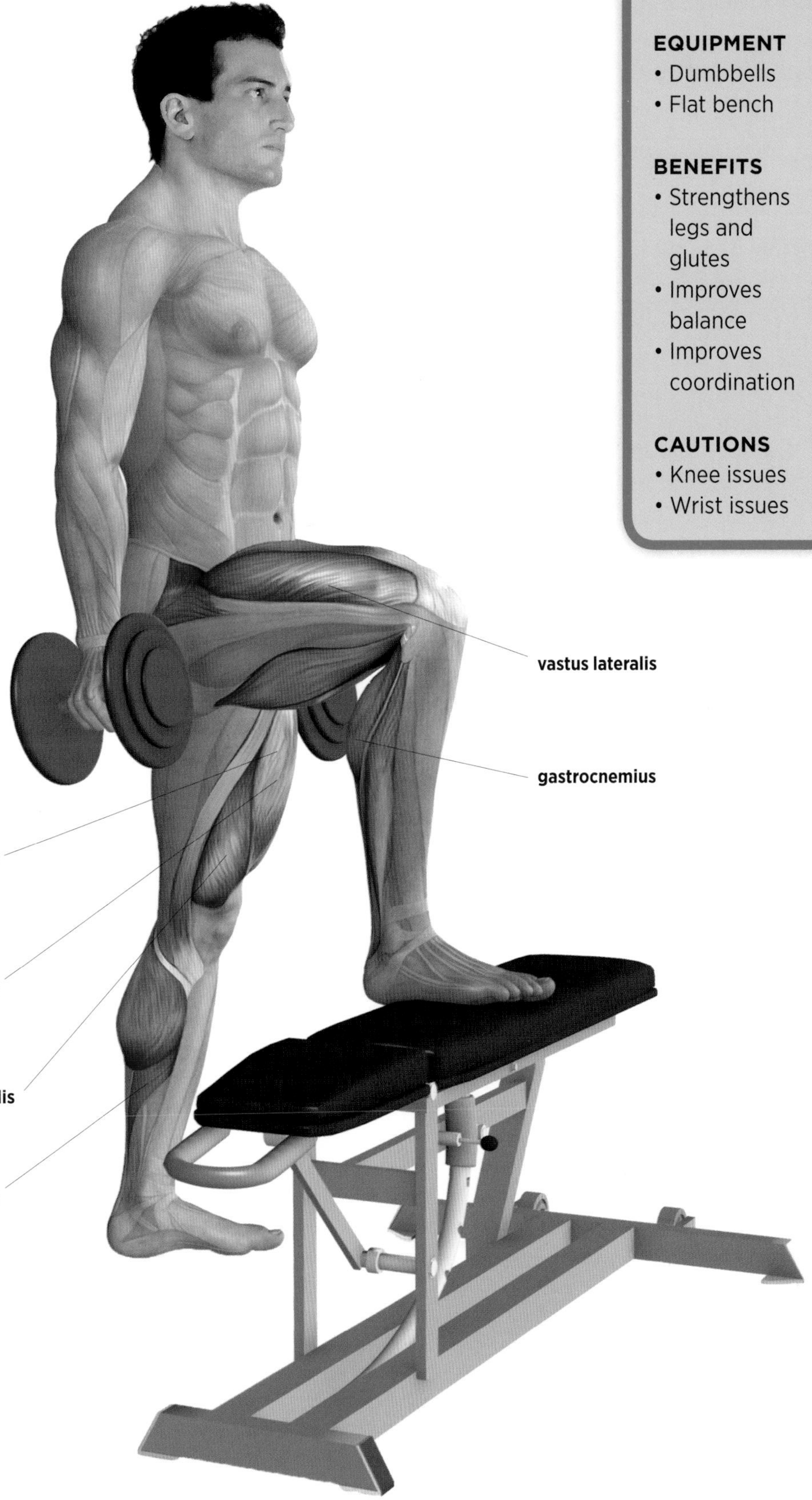

FACT FILE

TARGETS
- Quadriceps
- Hamstrings
- Glutes
- Calves

EQUIPMENT
- Dumbbells
- Flat bench

BENEFITS
- Strengthens legs and glutes
- Improves balance
- Improves coordination

CAUTIONS
- Knee issues
- Wrist issues

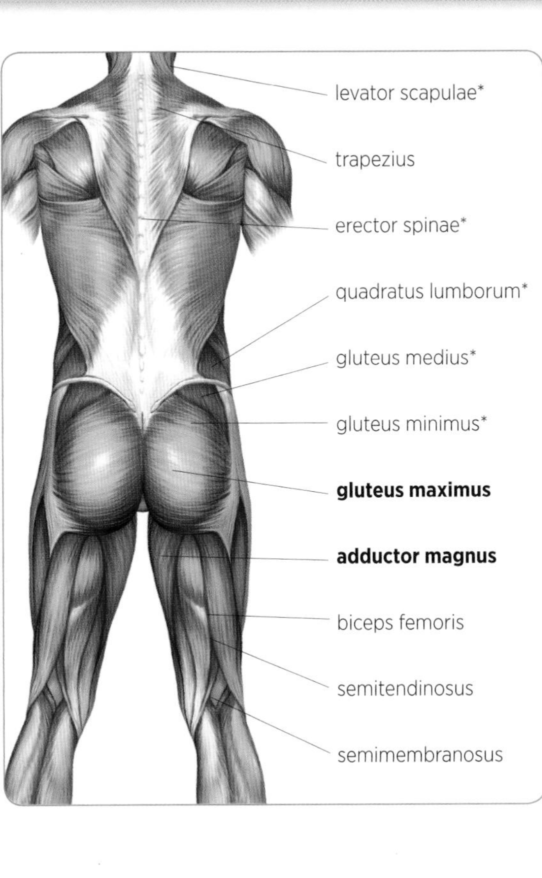

vastus lateralis

gastrocnemius

vastus intermedius*

rectus femoris

vastus medialis

soleus

Annotation Key

Bold text indicates target muscles
Light text indicates other working muscles
* indicates deep muscles

Dumbbell Lunge

The Dumbbell Lunge targets your quadriceps, hamstrings, and glutes. All lunges are great for toning your thighs and butt, but adding the dumbbells demands even more from your upper-leg and gluteal muscles.

HOW TO DO IT

- Stand with your feet planted about shoulder-width apart, and your arms at your sides with a dumbbell in each hand.
- Keeping your head up and your spine in a neutral position, take a big step forward with your right leg. At the same time, bend your knee to a 90-degree angle, and drop your thigh until it is parallel to the floor. Your left knee will drop behind you so that you are balancing on the toes of your left foot, creating a straight line from your spine to the back of your knee.
- Push through your right heel to stand upright, and then return to starting position. Repeat on the opposite side. Continue alternating sides for the recommended repetitions.

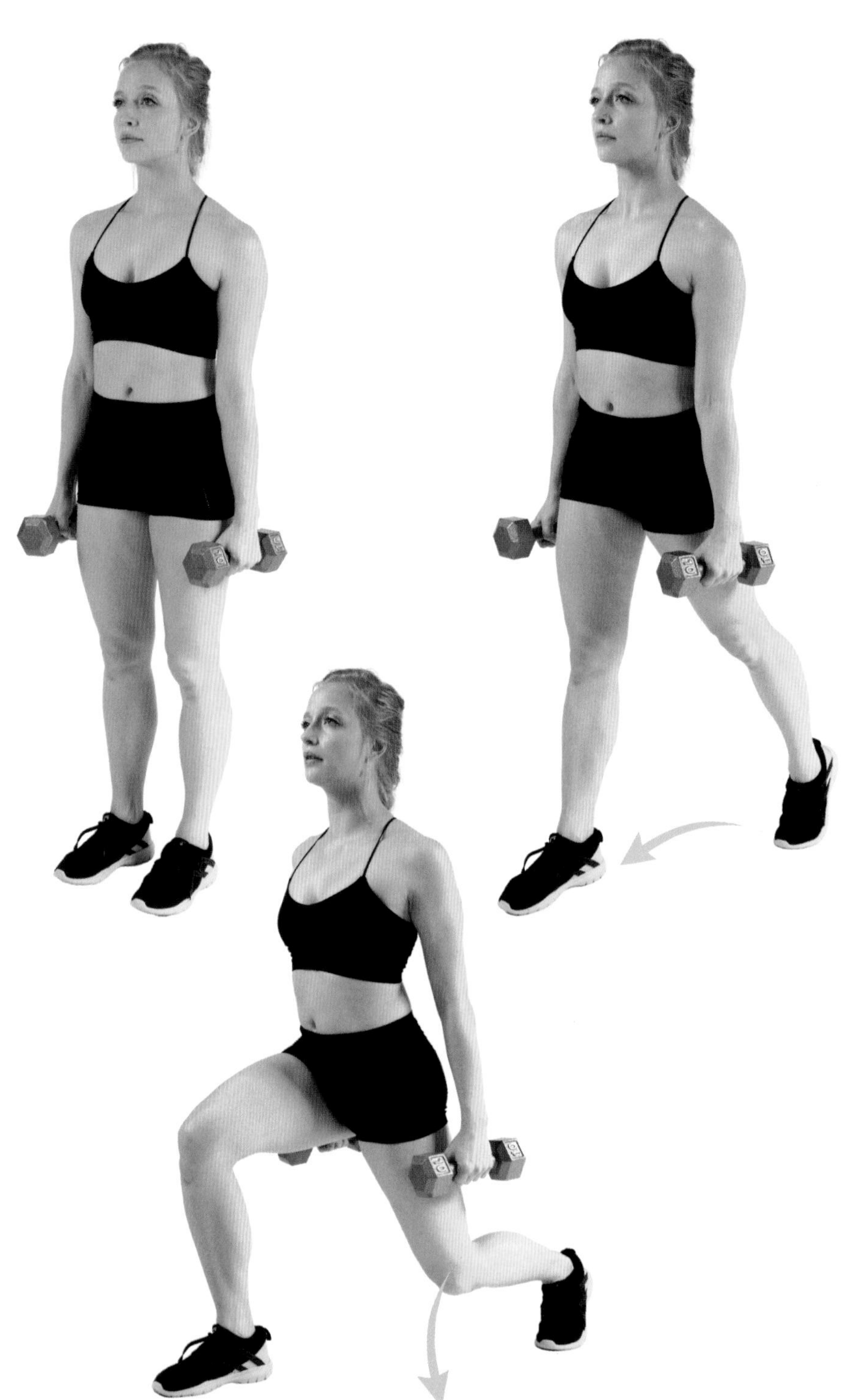

DO IT RIGHT

- Keep your body facing forward as you step one leg in front of you.
- Gaze forward.
- Make sure that your front knee is facing forward.
- Avoid turning your body to one side.
- Avoid allowing your front knee to extend beyond your foot.
- Avoid arching your back.

FACT FILE

TARGETS
- Quadriceps
- Glutes

EQUIPMENT
- Dumbbells

BENEFITS
- Strengthens and tones quadriceps and glutes

CAUTIONS
- Knee issues
- Wrist issues

Annotation Key

Bold text indicates target muscles
Light text indicates other working muscles
* indicates deep muscles

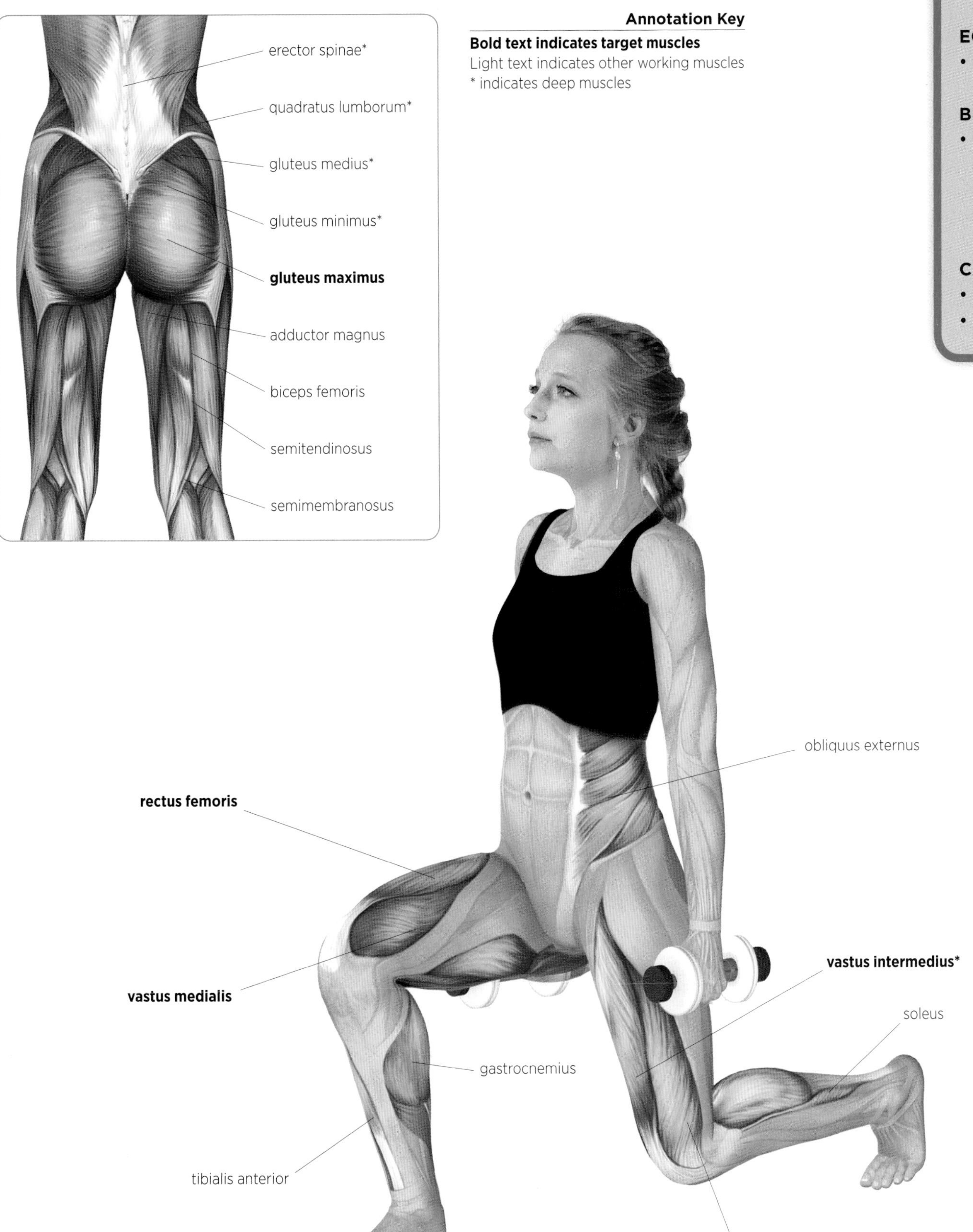

Kettlebell Single-Leg Russian Deadlift

The Kettlebell Single-Leg Russian Deadlift is an effective exercise to build strength and stability throughout your lower extremities and core. By focusing on one side at a time and offsetting balance, it facilitates hamstring, glute, and core strength and endurance.

FACT FILE

TARGETS
- Hamstrings
- Glutes
- Back

EQUIPMENT
- Kettlebell

BENEFITS
- Strengthens and tones back and abdominals
- Improves balance
- Improves coordination

CAUTIONS
- Lower-back pain

HOW TO DO IT

- Stand with your feet together with the kettlebell in your right hand hanging by your side.
- Pivoting at the hips and keeping your back in a neutral position, allow your left foot to travel back behind you and in the air, while you reach the kettlebell toward the floor in front of your planted right foot.
- Touch the kettlebell to the floor while your left leg should be extended behind you, nearly parallel to the floor and in a straight line with your back.
- Reverse the steps above to return to the starting position. Repeat for the recommended repetitions, and then repeat on the opposite side.

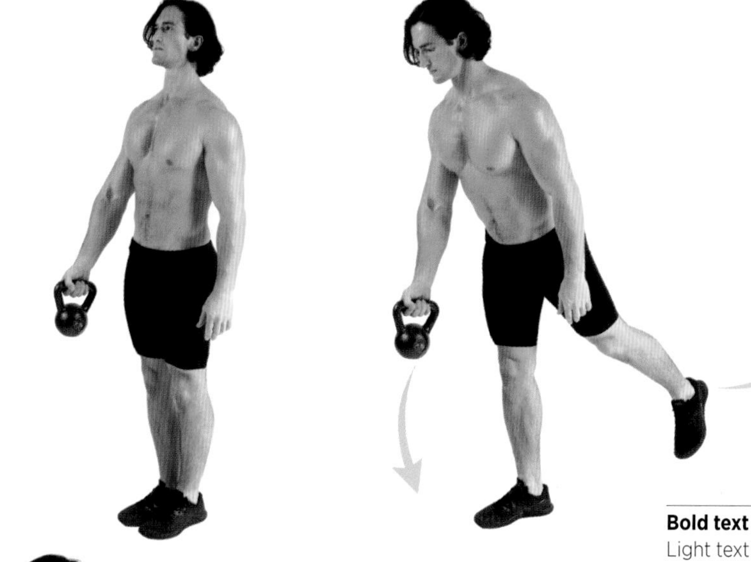

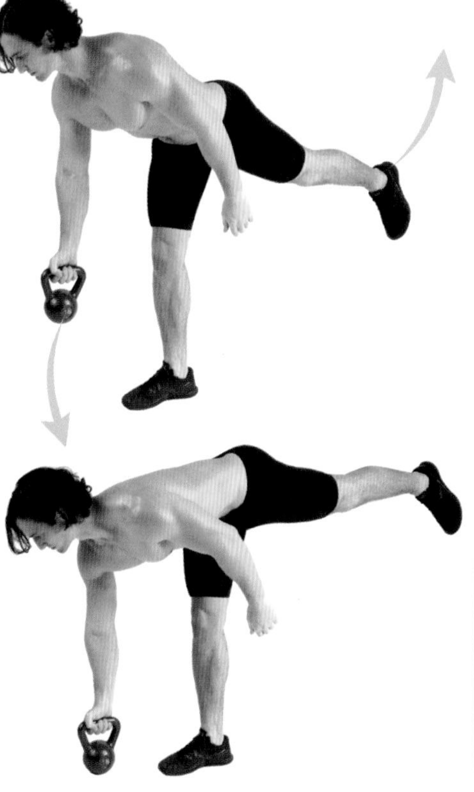

DO IT RIGHT

- Employ a full range of motion.
- Avoid hyperextending your knees past your toes.

Annotation Key
Bold text indicates target muscles
Light text indicates other working muscles
* indicates deep muscles

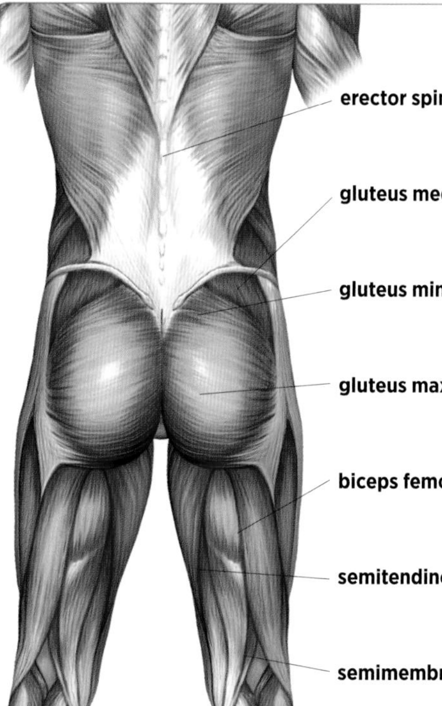

Goblet Squat

Your hand position—holding a weight in front of your chest as if your were clutching a goblet—gives this exercise its name. This full-body movement works your quads, calves, glutes, and core. It also gives your arms a workout and can improve your grip strength.

FACT FILE

TARGETS
- Quadriceps
- Calves
- Glutes
- Hamstrings
- Shoulders

EQUIPMENT
- Kettlebell

BENEFITS
- Strengthens legs, glutes, and shoulders

CAUTIONS
- Hip issues
- Knee issues

HOW TO DO IT

- Holding a kettlebell with both hands close to your chest, stand with your feet placed generously outside of shoulder-width apart with your toes pointing slightly outward.
- Squat down until your thighs are parallel to the floor, bringing your elbows to your thighs.
- Keeping your back flat, push through your heels back to the starting position. Repeat for the recommended repetitions.

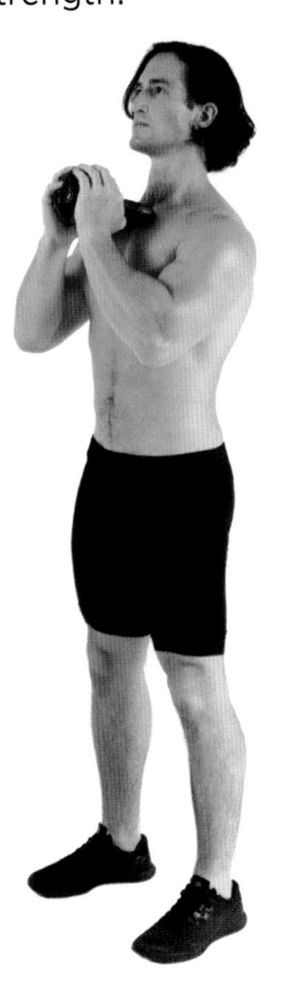

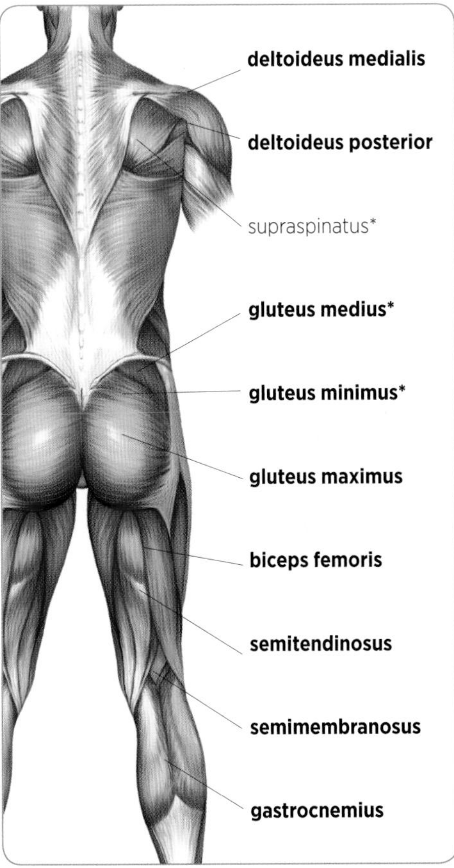

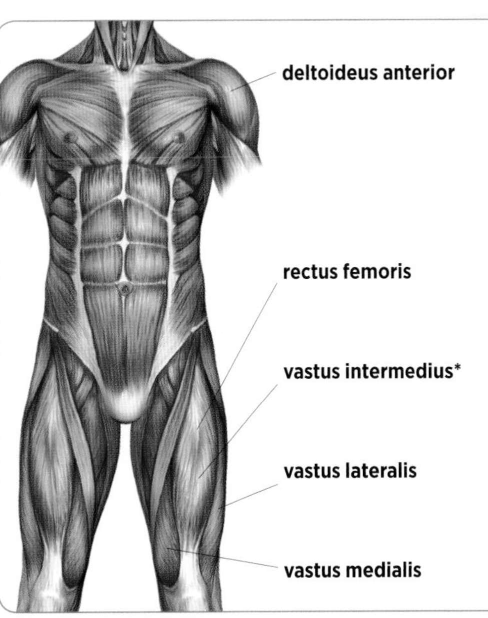

DO IT RIGHT

- Employ a full range of motion.
- Avoid hyperextending your knees past your toes.

Annotation Key

Bold text indicates target muscles
Light text indicates other working muscles
* indicates deep muscles

Plyo Goblet Squat

The Plyo Goblet Squat adds a burst of upward movement to the basic Goblet Squat (page 213). Just as the basic exercise does, it targets your quads, calves, glutes, and core. This plyometric boost will also train these muscles to produce power.

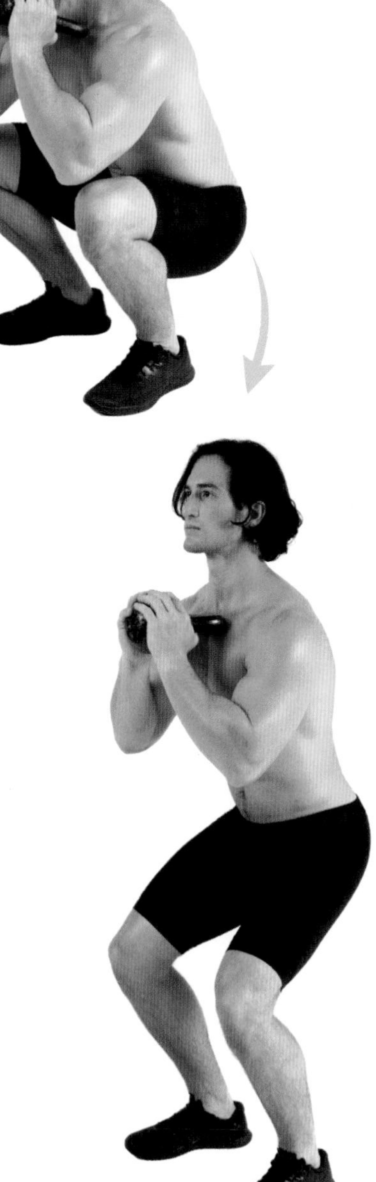

HOW TO DO IT

- Holding a kettlebell with both hands close to your chest, stand with your feet placed generously outside of shoulder-width apart with your toes pointing slightly outward.
- Squat down until your thighs are parallel to the floor, bringing your elbows to your thighs.
- Applying force with your legs, push through your heels to propel yourself upward into a jump, straightening your body.
- Land softly back into a half squat, and then rise to the starting position. Repeat for the recommended repetitions.

DO IT RIGHT

- Employ a full range of motion.
- Avoid hyperextending your knees past your toes.
- Land as softly as you can to avoid stress on your joints.

FACT FILE

TARGETS
- Quadriceps
- Calves
- Glutes
- Hamstrings
- Shoulders

EQUIPMENT
- Kettlebell

BENEFITS
- Strengthens legs, glutes, and shoulders
- Increases cardiovascular endurance
- Burn calories

CAUTIONS
- Hip issues
- Knee issues

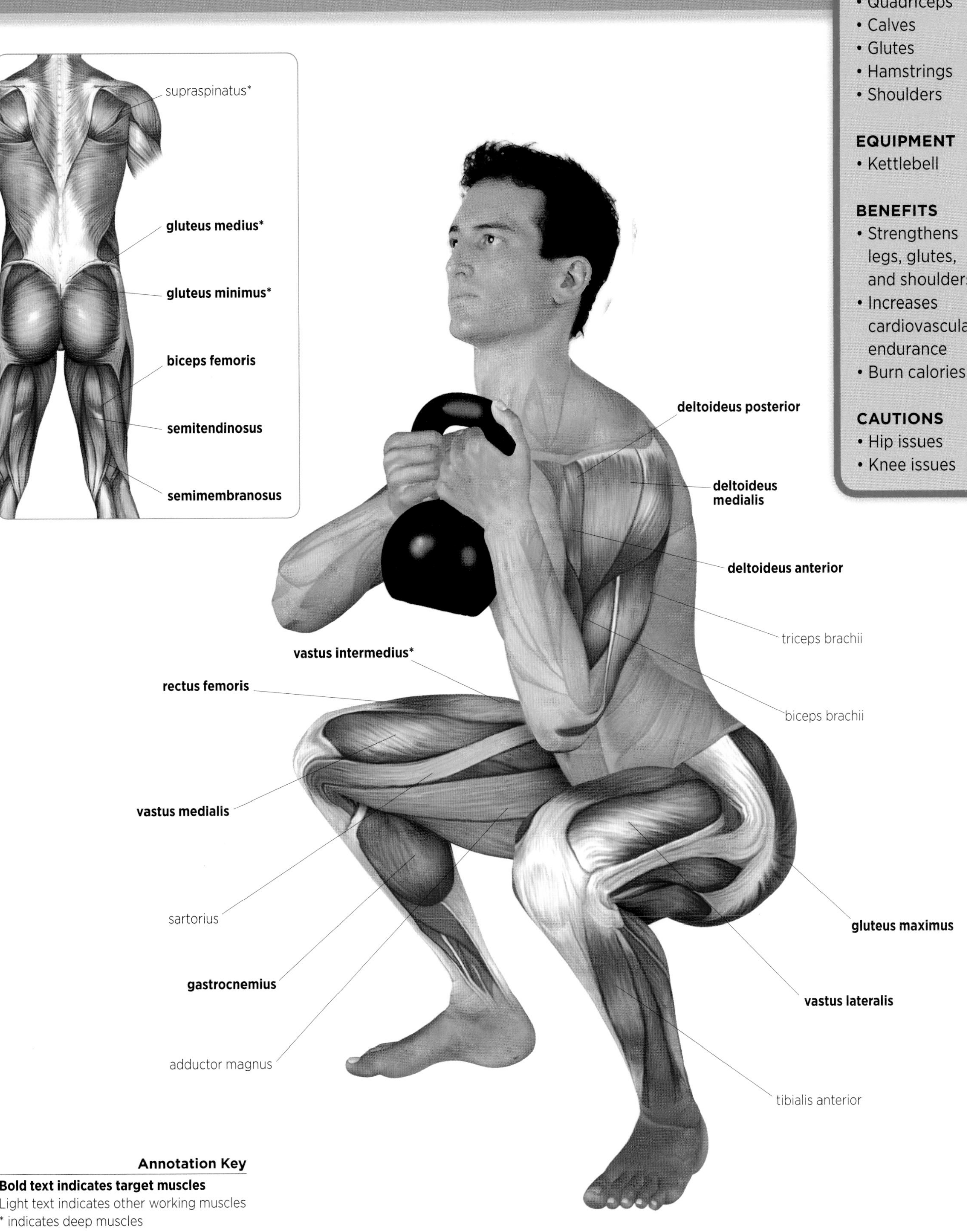

Annotation Key

Bold text indicates target muscles
Light text indicates other working muscles
* indicates deep muscles

Sumo Squat with Dumbbell

Foot placement plays an important role when performing a squat exercise. Also known as the Plié Dumbbell Squat, this squat variation uses a wide stance to home in on your outer glutes and inner thighs.

HOW TO DO IT

- Holding a dumbbell between your leg, stand with your feet turned out and planted wide beyond shoulder-width apart.
- Keeping your torso upright, bend your knees to lower into a squat position.
- Push through your heels to rise back into the starting position. Repeat for the recommended repetitions.

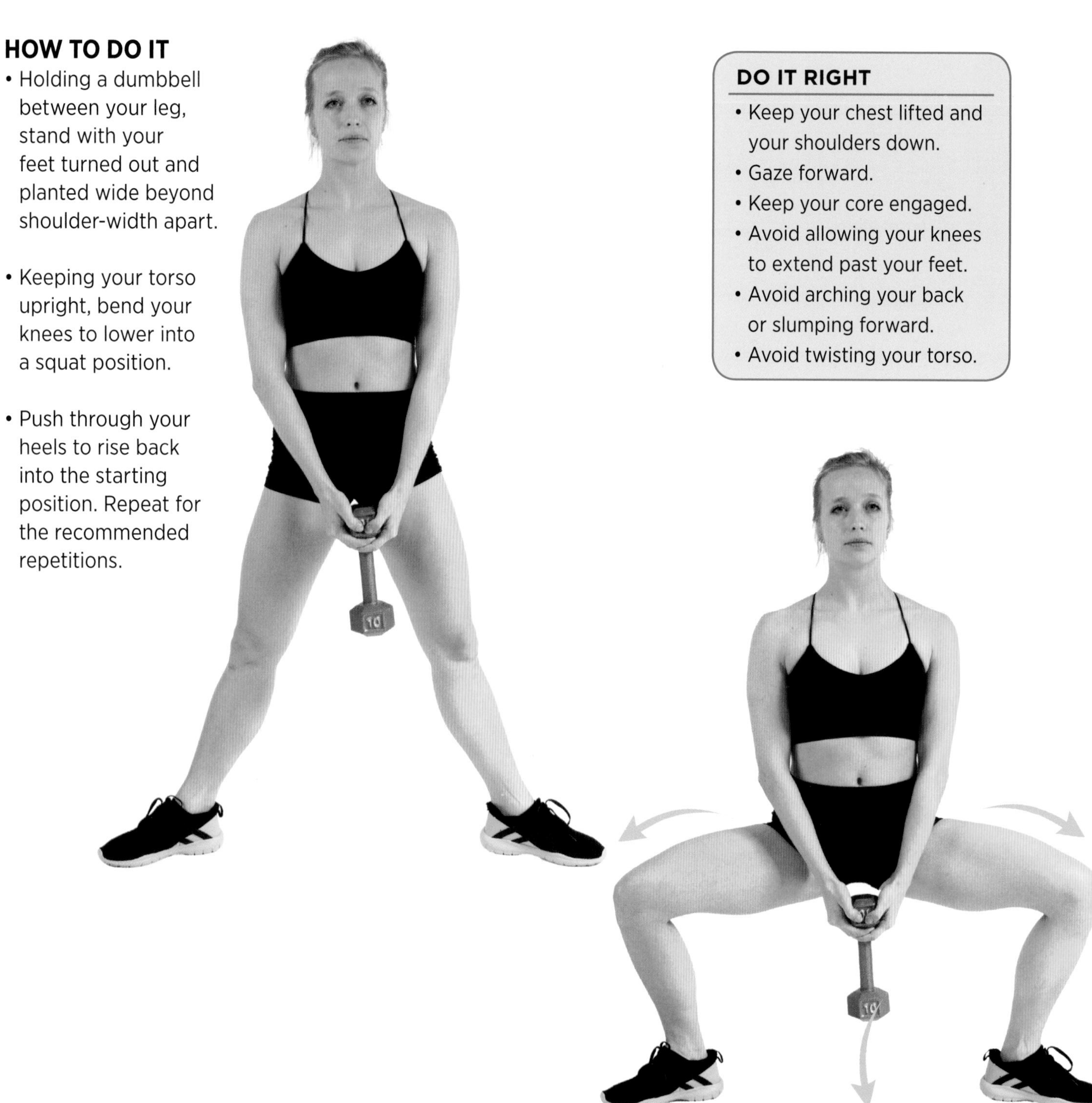

DO IT RIGHT

- Keep your chest lifted and your shoulders down.
- Gaze forward.
- Keep your core engaged.
- Avoid allowing your knees to extend past your feet.
- Avoid arching your back or slumping forward.
- Avoid twisting your torso.

FACT FILE

TARGETS
- Quadriceps
- Glutes
- Hip adductors

EQUIPMENT
- Dumbbell

BENEFITS
- Strengthens and tones quadriceps and glutes

CAUTIONS
- Knee issues
- Wrist issues

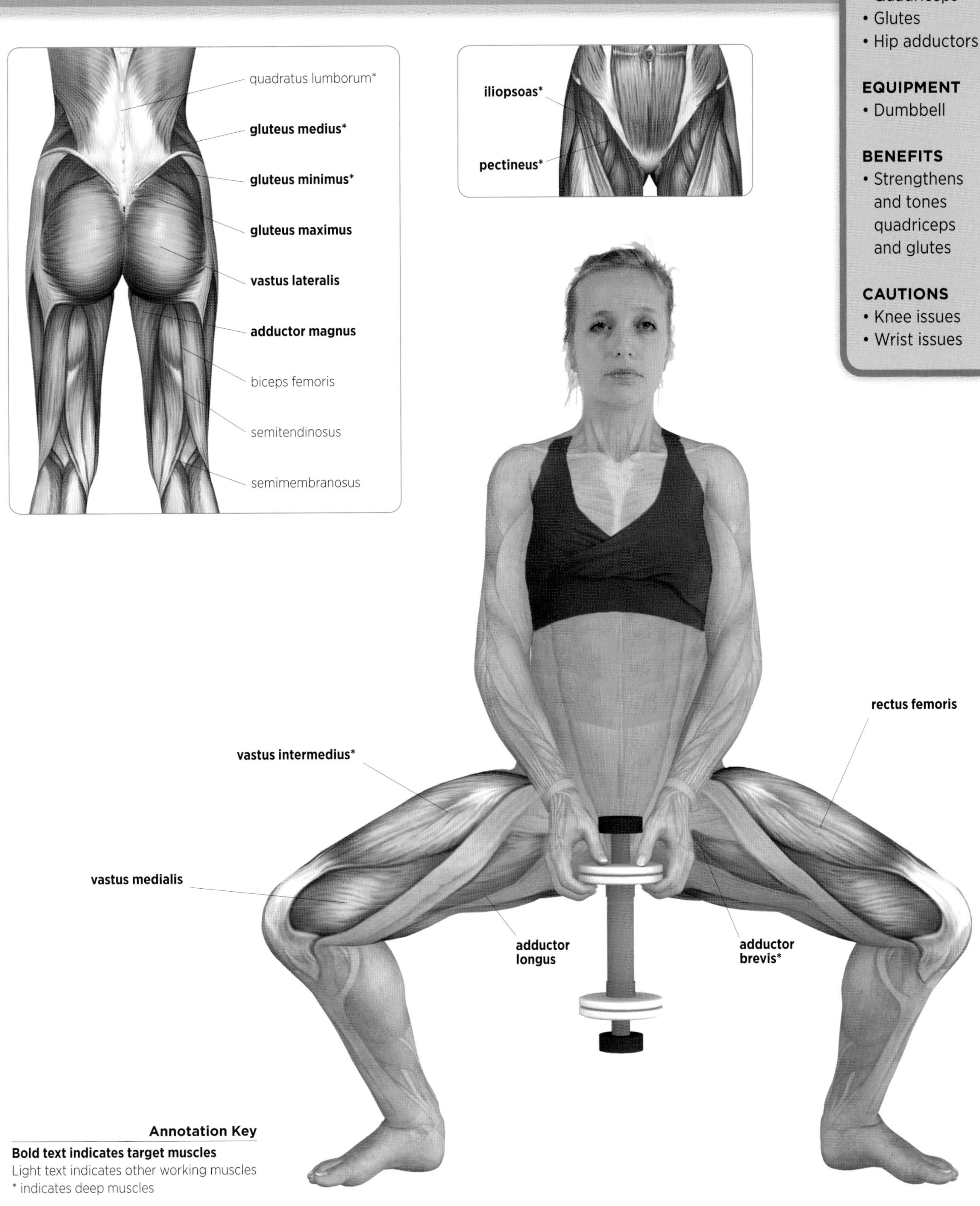

Annotation Key

Bold text indicates target muscles
Light text indicates other working muscles
* indicates deep muscles

Kettlebell Figure 8

The Kettlebell Figure strengthens your legs, abdominals, and arms and helps improve your coordination, balance, and body awareness. This fun exercise employs a complex movement pattern that will keep you stimulated.

HOW TO DO IT

- Stand with your feet placed generously outside of shoulder-width holding a kettlebell in your right hand between your legs. Bend forward slightly, keeping your back flat and pushing out your butt.
- Bring the kettlebell towards your left leg, and receive it in your left hand, which should come from behind your left leg.
- Repeat the movement with your left hand, passing the kettlebell from in front of your left leg to your right hand behind your right leg. This forms a figure 8 around your static legs.
- Repeat in both directions for the recommended repetitions.

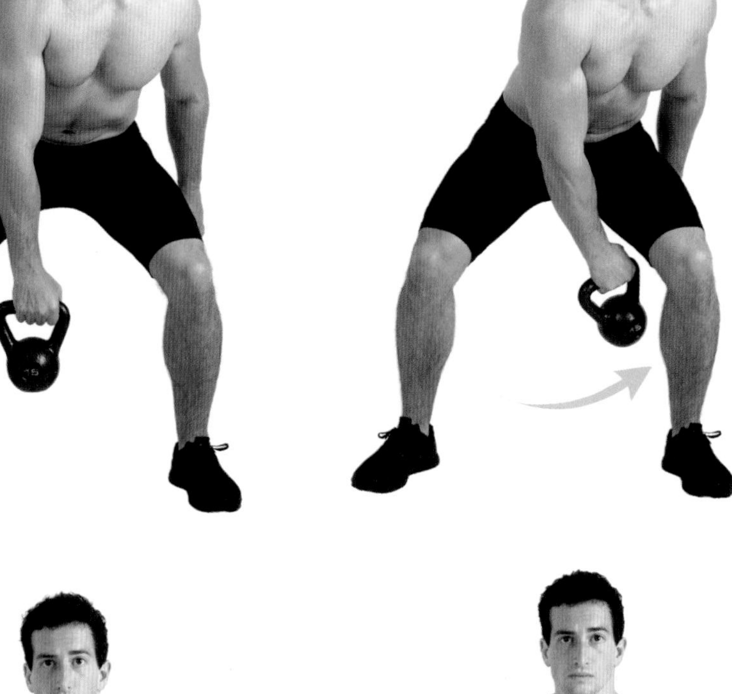

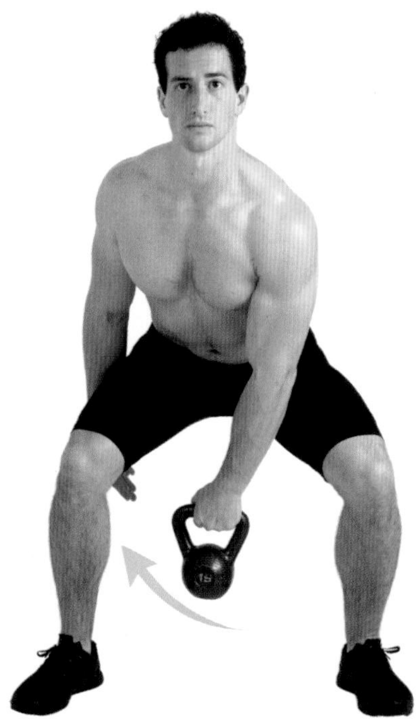

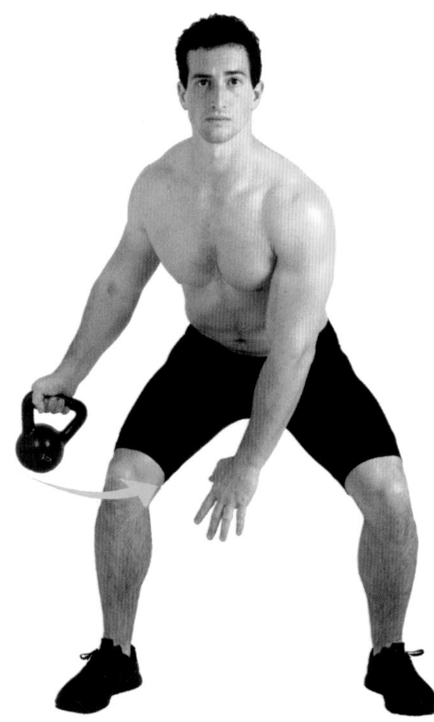

DO IT RIGHT

- Keep your back flat.
- Keep your core engaged.
- Keep your eyes pointed forward.
- Avoid bouncing excessively or relying on momentum.
- Make sure you pass the kettlebell from front to back.

FACT FILE

TARGETS
- Abdominals
- Hamstrings
- Shoulders

EQUIPMENT
- Kettlebell

BENEFITS
- Strengthens abdominals, legs, and arms
- Stabilizes core
- Increases cardiovascular endurance
- Improves coordination
- Burn calories

CAUTIONS
- Hip issues
- Knee issues

MODIFICATION

EASIER: Try the exercise without a kettlebell, just touching hand to hand.

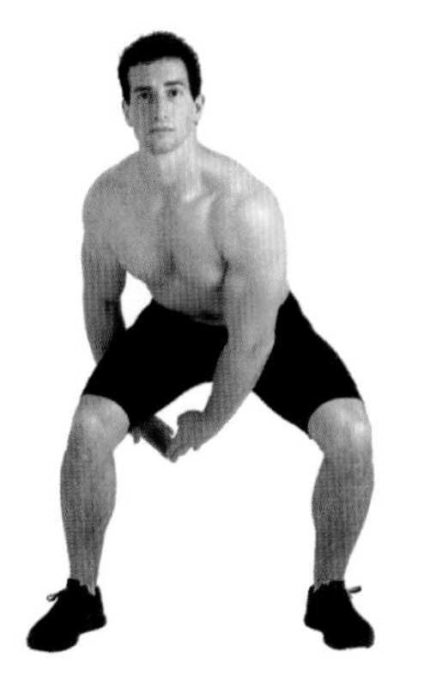

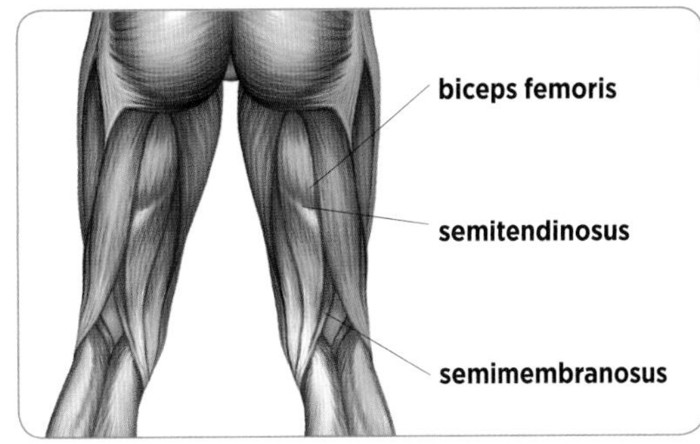

rectus abdominis

transversus abdominis*

rectus femoris

deltoideus medialis

deltoideus anterior

biceps brachii

triceps brachii

vastus intermedius*

vastus lateralis

vastus medialis

Annotation Key

Bold text indicates target muscles
Light text indicates other working muscles
* indicates deep muscles

Kettlebell Squat

The Kettlebell Squat is a powerful exercise that targets the large muscles groups of your lower body, including your quadriceps, hamstrings, and glutes. Using kettlebells while squatting works more muscles and challenges your balance.

HOW TO DO IT

- Stand with your feet hip-width apart holding a kettlebell in each hand.
- Push your hips backward to squat down until your thighs are parallel with the floor.
- Push through your heels to rise back into the starting position. Repeat for the recommended repetitions.

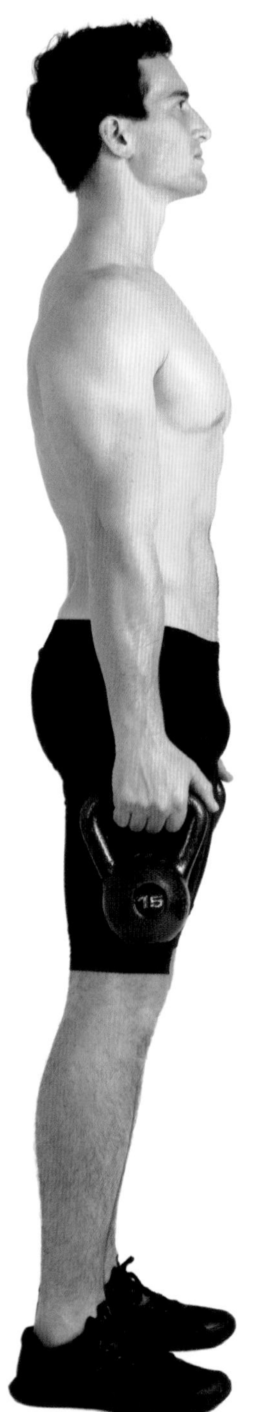

DO IT RIGHT

- Keep the weight on your heels and on the outside of your feet.
- Keep your neck elongated.
- Make sure your thighs are at least parallel with the floor during the squat.
- Breathe in as you descend; breathe out as you ascend.
- Avoid arching your back.

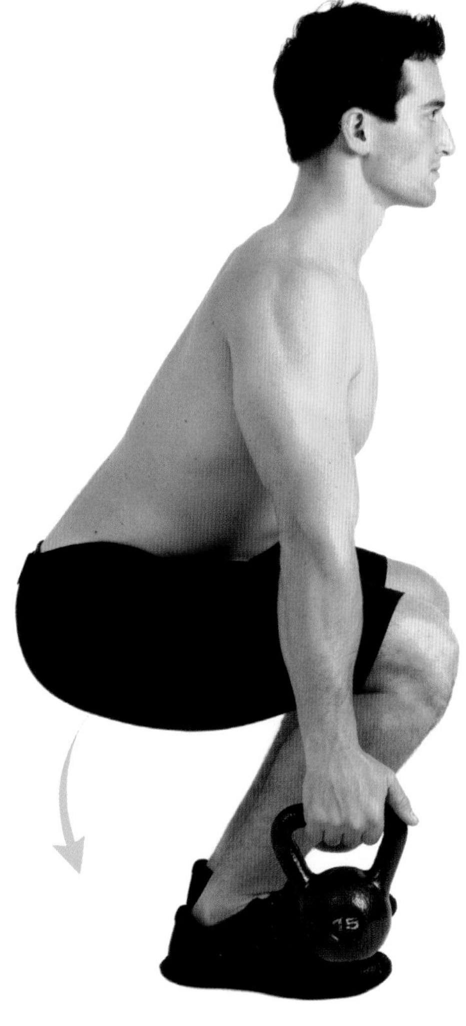

FACT FILE

TARGETS
- Quadriceps
- Hamstrings
- Glutes

EQUIPMENT
- Kettlebells

BENEFITS
- Strengthens and tones quadriceps, hamstrings, and glutes

CAUTIONS
- Knee issues
- Wrist issues

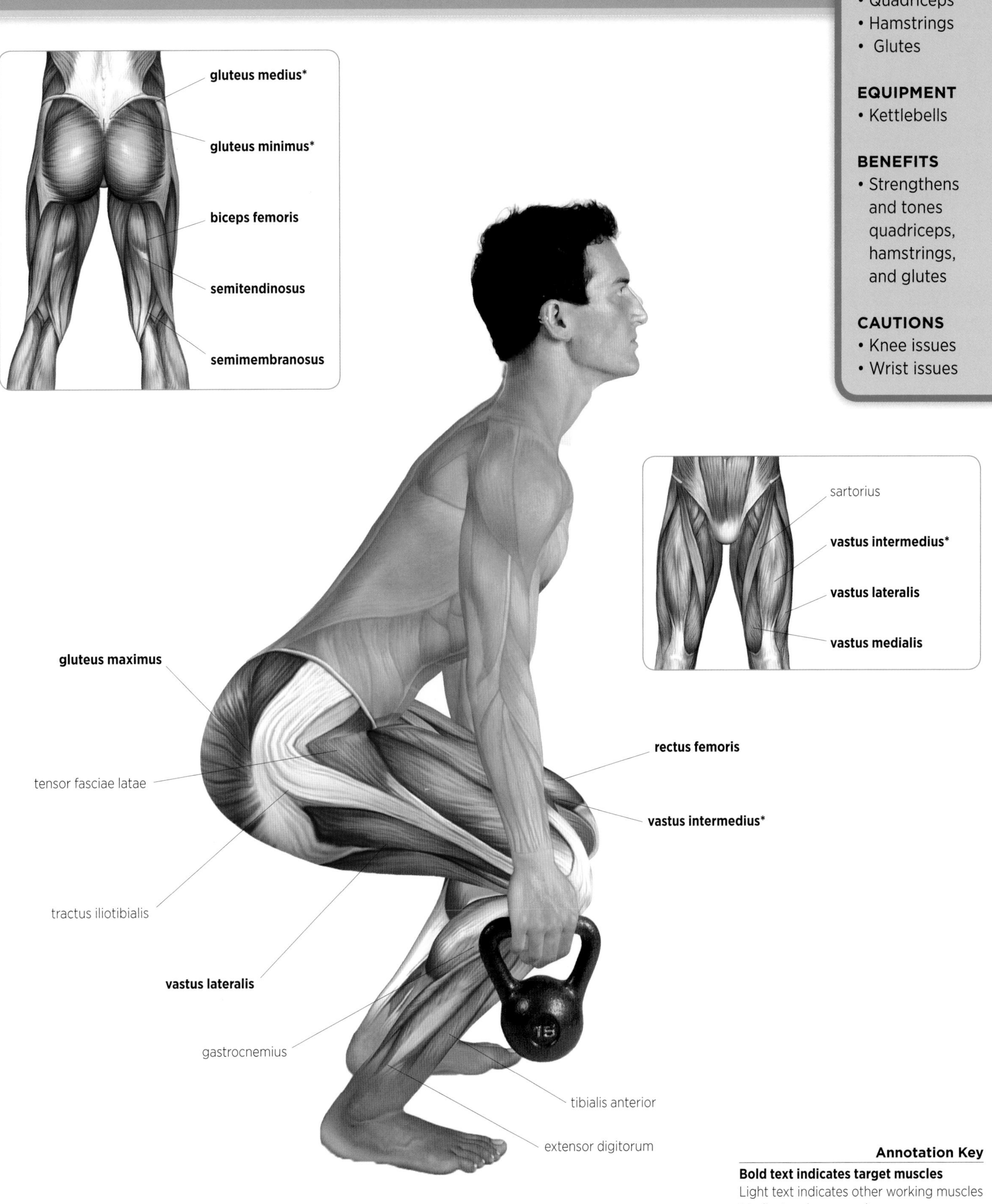

Annotation Key

Bold text indicates target muscles

Light text indicates other working muscles

* indicates deep muscles

Double Kettlebell Snatch

The Double Kettlebell Snatch can boast of multiple benefits: it builds strength, elevates heart rate, and increases mobility. Perform it quickly with lighter weights to reap maximum volume of oxygen benefits; use heavier weights at low speeds to promote full-body strength.

HOW TO DO IT

- Stand with your feet a little more than shoulder-width apart, holding a pair of kettlebells at your sides.
- Squat down, leaning forward slightly and sticking out your buttocks. Bring your arms between your legs so that the kettlebells are next to your inner thighs.
- In one swift, determined move, drive through your hips, and swing the kettlebells overhead.
- Lower your arms to the starting position, and then repeat for the recommended repetitions.

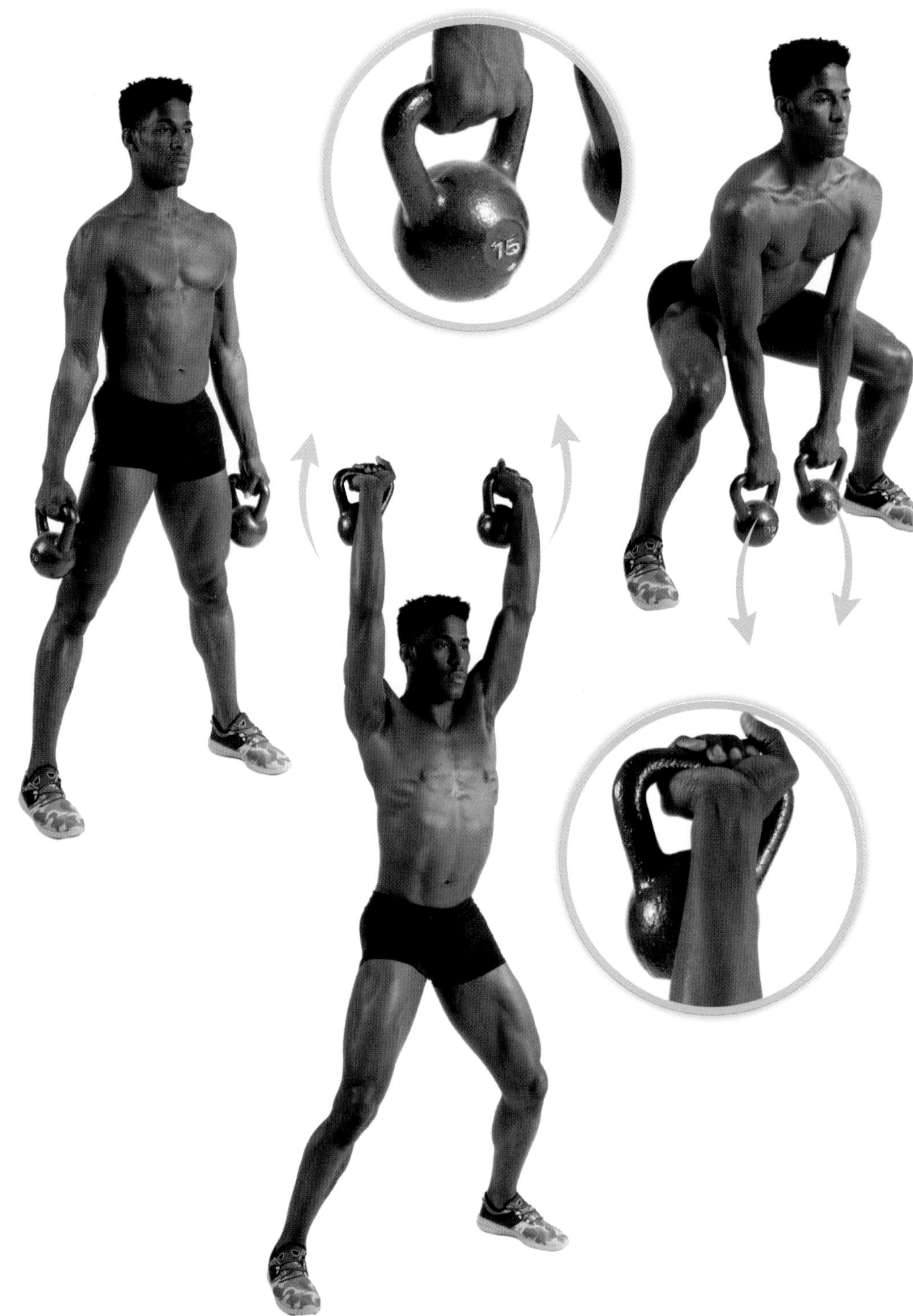

DO IT RIGHT

- As you swing the kettlebell upward, shrug your shoulders backward; this will pull the weights closer to your body, making them feel lighter when they reach the apex.
- Never use a weight heavier than you can safely control.

FACT FILE

TARGETS
- Deltoids
- Glutes
- Quads
- Hamstrings

EQUIPMENT
- Kettlebells

BENEFITS
- Strengthens upper body and lower body

CAUTIONS
- Shoulder issues
- Wrist issues

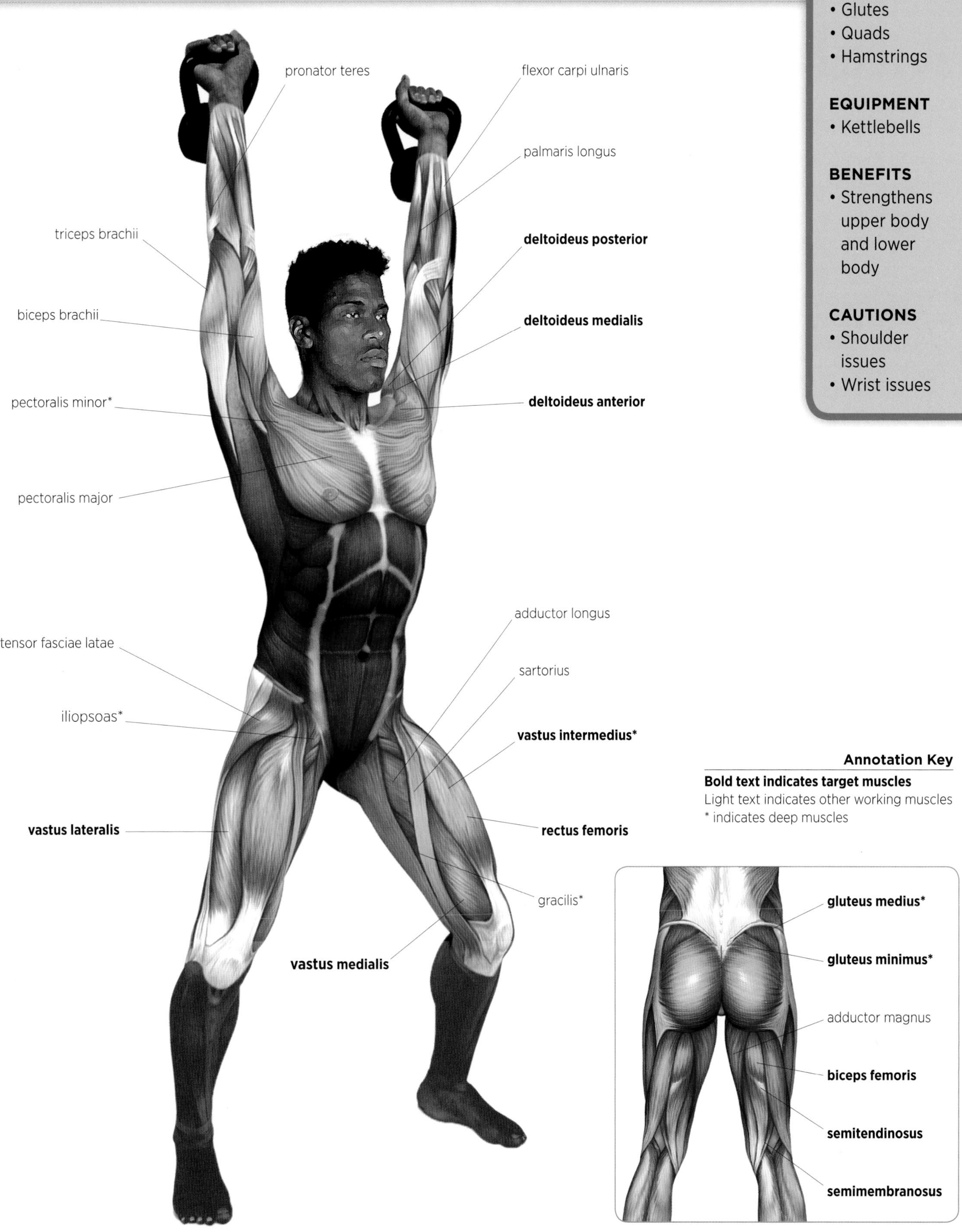

Annotation Key

Bold text indicates target muscles
Light text indicates other working muscles
* indicates deep muscles

Alternating Kettlebell Swing

Any Kettlebell Swing exercise has much to offer: it builds strength, increases aerobic and anaerobic capacity, decreases body fat, and gives you a cardio workout. In the Alternating Kettlebell Swing version, you use one arm at a time, which help develop core muscles and targets stabilizing muscles in your shoulders.

HOW TO DO IT

- Holding a kettlebell in your right hand, stand with your back straight and your legs bent.
- Stand up straight, swinging the kettlebell upward. At the top of the movement, pass the kettlebell to your left hand.
- Return to the starting position with your knees bent. Continue for the recommended repetitions, alternating the hand that begins the exercise holding the kettlebell.

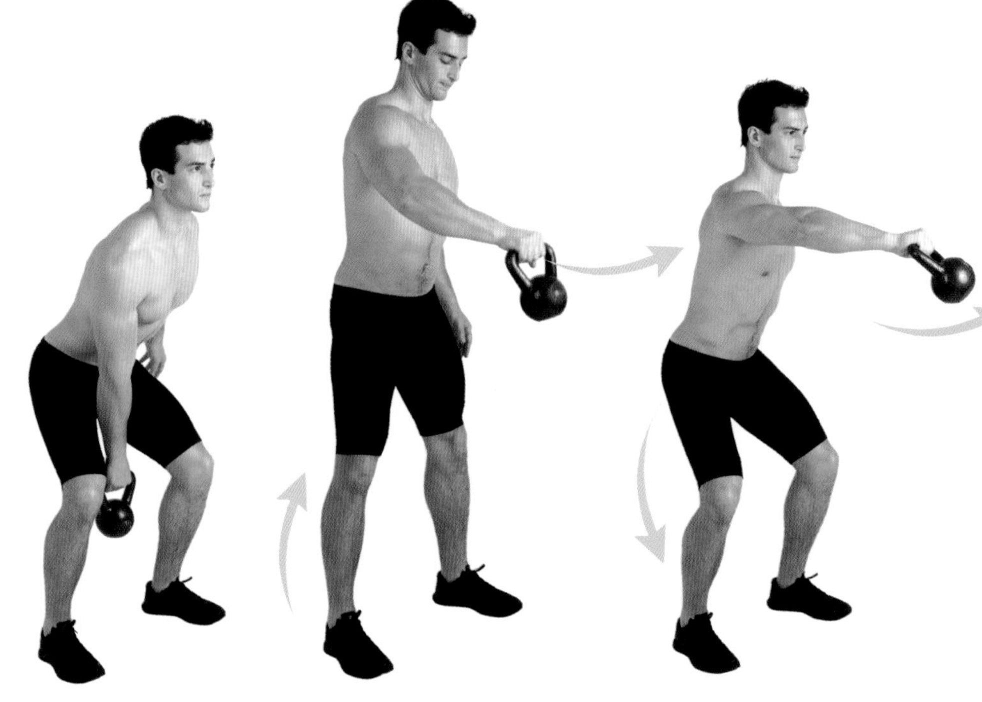

DO IT RIGHT

- Look for proper timing and tempo during repetitions.
- Keep your back flat.
- Strive for a full range of motion.
- Avoid swinging with excessive speed.
- Avoid bouncy repetitions or shallow or incomplete passes.

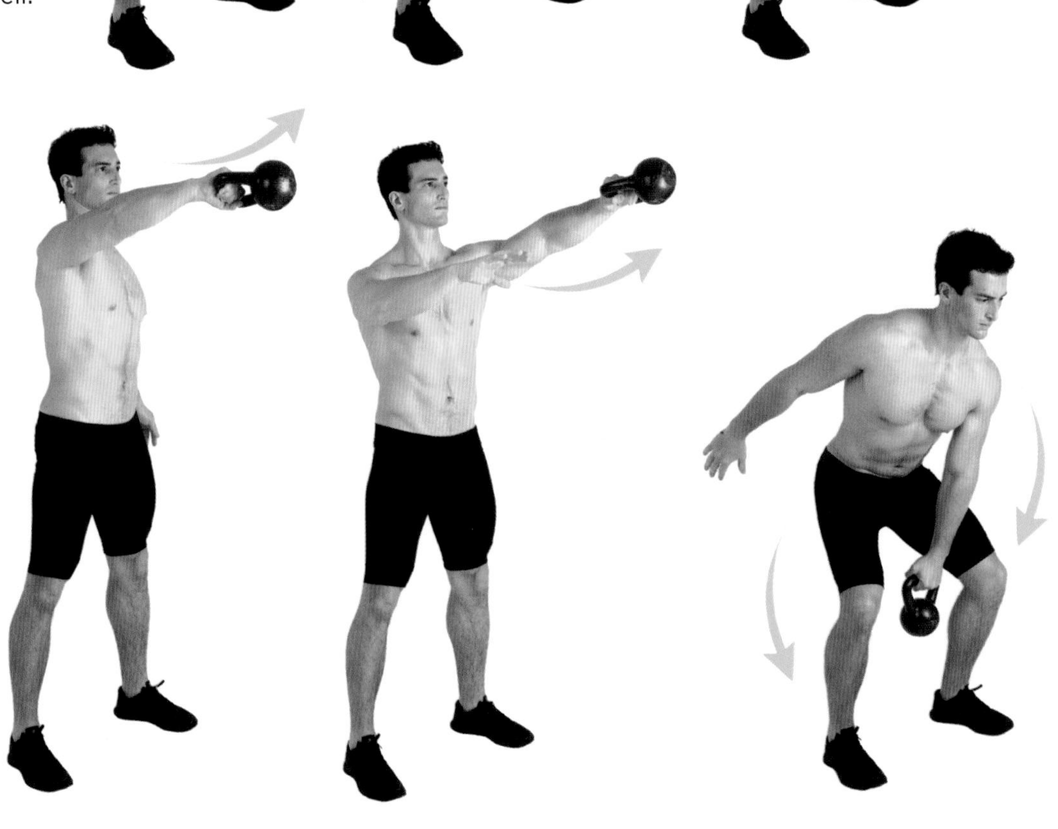

FACT FILE

TARGETS

- Abdominals
- Back
- Shoulders
- Hips
- Glutes
- Legs

EQUIPMENT

- Kettlebell

BENEFITS

- Strengthens upper and lower body
- Improves coordination
- Increases cardiovascular endurance

CAUTIONS

- Shoulder issues
- Wrist issues
- Lower-back pain

Annotation Key

Bold text indicates target muscles

Light text indicates other working muscles

* indicates deep muscles

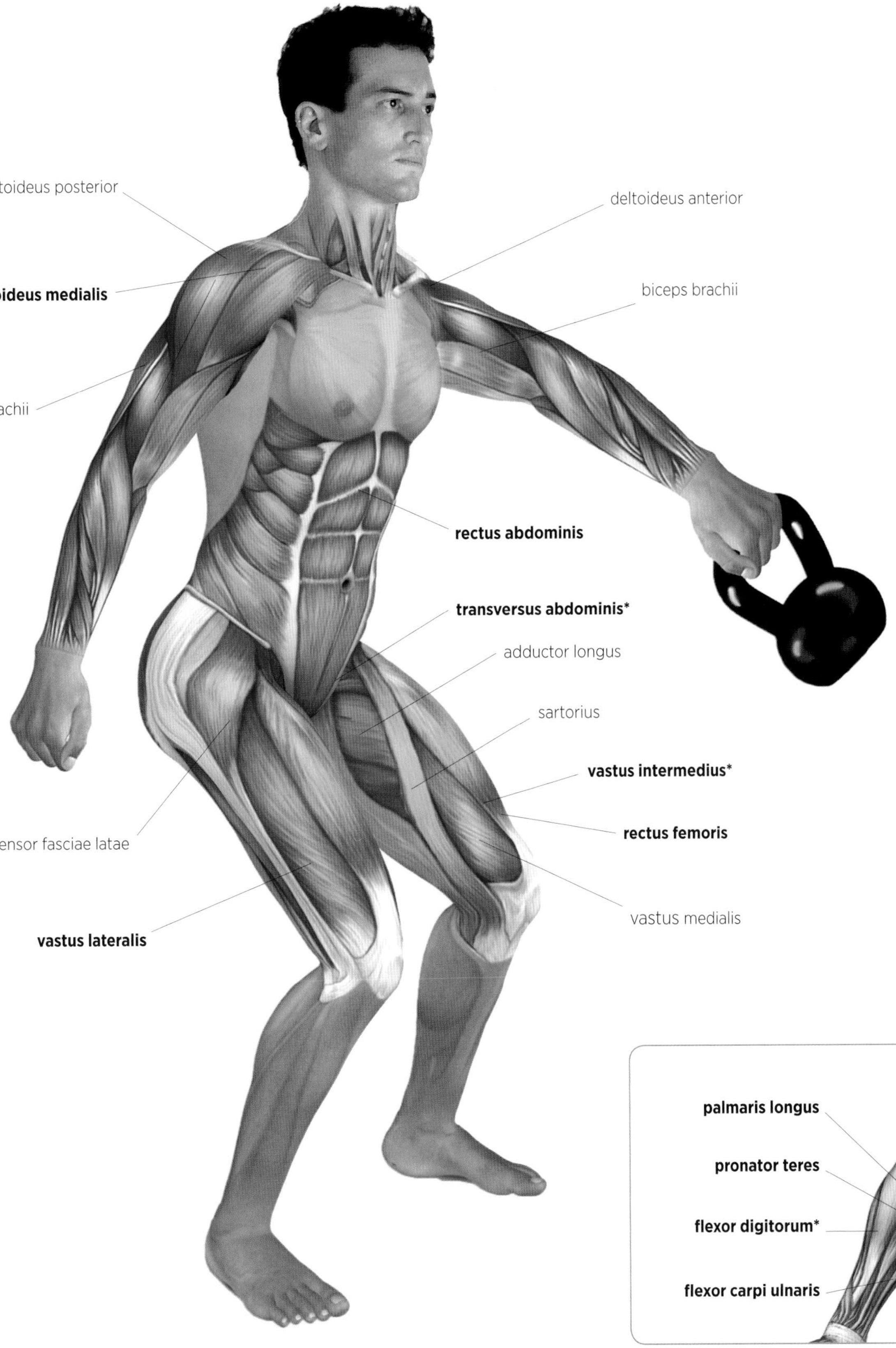

deltoideus posterior

deltoideus medialis

triceps brachii

deltoideus anterior

biceps brachii

rectus abdominis

transversus abdominis*

adductor longus

sartorius

vastus intermedius*

rectus femoris

tensor fasciae latae

vastus medialis

vastus lateralis

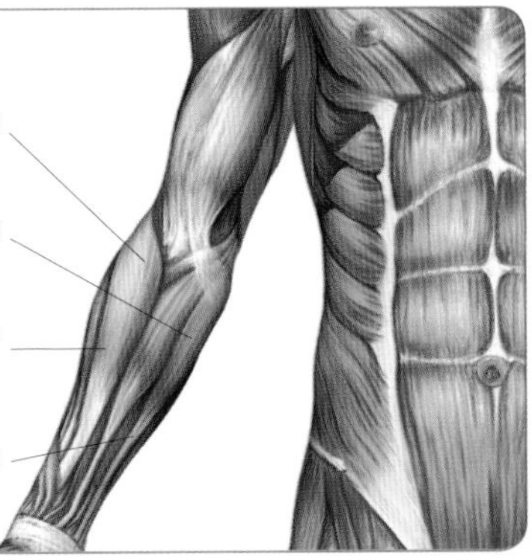

palmaris longus

pronator teres

flexor digitorum*

flexor carpi ulnaris

12-Count Body Builder

The 12-Count Body Builder effectively works your cardiovascular system by using multiple muscle systems. It is also a great exercise to strengthen just about your entire body. As with other military-inspired movements, you perform it to a steady, counting beat.

HOW TO DO IT

- For count 1, grasp a set of dumbbells in your hands with your palms facing each other. Bend down, and place the dumbbells on the floor in front of you.
- Kick your feet backward into a high plank position while keeping your hands on the weights. This is count 2.

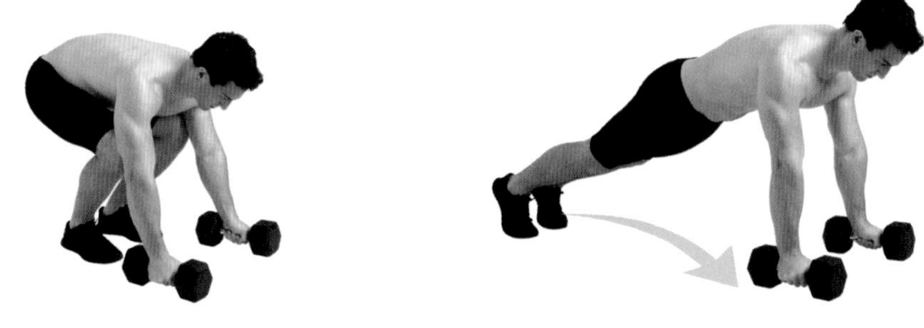

- Push downward into a push-up until your chest touches the dumbbells for count 3.
- Press back up to straighten your arms to again assume a high plank for count 4.
- Spread your legs for count 5.
- Close your legs for count 6.

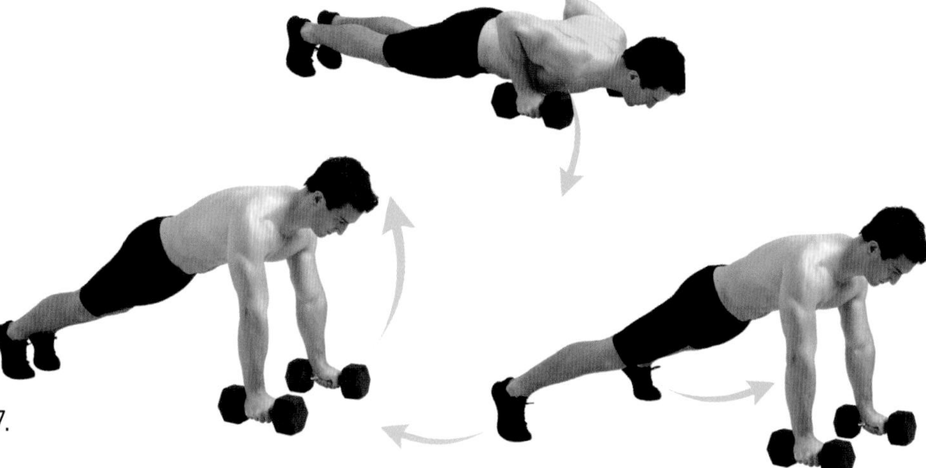

- Jump both knees to your chest for count 7.
- Stand for count 8.
- Lift the weights to your shoulders, and perform a biceps curl for count 9.
- Lower the weights to your sides for count 10.
- Raise the weights over your head for count 11.
- Lower the weights to your sides for count 12. Each 1-to-12 count equals one repetition. Perform for the recommended repetitions.

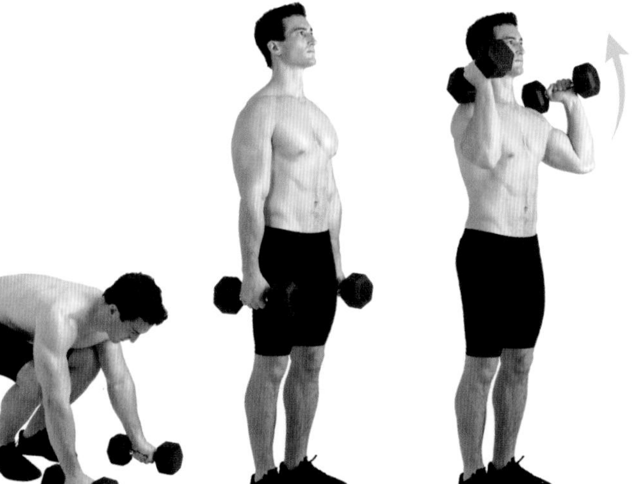

FACT FILE

TARGETS
- Abdominals
- Back
- Shoulders
- Hips
- Glutes
- Legs

EQUIPMENT
- Dumbbells

BENEFITS
- Strengthens the entire body
- Increases cardiovascular endurance
- Improves coordination

CAUTIONS
- Shoulder issues
- Wrist issues
- Lower-back pain

Annotation Key

Bold text indicates target muscles
Light text indicates other working muscles
* indicates deep muscles

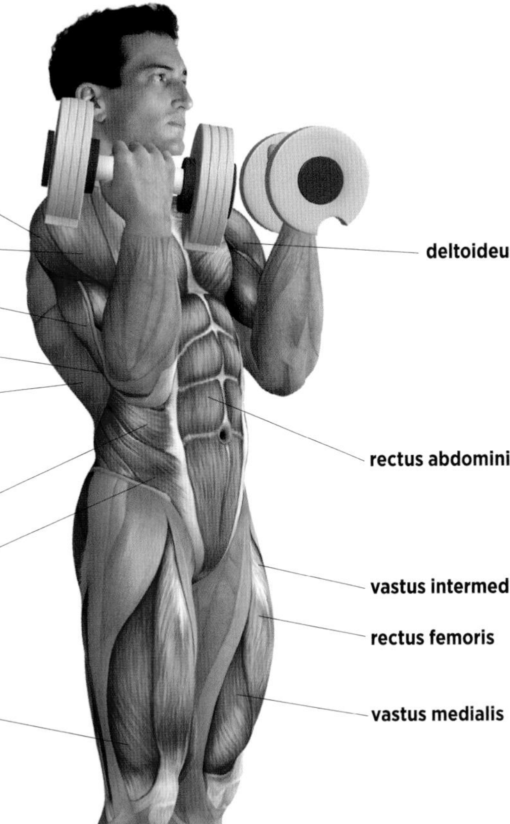

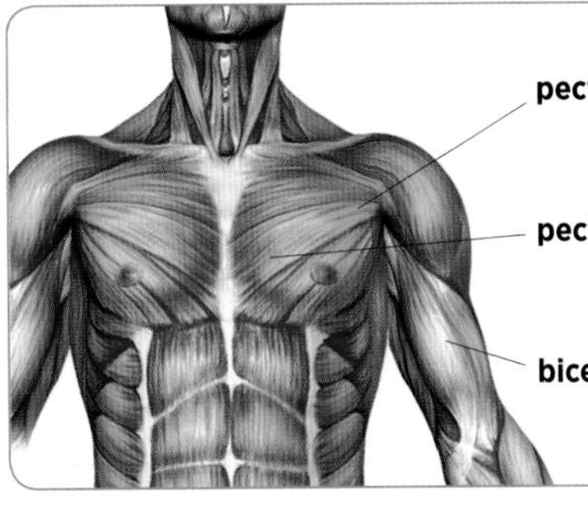

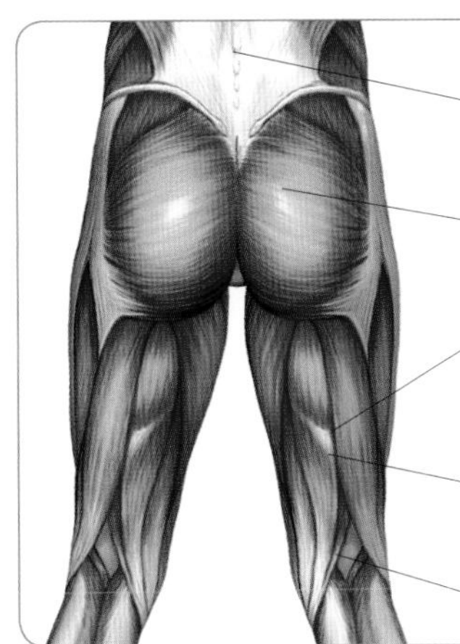

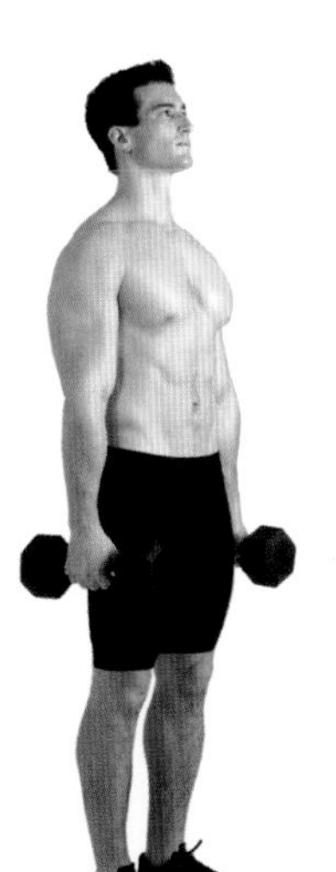

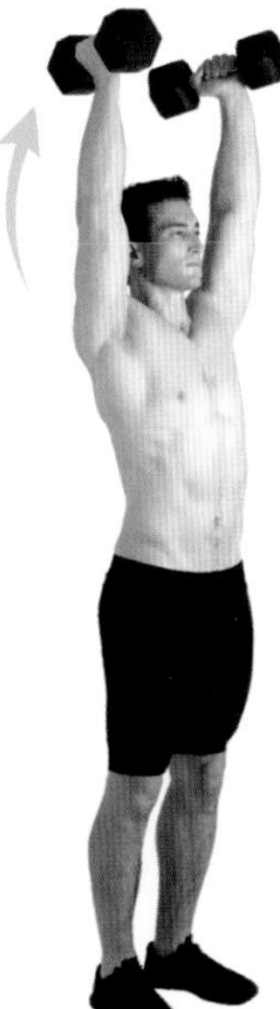

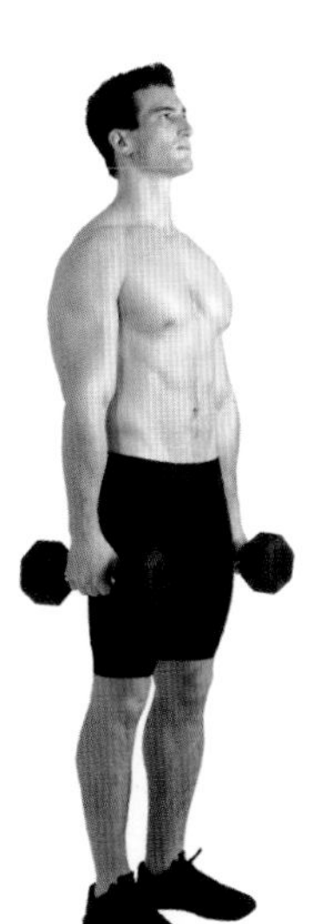

DO IT RIGHT
- Keep your hands close to your chest in the push-up position.
- Avoid resting your chest on the floor on count 3.

Split Squat with Overhead Press

A multipurpose exercise, the Split Squat with Overhead Press combines the single-leg strengthening move of a staggered-stance squat with the upper-body toning of an upward press. This exercise will challenge your quads, glutes, hamstrings, upper back, and shoulders.

HOW TO DO IT

- Stand with your right leg behind you with the ball of your foot resting on a step.
- With your elbows bent to form right angles, raise both arms to shoulder height. Position your hands as if your were grasping a bar using an overhand grip.
- Bend both knees into a split squat position. Simultaneously, extend your arms over your head.
- Return to the starting position, and then repeat on the opposite side. Repeat for the recommended repetitions.

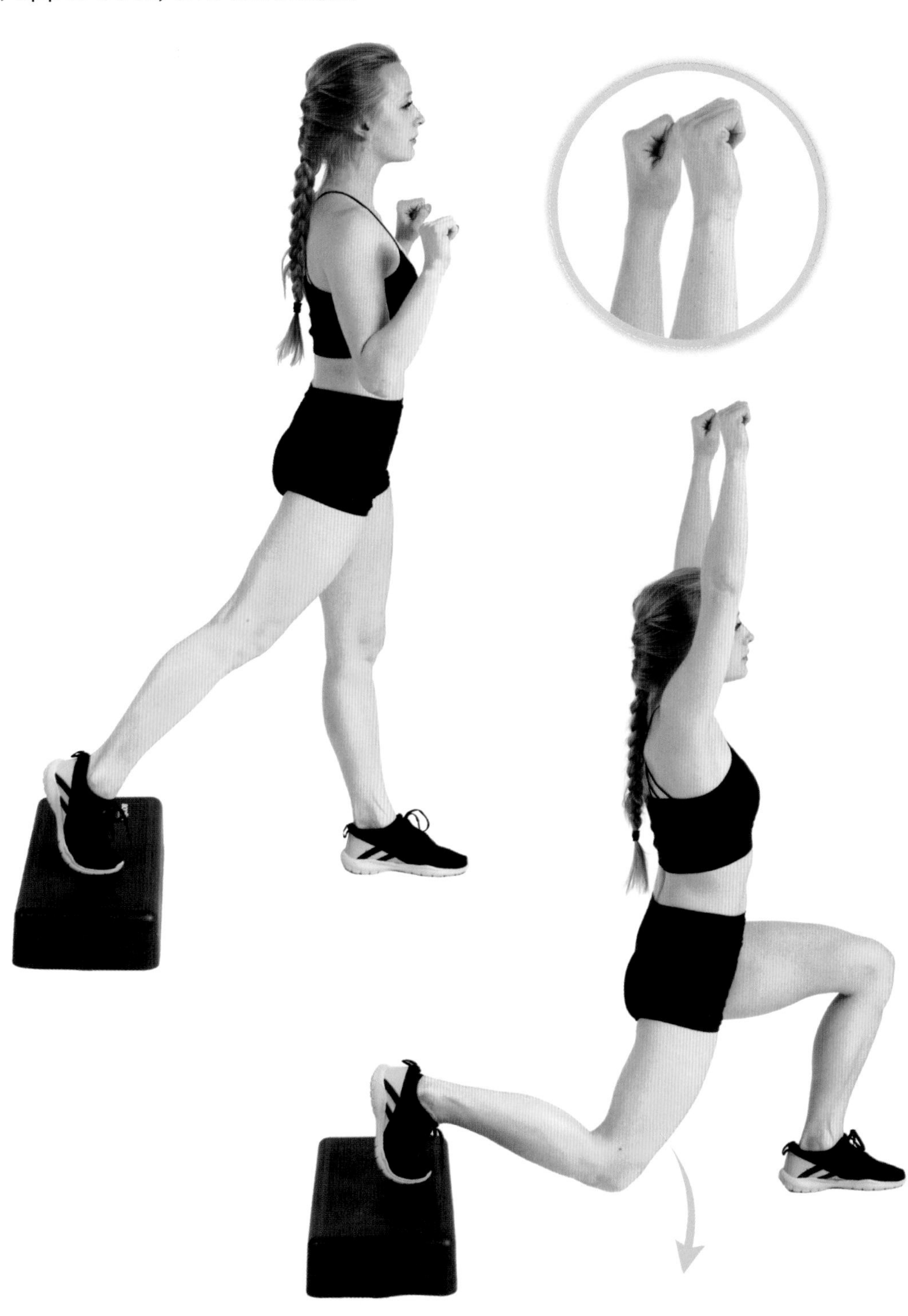

DO IT RIGHT

- Keep your back straight and your core upright.
- Press your shoulders back and down.
- Avoid arching your back as you raise your arms.
- Avoid letting your abdominals bulge outward.
- Avoid tensing your neck.

FACT FILE

TARGETS
- Glutes
- Quadriceps
- Hamstrings
- Shoulders
- Upper back

EQUIPMENT
- Aerobics step

BENEFITS
- Strengthens glutes, thighs, shoulders, and upper back
- Improves range of motion throughout body

CAUTIONS
- Shoulder issues
- Knee issues

Annotation Key
Bold text indicates target muscles
Light text indicates other working muscles
* indicates deep muscles

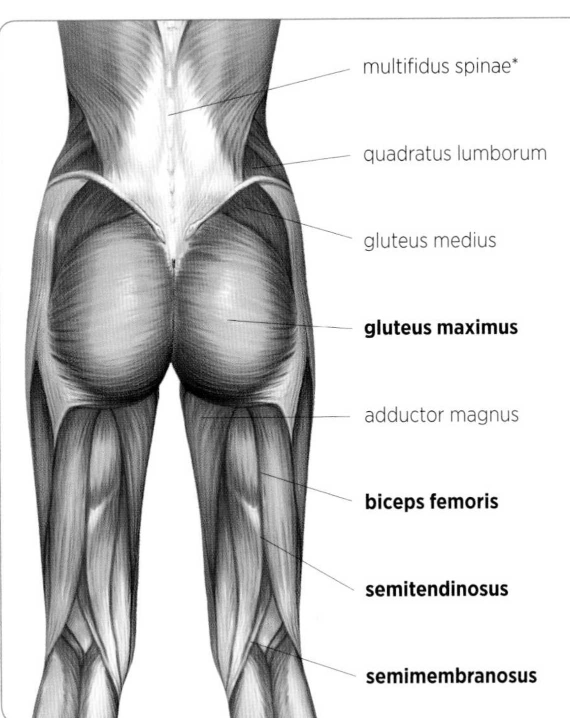

MODIFICATION

HARDER: Hold a pair of dumbbells above your head as your execute the exercise.

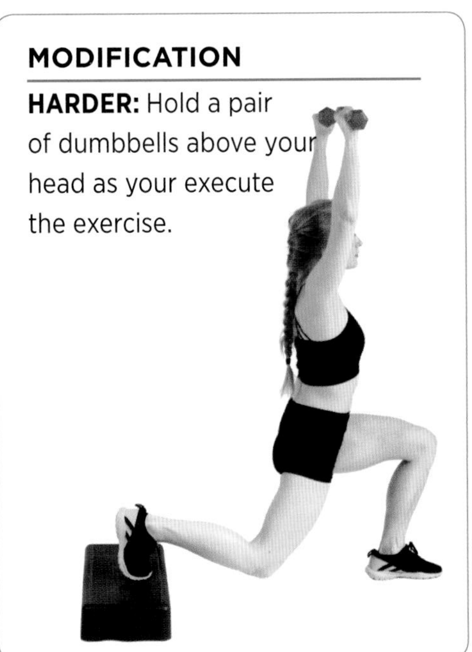

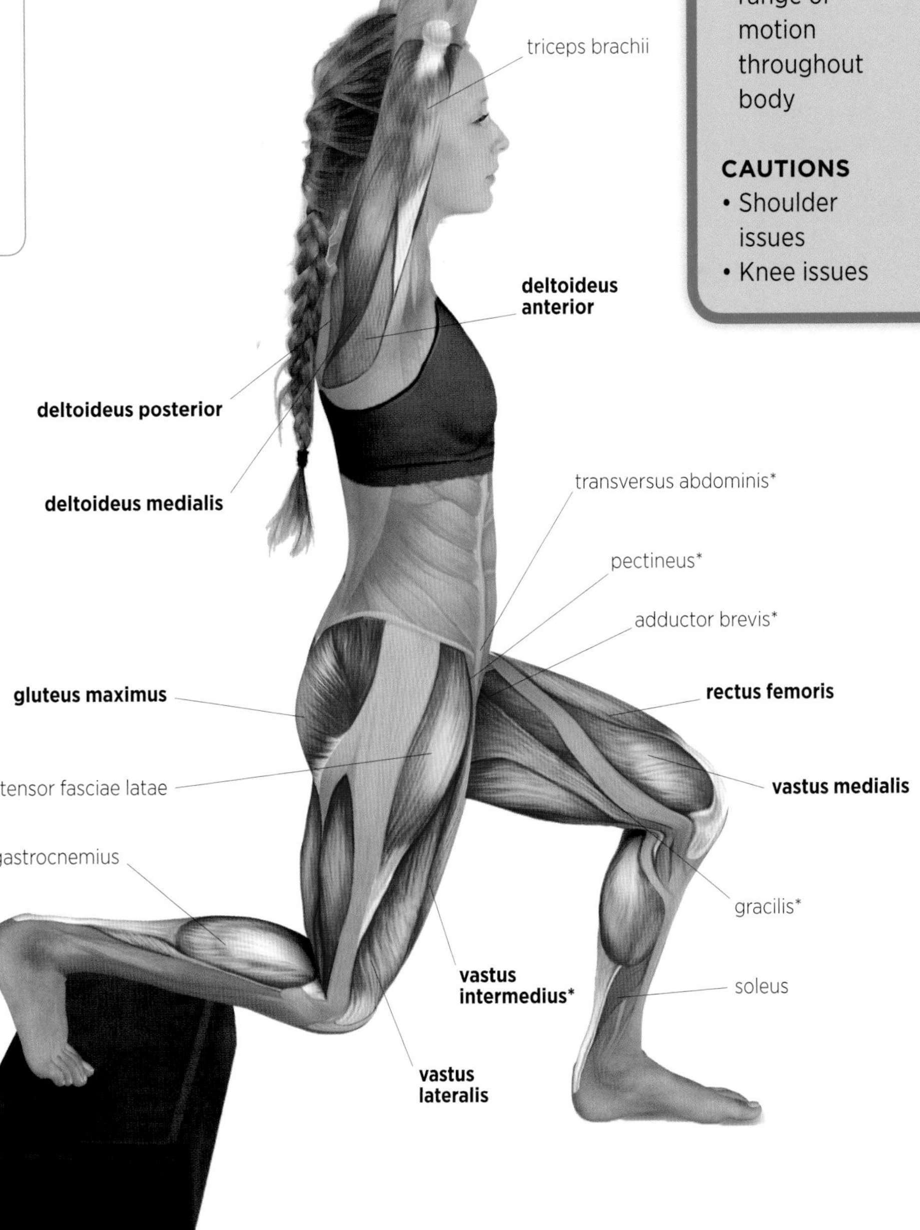

Lunge with Dumbbell Upright Row

It may look like a simple move, but the Lunge with Dumbbell Upright Row does a lot of work. The lunge portion of the exercise strengthens your lower body, whereas the row portion targets your front deltoids, upper back, forearms, biceps, and core.

HOW TO DO IT

- Stand holding a pair of dumbbells in each hand. Step your right leg forward.
- Bend your right knee until your thigh is parallel to the floor and you can feel the muscles of your rear thigh working. As you bend, simultaneously raise the dumbbells, with your elbows leading, until they are level with your shoulders.
- Push through your right heel to return to starting position. Repeat on the opposite side. Continue alternating sides for the recommended repetitions.

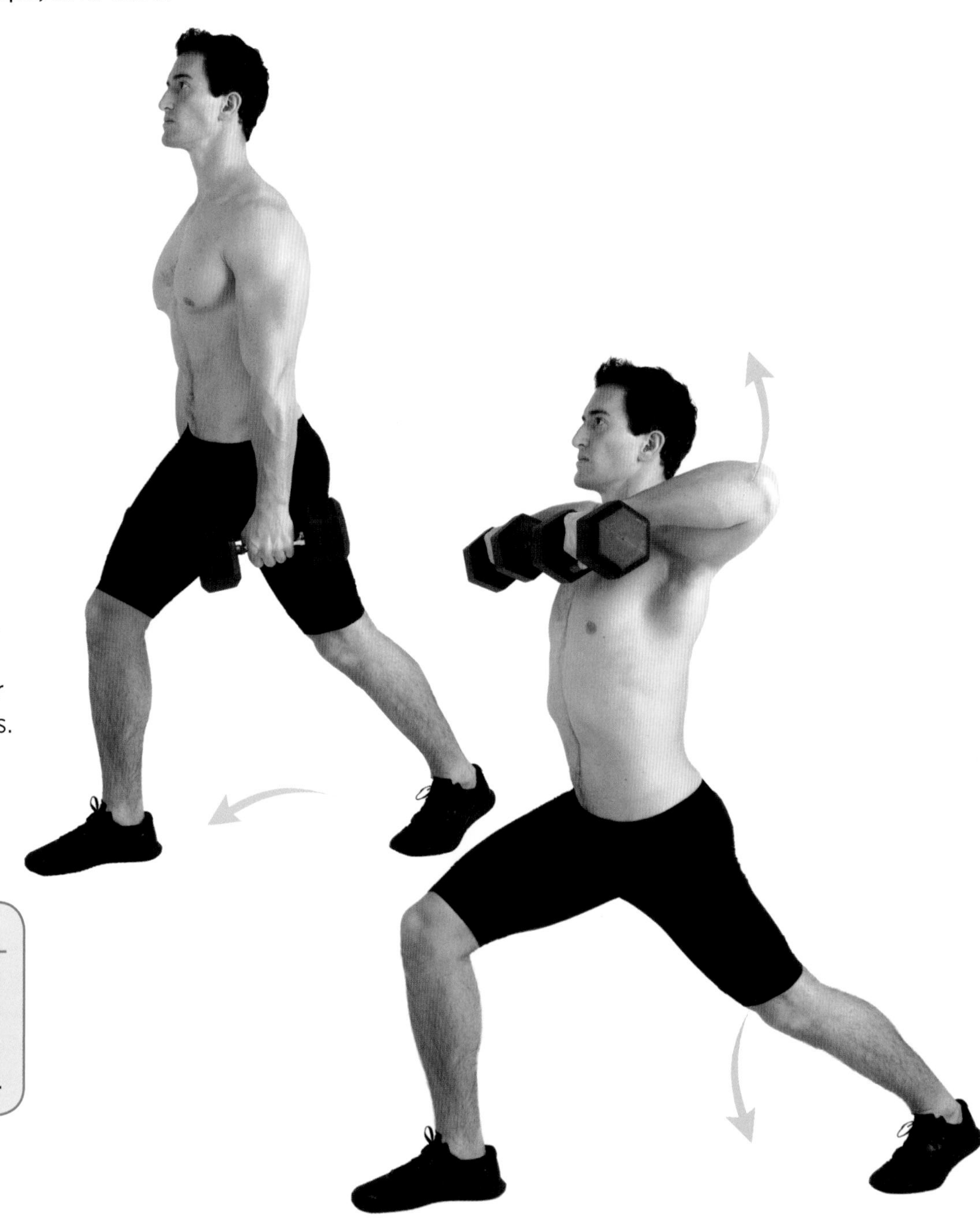

DO IT RIGHT

- Use your elbows to lead the upright row.
- Avoid hyperextending your knees past your toes.

FACT FILE

TARGETS
- Quadriceps
- Hamstrings
- Glutes
- Upper back
- Shoulders

EQUIPMENT
- Dumbbells

BENEFITS
- Strengthens glutes, thighs, shoulders, and upper back
- Increases leg and shoulder power.

CAUTIONS
- Knee issues
- Shoulder pain
- Elbow pain

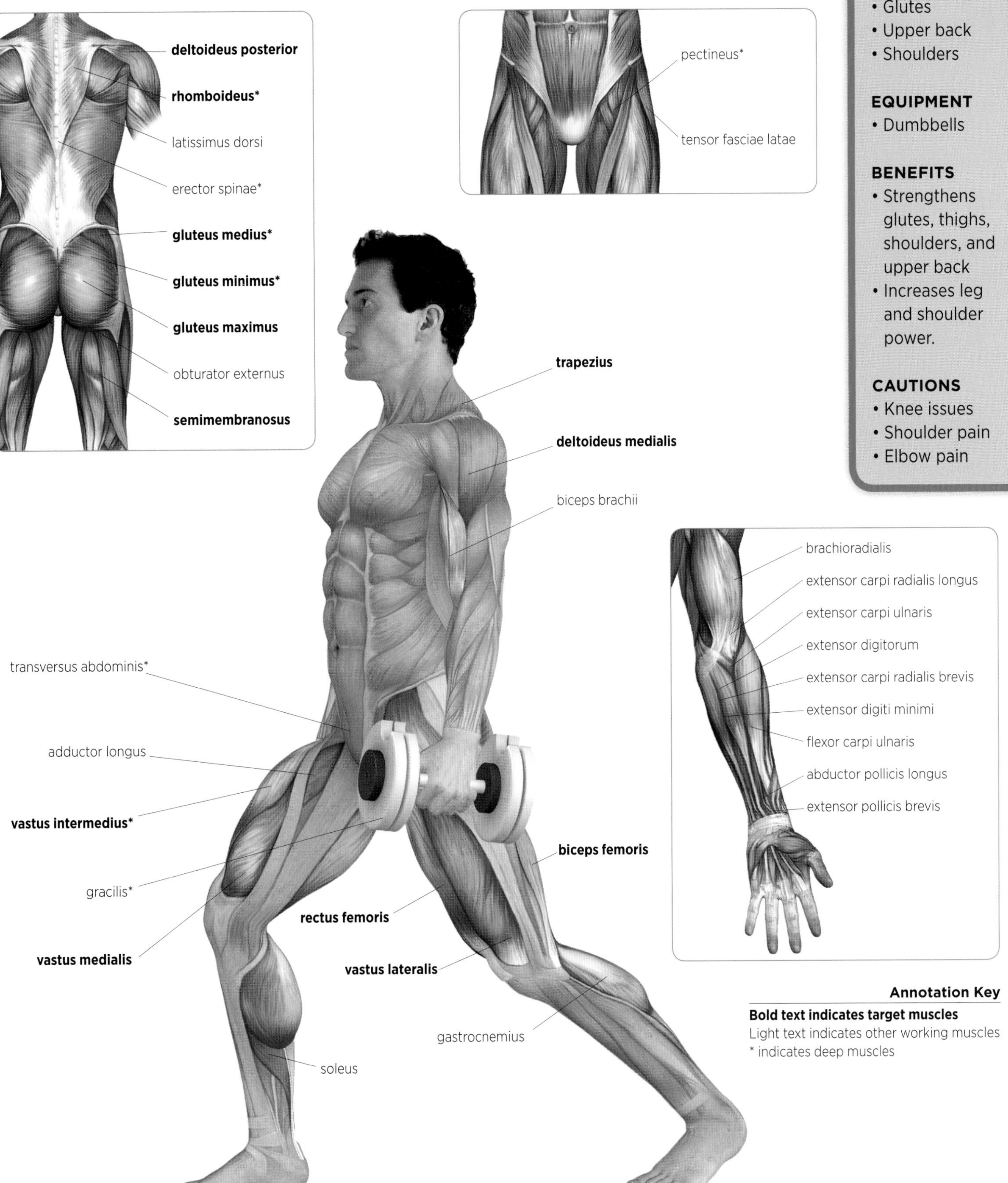

Annotation Key

Bold text indicates target muscles

Light text indicates other working muscles

* indicates deep muscles

Dumbbell Power Clean

The Dumbbell Power Clean calls into action multiple joints and increases the raw power, size, and strength throughout your shoulder girdle and upper back.

FACT FILE

TARGETS
- Shoulders
- Chest
- Back
- Glutes
- Quads

EQUIPMENT
- Dumbbells

BENEFITS
- Strengthens upper and lower body

CAUTIONS
- Wrist pain
- Shoulder issues

HOW TO DO IT
- Stand with your feet shoulder-width apart with a pair of dumbbells at your feet. Squat down, and grab the dumbbells with a wide, overhand grip so that they rest at the front of your thighs, your palms facing inward.
- Flip the dumbbells up until they are nearly touching your shoulders, and then reverse the movement to return to the starting position. Repeat for the recommended repetitions.

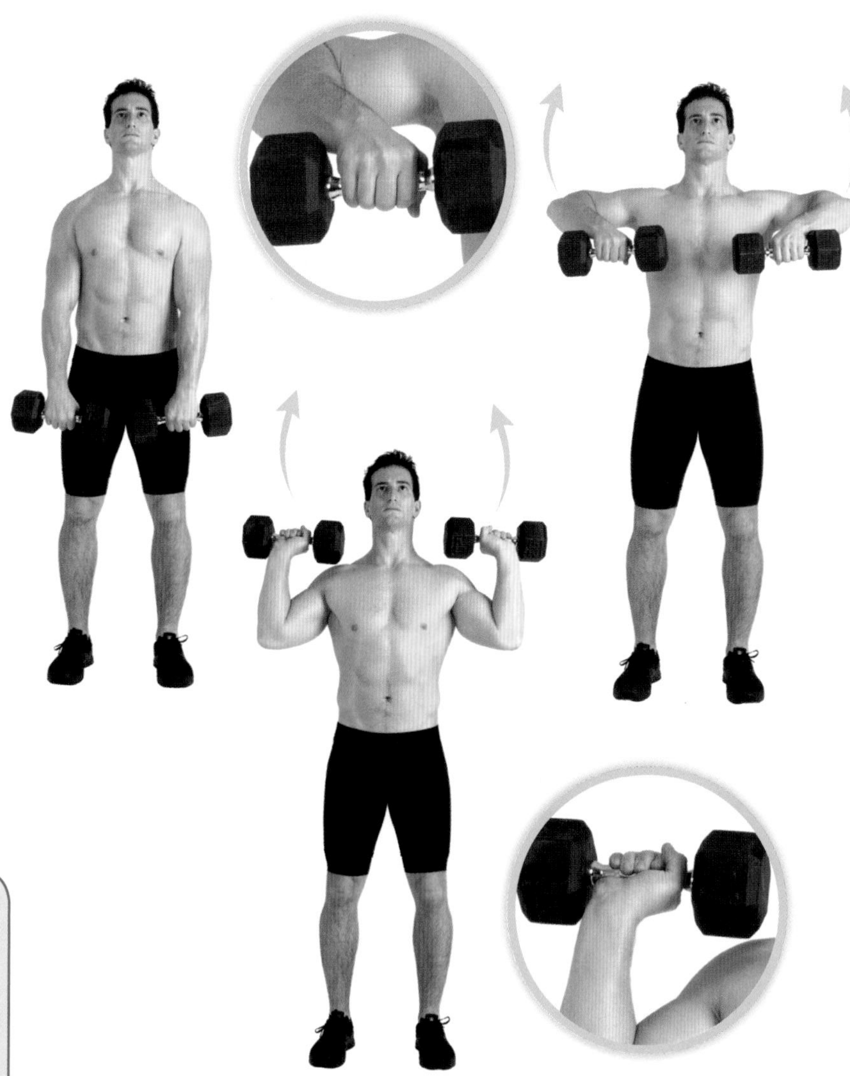

DO IT RIGHT
- Keep the dumbbells close to your body.
- Keep your back straight.
- Avoid placing too much stress on your wrists.
- Avoid excessive momentum; perform all steps with steady controlled movement.

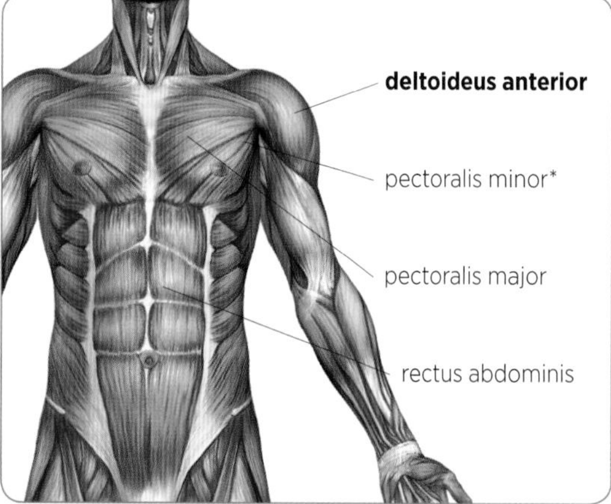

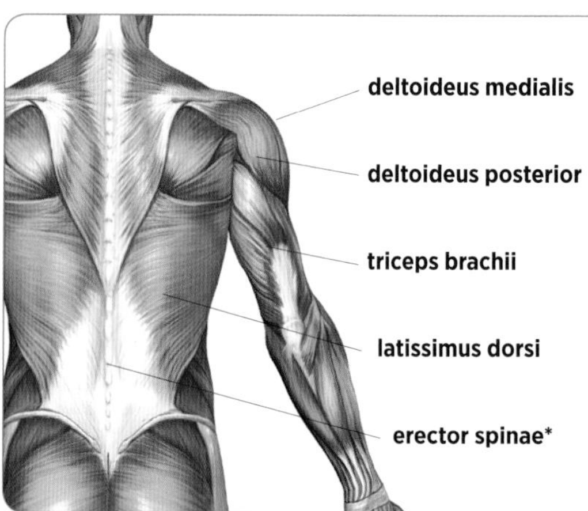

Annotation Key
Bold text indicates target muscles
Light text indicates other working muscles
* indicates deep muscles

Dumbbell Power Clean and Press

The Dumbbell Power Clean and Press works your major upper-body muscles, especially your shoulders, chest, and upper back. This advanced movement requires strength, timing, momentum, and proper technique.

FACT FILE

TARGETS
- Shoulders
- Chest
- Back
- Glutes
- Quads

EQUIPMENT
- Dumbbells

BENEFITS
- Strengthens upper and lower body

CAUTIONS
- Wrist pain
- Shoulder issues

HOW TO DO IT

- Stand with your feet shoulder-width apart with a pair of dumbbells at your feet. Squat down, and grab the dumbbells with a wide, overhand grip so that they rest at the front of your thighs, your palms facing inward.

- Flip the dumbbells up until they are nearly touching your shoulders.

- Press your arms upward to full lockout directly overhead, and then reverse all movements to return to the starting position. Repeat for the recommended repetitions.

DO IT RIGHT

- Keep the dumbbells close to your body.
- Keep your back straight.
- Avoid placing too much stress on your wrists.
- Avoid excessive momentum; perform all steps with steady controlled movement.

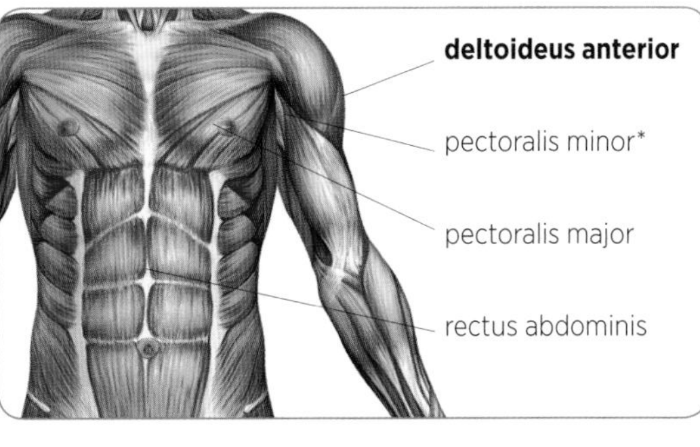

Annotation Key
Bold text indicates target muscles
Light text indicates other working muscles
* indicates deep muscles

deltoideus medialis
deltoideus posterior
triceps brachii
latissimus dorsi
erector spinae*

Kitchen Sink

This exercise includes everything and the kitchen sink! There is not one muscle this exercise spares, and—for this reason—it is an amazing full-body workout that will condition your cardiovascular system, aerobic endurance, and your muscular strength and endurance.

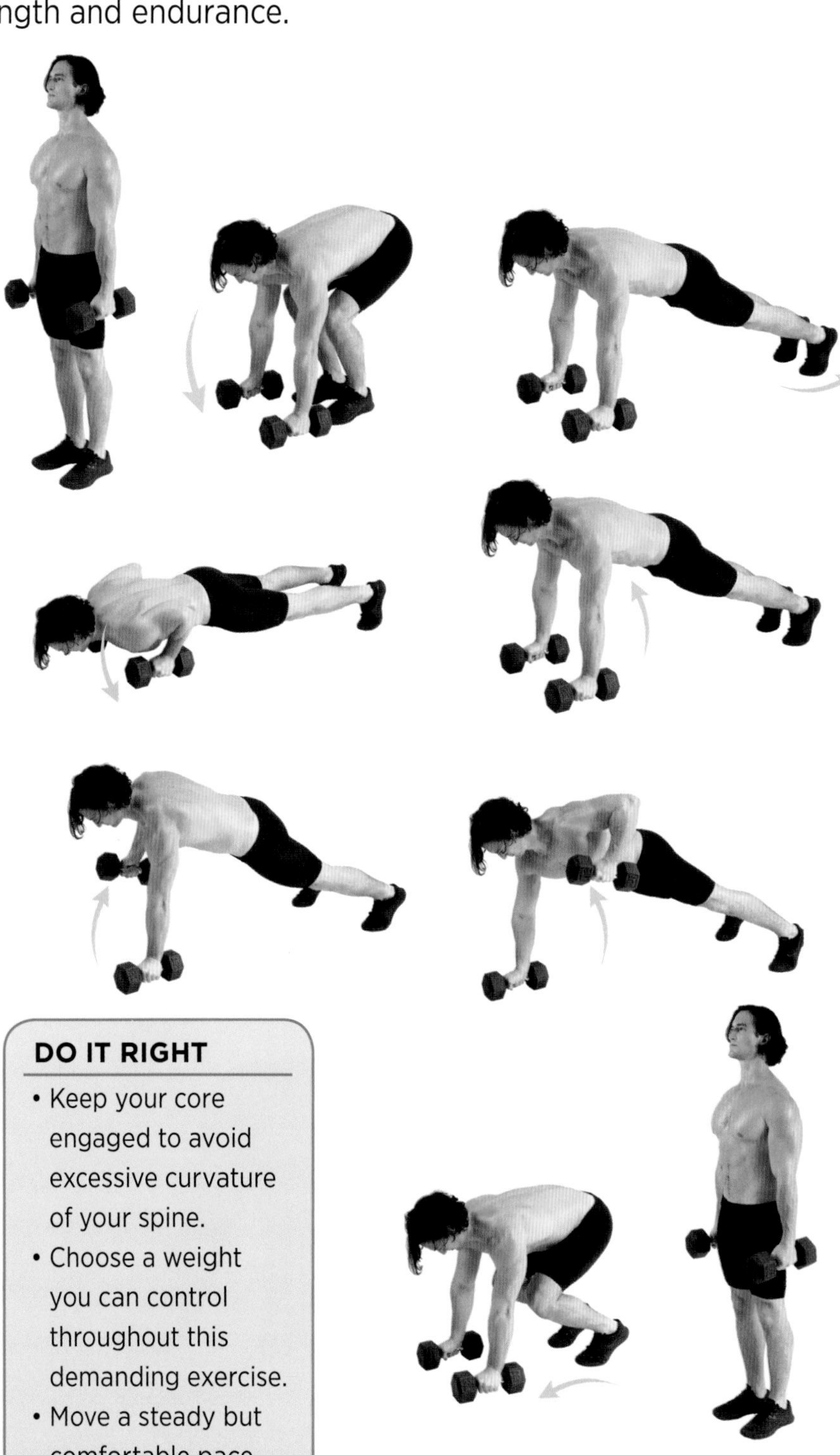

HOW TO DO IT

- Stand with your feet planted hip-width apart holding a pair of dumbbells in each hand.
- Bend at your waist, hips, and ankles to place your dumbbells on the floor in front of you.
- Supporting your weight through your arms on the dumbbells, kick your legs out behind you with your legs wider than hip-width apart to assume a high plank position.
- Bend your elbows, lowering your chest toward the floor to perform a push-up, and then return to the high plank position.
- Remaining in the high plank position, pull the kettlebell in your right hand up toward your chest while straightening your left arm and pushing that kettlebell into the floor. Lower your right arm, and then repeat the movement with the left.
- Hop your feet forward and underneath your hips, shifting your weight back and over your feet to return to a standing position, bringing the weights to the starting position.
- Bend your elbows, drawing the weights toward your shoulders to perform a biceps curl.
- Extend your arms overhead, before bringing the weights back down to your sides, to perform a shoulder press.
- Return to the starting position, and then repeat for the recommended repetitions.

DO IT RIGHT

- Keep your core engaged to avoid excessive curvature of your spine.
- Choose a weight you can control throughout this demanding exercise.
- Move a steady but comfortable pace.

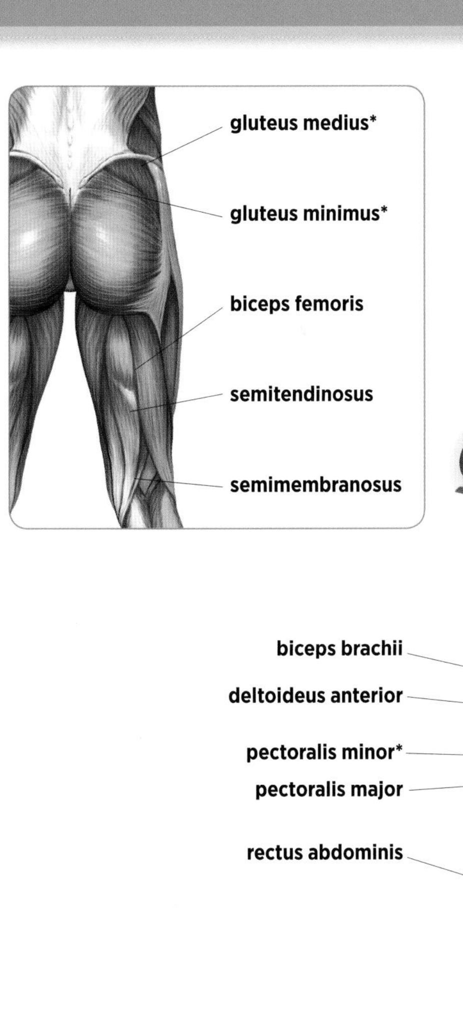

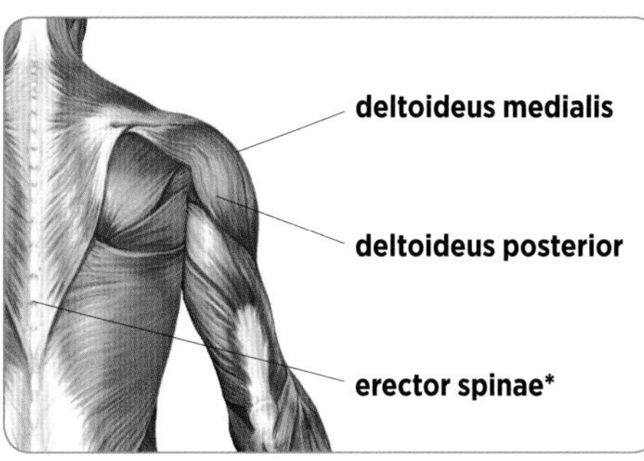

Annotation Key

Bold text indicates target muscles

Light text indicates other working muscles

* indicates deep muscles

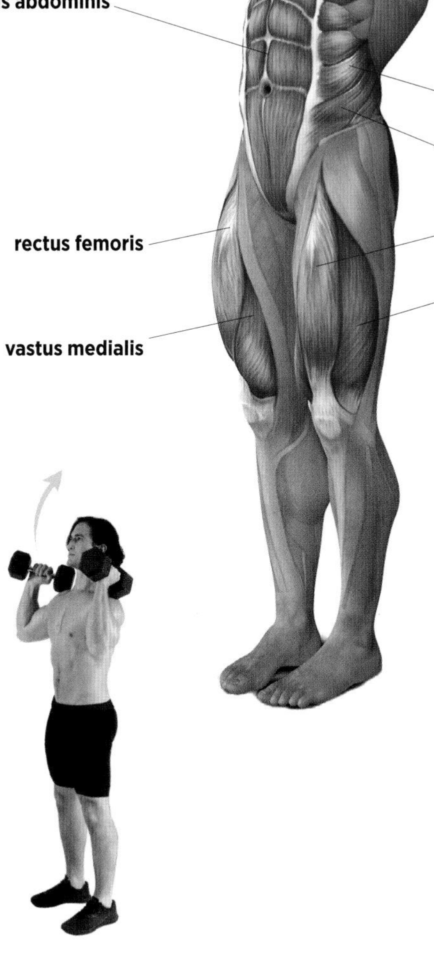

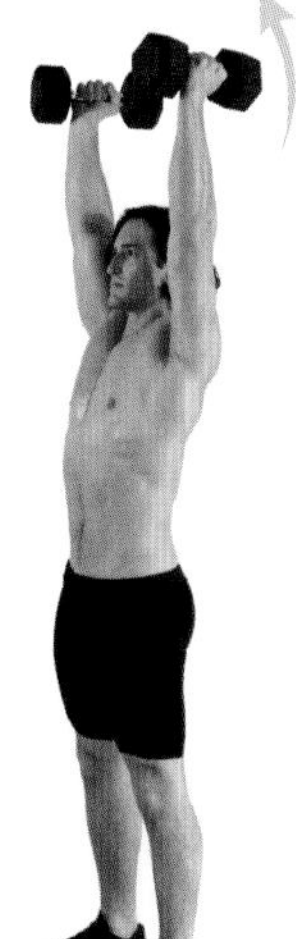

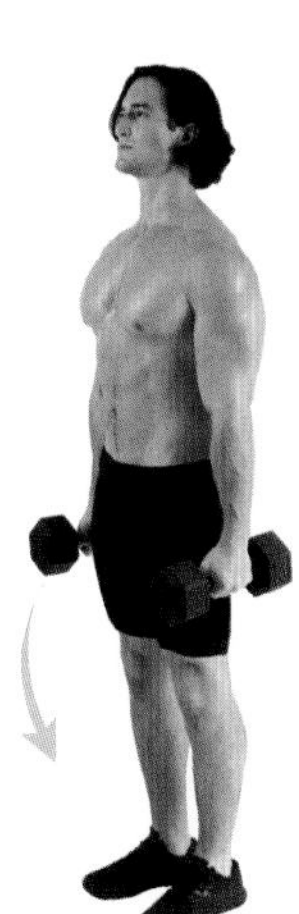

FACT FILE

TARGETS

- Deltoids
- Triceps
- Biceps
- Abdominals
- Back
- Pectorals
- Hip flexors
- Quadriceps
- Hamstrings
- Glutes

EQUIPMENT

- Dumbbells

BENEFITS

- Strengthens and tones abdominals, chest, arms, and legs
- Increases cardiovascular endurance
- Improves coordination

CAUTIONS

- Wrist issues
- Back issues
- Knee issues

Dumbbell Thruster

The compound movement of the Dumbbell Thruster requires high caloric expenditure and strengthens the upper body, core, and lower body. This exercise uses peripheral heart action, or the engagement of your upper- and lower-body musculature in succession, with little to no rest in between, making it great for your cardiovascular system.

HOW TO DO IT

- Stand with your feet hip-width apart with a dumbbell in each hand positioned at the level of your shoulders.
- Drop into a squat until the top of your thighs are parallel to the floor. Keep the weights on your shoulders with your elbows pointed forward.
- Keeping your back in a neutral position, press through your heels, extending your hips and legs to return to a standing position.
- Perform a shoulder press, extending your arms upward, driving the dumbbells overhead.
- Bend your elbows, lowering the weights to your shoulders, to return to the starting position. Repeat for the recommended repetitions.

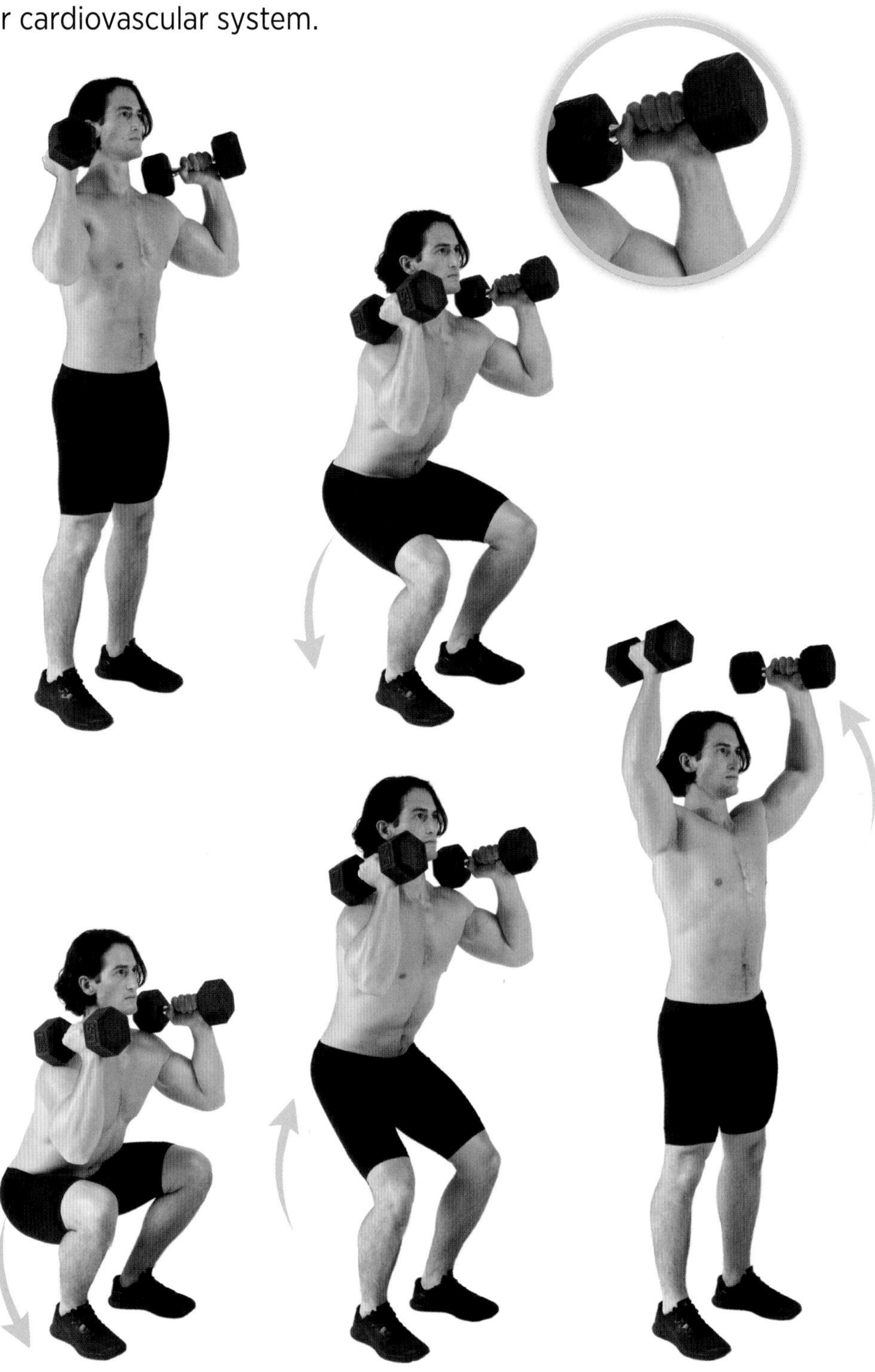

DO IT RIGHT

- Keep your back straight.
- Track your knees over your toes.
- Avoid caving in your knees or ankles.
- Keep your elbows positioned up and in front of your torso.

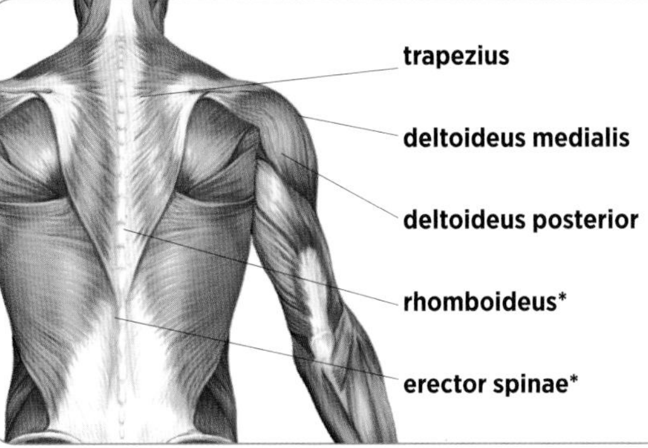

Annotation Key

Bold text indicates target muscles
Light text indicates other working muscles
* indicates deep muscles

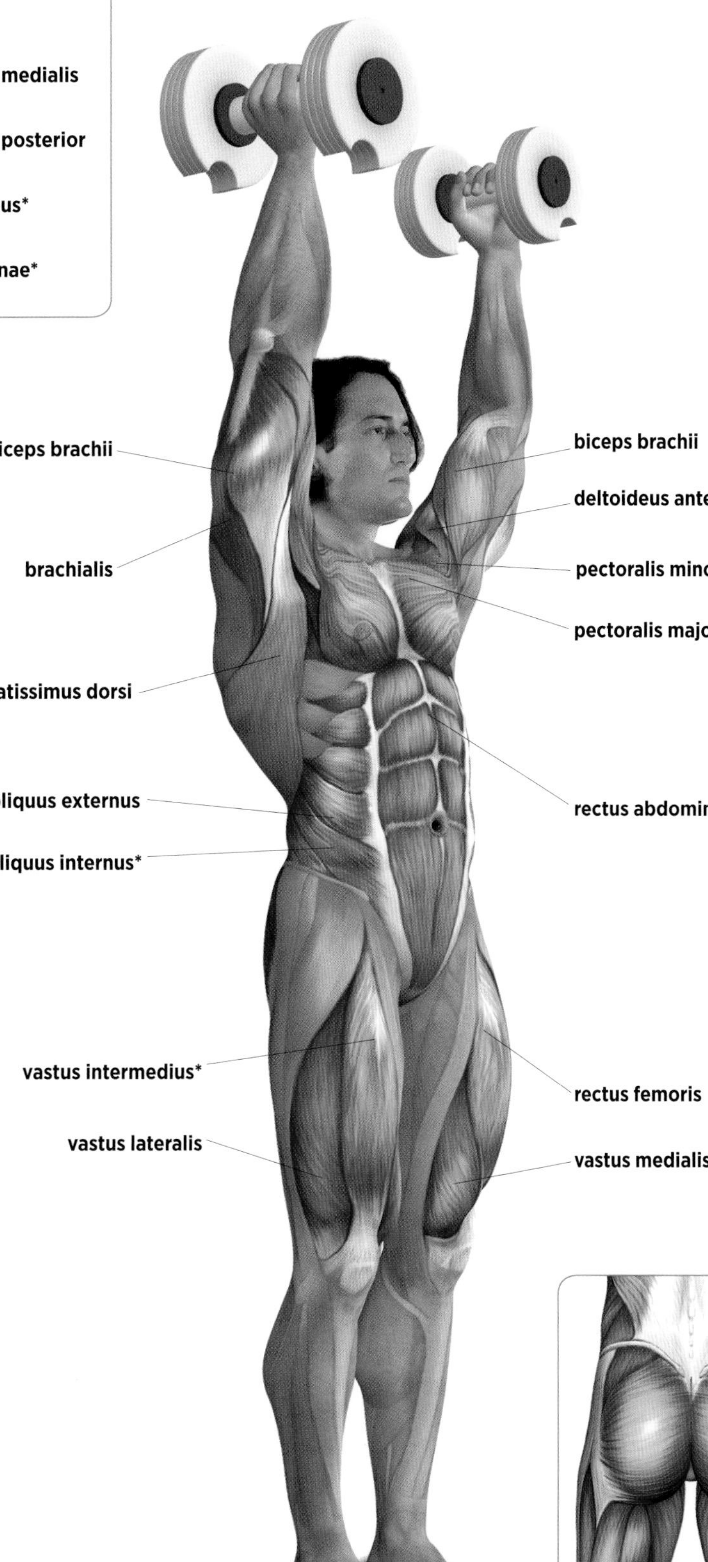

FACT FILE

TARGETS
- Triceps
- Deltoids
- Back
- Quadriceps
- Glutes

EQUIPMENT
- Dumbbells

BENEFITS
- Strengthens and tones back, arms, and legs
- Improves coordination
- Increases cardiovascular endurance

CAUTIONS
- Knee issues
- Lower-back issues

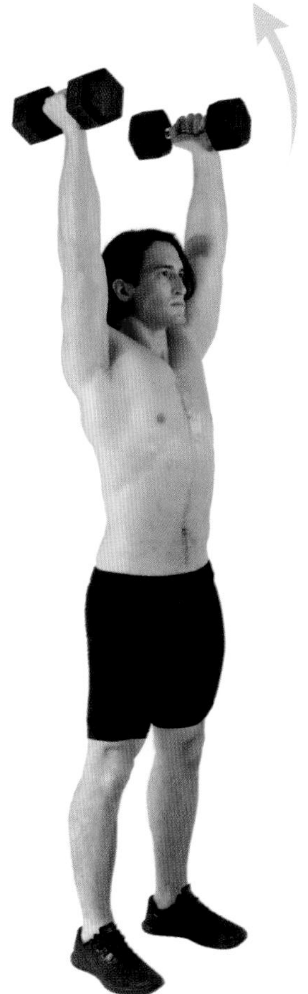

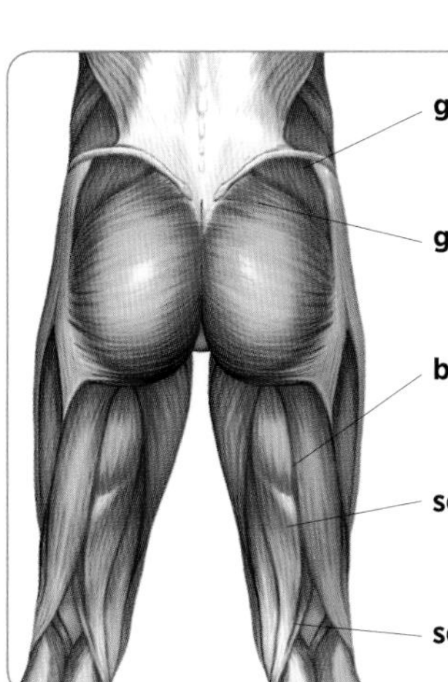

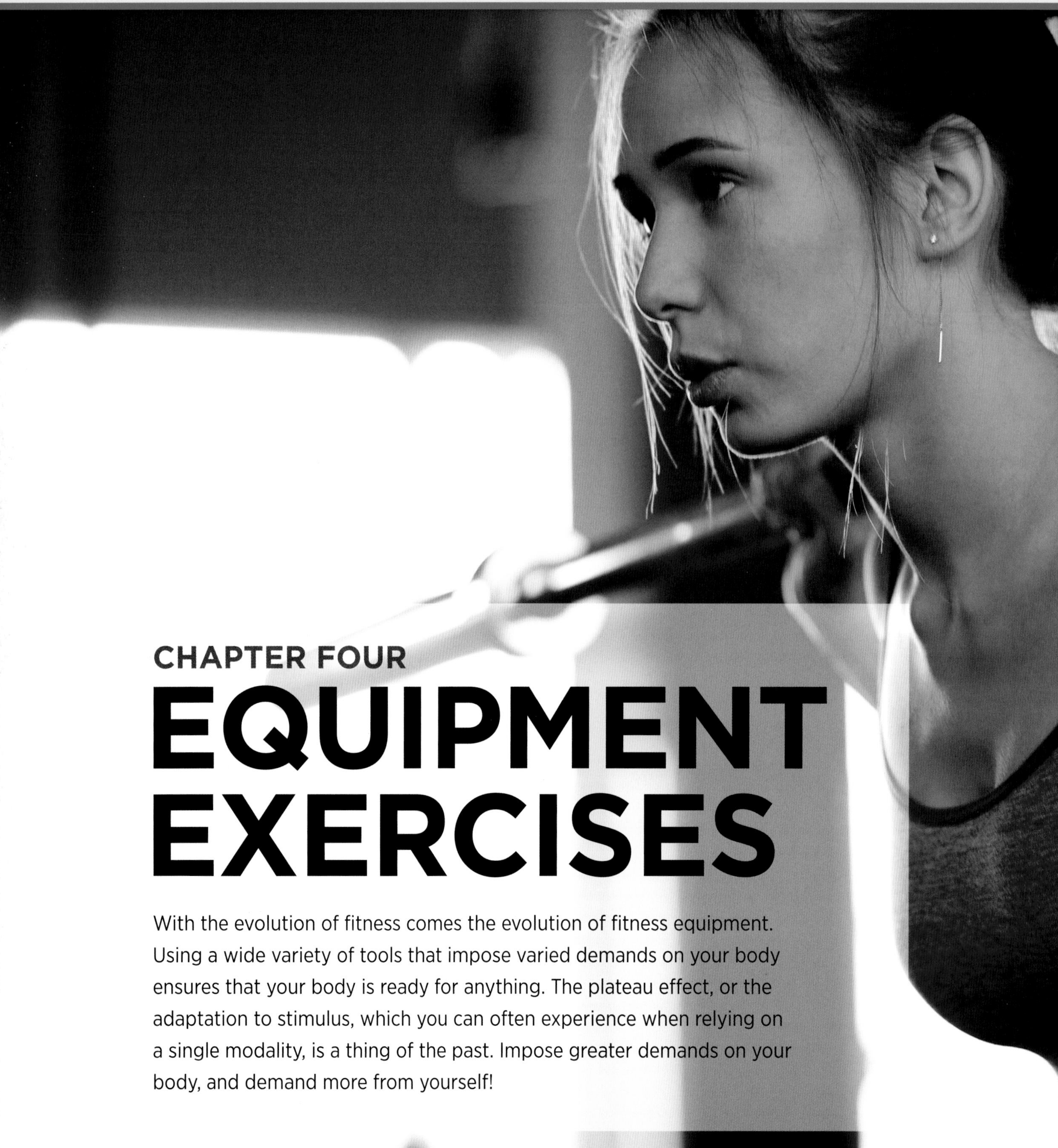

CHAPTER FOUR

EQUIPMENT EXERCISES

With the evolution of fitness comes the evolution of fitness equipment. Using a wide variety of tools that impose varied demands on your body ensures that your body is ready for anything. The plateau effect, or the adaptation to stimulus, which you can often experience when relying on a single modality, is a thing of the past. Impose greater demands on your body, and demand more from yourself!

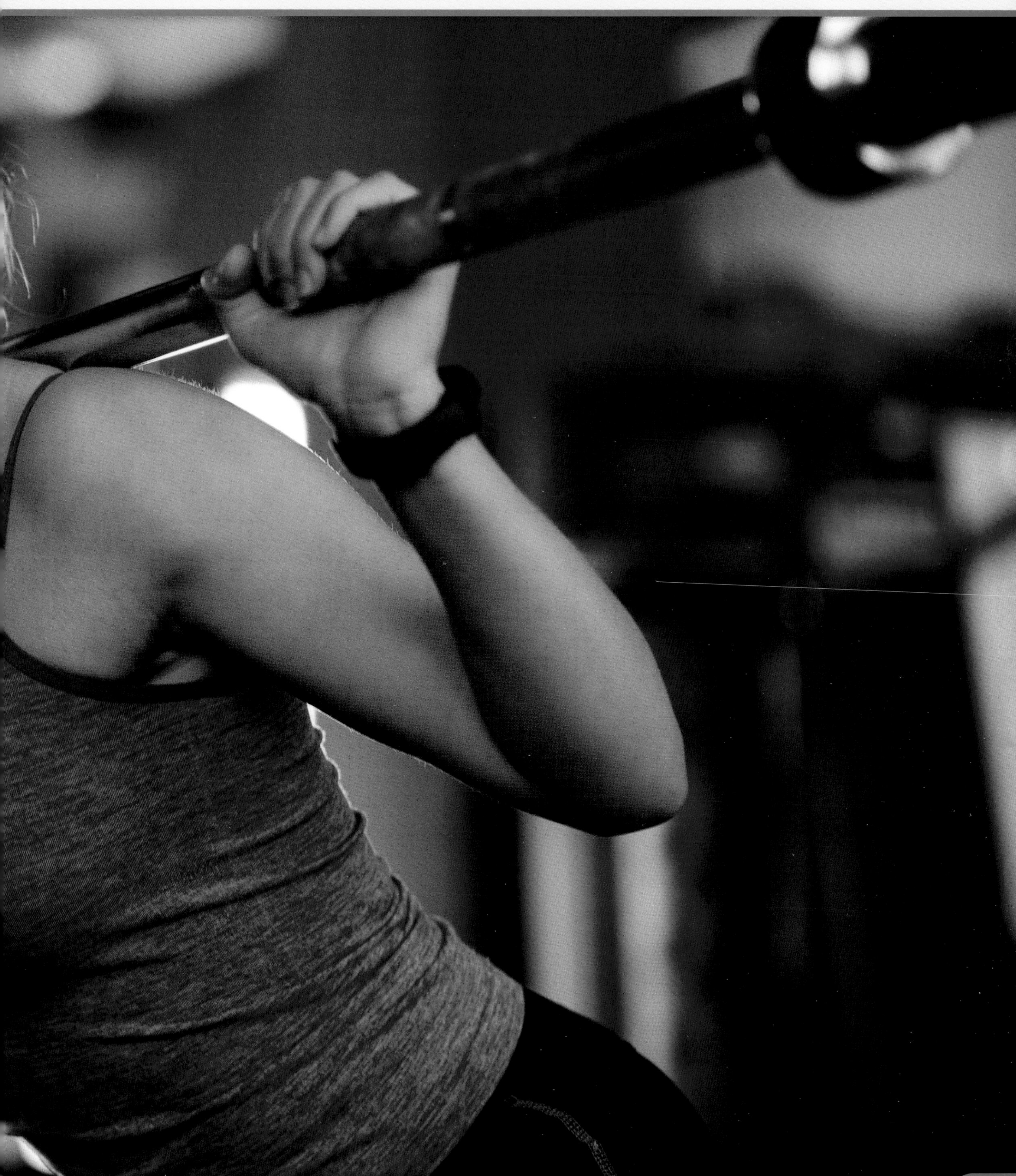

Barbell Deadlift

A body-building classic, the Barbell Deadlift increases power in your entire body. It benefits a wide range of muscle groups, including those of your lower and upper back, as well as your hamstrings and glutes. It will also engage your core.

HOW TO DO IT

- Place a barbell at your feet, and stand with your feet shoulder-width apart. Squat down to grasp the weight with both hands.
- Engaging your core, raise the barbell, hinging at the hips as you slowly rise to a standing position.
- Smoothly return the barbell to the floor, again hinging at the hips. Repeat for the recommended repetitions.

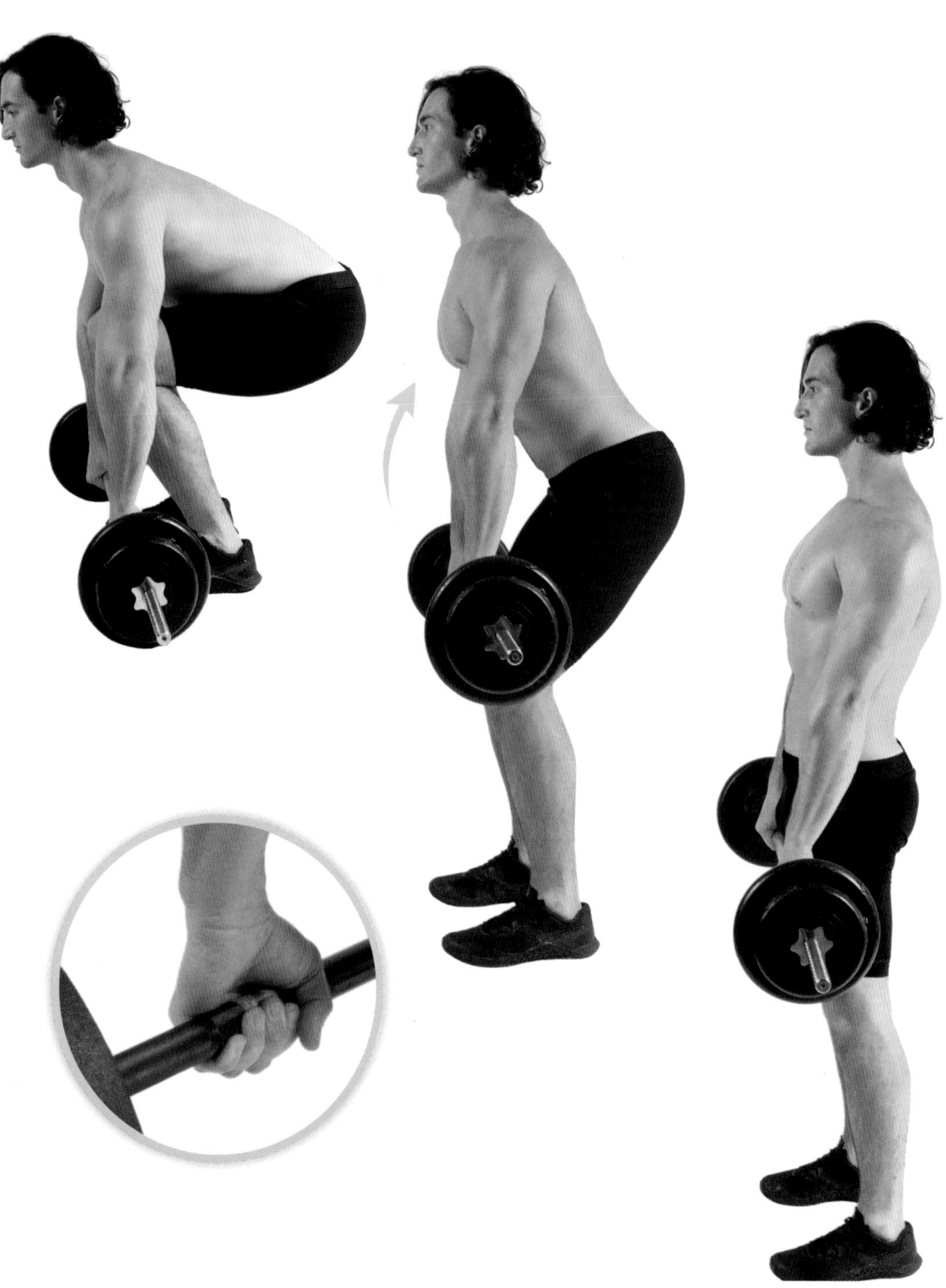

DO IT RIGHT

- Spend just as much time lowering the barbell as you spend lifting it.
- Engage your chest, core, and shoulder muscles.
- Gaze forward.
- Avoid letting your chest and shoulders collapse.
- Keep your shoulders down.
- Avoid jerky movements.
- Avoid arching your back.
- Avoid using a heavier weight than you can safely handle.

FACT FILE

TARGETS
- Back
- Glutes
- Legs

EQUIPMENT
- Barbell

BENEFITS
- Strengthens upper and lower back, hamstrings, and glutes

CAUTIONS
- Back pain

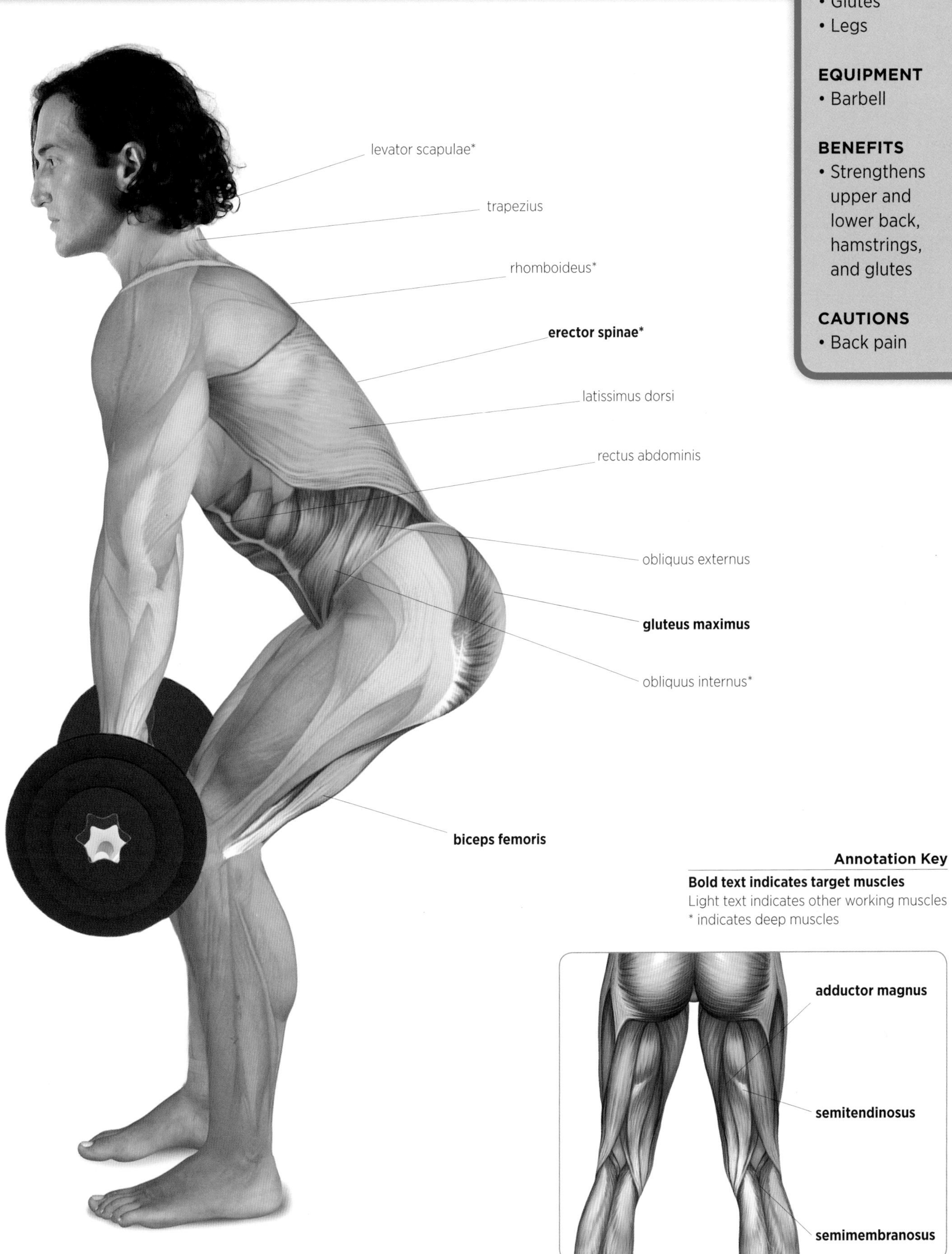

Annotation Key

Bold text indicates target muscles

Light text indicates other working muscles

* indicates deep muscles

Stiff-Legged Barbell Deadlift

The Stiff-Legged Barbell Deadlift targets numerous back muscles, including your erector spinae, rhomboids, trapezius, latissimus dorsi, and levator scapulae. It also works your hamstrings, glutes, and abdominals.

HOW TO DO IT

- Stand with your feet shoulder-width apart, grasping a barbell using an overhand grip.
- With your legs straight and your hips back, extend through your waist to lower the barbell to the floor.
- Raise the barbell back to the starting position, making sure to keep the barbell close to the front of your body. Repeat for the recommended repetitions.

DO IT RIGHT

- Move steadily and with control.
- Avoid rounding your back forward.
- Avoid using momentum to raise and lower the barbell.
- Avoid using a heavier weight than you can safely handle.

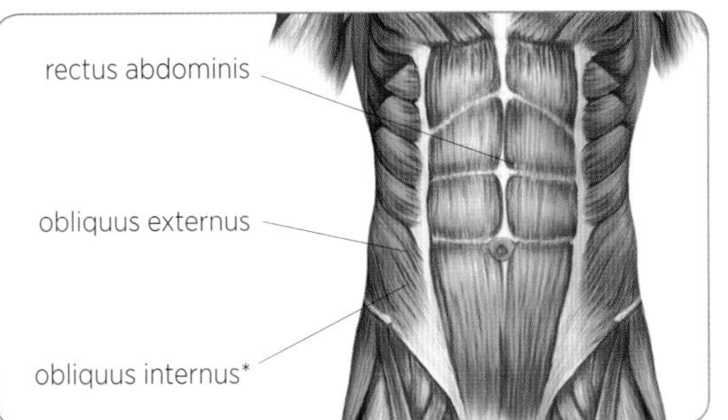

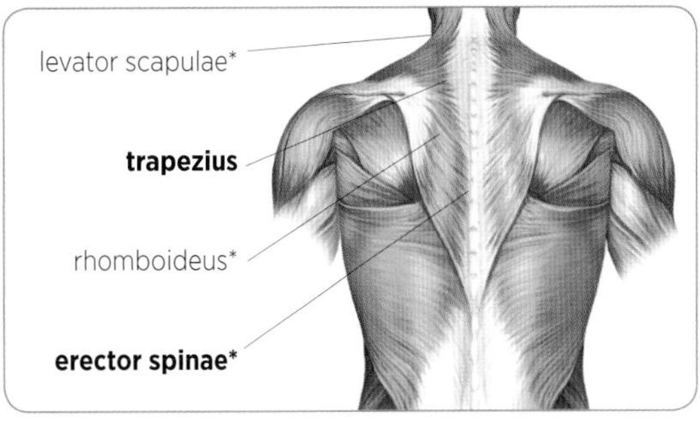

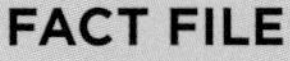

FACT FILE

TARGETS
- Back
- Hamstrings
- Glutes

EQUIPMENT
- Barbell

BENEFITS
- Strengthens upper and lower back, hamstrings, and glutes

CAUTIONS
- Lower-back issues

latissimus dorsi

gluteus maximus

semitendinosus

biceps femoris

semimembranosus

Annotation Key

Bold text indicates target muscles
Light text indicates other working muscles
* indicates deep muscles

Barbell Good Morning

The Barbell Good Morning is an effective exercise to help improve your back health. It strengthens your lower-back and core muscles, while also stretching your hamstrings. This is a very advanced exercise—execute it with caution and care. If you are unsure of how heavy your barbell should be, start with an extremely light weight.

HOW TO DO IT

- Standing with your feet parallel and shoulder-width apart, place a barbell on your shoulders with your hands an equal distance apart. Keep your head up to ensure a proper flat back.
- Keeping your back flat, legs stationary, and core braced, push your hips back, lowering your torso until it is nearly parallel to the floor.
- Raise your torso back to the starting position, and repeat for the recommended repetitions.

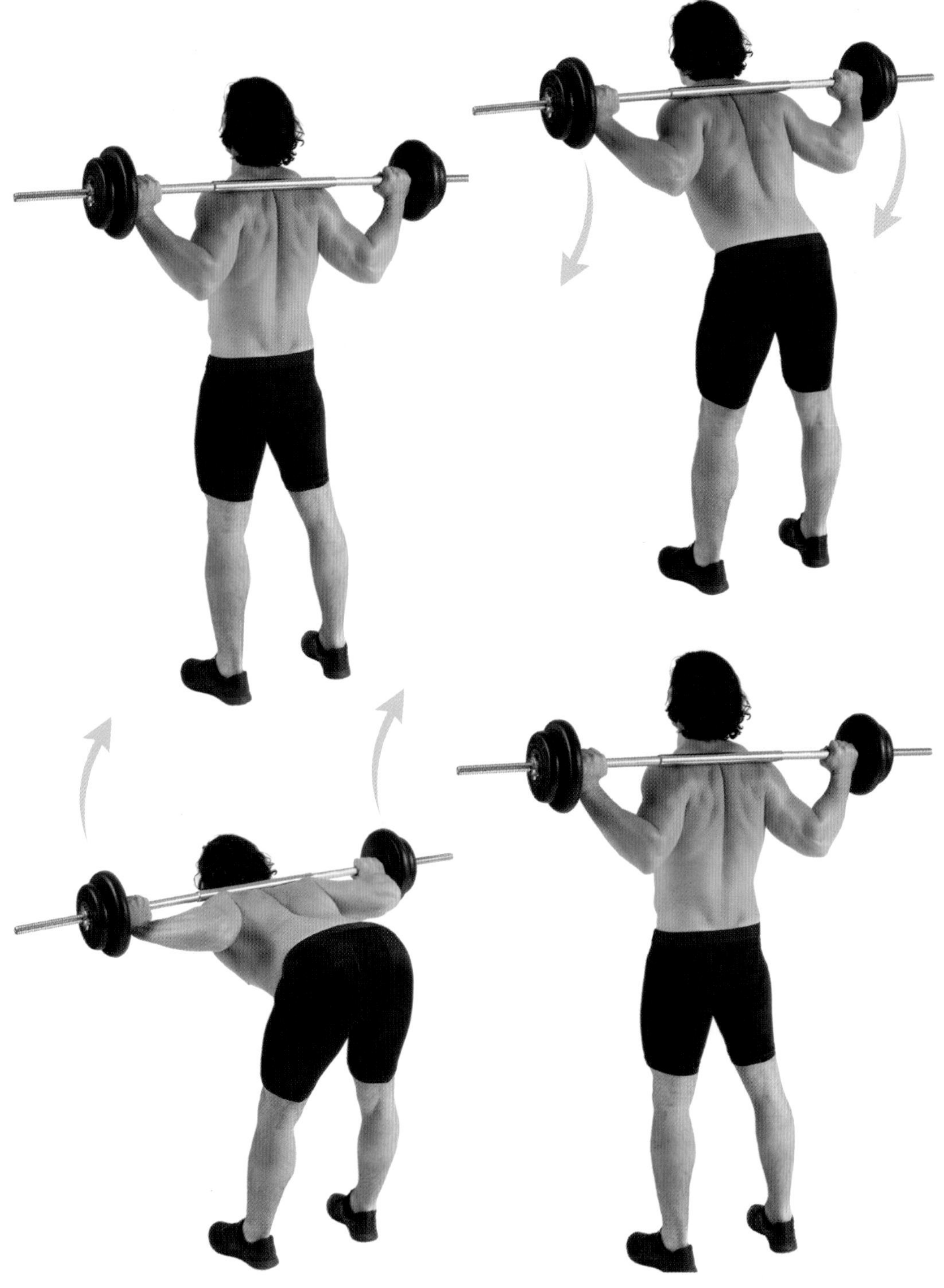

DO IT RIGHT

- Keep your head up throughout the movement.
- Move your torso up and down through an arc of about 90 degrees.
- Avoid bending your torso below parallel to the floor.
- Avoid using a heavier weight than you can safely handle.

FACT FILE

TARGETS
- Back
- Hamstrings
- Core

EQUIPMENT
- Barbell

BENEFITS
- Strengthens back and core
- Stretches hamstrings

CAUTIONS
- Shoulder issues
- Wrist issues
- Lower-back issues

Annotation Key

Bold text indicates target muscles

Light text indicates other working muscles

* indicates deep muscles

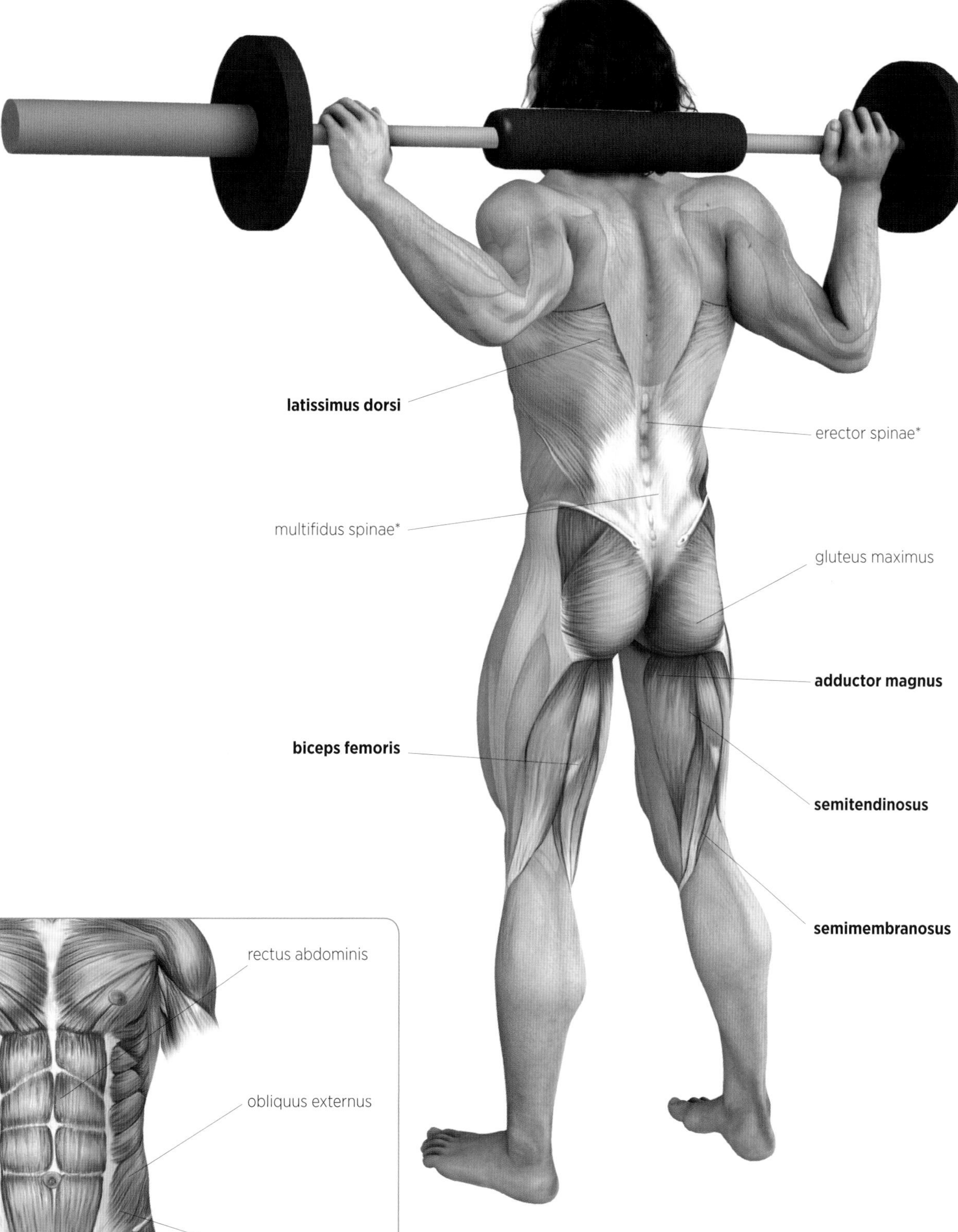

Barbell Bent-Over Row

A fundamental exercise that builds your back muscles, the Barbell Bent-Over Row also calls for you to engage your core, hips, and arms. This body-building staple is great for your shoulders, too, helping you to learn proper scapular retraction, which occurs when you squeeze your shoulder blades.

HOW TO DO IT

- Stand with your feet parallel and shoulder-width apart, your knees slightly bent, and your midfoot under the bar. Bend over to grab the bar with your hands about shoulder-width apart and your palms facing inward.
- Keeping your torso stationary, exhale and lift the barbell toward your chest. At the top of the movement, squeeze your back muscles, and hold for a slight pause.
- Inhale and slowly lower the barbell back to the starting position. Repeat for the recommended repetitions.

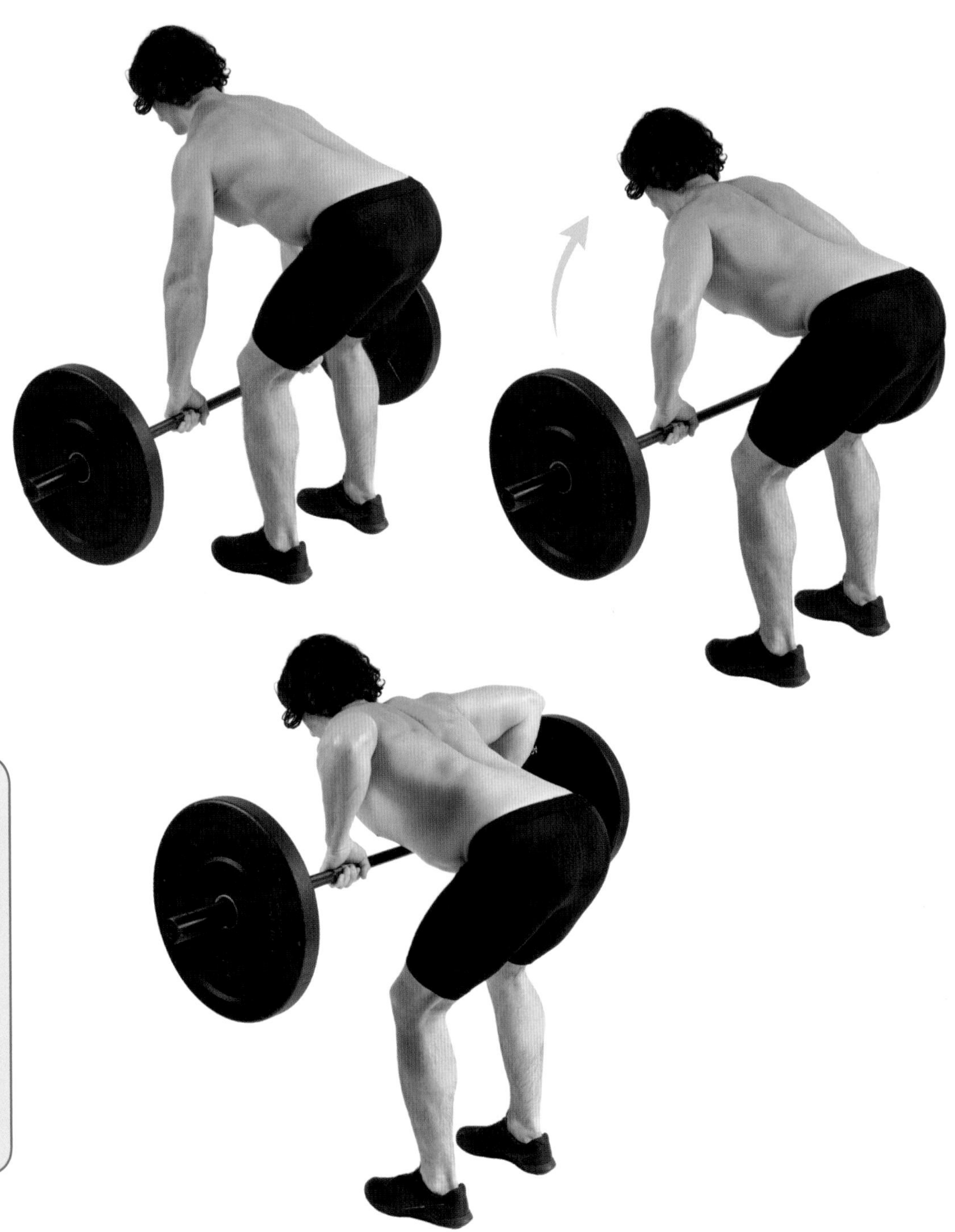

DO IT RIGHT

- Keep your torso horizontal.
- Let your upper-back muscles do most of the work.
- Avoid allowing your lower back to sag.
- Rest the barbell on the floor between repetitions, if necessary.
- Avoid using a heavier weight than you can safely handle.

FACT FILE

TARGETS
- Back
- Deltoids

EQUIPMENT
- Barbell

BENEFITS
- Strengthens back
- Stabilizes shoulders

CAUTIONS
- Shoulder issues
- Wrist issues
- Lower-back issues

Annotation Key

Bold text indicates target muscles

Light text indicates other working muscles

* indicates deep muscles

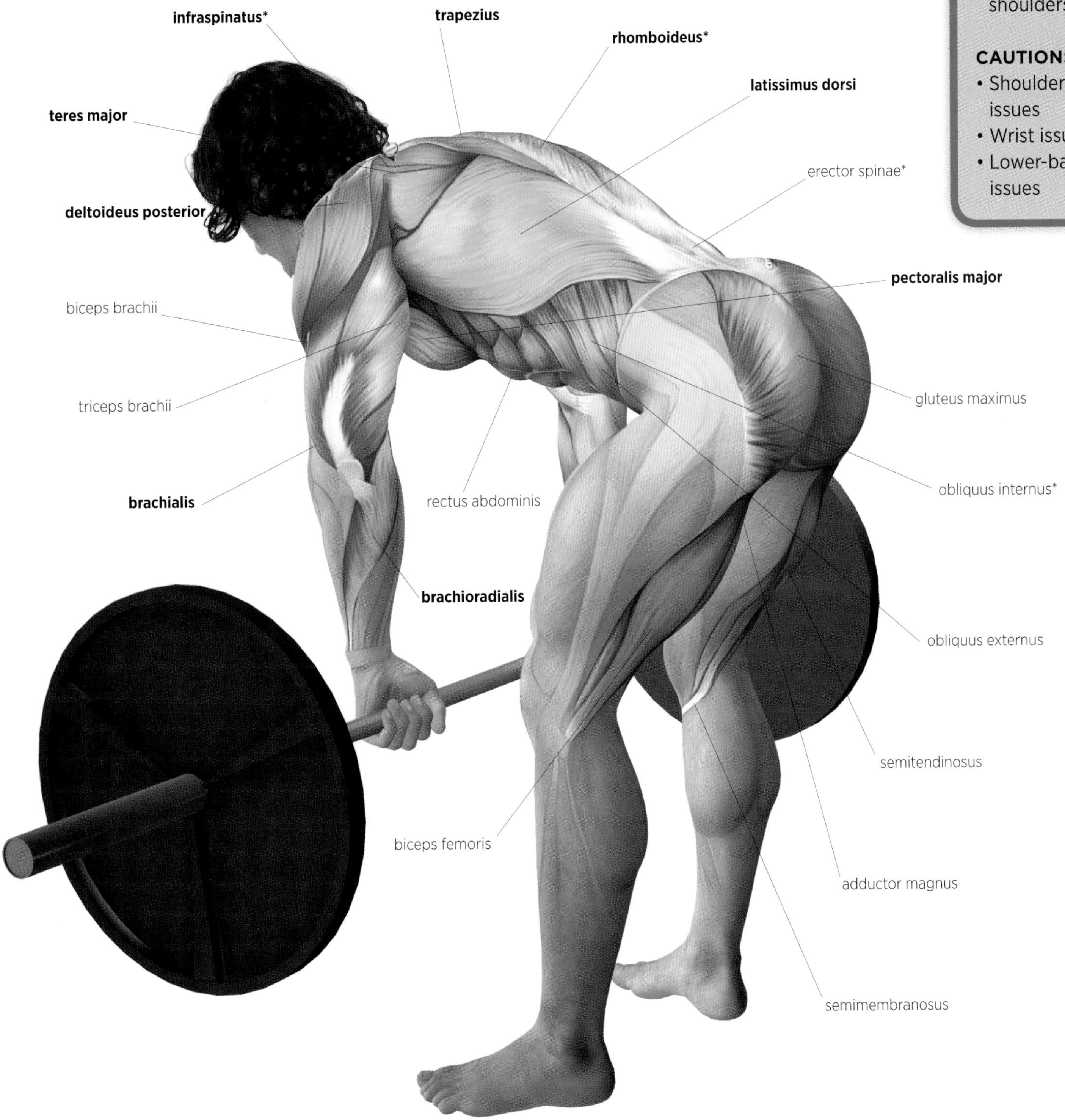

Barbell Upright Row

Performing the Barbell Upright Row will increase the power and mass of your trapezius muscle. It also targets your front deltoids, upper back, forearms, biceps, and core. Swap the barbell for a very light bar to make the exercise less challenging.

HOW TO DO IT

- Standing with your feet parallel and shoulder-width apart, holding a barbell with a relatively close grip and letting it hang at arm's length in front of you.

- Keeping your body erect, pull the barbell straight up.

- When the barbell is nearly touching your chin, lower it back to the starting position. Repeat for the recommended repetitions.

DO IT RIGHT

- Keep the barbell close to your body, and lead with your elbows.
- Avoid hitting your chin with the barbell.
- Avoid using a heavier weight than you can safely handle.

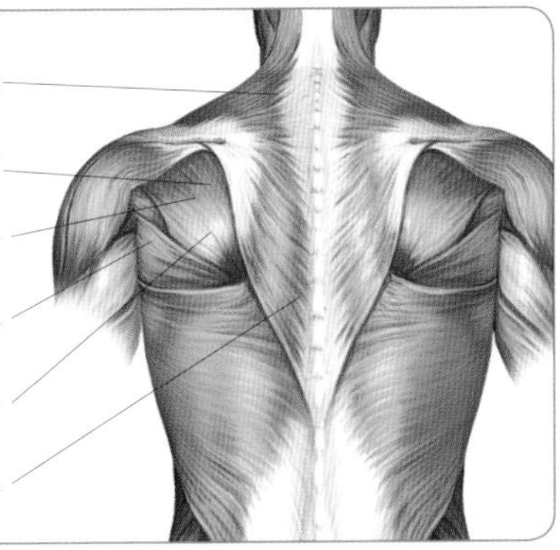

trapezius

infraspinatus*

supraspinatus*

teres major

subscapularis*

rhomboideus*

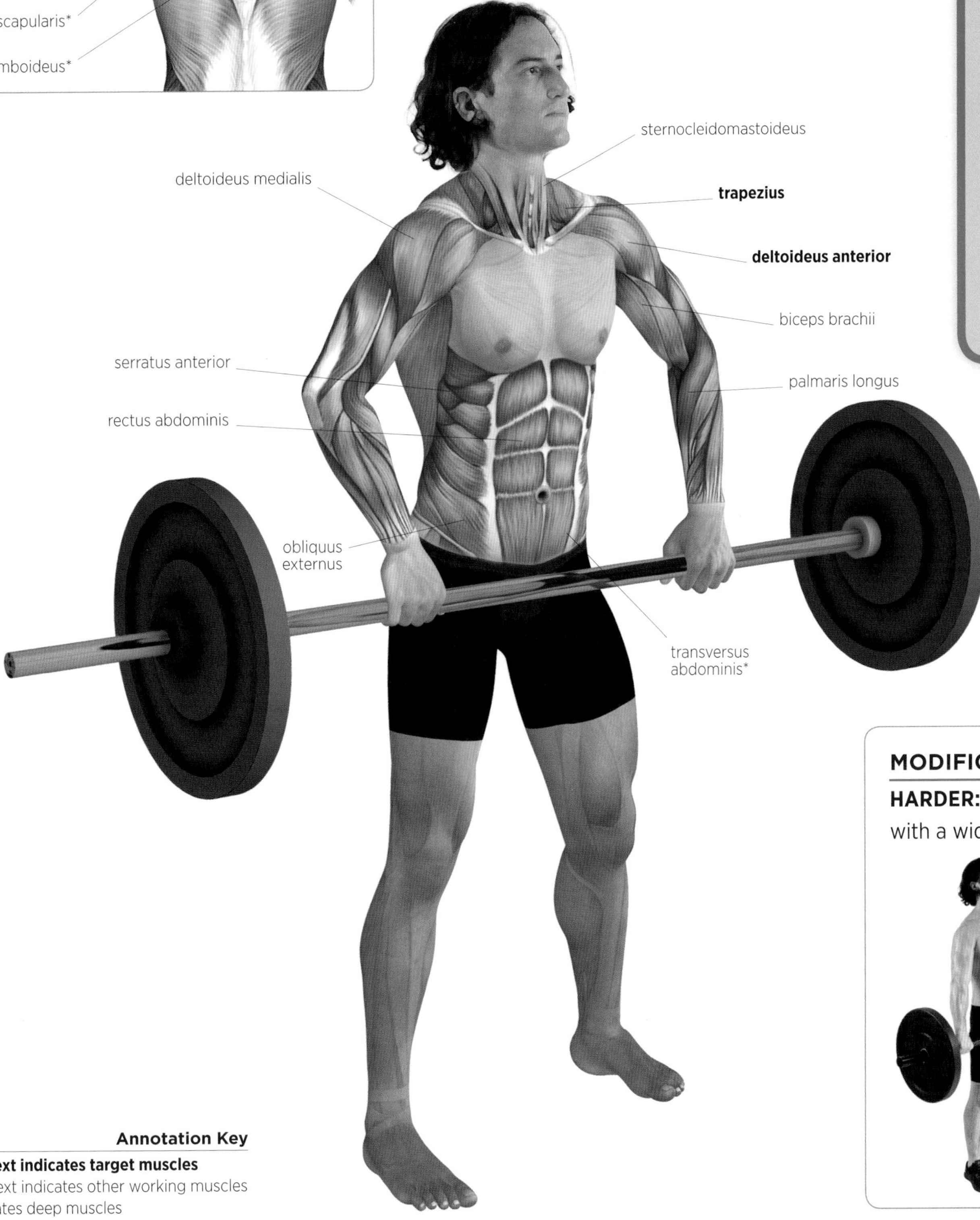

sternocleidomastoideus

deltoideus medialis

trapezius

deltoideus anterior

biceps brachii

serratus anterior

palmaris longus

rectus abdominis

obliquus externus

transversus abdominis*

Annotation Key

Bold text indicates target muscles
Light text indicates other working muscles
* indicates deep muscles

FACT FILE

TARGETS
- Upper back
- Front deltoids
- Forearms
- Biceps
- Core

EQUIPMENT
- Barbell

BENEFITS
- Strengthens upper back, shoulders, arms, and core

CAUTIONS
- Shoulder issues
- Wrist issues
- Lower-back issues

MODIFICATION

HARDER: Hold the bar with a wider grip.

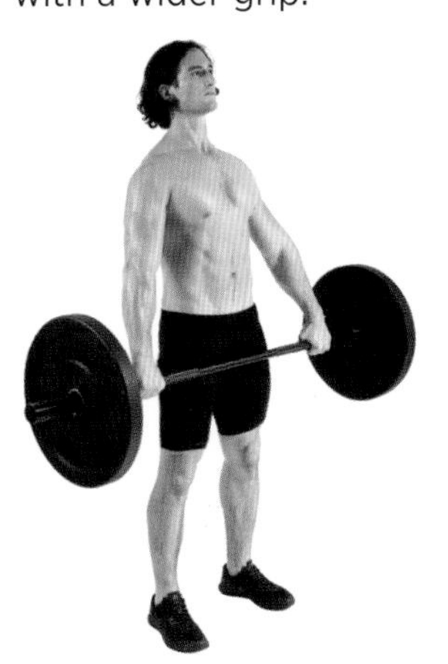

Wide-Grip High Pull

The Wide-Grip High Pull targets your upper back, legs, forearms, and core to increase strength and mass in your upper body and thighs. Use a lighter barbell to make the exercise easier, or move your feet closer together to add an extra degree of difficulty.

HOW TO DO IT

- Stand in front of a barbell with your feet hip-width apart; your shins should be close to the bar. Bend your legs until your thighs are nearly parallel to the floor, and then grab the barbell with a grip that is just beyond shoulder-width. Keeping a flat back, straighten your knees to stand up.
- Pull the barbell up to your shoulders.
- Lower the barbell back to the starting position. Repeat for the recommended repetitions.

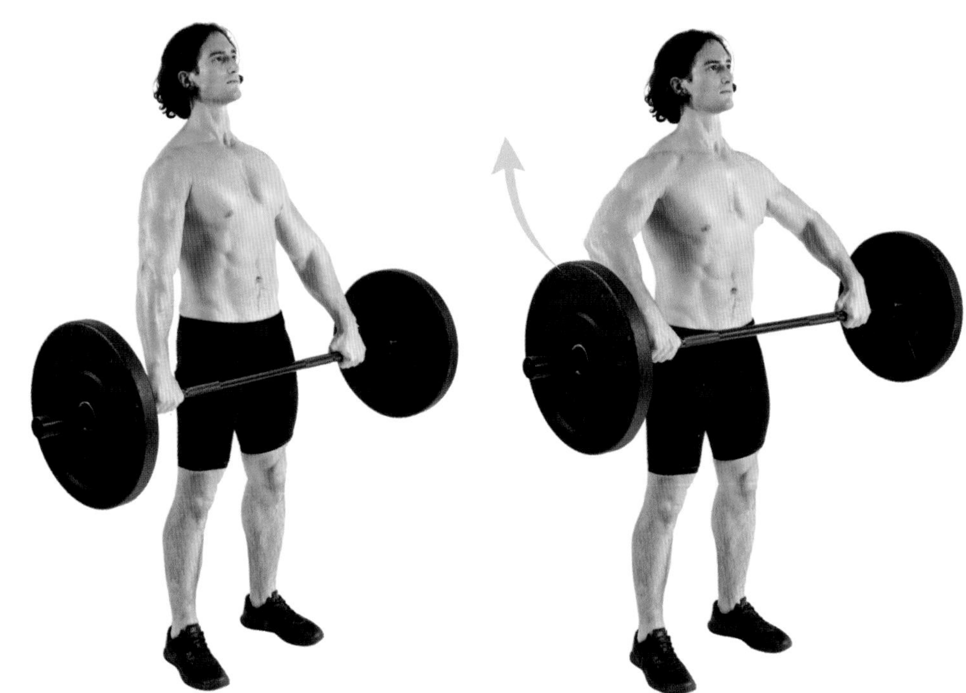

DO IT RIGHT

- Keep your back straight.
- Avoid performing the exercise with excessive speed: move with control.
- Avoid using a heavier weight than you can safely handle.

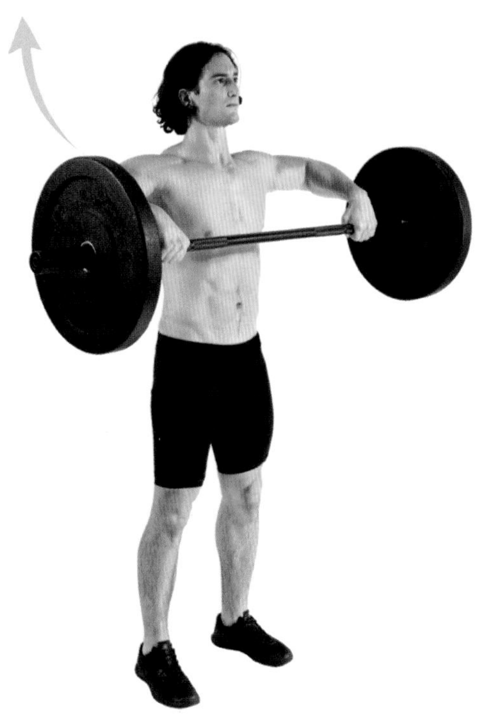

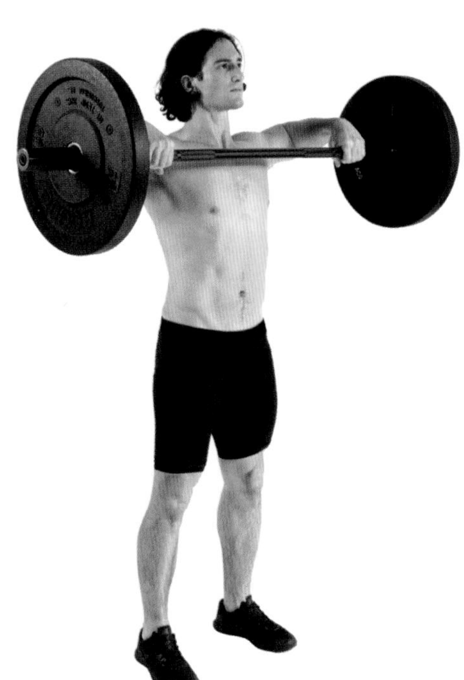

FACT FILE

TARGETS
- Upper back
- Legs
- Forearms
- Core

EQUIPMENT
- Barbell

BENEFITS
- Strengthens back, legs, arms, and core

CAUTIONS
- Shoulder issues
- Wrist issues
- Lower-back issues

Annotation Key

Bold text indicates target muscles
Light text indicates other working muscles
* indicates deep muscles

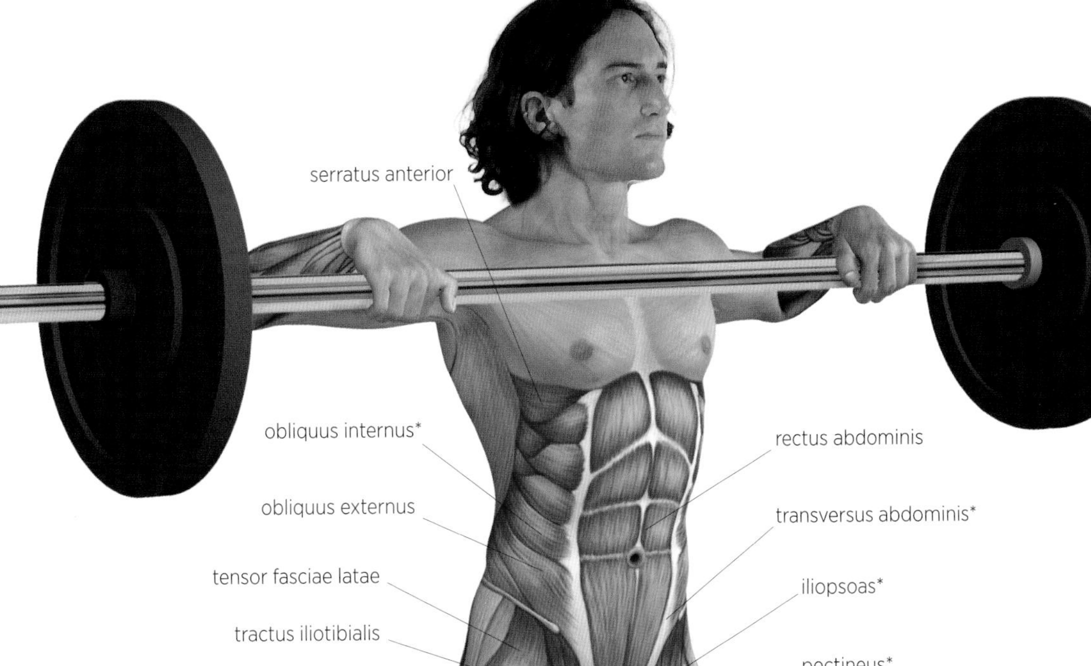

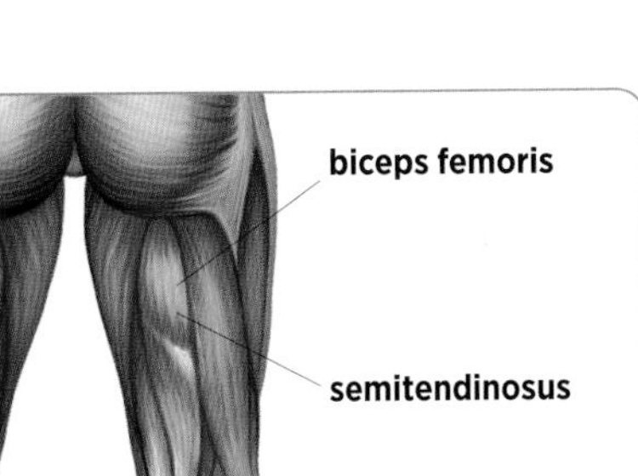

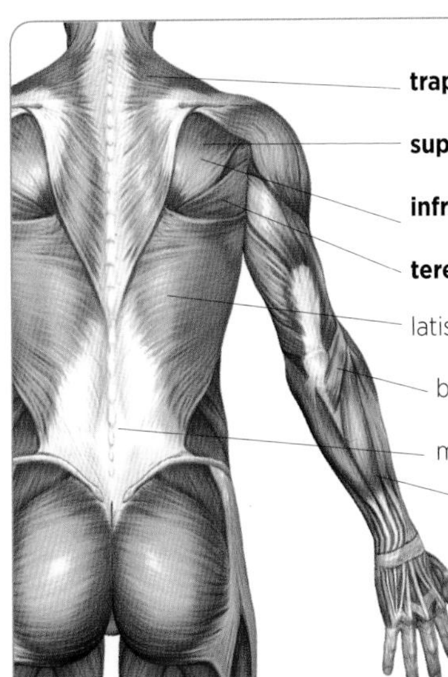

Medicine Ball Pullover on Swiss Ball

Pullover exercises work two opposing muscle groups in your back and chest, specifically your pectoral, latissimus dorsi, and serratus muscles. The Medicine Ball Pullover on Swiss Ball also adds an element of instability that will engage your core.

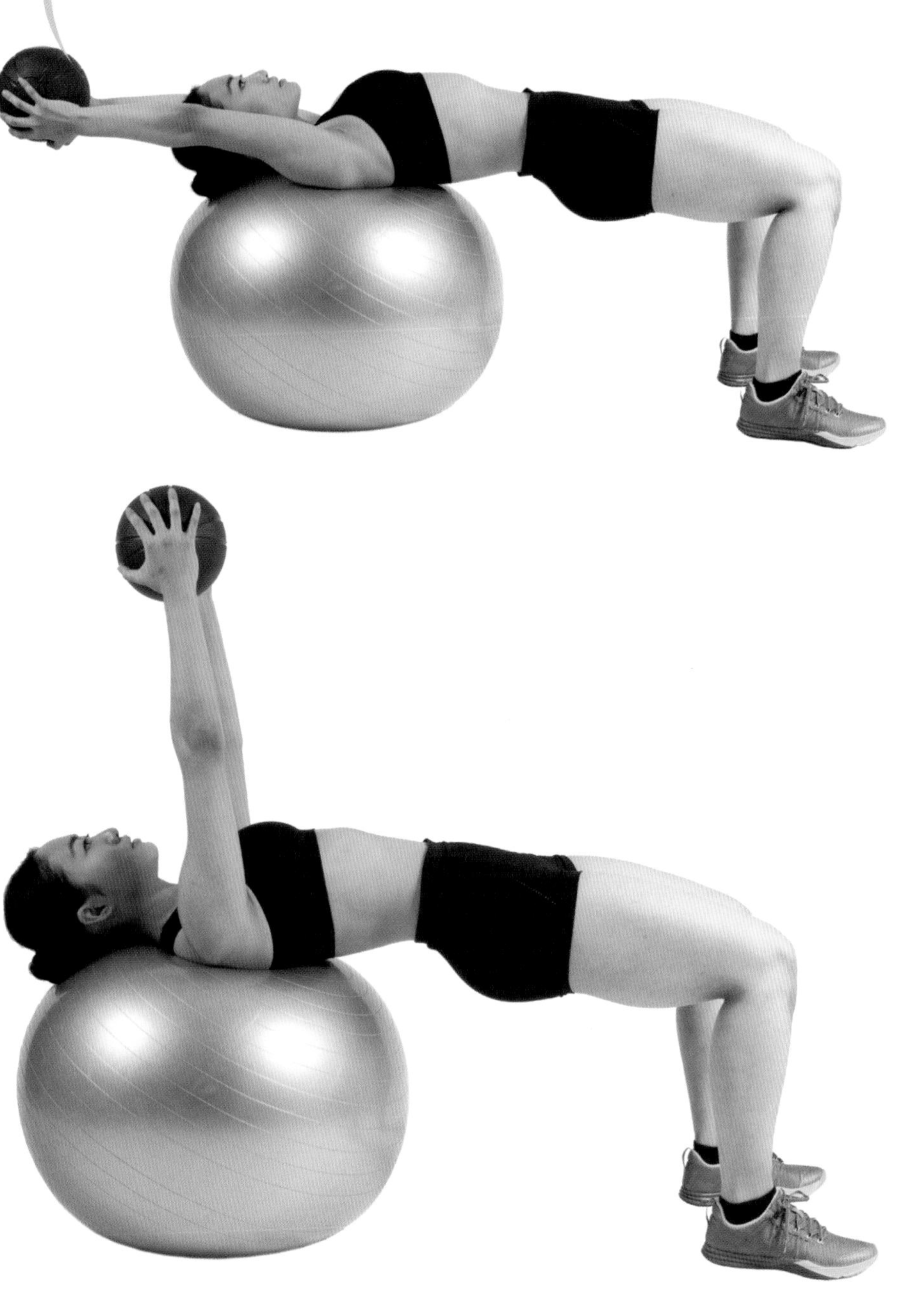

HOW TO DO IT

- Lie faceup on a Swiss ball with your upper back, neck, and head supported. Bend your knees to right angles, and plant your feet a little wider than shoulder-width apart. Grasp a medicine ball with both hands, and extend your arms behind you, level with your shoulders so that your body forms a straight line from knees to fingertips.

- Keeping your body stable and your arms as straight as possible, raise your arms upward so they are perpendicular to your body.

- Return your arms to the starting position. Repeat for the recommended repetitions.

DO IT RIGHT

- Keep your arms directly above your shoulders when lifting the weights overhead.
- Keep your torso stable and your feet planted.
- Engage your abdominals.
- Lift your buttocks and pelvis.
- Move smoothly and with control; avoid rushing through the exercise.
- Avoid locking your arms when they are extended behind your head.
- Avoid arching your back.

FACT FILE

TARGETS
- Upper back
- Chest
- Core

EQUIPMENT
- Medicine ball
- Swiss ball

BENEFITS
- Strengthens back
- Stabilizes core and upper body

CAUTIONS
- Shoulder issues
- Wrist issues

Annotation Key
Bold text indicates target muscles
Light text indicates other working muscles
* indicates deep muscles

MODIFICATION

SIMILAR DIFFICULTY: Instead of using a medicine ball, grasp a dumbbell in each hand.

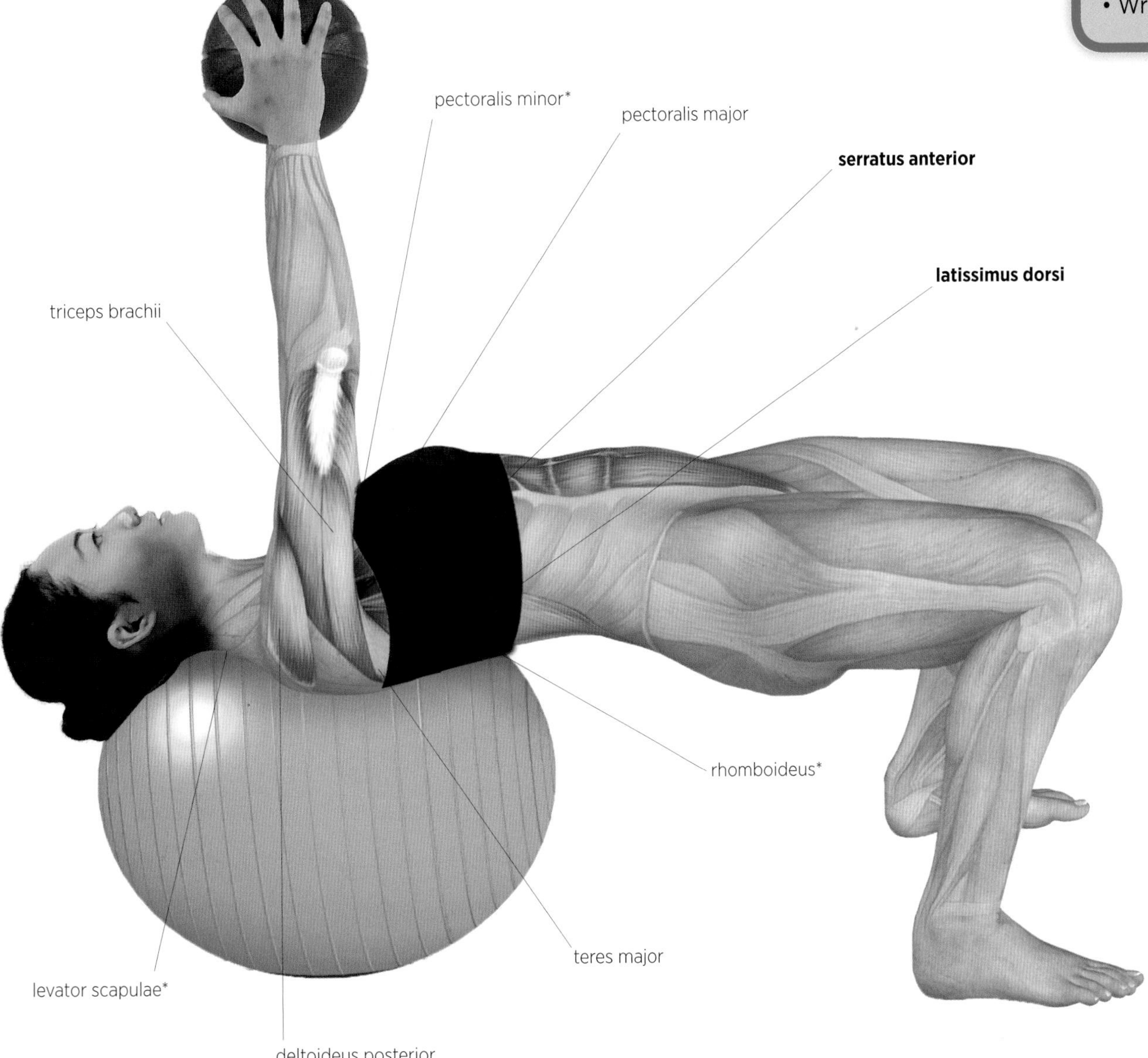

Barbell Curl

The granddaddy of biceps exercises, you will find the Barbell Curl in many arm-building workouts. It effectively targets your biceps, while relying on other arm and shoulder muscles as stabilizers.

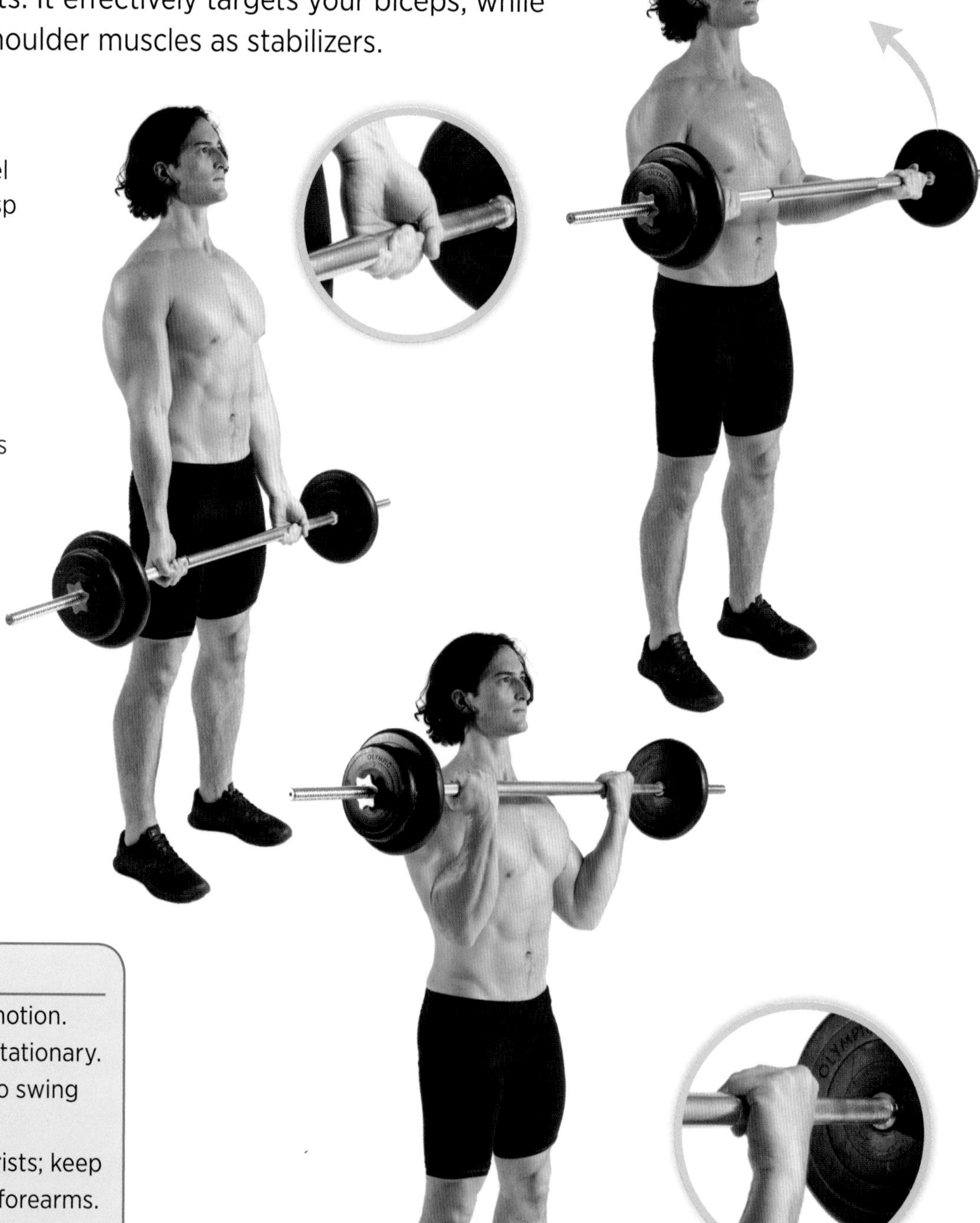

HOW TO DO IT

- Standing with your feet parallel and shoulder-width apart, grasp a barbell with an underhand grip, your hands positioned shoulder-width apart.
- Keep your elbows as close to the sides of your body as possible. With your upper arms stationary, bend your arms at the elbow and curl the barbell up toward your upper chest.
- When the barbell is at the top of the movement, pause and then slowly lower it back down. Repeat for the recommended repetitions.

DO IT RIGHT

- Employ a full range of motion.
- Keep your upper arms stationary.
- Avoid using your back to swing the barbell upward.
- Avoid bending at the wrists; keep them aligned with your forearms.
- Avoid raising your shoulders.
- Avoid using a heavier weight than you can safely handle.

FACT FILE

TARGETS
- Biceps
- Elbow flexors

EQUIPMENT
- Barbell

BENEFITS
- Strengthens arms

CAUTIONS
- Wrist issues

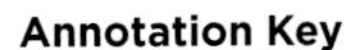

Annotation Key

Bold text indicates target muscles

Light text indicates other working muscles

* indicates deep muscles

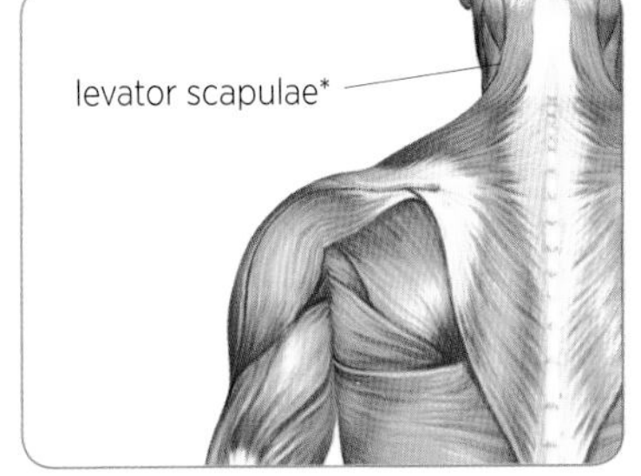

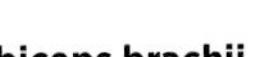

Plate Curl

Mix up you arm routine with this variation of a biceps curl. Use a 10-pound, 25-pound, or 45-pound plate, depending on your strength and number of repetitions.

HOW TO DO IT

- Stand with your feet parallel and shoulder-width apart, with your knees soft and your pelvis slightly tucked in. Grip a weight plate with both hands using a hammer-grip position. Keep your upper arms stationary, your elbows close to your torso, and your shoulders down and back away from your ears.

- Curl the plate up toward your chest, pausing slightly at the top of the range of movement.

- Slowly lower the plate back to the starting position. Repeat for the recommended repetitions.

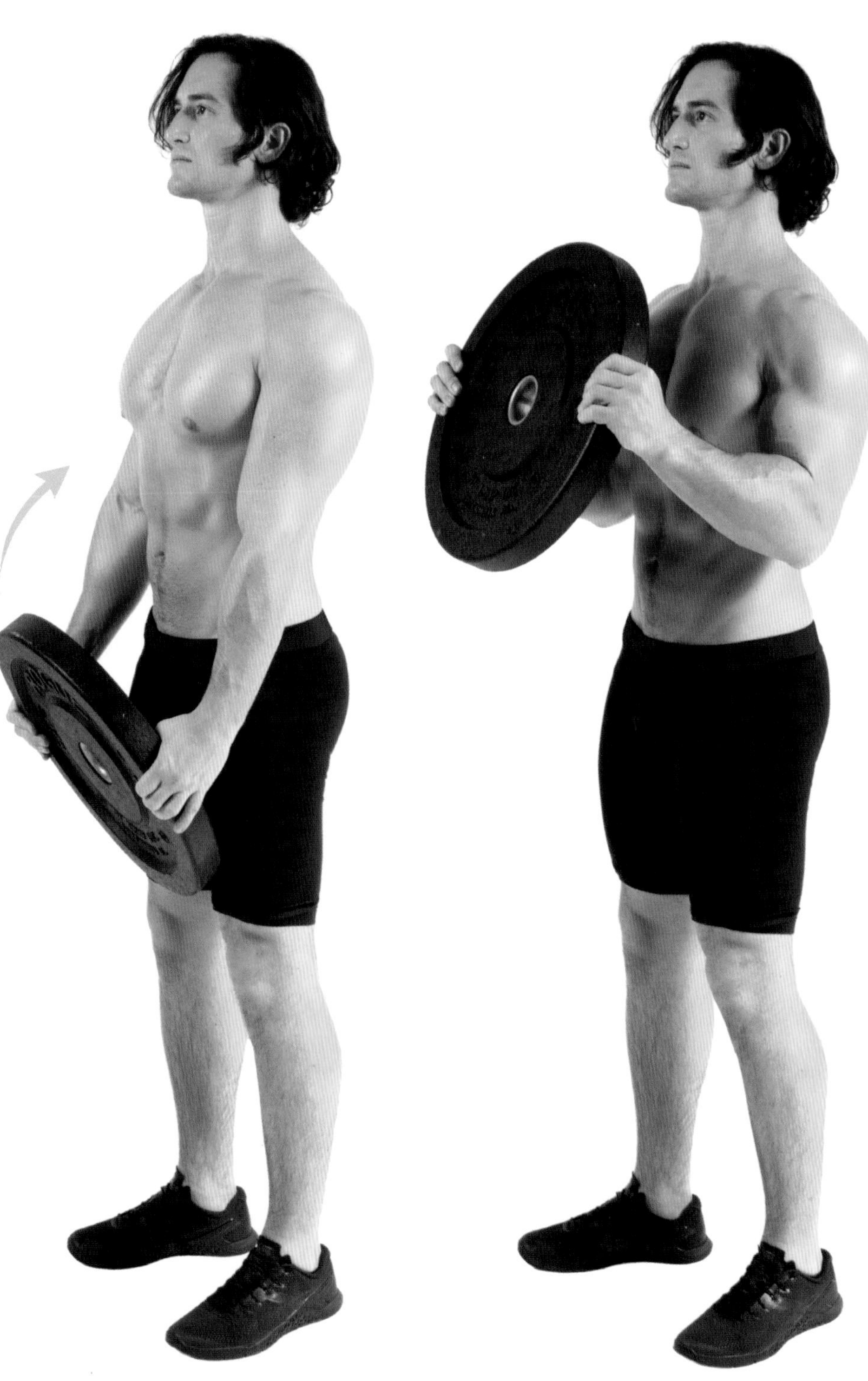

DO IT RIGHT

- Move the plate in a smooth, even arc as you curl it upward and lower it back to the starting position.
- Avoid using your back to lift the plate—concentrate on isolating your biceps.
- Avoid using a heavier weight than you can safely handle.

FACT FILE

TARGETS
- Biceps
- Elbow flexors

EQUIPMENT
- Weight plate

BENEFITS
- Strengthens arms

CAUTIONS
- Wrist issues

Annotation Key

Bold text indicates target muscles
Light text indicates other working muscles
* indicates deep muscles

levator scapulae*
trapezius
deltoideus anterior
biceps brachii
brachialis
brachioradialis

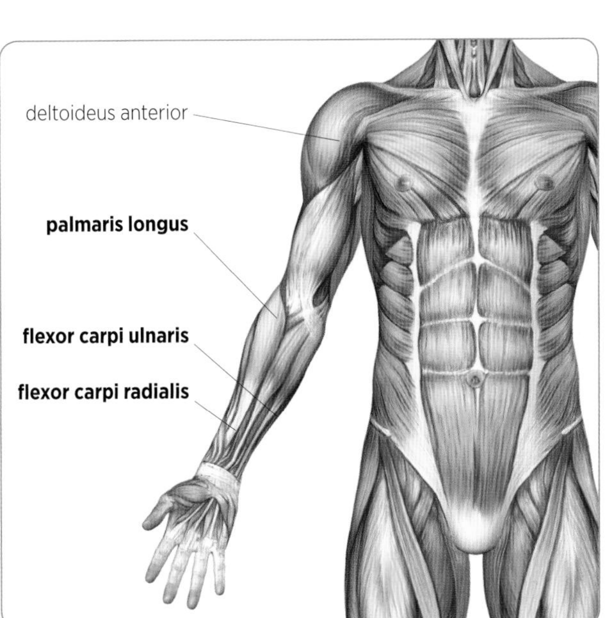

Front Plate Raise

An isolation exercise, the Front Plate Raise calls for you to flex your shoulders while holding a weight for resistance. It primarily works your front deltoids, with assistance from the serratus anterior, biceps brachii, and pectoralis major. Use a 10-pound, 25-pound, or 45-pound plate, depending on your strength and number of repetitions.

HOW TO DO IT

- Stand with your feet parallel and shoulder-width apart, with your knees soft and your pelvis slightly tucked in. Grip a weight plate with both hands using a hammer-grip position. Keep your upper arms stationary, your elbows close to your torso, and your shoulders down and back away from your ears.

- Raise the plate to shoulder height.

- Slowly lower the plate back to the starting position. Repeat for the recommended repetitions.

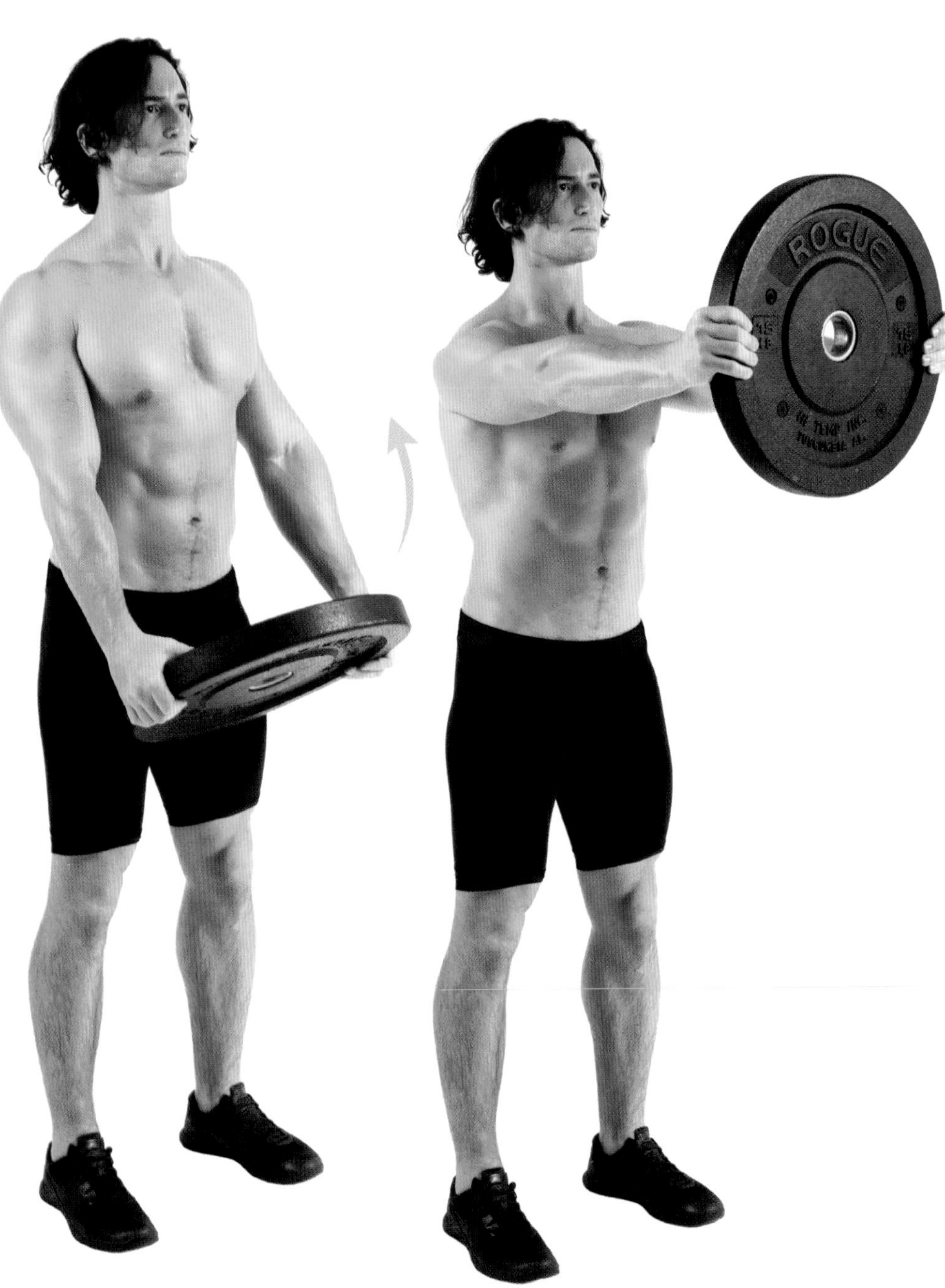

DO IT RIGHT

- Move the plate with steady, controlled movement.
- Avoid hyperextending your elbows while lifting the weight.
- Avoid allowing your shoulders to rotate inward.
- Avoid using a heavier weight than you can safely handle.

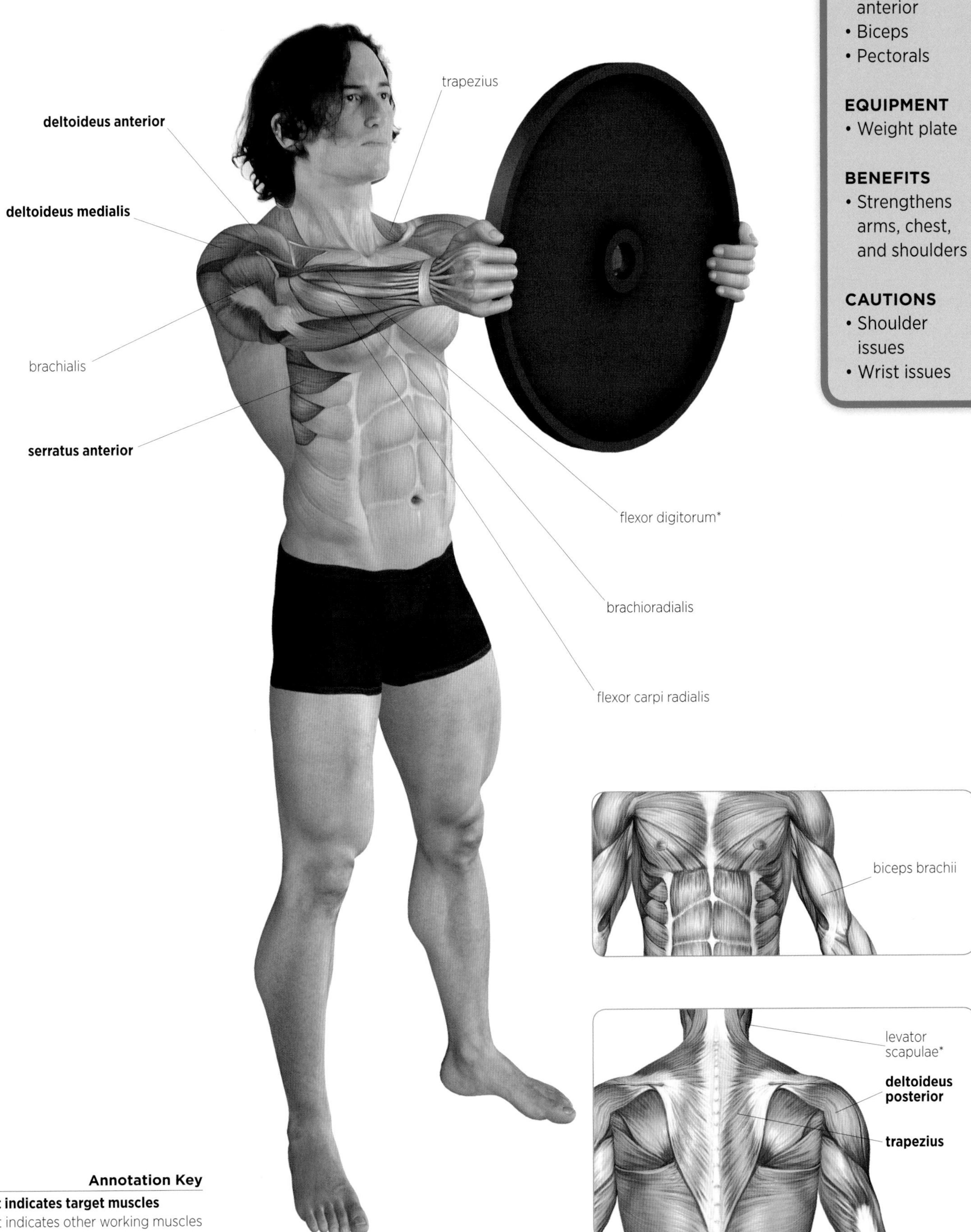

FACT FILE

TARGETS
- Front deltoids
- Serratus anterior
- Biceps
- Pectorals

EQUIPMENT
- Weight plate

BENEFITS
- Strengthens arms, chest, and shoulders

CAUTIONS
- Shoulder issues
- Wrist issues

Annotation Key

Bold text indicates target muscles

Light text indicates other working muscles

* indicates deep muscles

Skull Crusher

Also known as Triceps Extension and Nose Breaker, the Skull Crusher is a primary strength exercise that homes in on your triceps. It gets its name for the part of the body it might break if you lose control, so be sure to use only a weight you can safely handle, and work with a spotter.

HOW TO DO IT

- Sit on the edge of a flat bench with a barbell on your lap, grasping the bar with your palms facing down and your hands positioned slightly less than shoulder-width apart. Carefully begin to lower your body onto the bench. Press the bar straight upward until your arms are straight above your chest.

- While keeping your upper arms and elbows stationary, slowly lower the bar backward until it nearly touches your forehead.

- Concentrate on engaging your triceps to lift the bar back to the starting position. Repeat for the recommended repetitions.

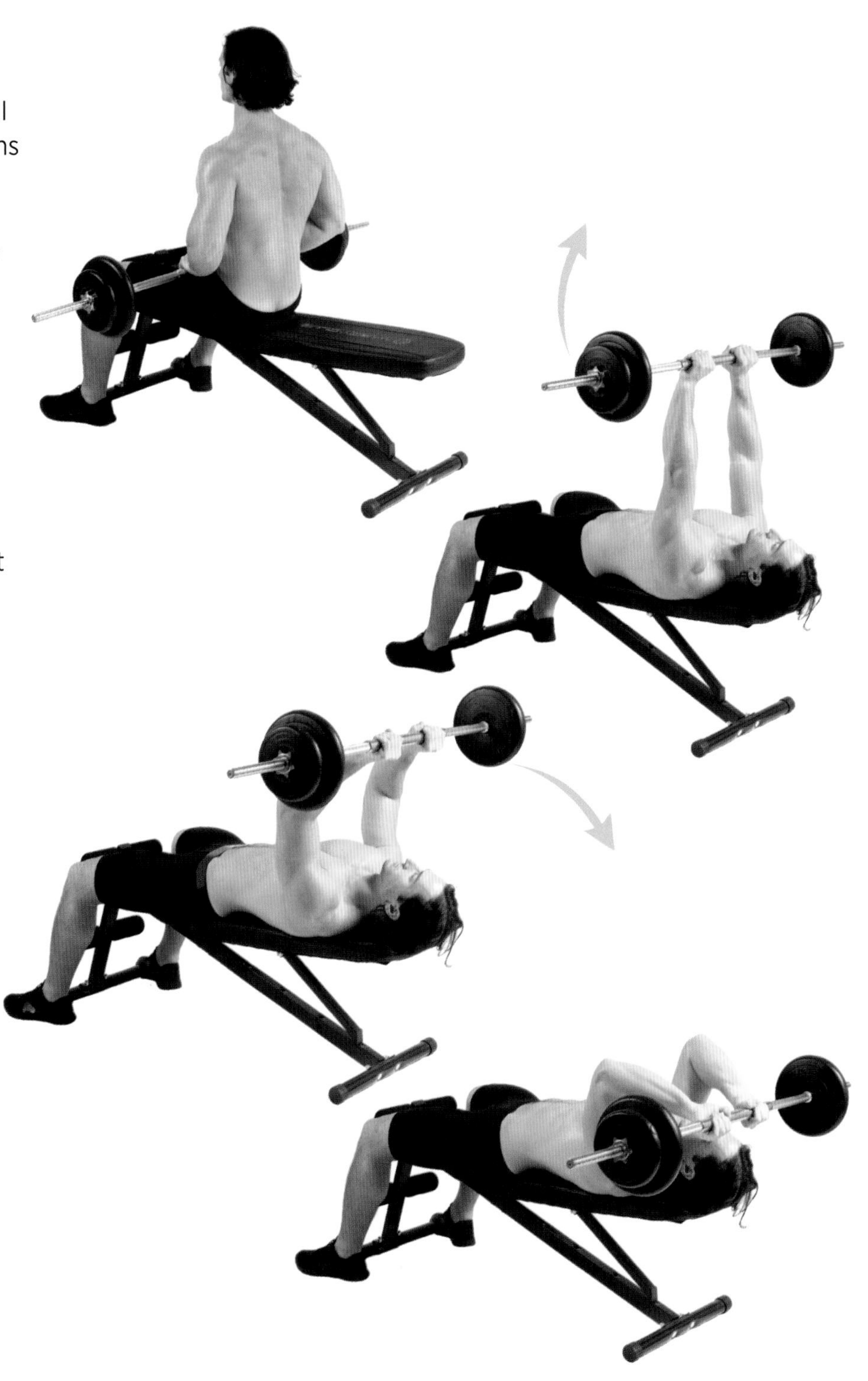

DO IT RIGHT

- Keep your lower back and glutes in contact with the bench.
- Point your elbows forward.
- Avoid tensing your neck or jaw.
- Inhale as you lower the barbell toward your forehead, and exhale as you lift it back to the starting position.
- Slow the barbell's descent as it approaches your forehead.
- When you are finished with this exercise, bend your elbows and lower the barbell toward your chest, and lift your body back to the starting position, gently placing the barbell back onto your thighs.
- Avoid using a heavier weight than you can safely handle.

FACT FILE

TARGETS
- Triceps

EQUIPMENT
- Barbell
- Flat bench

BENEFITS
- Strengthens upper arms

CAUTIONS
- Shoulder issues
- Wrist issues

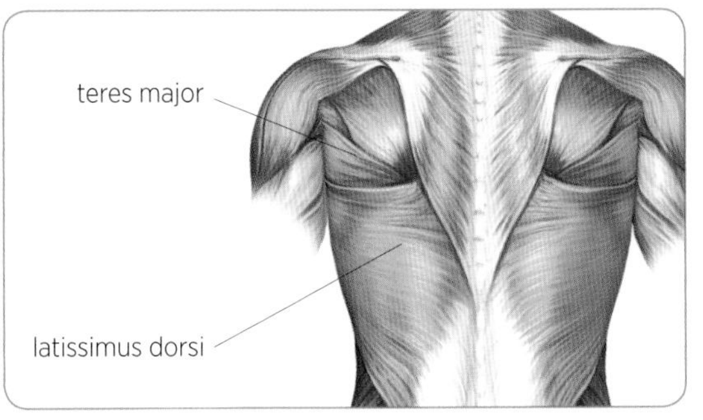

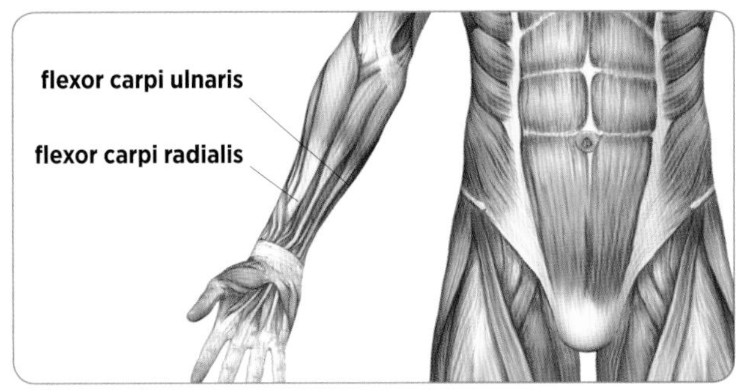

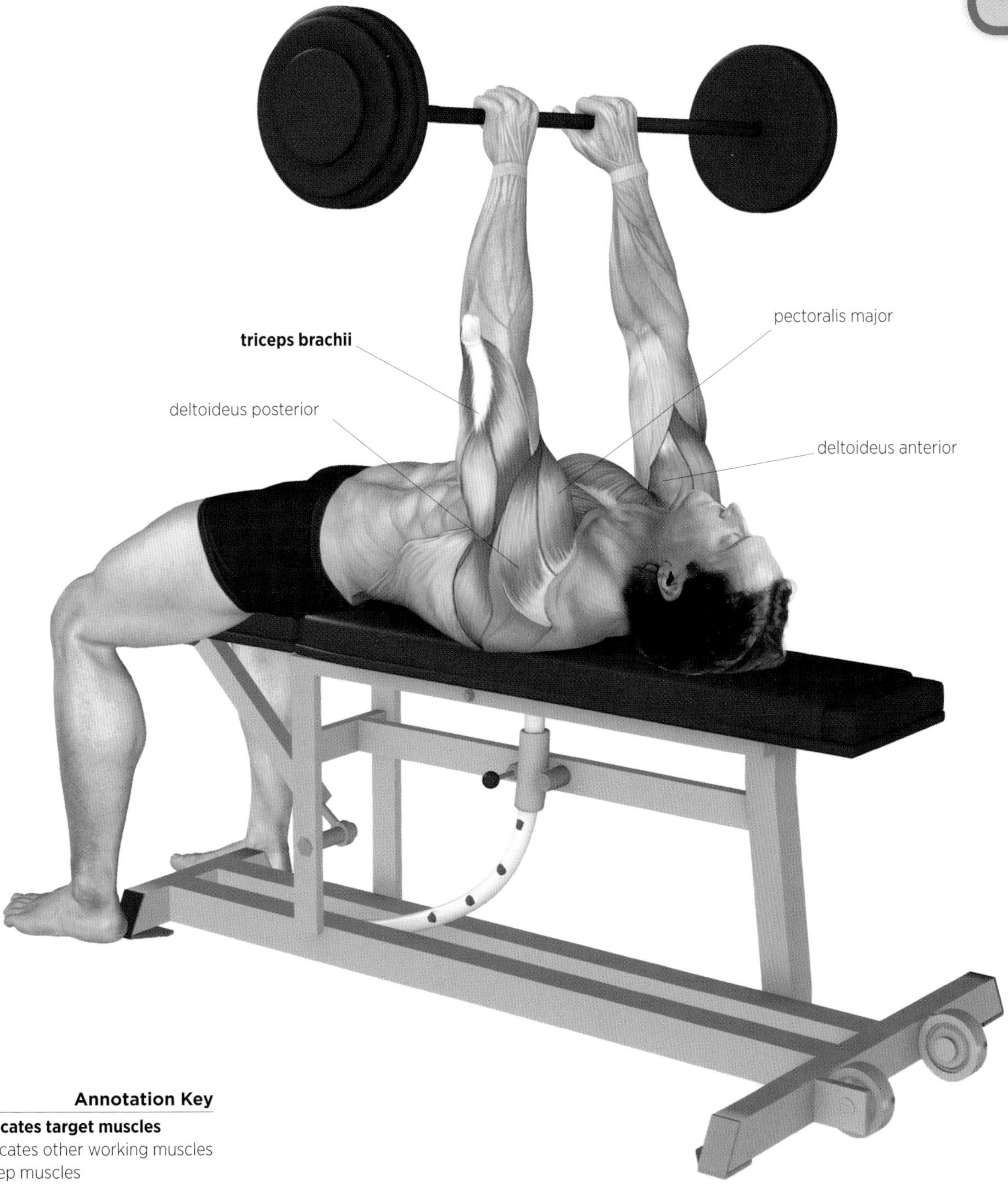

teres major
latissimus dorsi

flexor carpi ulnaris
flexor carpi radialis

triceps brachii
pectoralis major
deltoideus posterior
deltoideus anterior

Annotation Key

Bold text indicates target muscles

Light text indicates other working muscles

* indicates deep muscles

Barbell Full Raise

The Barbell Full Raise is beautiful in its simplicity and effectiveness. This exercise will condition your shoulders, upper back, and core musculature. Try it with just an unloaded bar until you gain enough strength to lift a full load.

HOW TO DO IT

- Standing with your feet parallel and hip-width apart, grasp a bar with an overhand grip just outside shoulder-width with your palms facing inward.
- Keeping your arms straight and your core engaged, press the bar overhead.
- Lower your arms, bringing the bar back to the starting position. Repeat for the recommended repetitions.

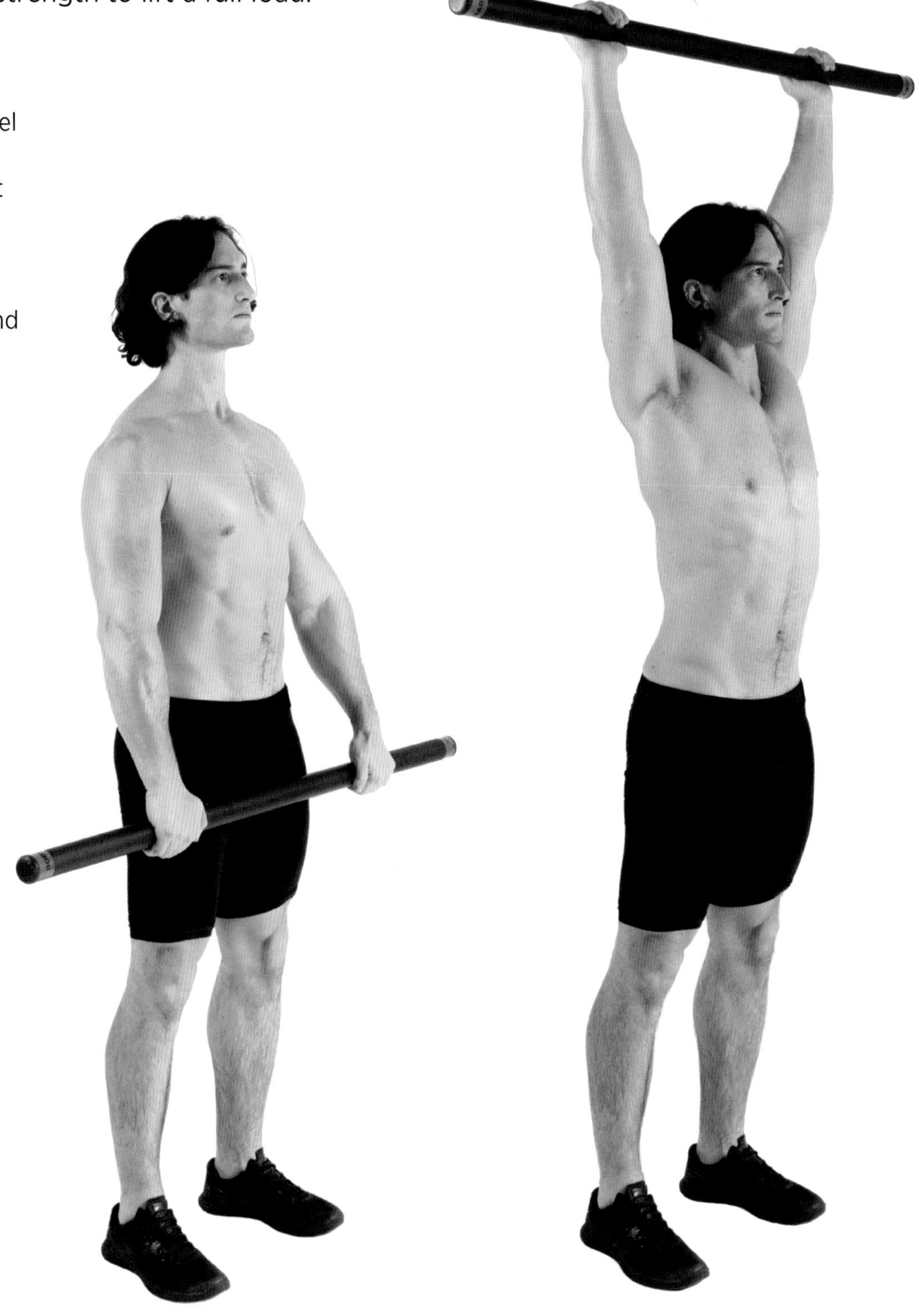

DO IT RIGHT

- Keep your back in a neutral position.
- Avoid excessive trunk movement.
- Avoid using a heavier weight than you can safely handle.

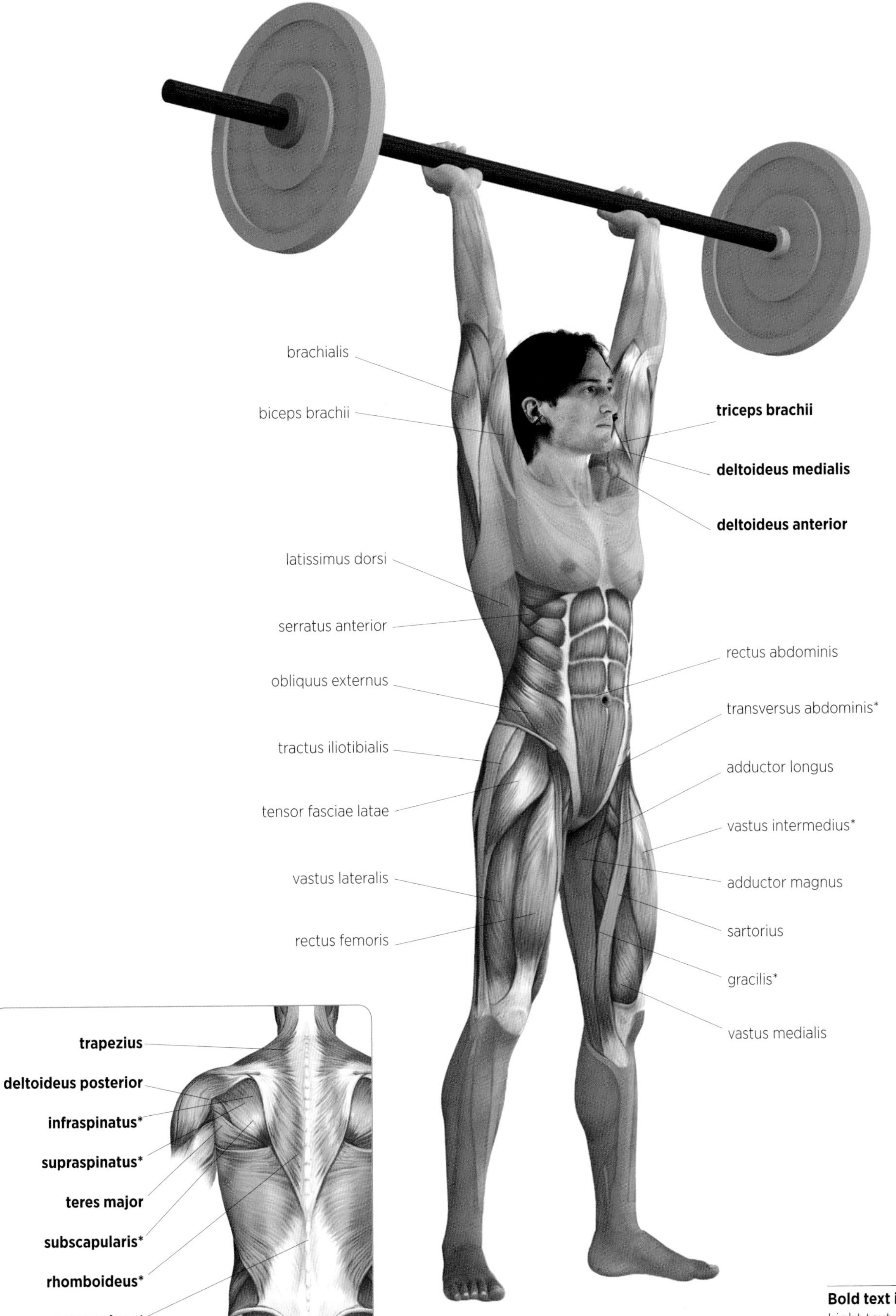

FACT FILE

TARGETS
- Deltoids
- Abdominals
- Back

EQUIPMENT
- Barbell

BENEFITS
- Strengthens and tones arms, back, shoulders, and abdominals

CAUTIONS
- Shoulder issues
- Wrist issues

Annotation Key

Bold text indicates target muscles

Light text indicates other working muscles

* indicates deep muscles

Barbell Hang Clean

The Barbell Hang Clean is a high-energy, demanding exercise. This power movement will condition your arms, upper and lower back, and core, with a cardiovascular component that will get your heart pumping.

HOW TO DO IT

- Standing with your feet parallel and hip-width apart, grasp a barbell with an overhand grip just outside shoulders-width with palms facing inward.
- Hinging at your hips, drop the bar down to just above your knees.
- In one explosive motion, extend your hips and pull the bar to shoulder level by shrugging your shoulders, drawing your elbows upward.
- Catch the bar on your shoulders with your elbows pointed forward.
- Lower your arms, bringing the bar back to the starting position. Repeat for the recommended repetitions.

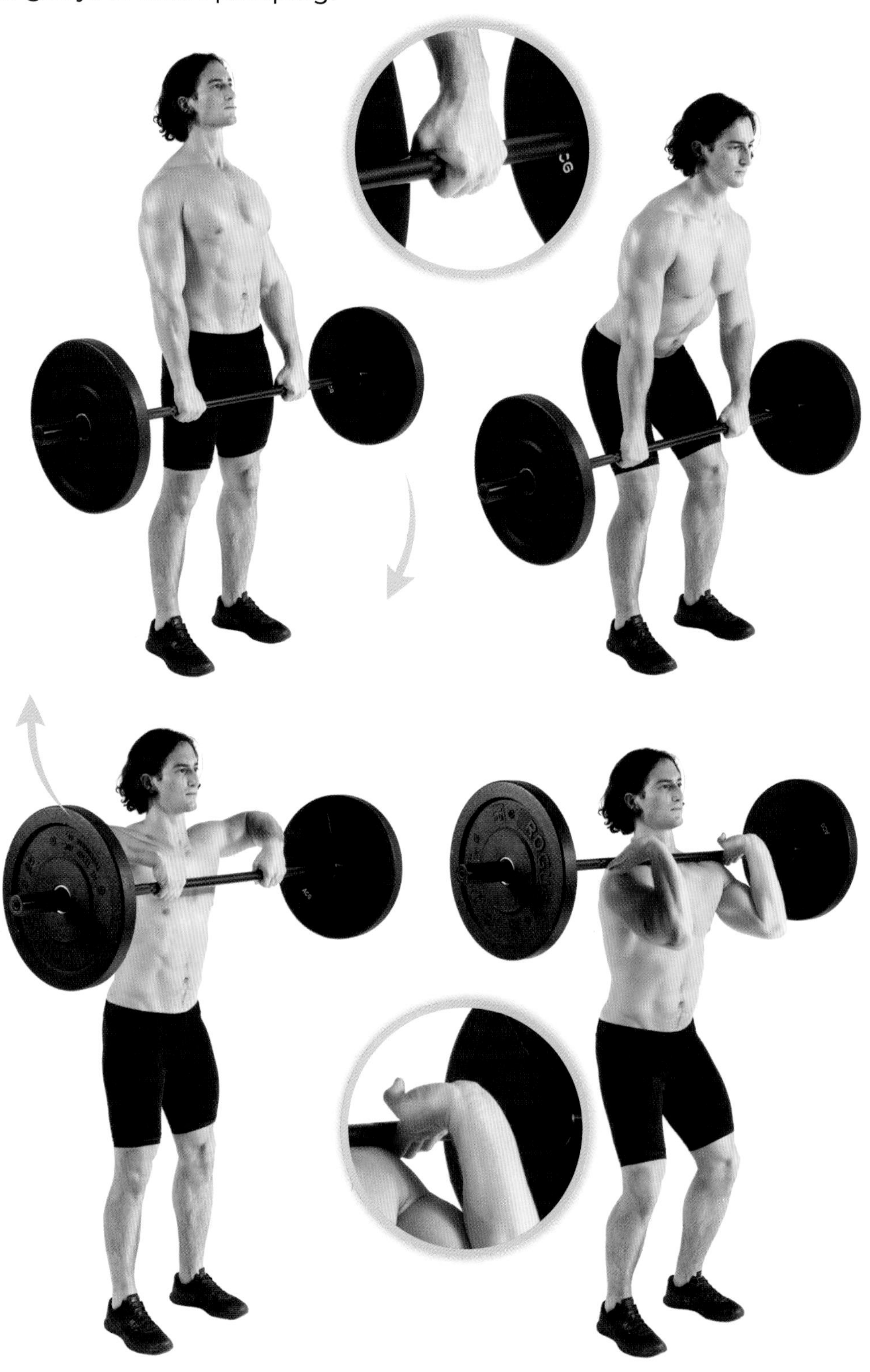

DO IT RIGHT

- Keep your back in a neutral position.
- Make sure to bend your knees, keeping your weight back on your heels to keep your center of gravity beneath you.
- Avoid using a heavier weight than you can safely handle.

latissimus dorsi
erector spinae*
multifidus spinae*

biceps femoris
semitendinosus
semimembranosus

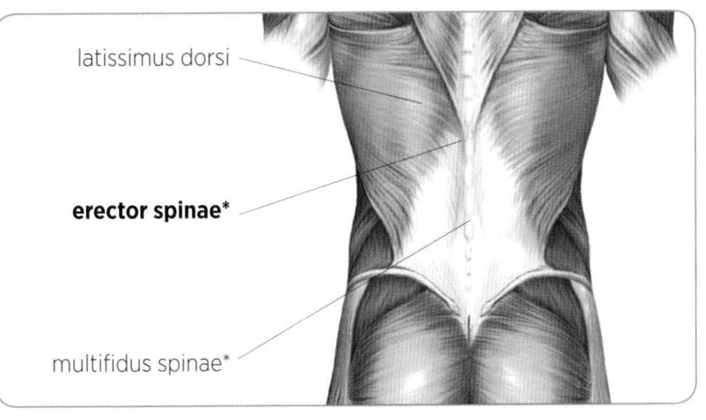

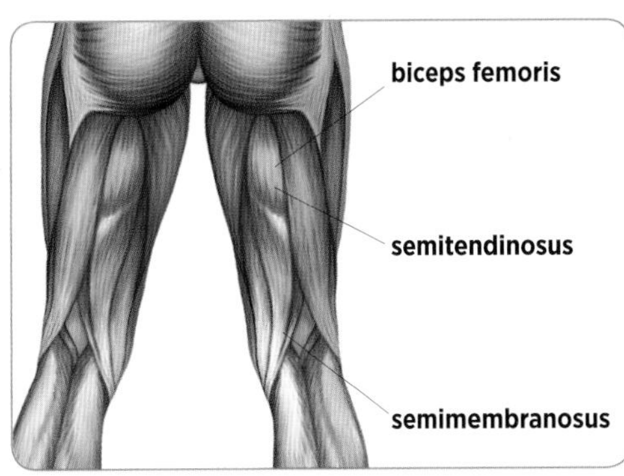

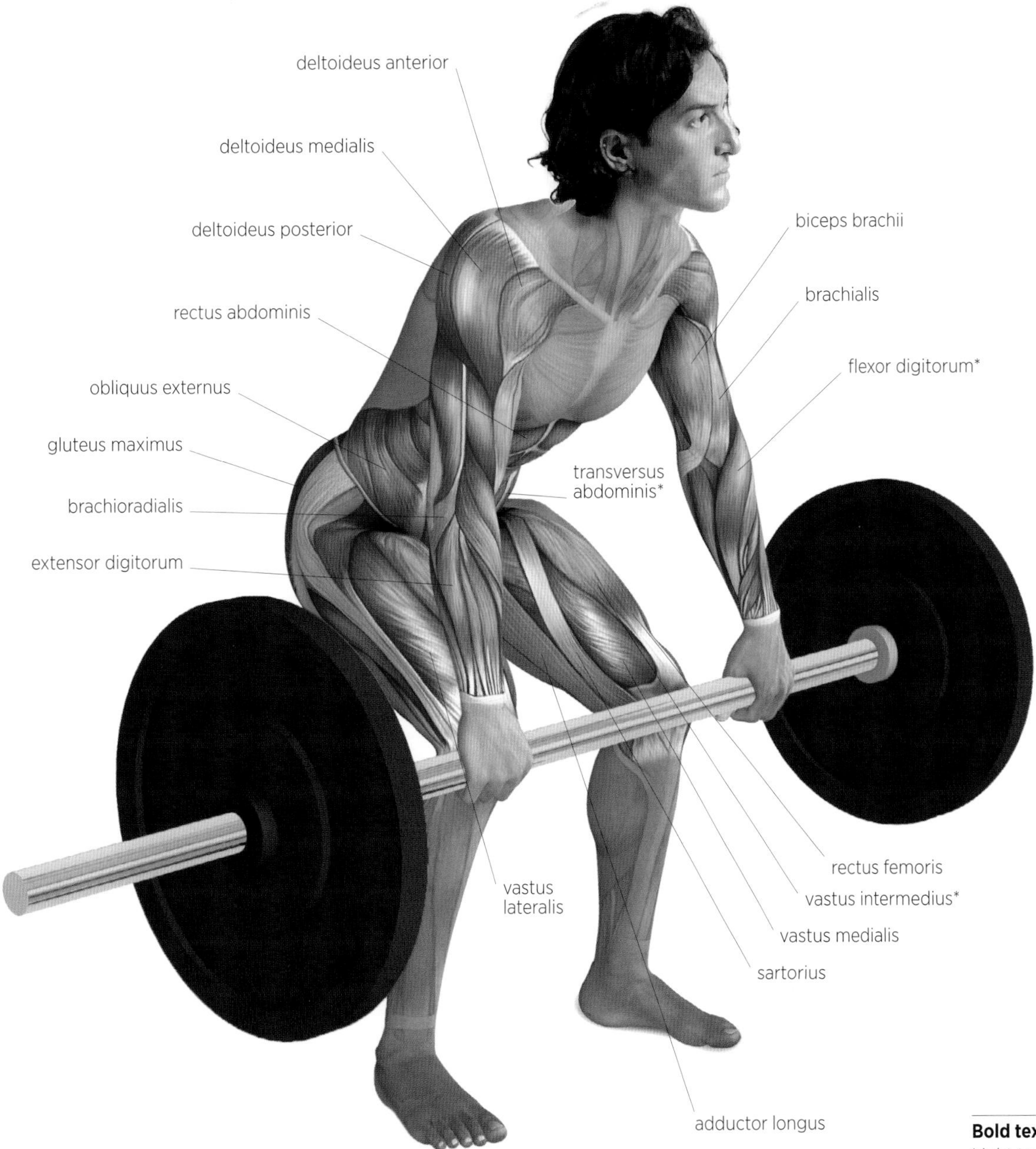

deltoideus anterior
deltoideus medialis
deltoideus posterior
rectus abdominis
obliquus externus
gluteus maximus
brachioradialis
extensor digitorum
biceps brachii
brachialis
flexor digitorum*
transversus abdominis*
vastus lateralis
rectus femoris
vastus intermedius*
vastus medialis
sartorius
adductor longus

FACT FILE

TARGETS
- Biceps
- Deltoids
- Back
- Quadriceps
- Glutes

EQUIPMENT
- Barbell

BENEFITS
- Strengthens and tones arms, back, shoulders, and core
- Increases cardiovascular endurance
- Improves coordination

CAUTIONS
- Wrist issues
- Shoulder/ rotator cuff issues
- Lower-back issues

Annotation Key

Bold text indicates target muscles
Light text indicates other working muscles
* indicates deep muscles

Battle Rope Side-to-Side Swing

Working with battle ropes provides you with powerful strength training and high-energy cardio, and helps build speed and agility. Moves such as Battle Rope Side-to-Side Swings target your arms and shoulders and also call for your obliques to kick in with a strong contribution from your trapezius, quadriceps, and hamstrings.

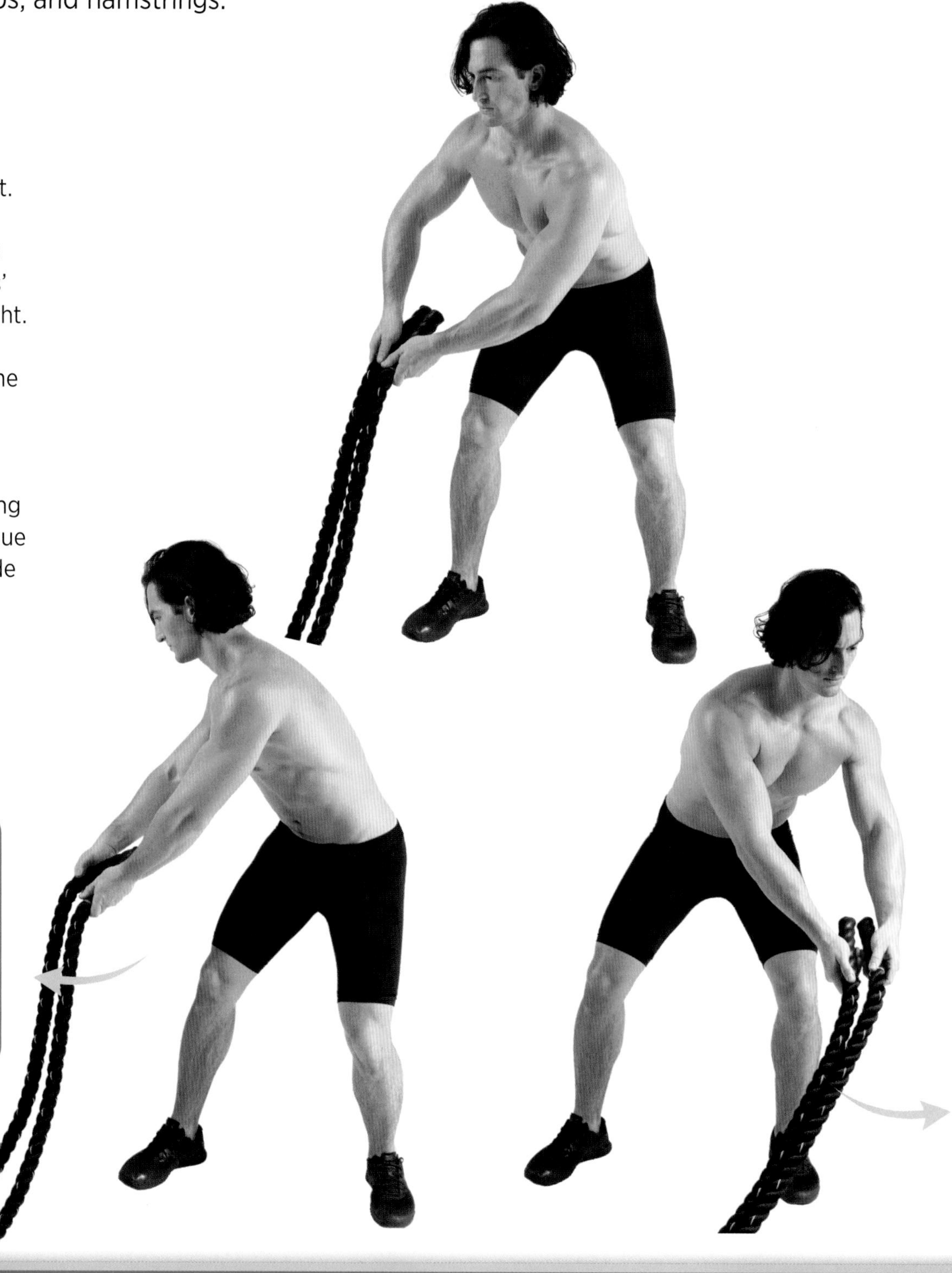

HOW TO DO IT

- Stand with your feet wider than shoulder-width apart and your knees slightly bent. Take a battle rope in each hand, and bring your hands together, keeping the ropes' handles at about waist height.
- Engage your core, and in one forceful motion, swing the ropes to the right.
- Reverse the motion, swinging the ropes to the left. Continue swinging the ropes from side to side while maintaining a strong, tight, and braced stance. Repeat for the recommended repetitions.

DO IT RIGHT

- Keep your feet planted in one place.
- Keep your core engaged.
- Move forcefully and with control, maintaining a steady rhythm.

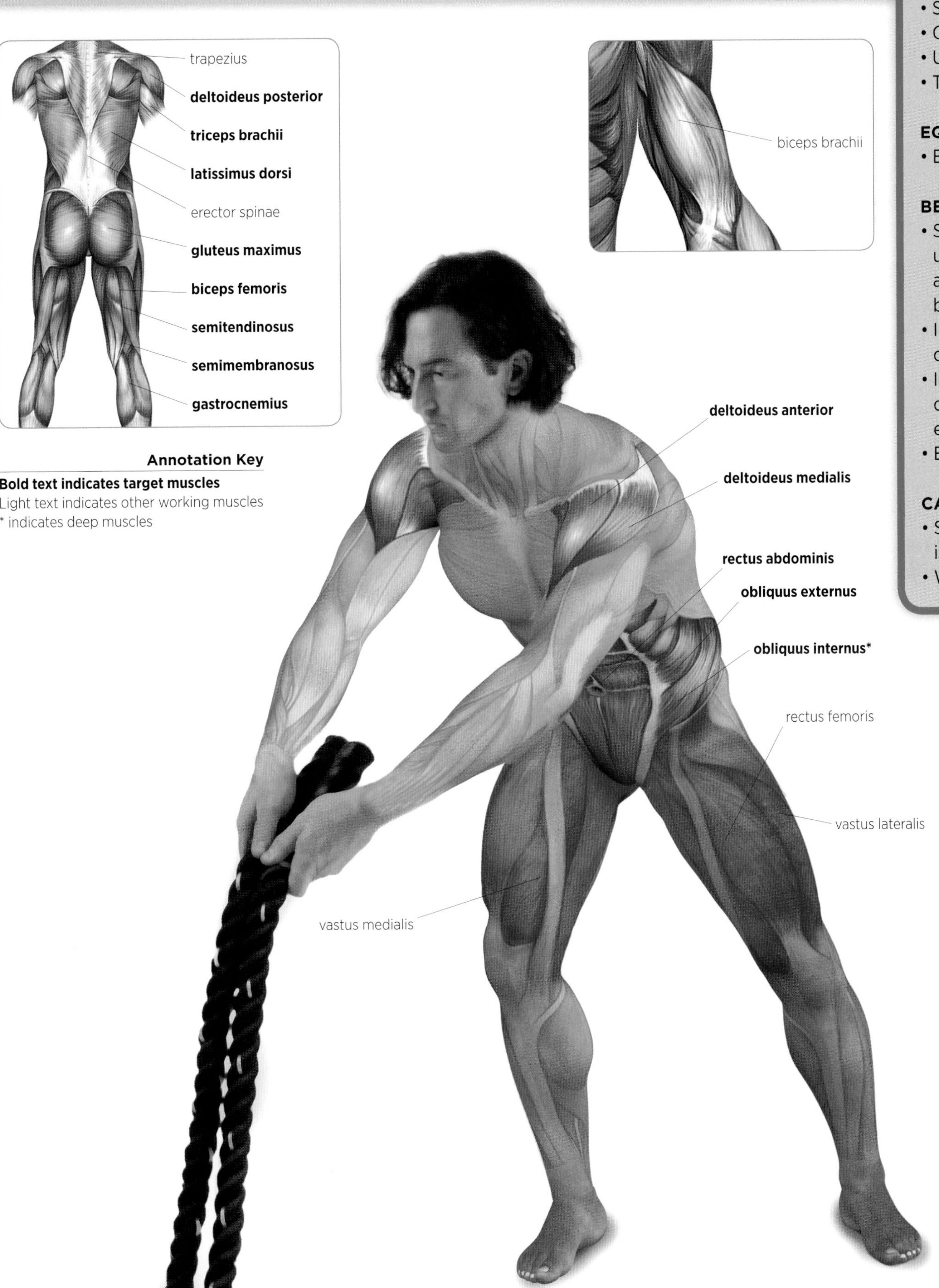

Annotation Key

Bold text indicates target muscles
Light text indicates other working muscles
* indicates deep muscles

FACT FILE

TARGETS

- Arms
- Shoulders
- Obliques
- Upper back
- Thighs

EQUIPMENT

- Battle ropes

BENEFITS

- Strengthens upper body and lower body
- Improves coordination
- Increases cardiovascular endurance
- Burns calories

CAUTIONS

- Shoulder issues
- Wrist issues

Medicine Ball Throw

Simple to execute, the Medicine Ball Throw still has much to offer. It trains multiple muscles, including your shoulders, and helps you develop coordination, balance, and power while working on core stability and strength. Try this as a game of catch with a partner.

HOW TO DO IT

- Stand holding a weighted medicine ball. To prepare to throw the ball, step your right foot forward. Keeping your torso stable, raise the ball until it is positioned above your right shoulder.
- Lift your left leg as you throw the ball forward.
- Retrieve the ball (or have a partner toss it back to you). Repeat with your left leg leading, and then continue alternating sides for the recommended repetitions.

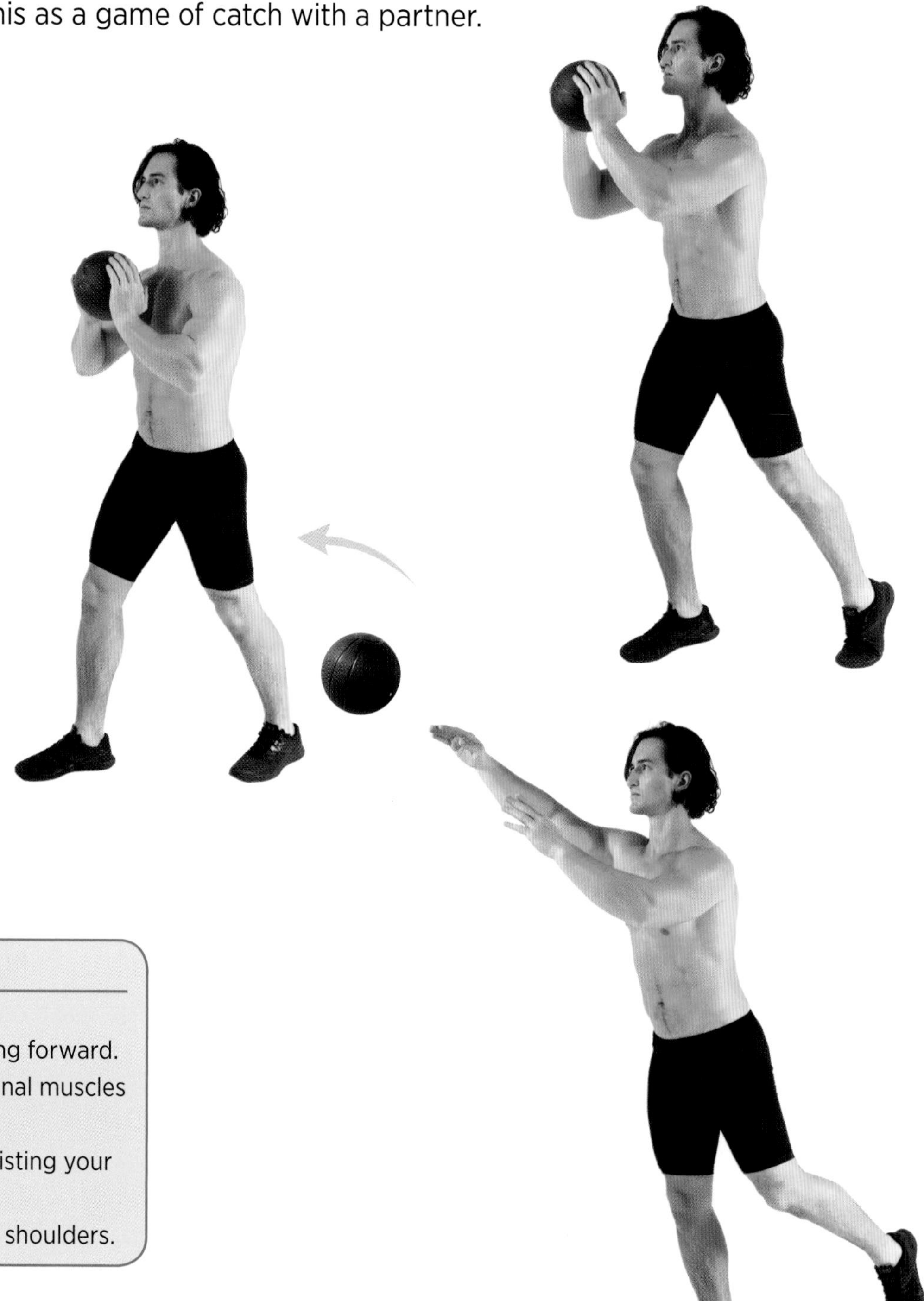

DO IT RIGHT

- Gaze forward.
- Keep your torso facing forward.
- Engage your abdominal muscles as you throw.
- Avoid excessively twisting your torso to either side.
- Avoid hunching your shoulders.

FACT FILE

TARGETS
- Shoulders
- Abdominals
- Glutes
- Thighs

EQUIPMENT
- Medicine ball

BENEFITS
- Strengthens shoulders and upper back
- Stabilizes core
- Improves balance and coordination
- Increases core rotational ability and range of upper-body motion

CAUTIONS
- Shoulder issues
- Wrist issues

Annotation Key

Bold text indicates target muscles
Light text indicates other working muscles
* indicates deep muscles

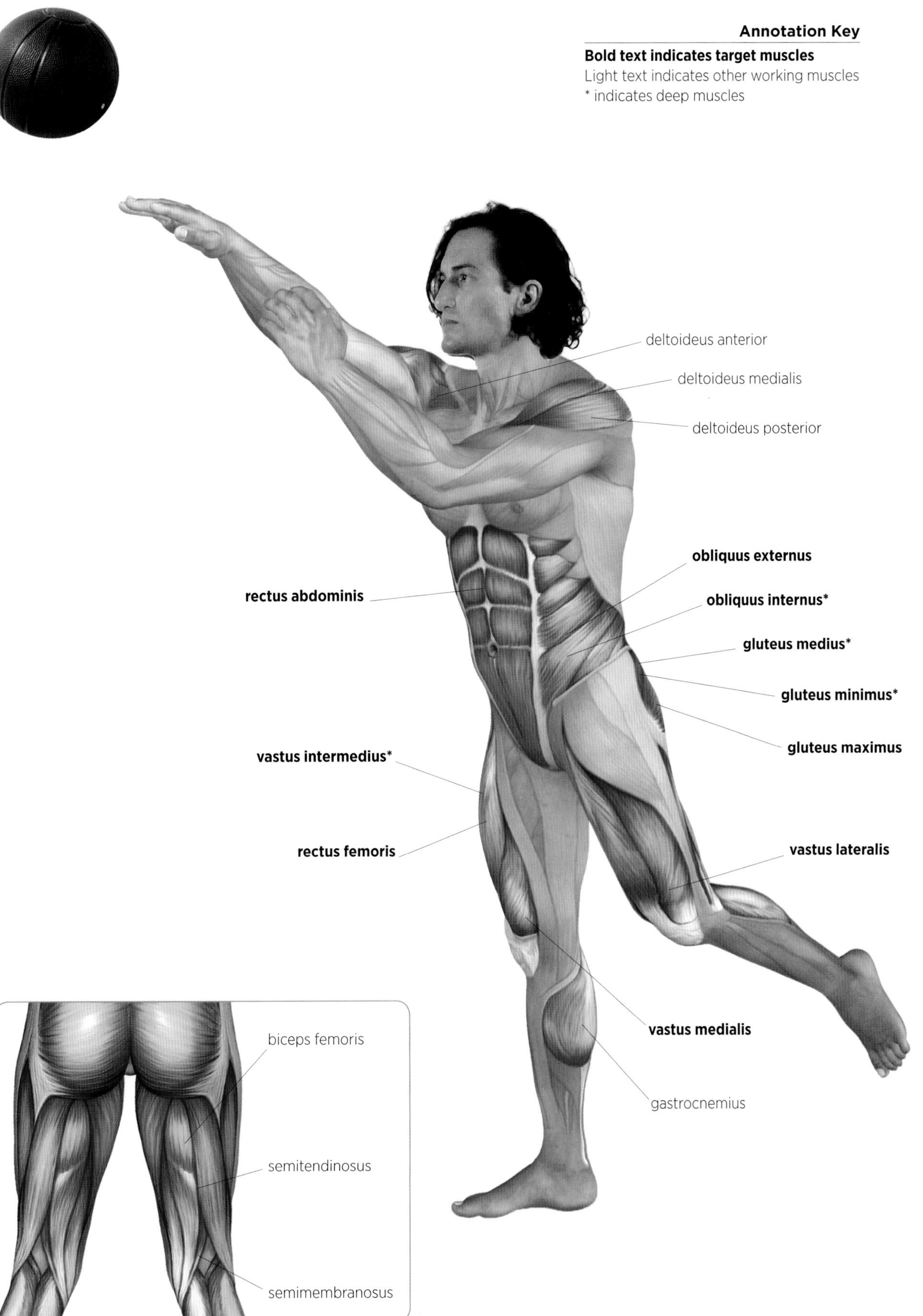

Barbell Bench Press

Arguably the best-known of all equipment-based exercises, the Barbell Bench Press is a go-to exercise for developing chest strength. It works many of the major upper-body muscle groups.

HOW TO DO IT

- Lie faceup with your back flat on a bench with your feet firmly on the floor and a barbell resting on the bench's rack. Grasp the bar with an overhand grip, your hands shoulder-width apart, and unrack it.
- On an inhale, lower the bar with a slow, controlled movement to your nipple line.
- Exhale as you press the barbell upward until your arms are fully extended.
- Carefully lower back to the starting position. Repeat for the recommended repetitions.

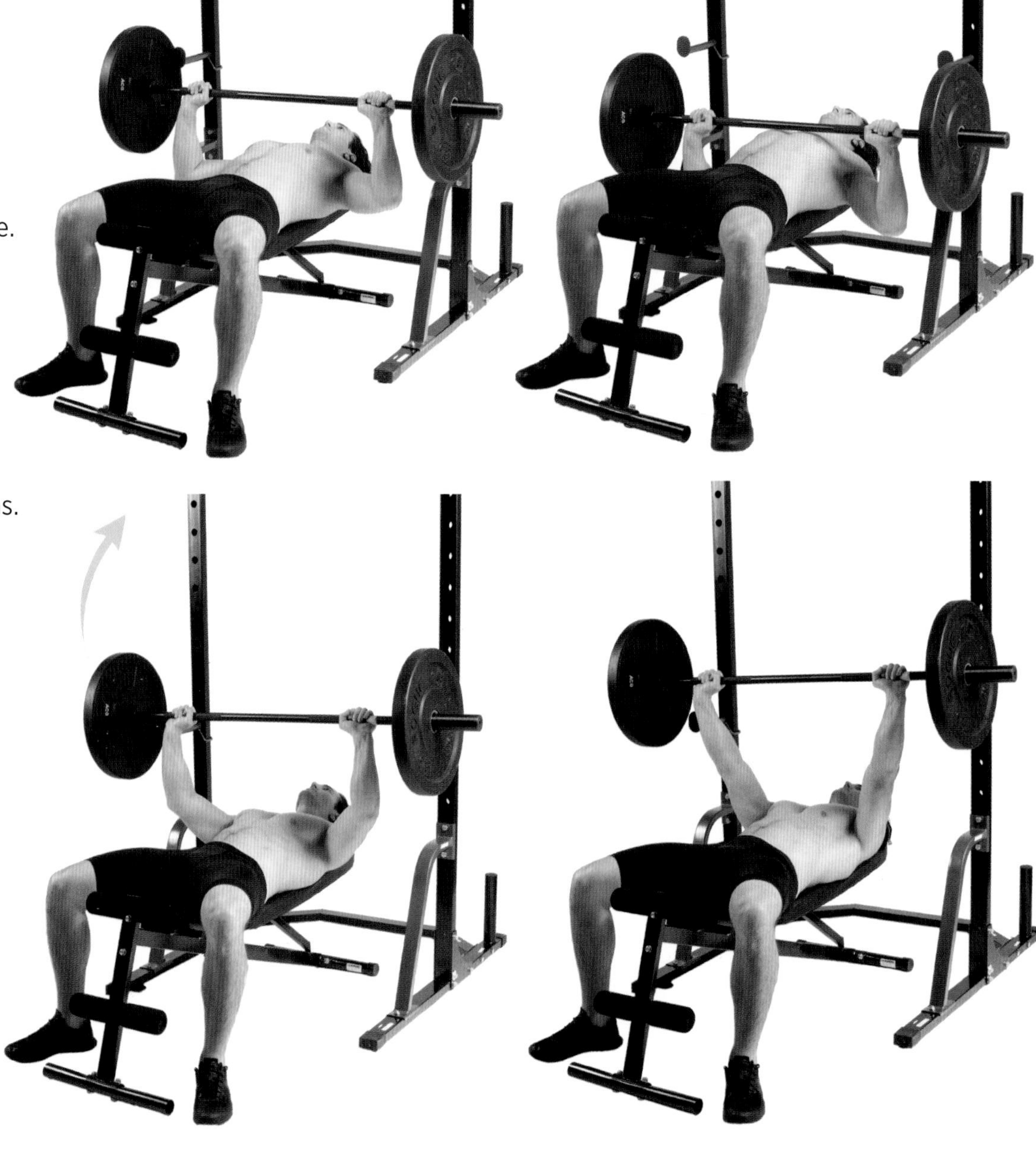

DO IT RIGHT

- Thrust your chest outward to complete the movement.
- Avoid bouncing the weight off your chest.
- Avoid using a heavier weight than you can safely handle.

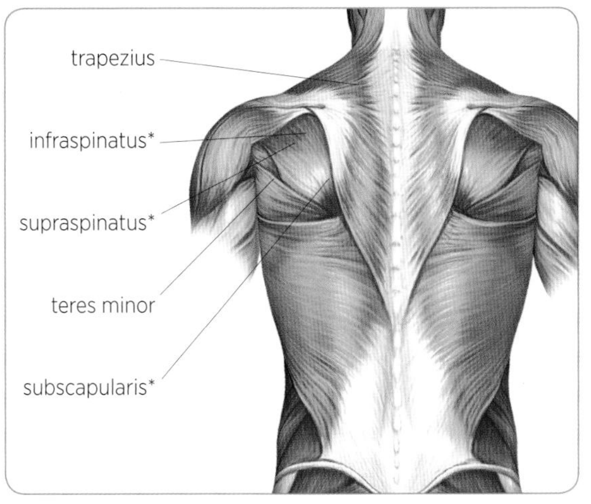

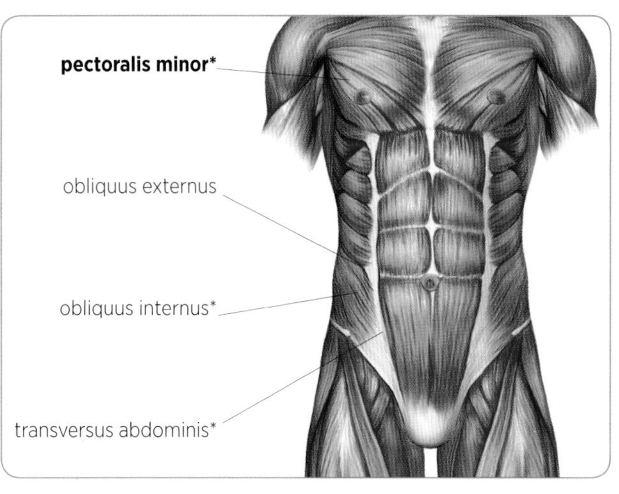

FACT FILE

TARGETS

- Pectorals
- Front deltoids
- Triceps
- Abdominals
- Upper back

EQUIPMENT

- Barbell
- Flat bench
- Barbell rack

BENEFITS

- Strengthens chest, arms, shoulders, and abdominals
- Increases chest power and mass

CAUTIONS

- Shoulder issues
- Wrist issues
- Elbow issues
- Lower-back issues

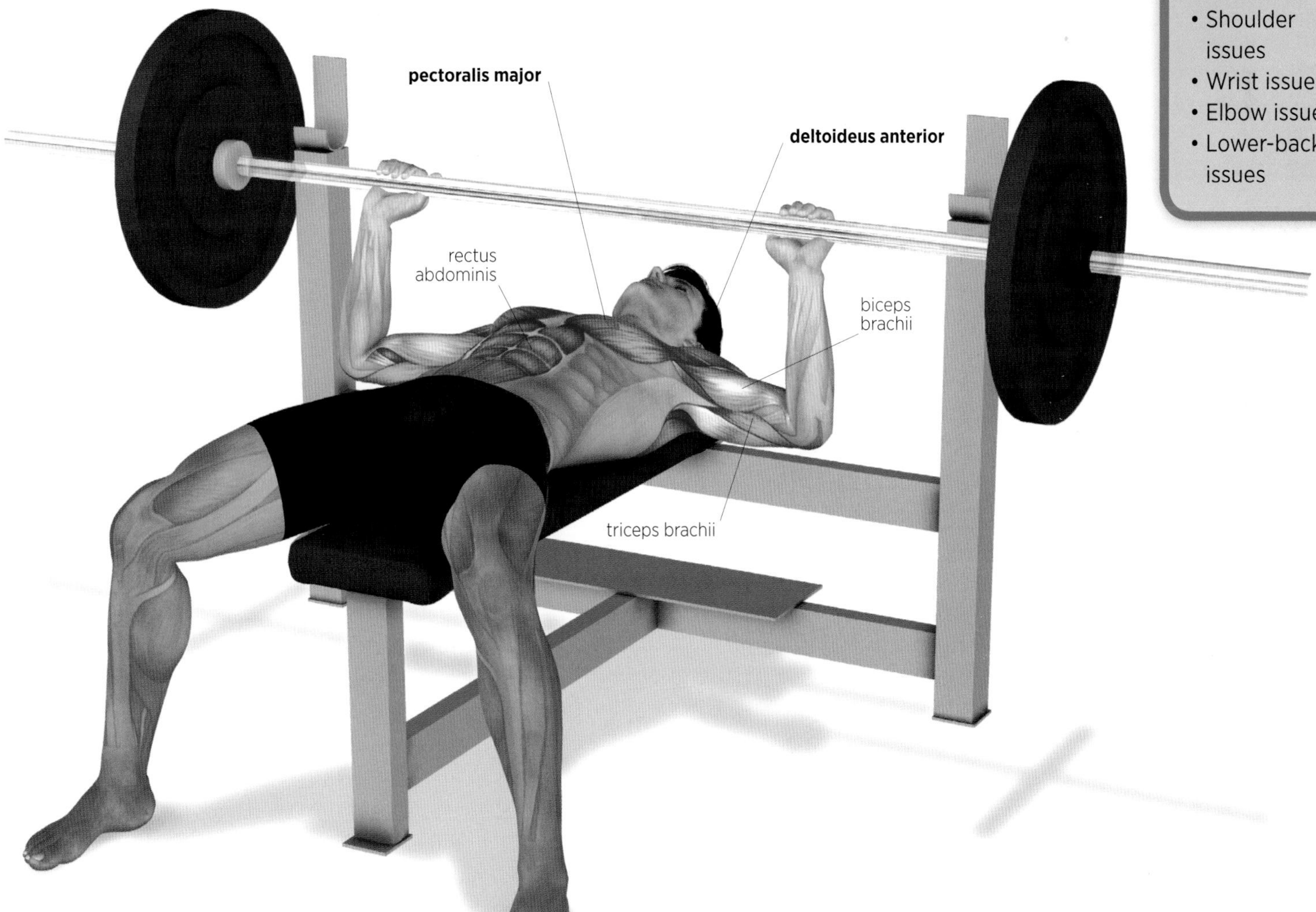

pectoralis major

deltoideus anterior

rectus abdominis

biceps brachii

triceps brachii

Annotation Key

Bold text indicates target muscles
Light text indicates other working muscles
* indicates deep muscles

Push-Up Hand Walk-Over

The Push-Up Hand Walk-Over adds a dynamic element to the basic push-up. As with any push-up, this variation targets your pectorals and triceps. The added lateral movement also challenges your shoulder and core stabilizers.

DO IT RIGHT

- Keep your hands aligned under your shoulders.
- Avoid dipping your shoulders to one side.
- Avoid shifting your hips as your hands walk.
- Avoid craning your neck.

HOW TO DO IT

- Begin in a high plank position, balancing on your toes with your feet together and with your right hand on the floor and your left on an elevated box or step.
- Keeping your torso rigid and your legs straight, bend your elbows to lower your chest toward the floor to perform a push-up.
- Push back up, straightening your elbows to return to the starting position.
- Lift your right hand off the floor, and place it beside your left on the top of the box.
- Lift your left hand off the box, placing it on the floor about one shoulder-width to the left, again assuming a high plank position.
- Bend your elbows to perform another push-up, this time on the other side of the box.
- Return to the top of the box. Continue alternating sides for the recommended repetitions.

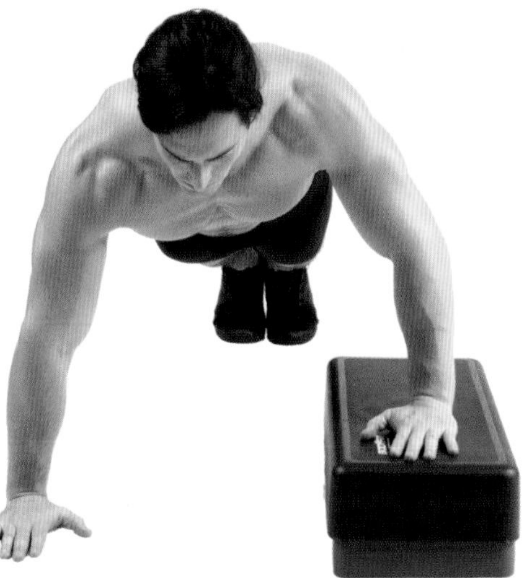

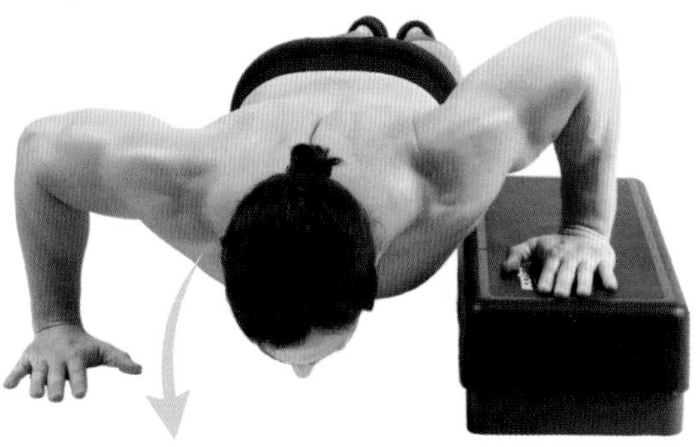

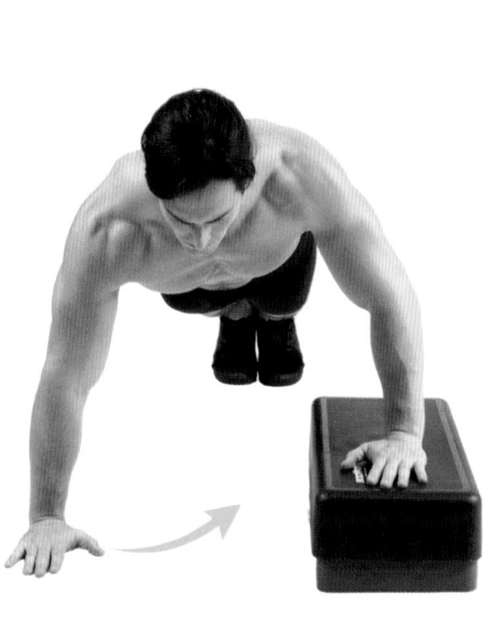

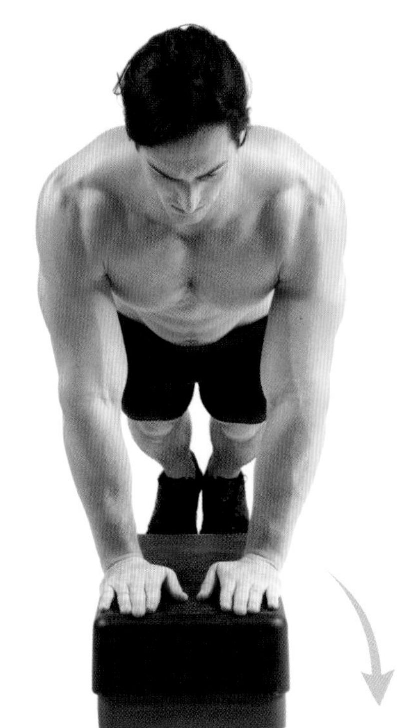

FACT FILE

TARGETS
- Chest
- Shoulders
- Back
- Arms
- Legs

EQUIPMENT
- Step or box

BENEFITS
- Strengthens pelvic, trunk, and shoulder stabilizers
- Stabilizes entire body

CAUTIONS
- Shoulder issues
- Back issues
- Neck pain

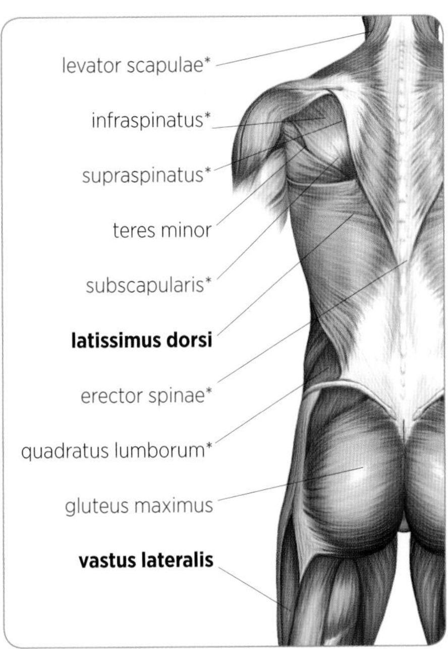

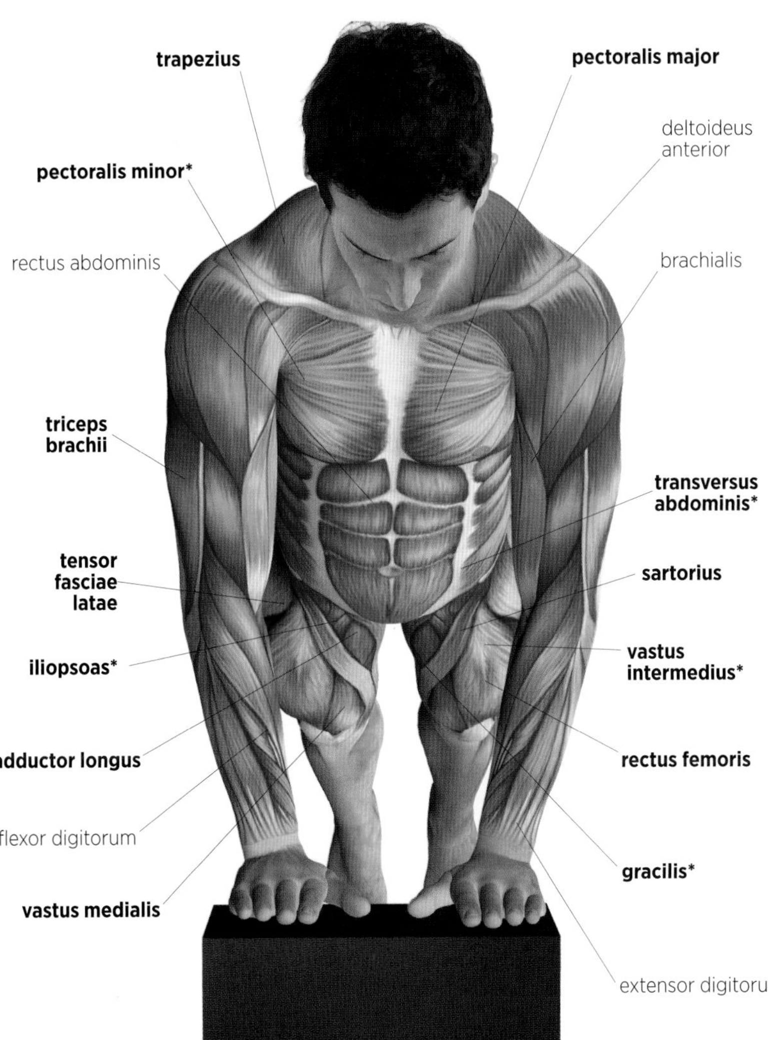

Annotation Key

Bold text indicates target muscles

Light text indicates other working muscles

* indicates deep muscles

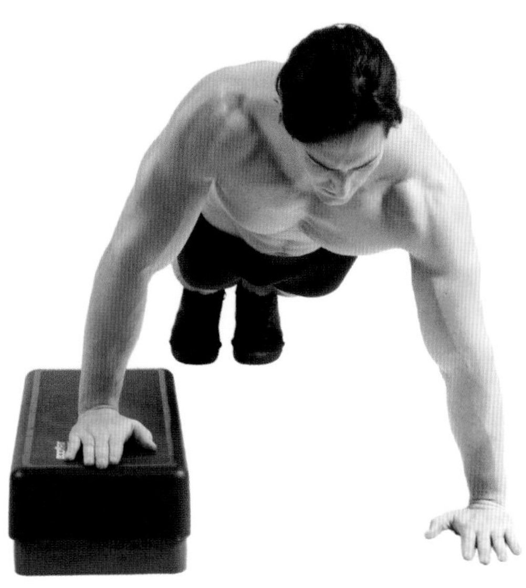

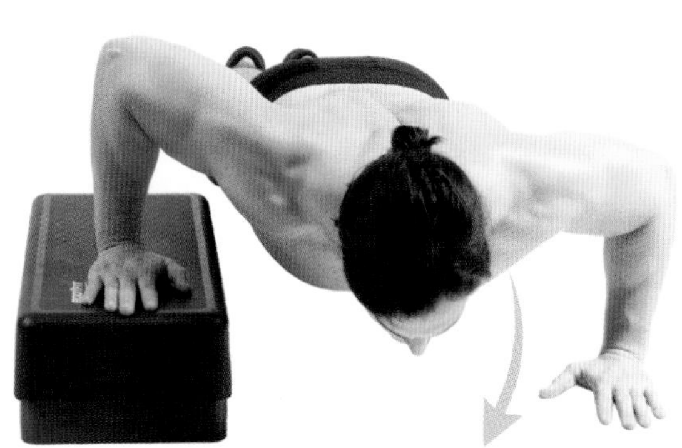

Roller Push-Up

Another one of the push-up's countless variations, the Roller Push-Up is great for a chest workout. It relies on a foam roller's unstable surface to also help improve shoulder and core function, calling for contributions from your rotator cuff and shoulder stabilizers, as well as your abdominals.

HOW TO DO IT

- Kneel on the floor with a foam roller placed crosswise in front of you. Place your hands on roller with your fingers pointed away from you. Press into a high plank position, balancing on your toes with your feet together.
- Keep your hips level with your shoulders, and without allowing your shoulders to sink, bend your elbows to lower your chest toward the roller. Avoid any roller movement throughout the motion.
- Press upward, straightening your elbows, and maintaining a straight spine to return to the starting position. Repeat for the recommended repetitions.

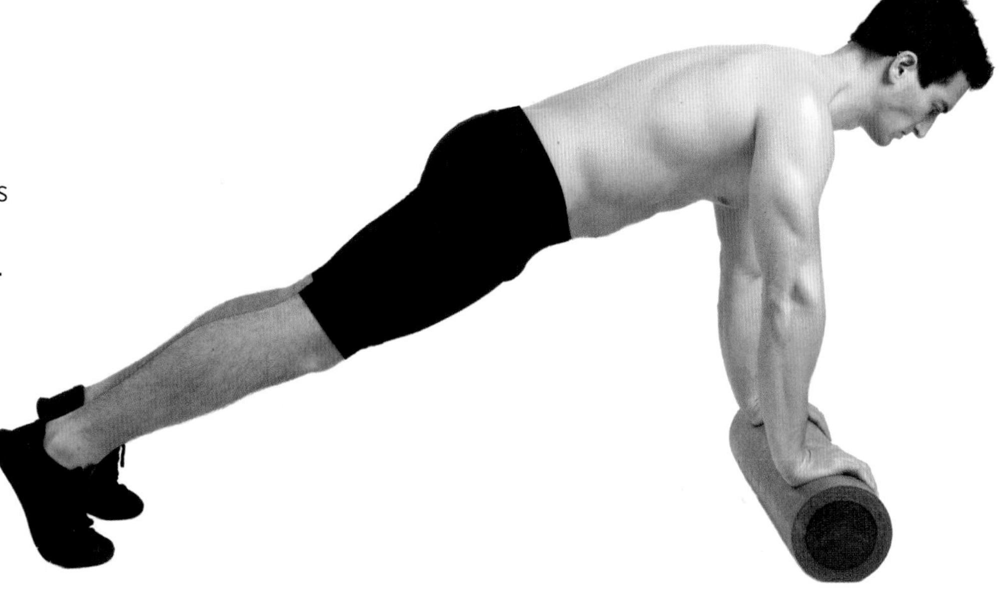

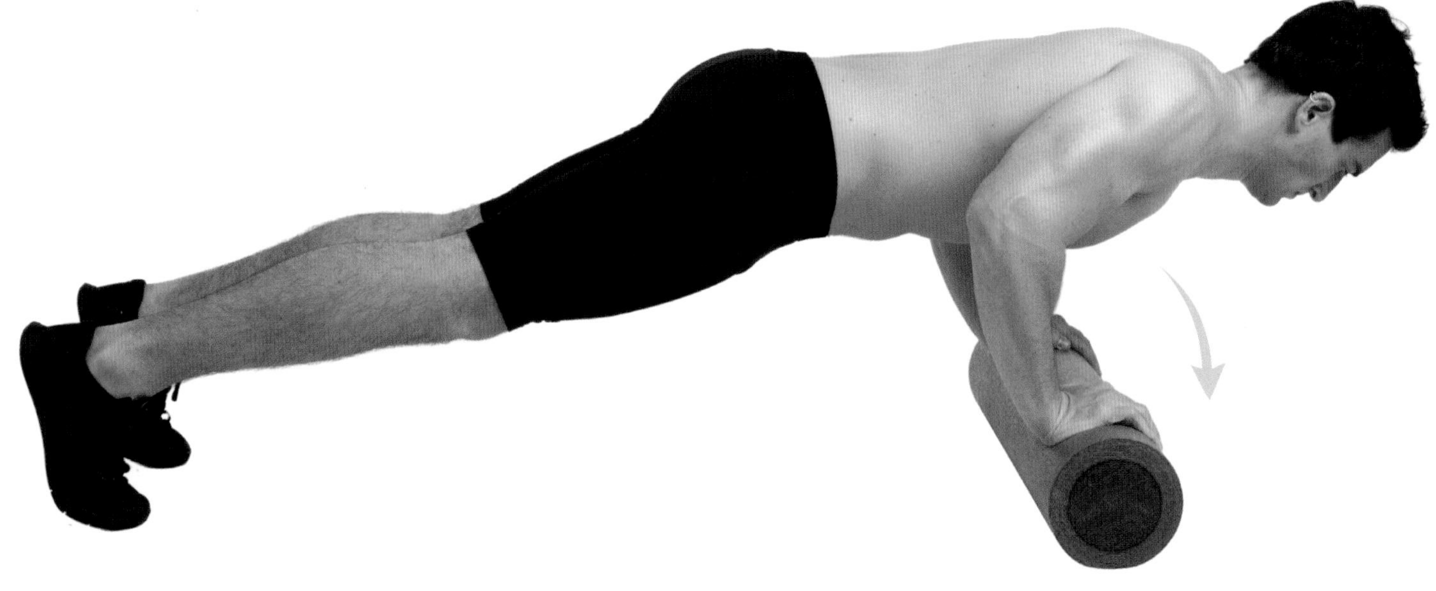

FACT FILE

TARGETS
- Chest
- Triceps
- Shoulder stabilizers
- Abdominals

EQUIPMENT
- Foam roller

BENEFITS
- Strengthens chest and shoulders
- Improves core, pelvic, and shoulder stability

CAUTIONS
- Wrist issues
- Shoulder pain
- Lower-back issues

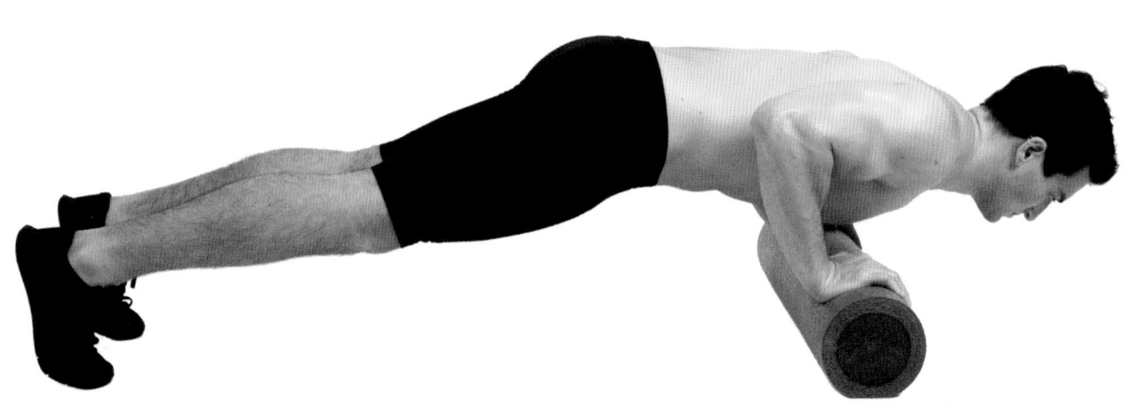

DO IT RIGHT
- Keep your neck and shoulders relaxed.
- Maintain a single plane of movement, with your body forming a straight line from shoulders to ankle.
- Keep the roller still; avoid pushing it forward or dragging it backward.
- Avoid lifting your shoulders toward your ears.
- Avoid bending your knees.

levator scapulae*
infraspinatus*
supraspinatus*
teres minor
teres major
subscapularis

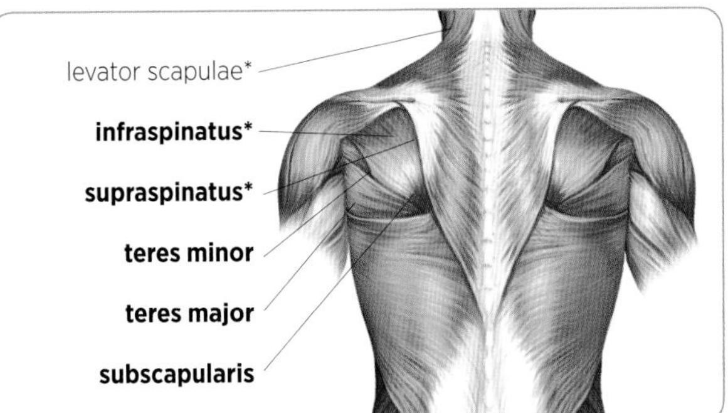

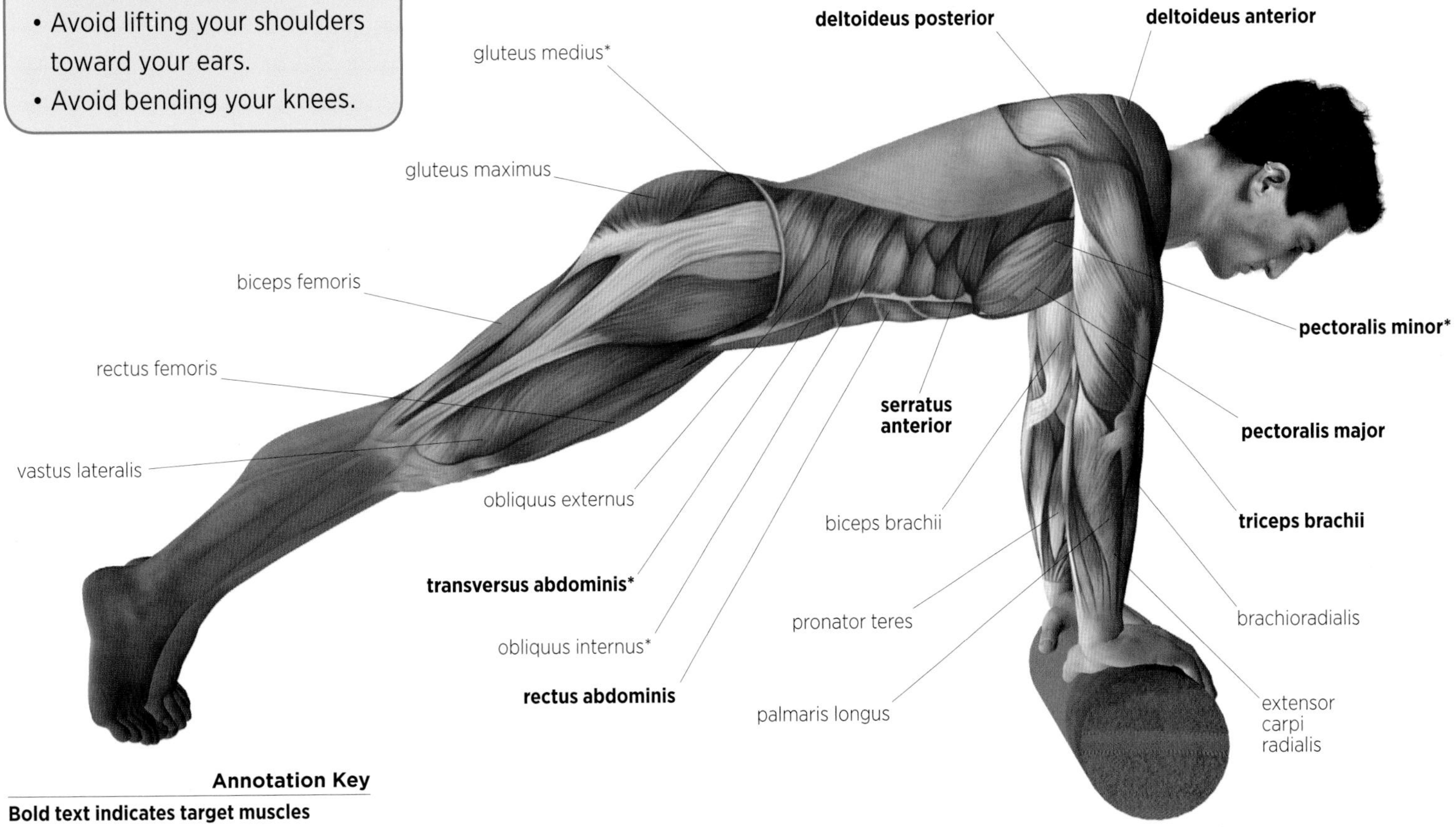

deltoideus posterior
deltoideus anterior
gluteus medius*
gluteus maximus
biceps femoris
rectus femoris
vastus lateralis
obliquus externus
transversus abdominis*
obliquus internus*
rectus abdominis
serratus anterior
biceps brachii
pronator teres
palmaris longus
pectoralis minor*
pectoralis major
triceps brachii
brachioradialis
extensor carpi radialis

Annotation Key
Bold text indicates target muscles
Light text indicates other working muscles
* indicates deep muscles

Plate Push-Up

The Plate Push-Up adds an extra level of resistance beyond your body weight to amplify the benefits of this standard chest exercise. Use a 10-pound, 25-pound, or 45-pound plate, depending on your strength and number of repetitions.

HOW TO DO IT

- Begin in a high plank position, balancing on your toes with your feet together.
- To prevent irritation and discomfort, have a training partner place a towel on your upper- to middle-back region before placing the weight plate on your upper back between your shoulder blades.
- Bend your elbows to lower your chest toward the floor, maintaining a single plane from shoulder to feet.
- Push back up into the high plank starting position, and then repeat for the recommended repetitions.

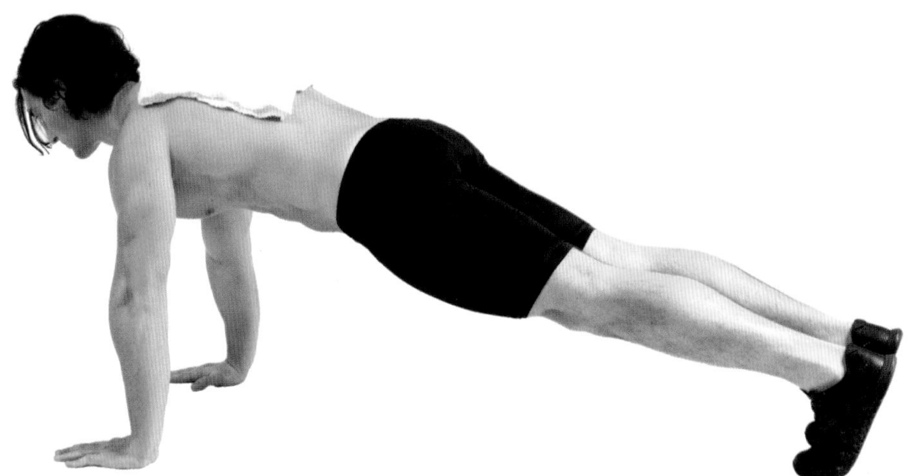

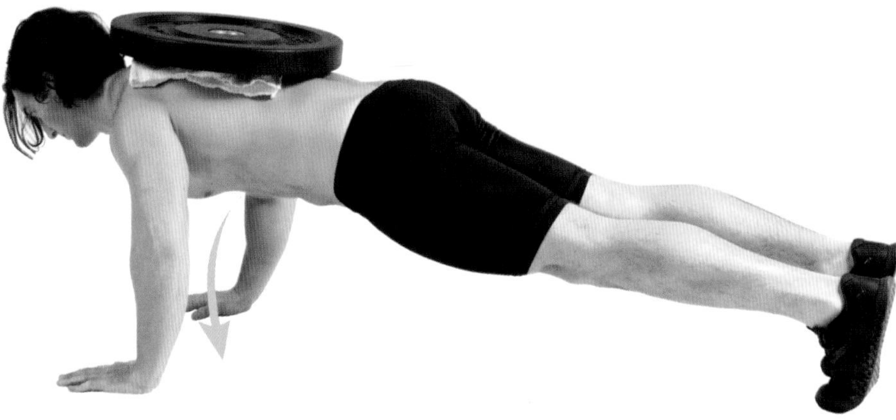

DO IT RIGHT

- Keep your neck and shoulders relaxed.
- Maintain a single plane of movement, with your body forming a straight line from shoulders to ankle.
- Avoid lifting your shoulders toward your ears.
- Avoid bending your knees.
- Avoid pointing your elbows to the side.
- Avoid hyperextending your arms at the top range of the movement.

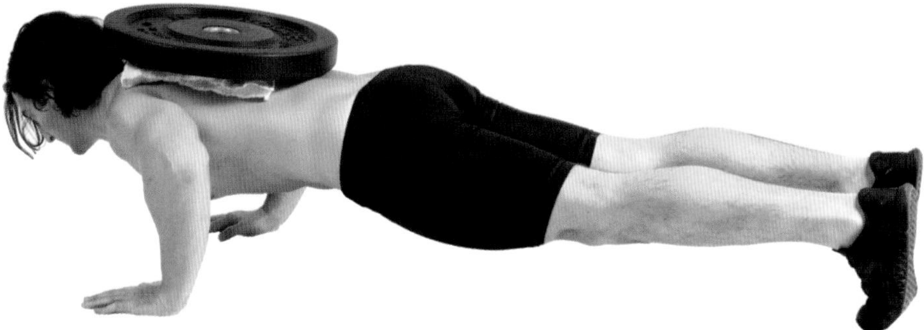

FACT FILE

TARGETS
- Chest
- Triceps
- Shoulder stabilizers
- Abdominals

EQUIPMENT
- Weight plate
- Towel

BENEFITS
- Strengthens upper, middle, and lower chest and arms
- Stabilizes shoulders

CAUTIONS
- Shoulder issues
- Wrist issues
- Lower-back issues

Annotation Key

Bold text indicates target muscles
Light text indicates other working muscles
* indicates deep muscles

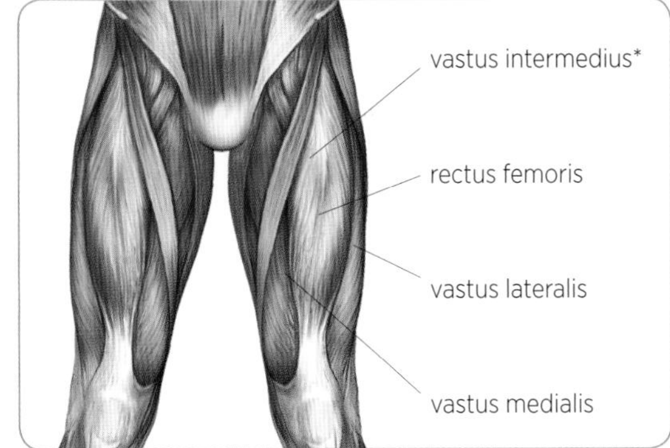

serratus anterior
obliquus externus
obliquus internus*
deltoideus anterior
triceps brachii
rectus abdominis
pectoralis major
biceps brachii
pectoralis minor*

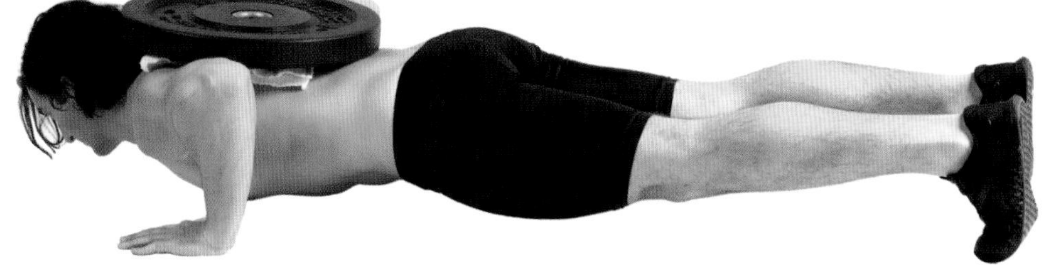

Two-Level Push-Up

The explosive Two-Level Push-Up takes your fitness to another level. This plyometric exercise uses a higher power movement to target your chest in a way that will improve power, strength, and coordination.

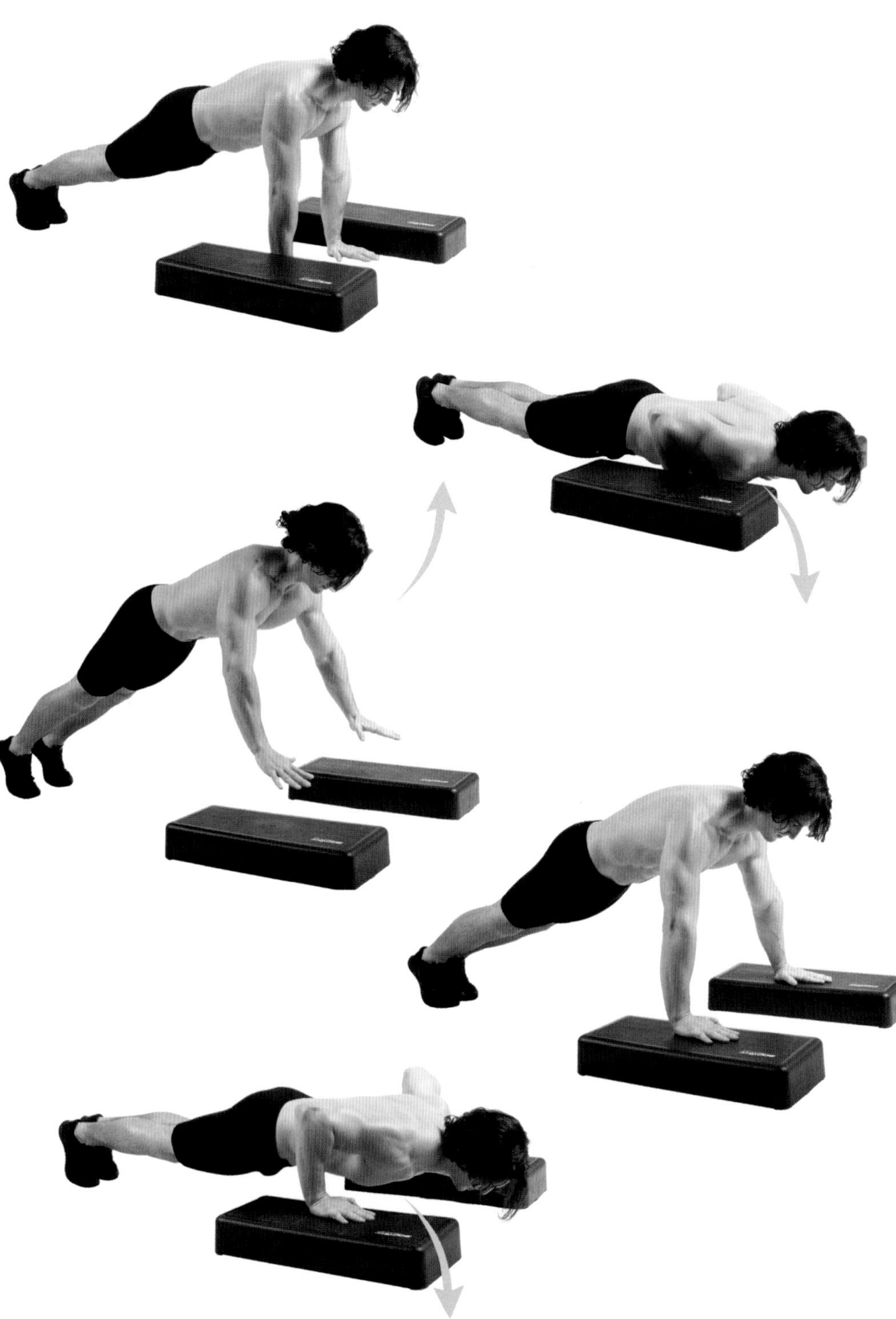

HOW TO DO IT

- Place two aerobics steps or low boxes on the floor. Position your palms shoulder-width apart between the steps, and assume a high plank position, balancing on your toes with your feet together and your back in a neutral position.

- Keeping your torso rigid and your legs straight, bend your elbows to lower your chest toward the floor to perform a push-up.

- In one explosive movement, press up from the floor, extending your arms dynamically to elevate your body with enough velocity to allow yourself to place your hands on the steps on either side of your torso.

- In a high plank position on the steps, repeat the steps above, performing a push-up on the steps, and then catching yourself once again on the floor between the equipment. Repeat for the recommended repetitions.

DO IT RIGHT

- Keep your back straight.
- Avoid any excessive arching in the spine.
- Bend your elbows to absorb the shock of landing.

deltoideus medialis
deltoideus posterior
erector spinae*

pectoralis minor*
rectus abdominis

FACT FILE

TARGETS
- Pectorals
- Deltoids
- Abdominals
- Triceps

EQUIPMENT
- Boxes or steps

BENEFITS
- Strengthens and tones abdominals, chest, and arms
- Increases cardiovascular endurance
- Improves coordination

CAUTIONS
- Shoulder issues
- Wrist issues
- Elbow issues

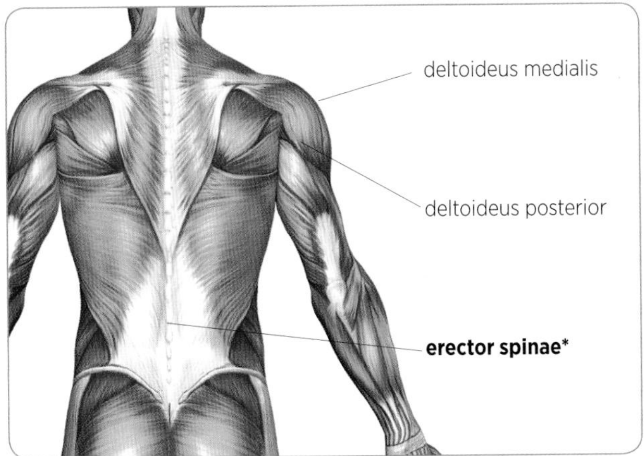

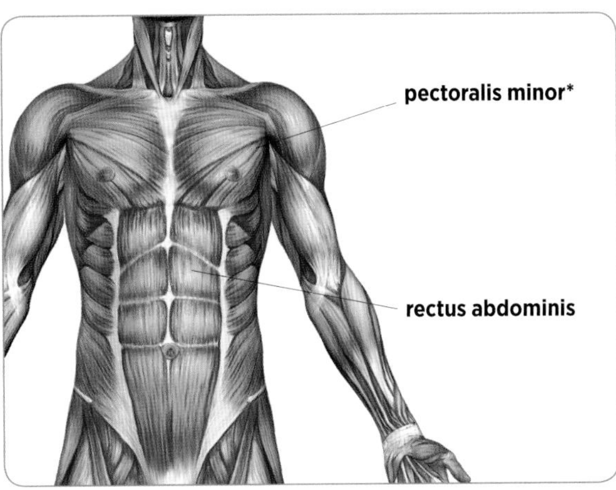

latissimus dorsi
obliquus externus
obliquus internus*
deltoideus anterior
pectoralis major
biceps brachii
triceps brachii
rectus femoris

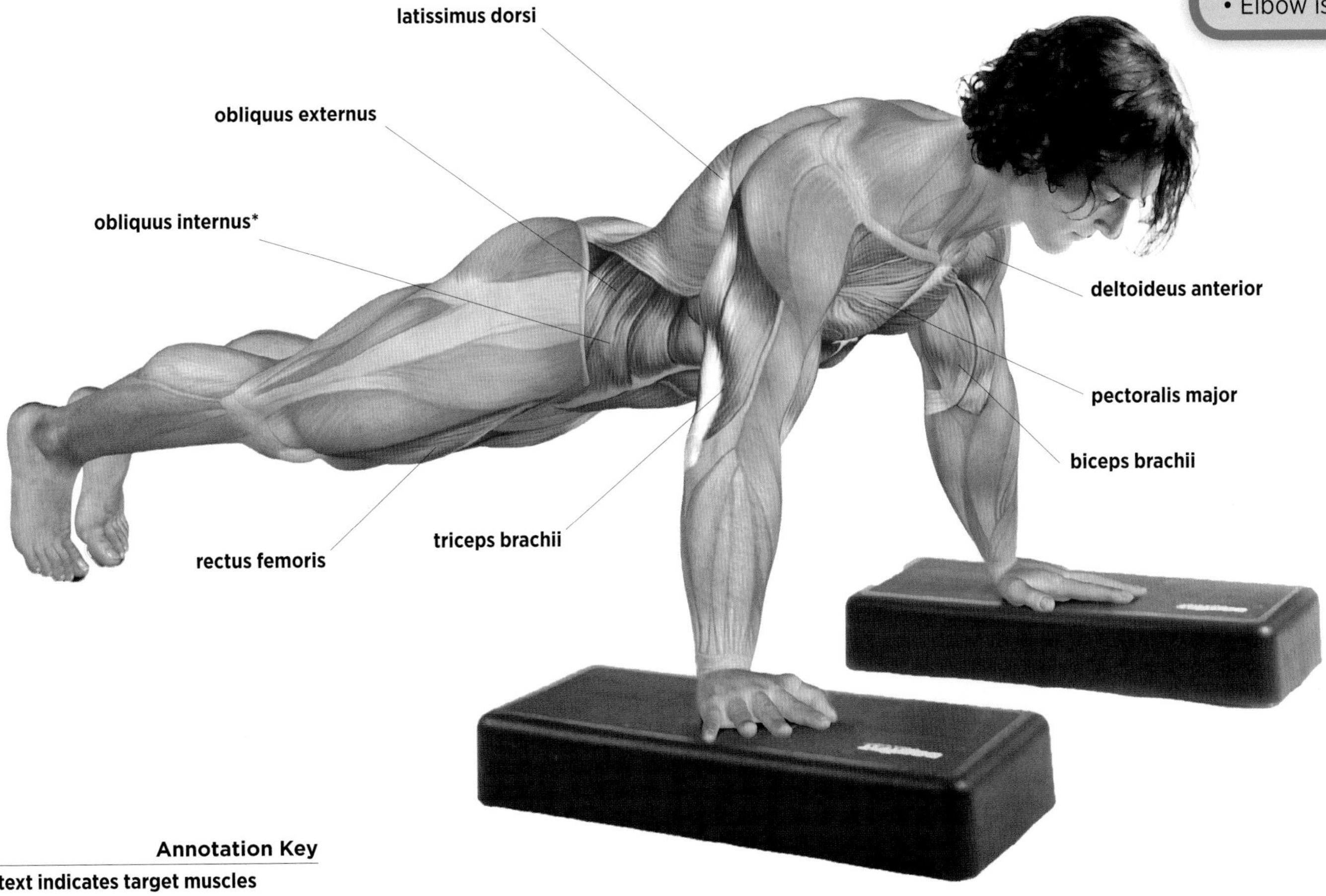

Annotation Key

Bold text indicates target muscles
Light text indicates other working muscles
* indicates deep muscles

Single-Arm Medicine Ball Push-Up

The Single-Arm Medicine Ball Push-Up goes beyond the traditional push-up, working you even harder to increase your strength, range of motion, balance, and stability.

FACT FILE

TARGETS
- Chest
- Triceps
- Shoulder stabilizers
- Abdominals

EQUIPMENT
- Medicine ball

BENEFITS
- Strengthens chest and shoulders
- Improves core, pelvic, and shoulder stability
- Improves coordination

CAUTIONS
- Wrist issues
- Shoulder issues
- Lower-back issues

HOW TO DO IT

- Begin in a high plank position, balancing on your toes with your feet together. Place a medicine ball beneath your left hand.

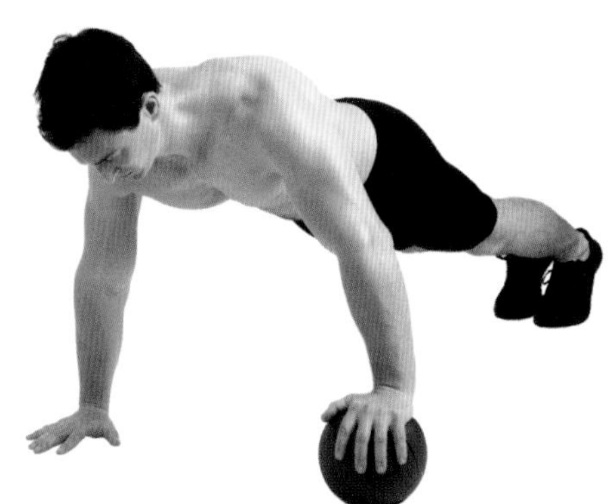

- Bend your elbows to lower your chest toward the floor, maintaining a single plane from shoulder to feet.

- Push your back up, with arms to full extension. Once at the top, pass the ball to your right hand, and perform the movement again. Continue alternating sides for the recommended repetitions.

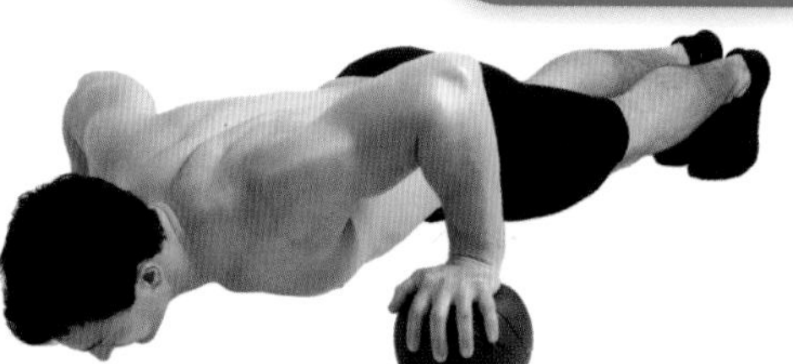

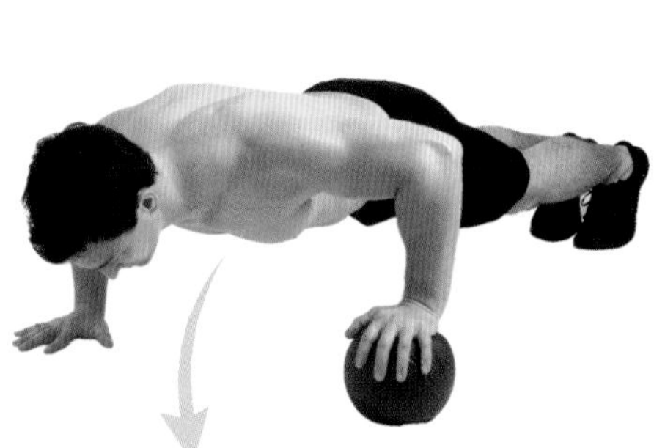

DO IT RIGHT

- Keep your core engaged.
- Stabilize your torso and keep your body straight as you pass the ball back and forth at the top of the movement.
- Avoid excessive speed; move slowly and with control.
- Avoid shallow or bouncy repetitions.
- Avoid allowing your lower back to dip too far.

Annotation Key
Bold text indicates target muscles
Light text indicates other working muscles
* indicates deep muscles

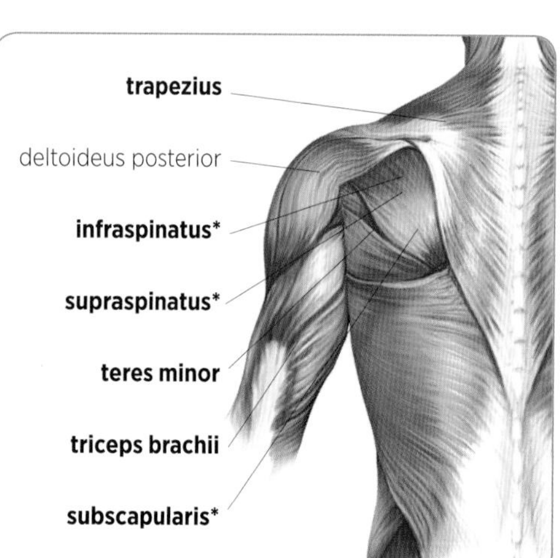

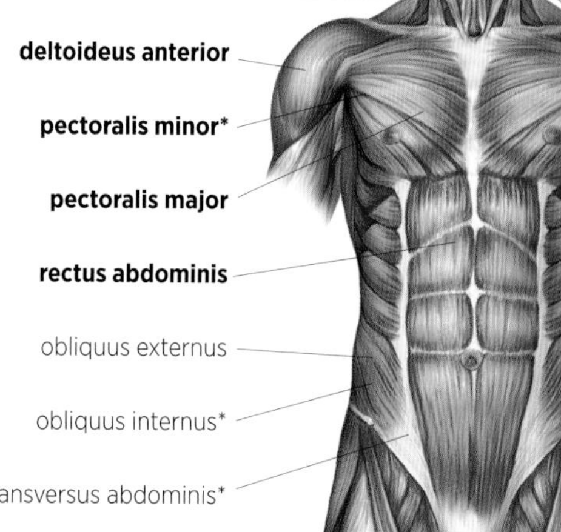

Triangle Push-Up with Medicine Ball

A Triangle-Push-Up really focuses on your triceps, as well as your pectorals. This version, performed on a medicine ball, is even more taxing, calling for you to keep your balance as you move up and down.

HOW TO DO IT

- Begin in a high plank position, balancing on your toes with your feet planted shoulder-width apart, and with your hands on either side of a medicine ball, forming a triangle directly beneath your chest.

- Engage your abdominals, and bend your elbows to lower your chest toward the ball, maintaining a single plane from shoulders to feet.

- Push your back up, with arms to full extension, to return to the starting position. Repeat for the recommended repetitions.

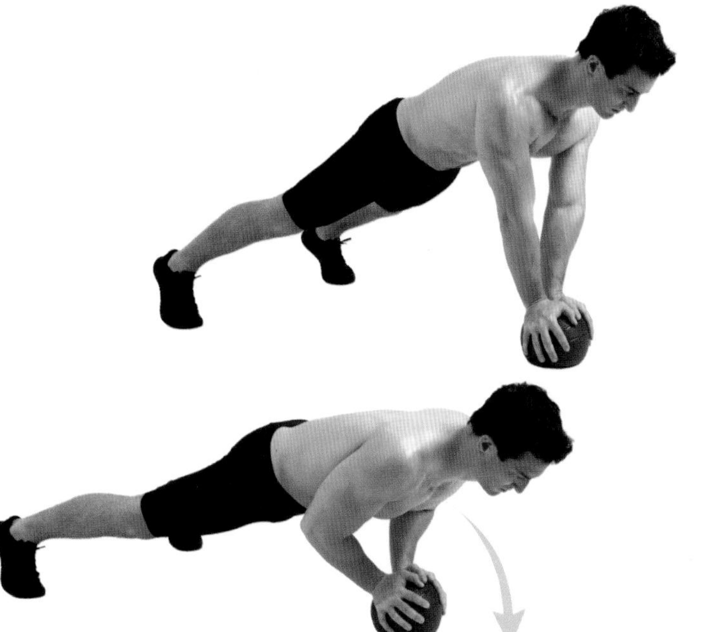

DO IT RIGHT

- Keep your core engaged.
- Avoid excessive speed; move slowly and with control.
- Avoid shallow or bouncy repetitions.
- Avoid allowing your lower back to dip too far.

Annotation Key

Bold text indicates target muscles
Light text indicates other working muscles
* indicates deep muscles

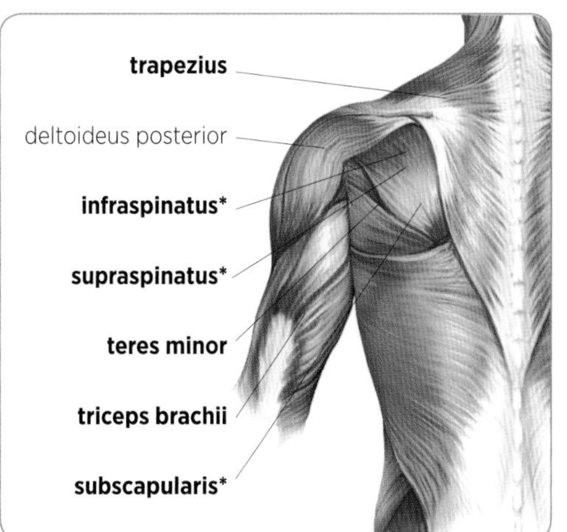

deltoideus anterior
pectoralis minor*
pectoralis major
rectus abdominis
obliquus externus
obliquus internus*
transversus abdominis*

FACT FILE

TARGETS

- Triceps
- Chest
- Shoulder stabilizers
- Abdominals

EQUIPMENT

- Medicine ball

BENEFITS

- Strengthens chest and shoulders
- Improves core, pelvic, and shoulder stability

CAUTIONS

- Wrist issues
- Shoulder issues
- Lower-back issues

Floor Wiper

The Floor Wiper builds upper-body strength while simultaneously building core strength, both linearly and diagonally. This means that all your abdominal muscle fibers are engaged dynamically, while an isometric stress is placed on your upper extremities to give you a great upper-body workout, all while you're lying down.

HOW TO DO IT

- Lie faceup with your legs extended and feet together. Place your hands shoulder-width apart on the bar with your arms extended, placing the bar directly over your chest.
- Flexing at your hips, engage your abdominals to bring your legs up.
- Keeping your legs straight, direct your feet toward the left end of the bar.
- Lower both legs down toward the floor in the center without making contact with the floor.
- Keeping your legs straight, direct your feet toward the right end of the bar.
- Continue alternating sides without letting your feet touch the floor. Repeat for the recommended repetitions.

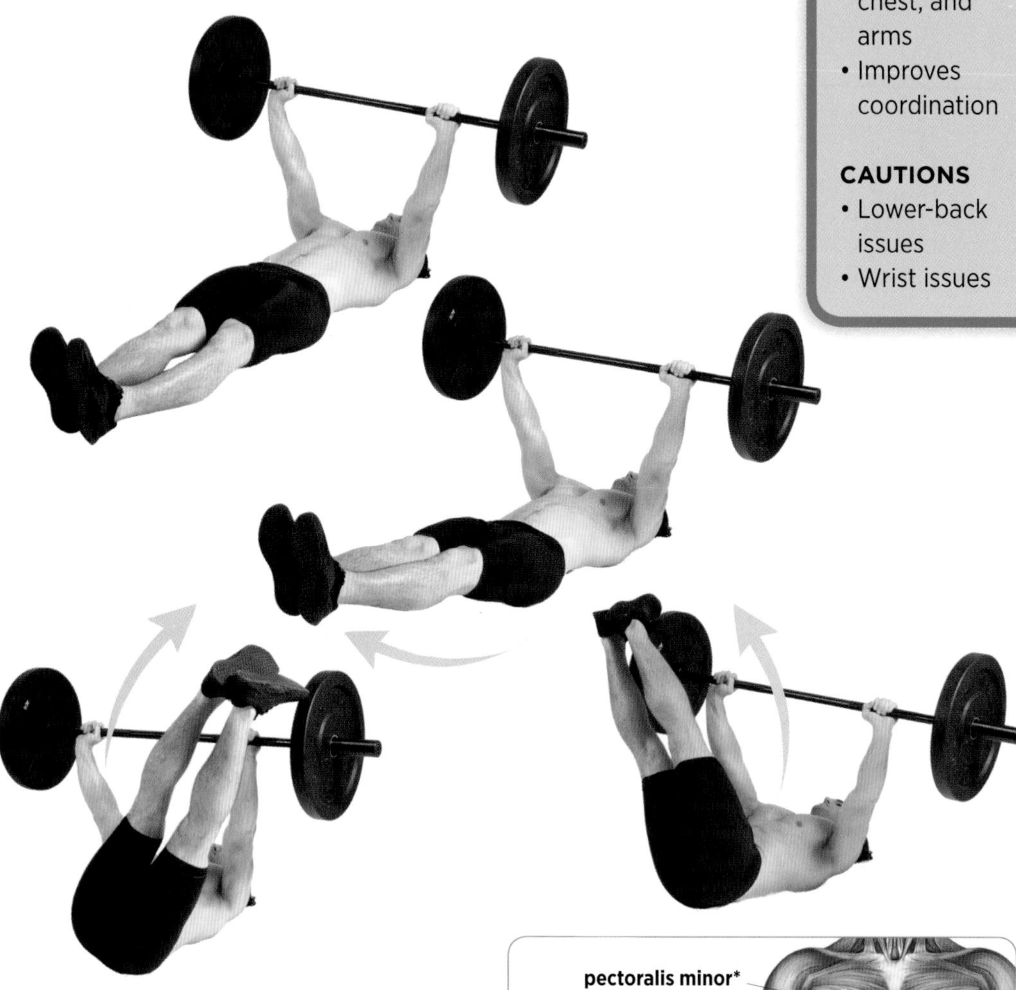

DO IT RIGHT

- Keep your arms and legs straight and feet together.
- Keep your core engaged.
- Keep you back grounded on the floor.

triceps brachii

pectoralis minor*
pectoralis major
rectus abdominis
obliquus externus
obliquus internus*
transversus abdominis*
iliopsoas*
pectineus*
rectus femoris

Annotation Key
Bold text indicates target muscles
Light text indicates other working muscles
* indicates deep muscles

FACT FILE

TARGETS
- Abdominals
- Pectorals
- Triceps
- Hip flexors

EQUIPMENT
- Barbell

BENEFITS
- Strengthens and tones abdominals, chest, and arms
- Improves coordination

CAUTIONS
- Lower-back issues
- Wrist issues

Medicine Ball Core Twist

The Medicine Ball Core Twist is a fundamental resistance exercise that builds abdominal core and upper-body strength with a simple movement. It will help hone your balance, endurance, and postural stability.

FACT FILE

TARGETS
- Abdominals
- Deltoids
- Biceps

EQUIPMENT
- Medicine ball

BENEFITS
- Strengthens and tones abdominals, shoulders, and arms
- Warms up muscles
- Improves balance

CAUTIONS
- Severe back pain

HOW TO DO IT
- Stand with your feet hip-width apart and hold a large medicine ball with your arms extended in front of you, centered with your chest.
- Twisting your torso, rotate as far to the left as possible, keeping the medicine ball at chest level.
- Reverse direction, rotating your torso to the right, bringing the ball in a smooth line at chest level.
- Continue alternating sides, passing through center. Repeat for the recommended repetitions.

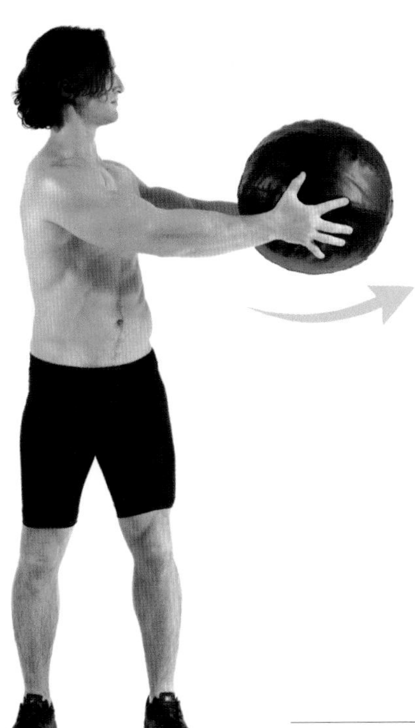

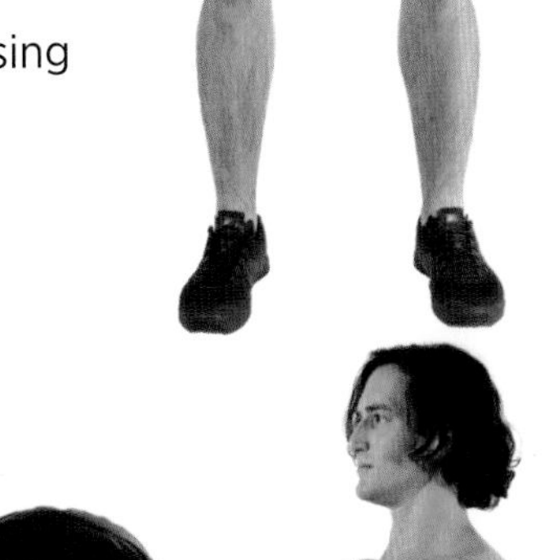

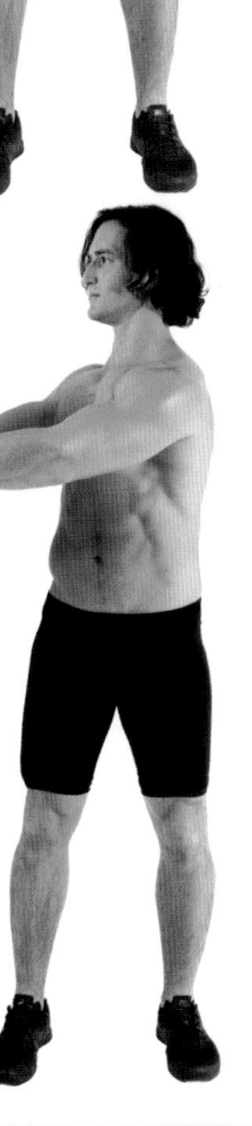

DO IT RIGHT
- Keep your arms straight, with a slight bend at your elbows.
- Keep your core engaged.
- Avoid any excessive trunk sway.
- Exaggerate the twisting motions, avoiding any small movements.

Annotation Key

Bold text indicates target muscles

Light text indicates other working muscles

* indicates deep muscles

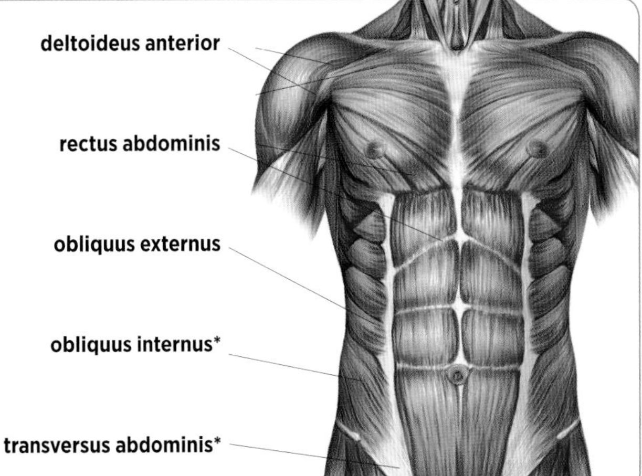

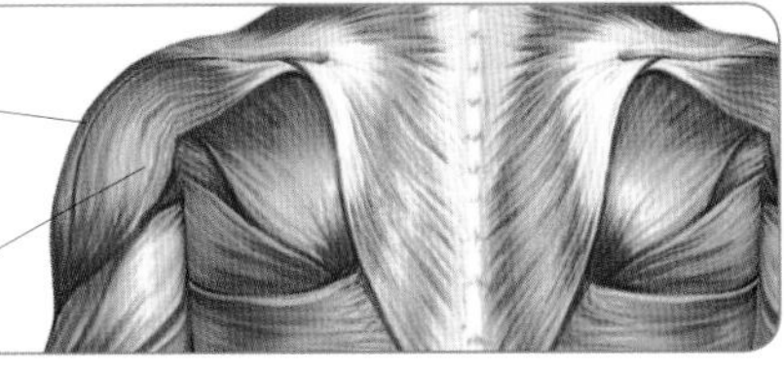

Rope Pull-Down

Also known as the Kneeling Cable Crunch, this move takes the standard crunch and adds resistance to it. It is a very effective core-strengthening exercise suitable for all levels.

HOW TO DO IT

- Kneel in front of a cable system with a rope attached. Select an appropriate weight resistance, and then grasp the rope with both hands, reaching overhead. Your torso should be upright in the starting position.
- Flex your spine, attempting to bring your rib cage to your legs as you pull the cable down so that your wrists rest against your head.
- Pause at the bottom of the motion, and then slowly return to the starting position. Repeat for the recommended repetitions.

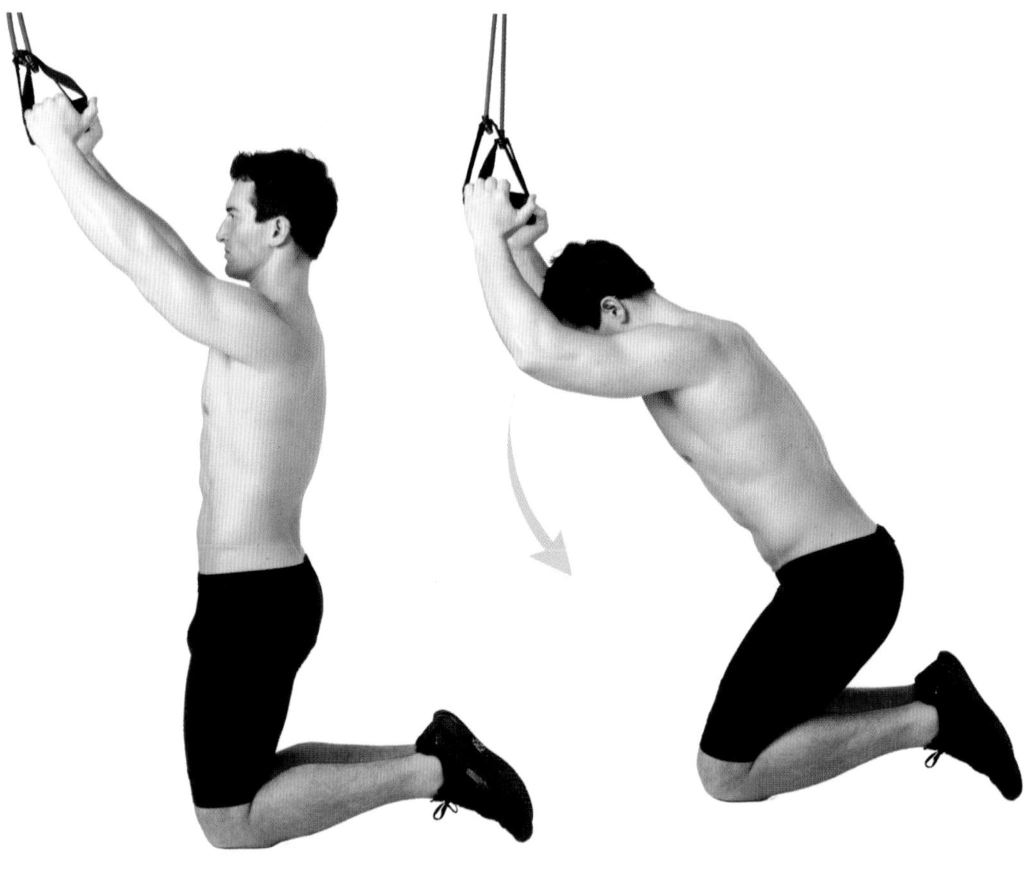

DO IT RIGHT

- Look for the movement to occur in your waist.
- Maintain a full range of motion.
- Avoid shifting your hips once movement begins.
- Avoid pulling down with your arms; let your abdominals drive the movement.

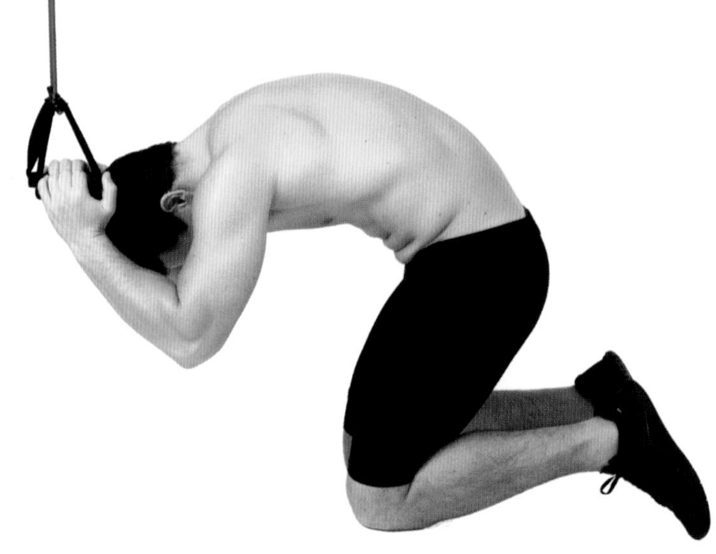

FACT FILE

TARGETS
- Upper abdominals
- Obliques

EQUIPMENT
- Cable machine
- Rope attachment

BENEFITS
- Strengthens abdominals

CAUTIONS
- Shoulder issues
- Wrist issues
- Knee issues

MODIFICATION

HARDER: Follow previous instructions, but add a twist to the movement, aiming your elbow for the opposite knee.

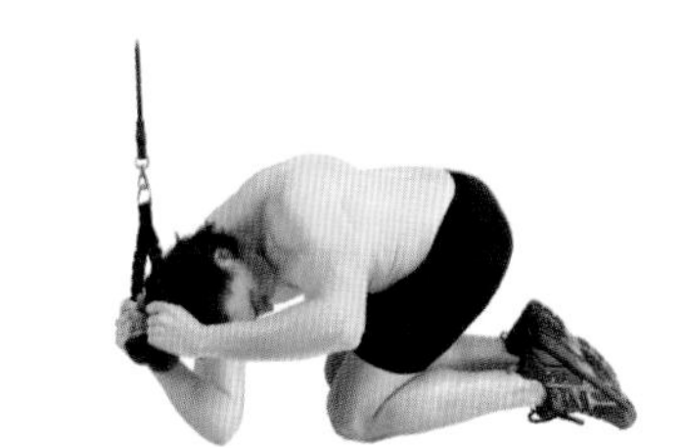

Annotation Key

Bold text indicates target muscles

Light text indicates other working muscles

* indicates deep muscles

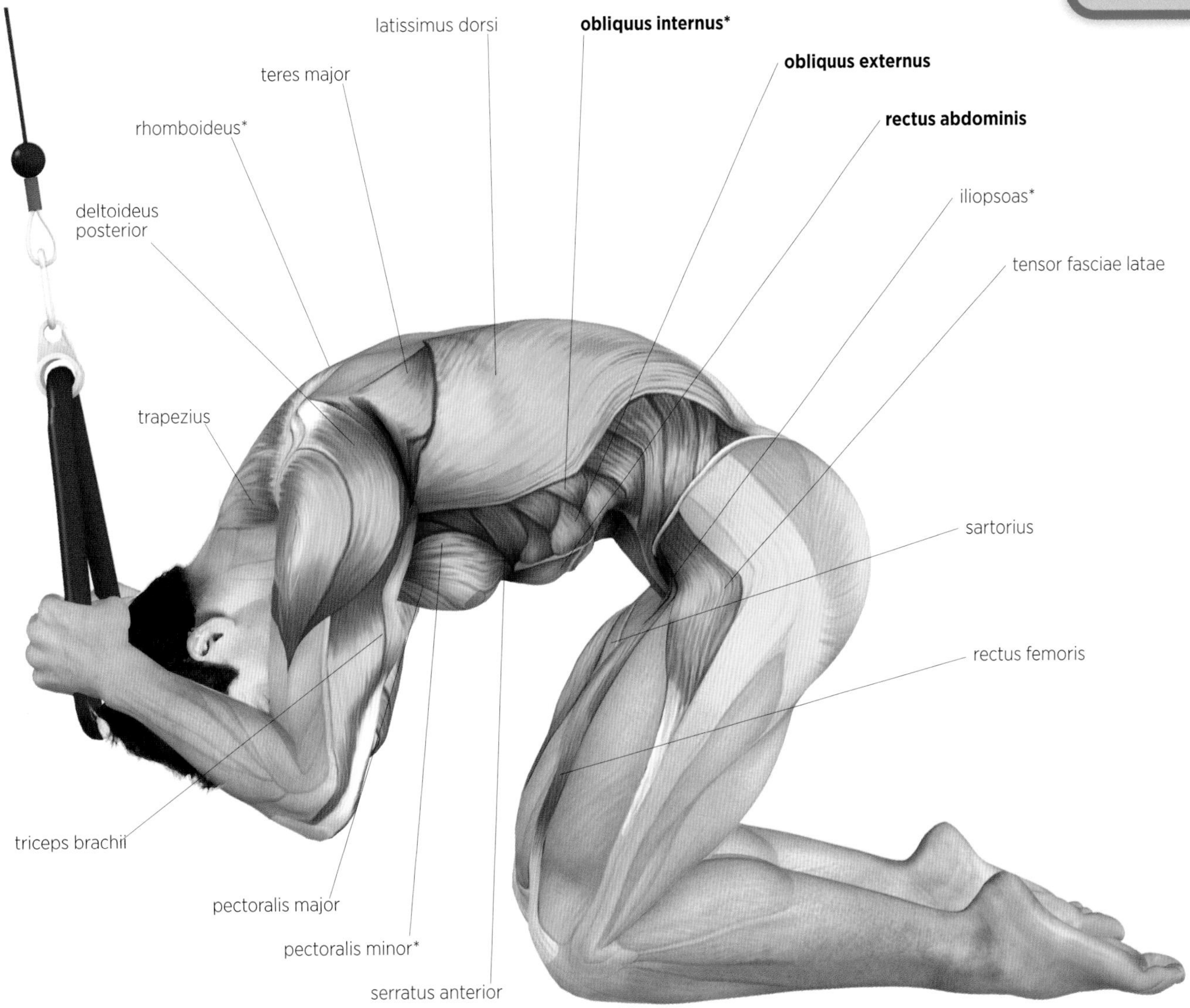

latissimus dorsi

obliquus internus*

obliquus externus

rectus abdominis

teres major

rhomboideus*

deltoideus posterior

iliopsoas*

tensor fasciae latae

trapezius

sartorius

rectus femoris

triceps brachii

pectoralis major

pectoralis minor*

serratus anterior

Figure 8

Target your obliques with the Figure 8, which takes you through a graceful pattern of movement. It also works your shoulders.

HOW TO DO IT

- Stand with your feet hip-width apart or slightly wider. Grasp a medicine ball in both hands, and hold it in front of your torso.
- Shift your weight to the right. In a smooth, controlled movement, extend both arms and bring the medicine ball toward the lower right side of your body.
- Continue shifting your weight to the right as you raise the ball toward the upper-right side of your body.
- In a Figure 8 motion, bring the ball diagonally toward the lower-left side of your body, and then raise it to the upper left as you shift your weight onto your left leg.
- Repeat for the recommended repetitions, and then repeat all steps, moving in the opposite direction.

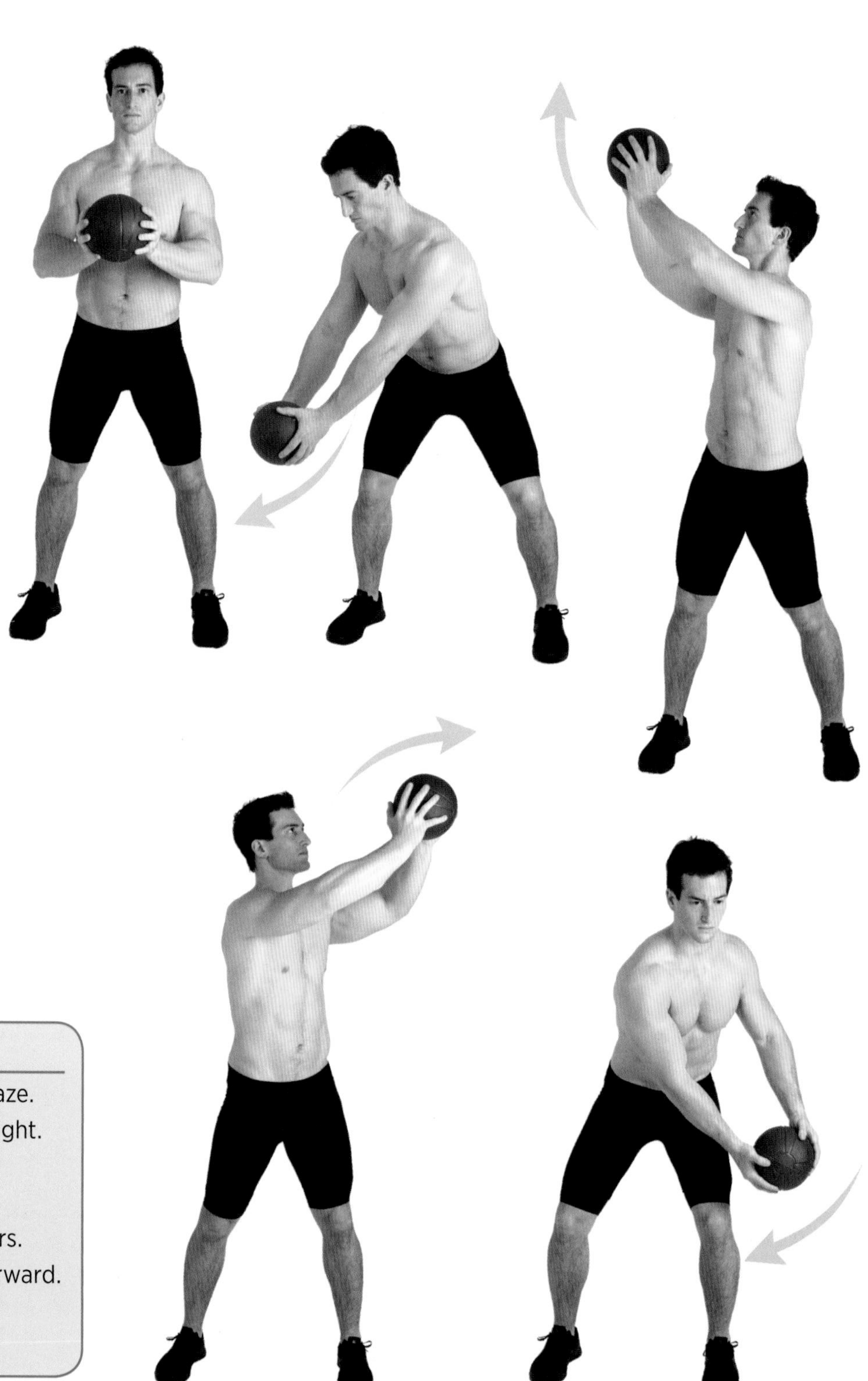

DO IT RIGHT

- Follow the ball's movement with your gaze.
- Keep your abdominals contracted and tight.
- Firmly anchor both feet to the floor.
- Avoid straining your neck.
- Avoid tensing or hunching your shoulders.
- Avoid arching your back or hunching forward.
- Move smoothly and with control; avoid rushing through the exercise.

Annotation Key

Bold text indicates target muscles

Light text indicates other working muscles

* indicates deep muscles

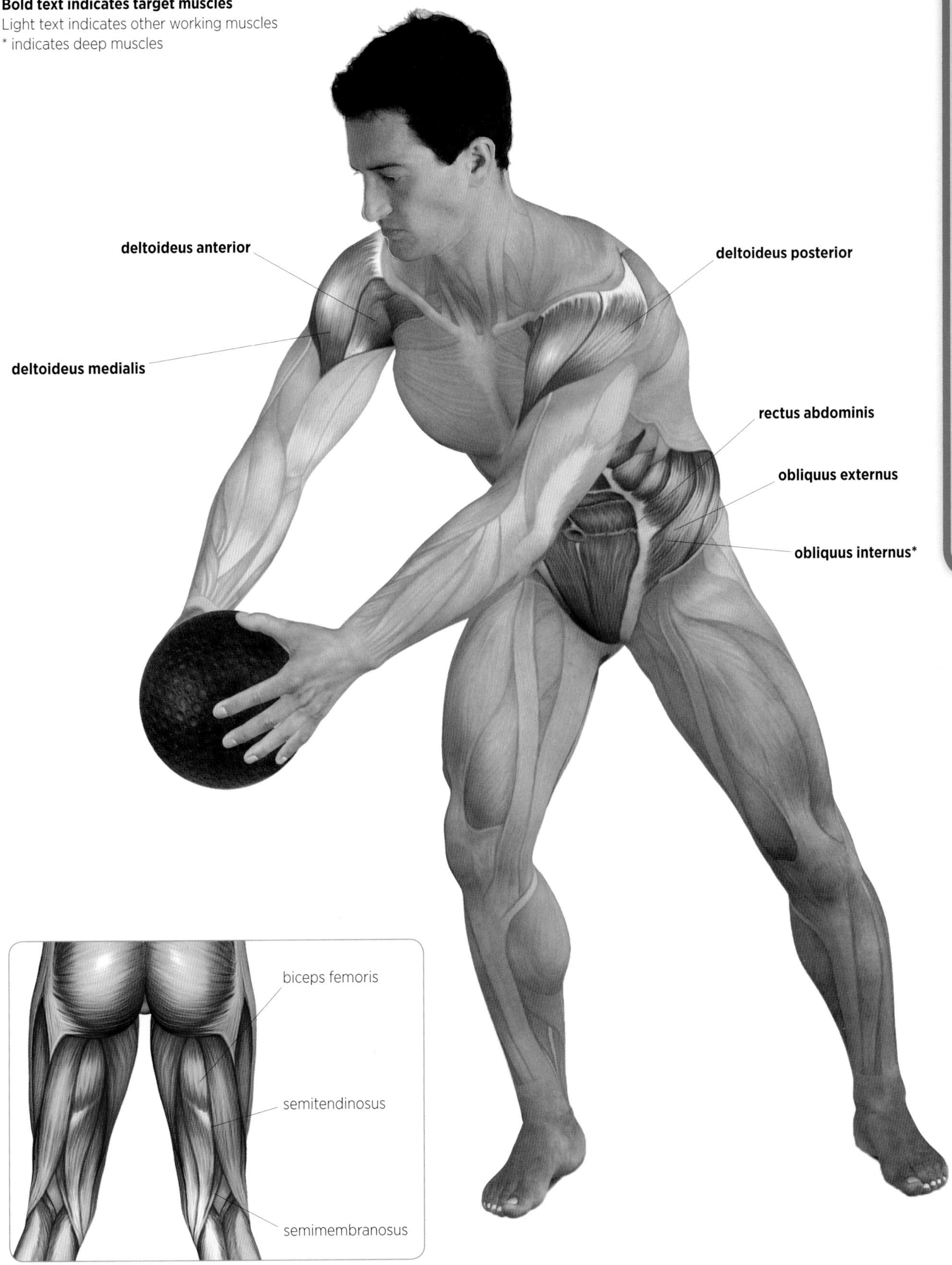

deltoideus anterior

deltoideus medialis

deltoideus posterior

rectus abdominis

obliquus externus

obliquus internus*

biceps femoris

semitendinosus

semimembranosus

FACT FILE

TARGETS
- Core
- Shoulders
- Spine

EQUIPMENT
- Medicine ball

BENEFITS
- Improves coordination, flexibility, and range of motion
- Strengthens and tones core and shoulders
- Stabilizes core
- Stretches spine

CAUTIONS
- Shoulder issues
- Lower-back pain

Medicine Ball Woodchop

The Medicine Ball Woodchop is a take on a classic gym exercise. Perform this version to strengthen your abdominals, especially your obliques. This exercise also works your arm, shoulder, and spinal muscles.

HOW TO DO IT

- Stand with your feet shoulder-width apart, holding a medicine ball with both hands to the right side of your head.
- Twist your torso toward the left while lowering the medicine ball to the outside of your left leg.
- Return to the starting position, and then repeat for the recommended repetitions.
- Repeat all steps, moving in the opposite direction.

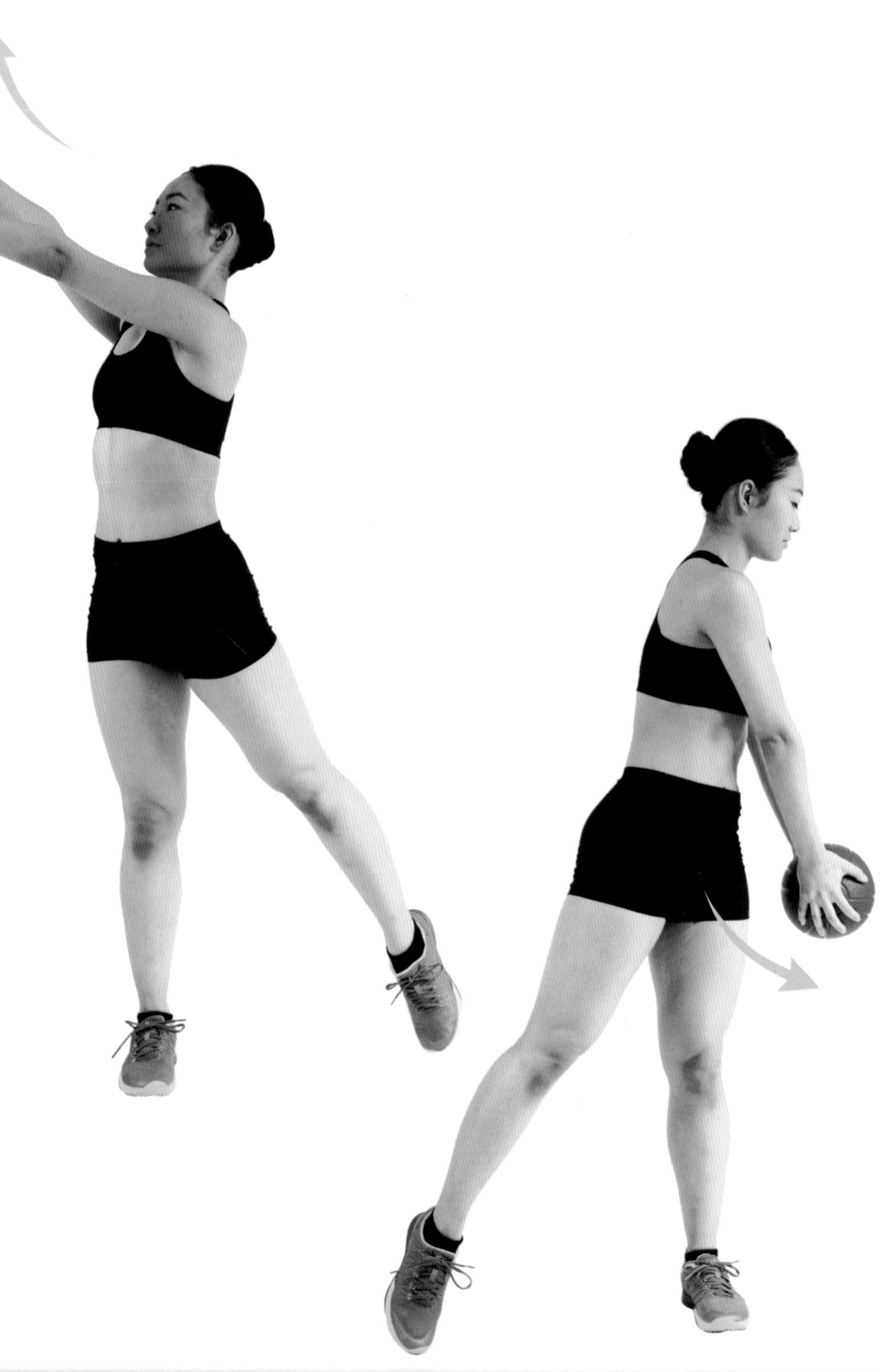

DO IT RIGHT

- Perform the positive portion of the exercise (swinging) aggressively and the negative portion (the wind-up) in a slow, controlled fashion.
- Follow the ball's movement with your gaze.
- Keep your abdominals contracted and tight.
- Avoid twisting too violently from side to side; this can throw your back out.

FACT FILE

TARGETS
- Obliques
- Abdominals
- Spine

EQUIPMENT
- Medicine ball

BENEFITS
- Improves flexibility and range of motion
- Strengthens and tones core and shoulders
- Stabilizes core
- Stretches spine

CAUTIONS
- Shoulder issues
- Lower-back pain

Annotation Key

Bold text indicates target muscles
Light text indicates other working muscles
* indicates deep muscles

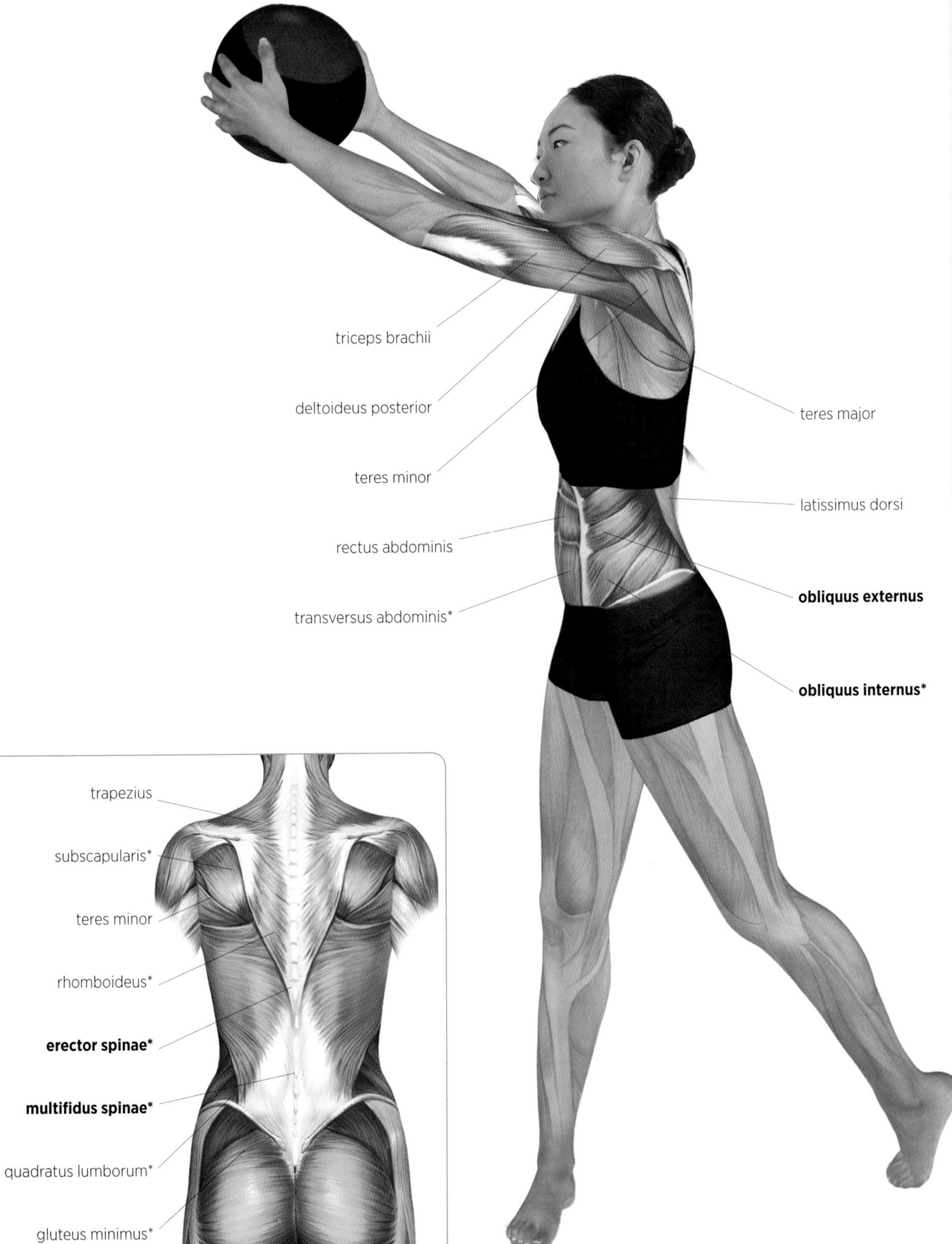

Pullover Pass

The Pullover Pass effectively helps you develop explosive strength in your abdominals. It also works your spinal muscles. Perform this as a game of catch with a workout partner.

HOW TO DO IT

- Lie faceup with your knees bent and your feet flat on the floor. Hold a medicine ball behind your head.
- Contracting your abdominals, quickly sit up and pass the ball to a partner.
- Receive the ball back, and gently return to the starting position. Repeat for the recommended repetitions.

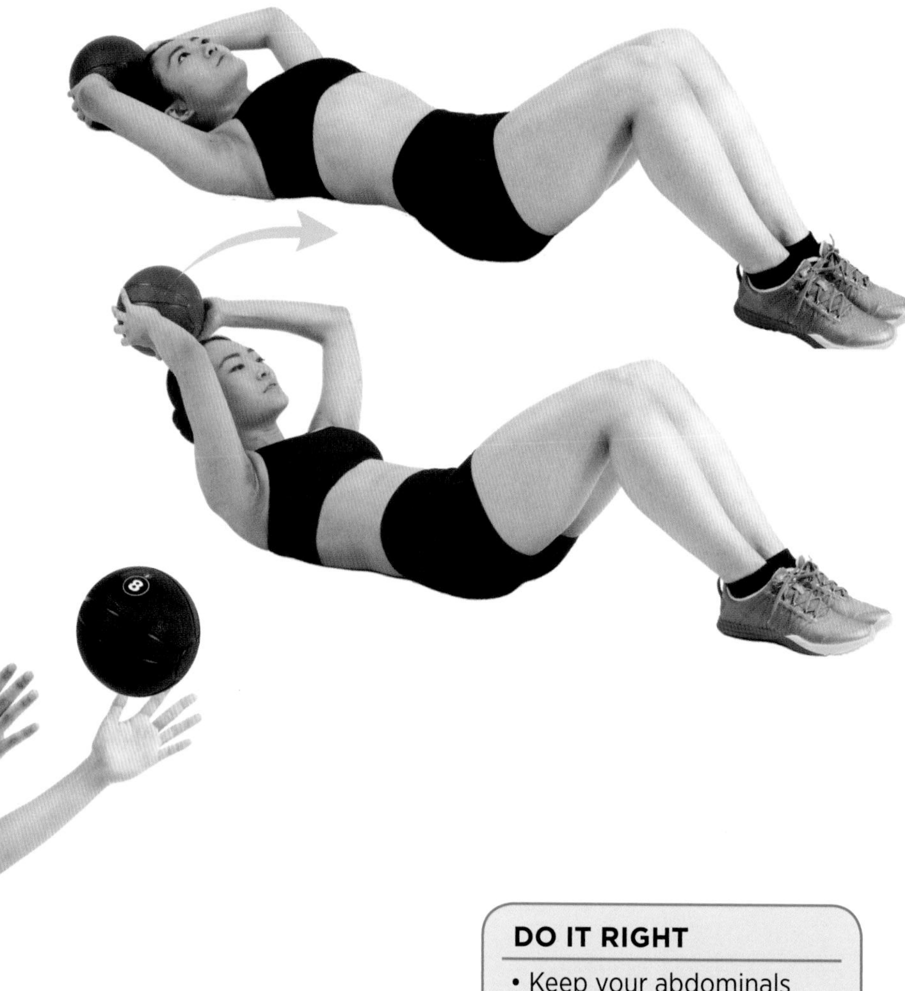

DO IT RIGHT

- Keep your abdominals contracted and tight.
- Follow the ball's movement with your gaze.
- Avoid straining your neck.

FACT FILE

TARGETS
- Abdominals
- Spine

EQUIPMENT
- Medicine ball

BENEFITS
- Strengthens abdominals and spine

CAUTIONS
- Shoulder issues
- Lower-back pain

Annotation Key

Bold text indicates target muscles

Light text indicates other working muscles

* indicates deep muscles

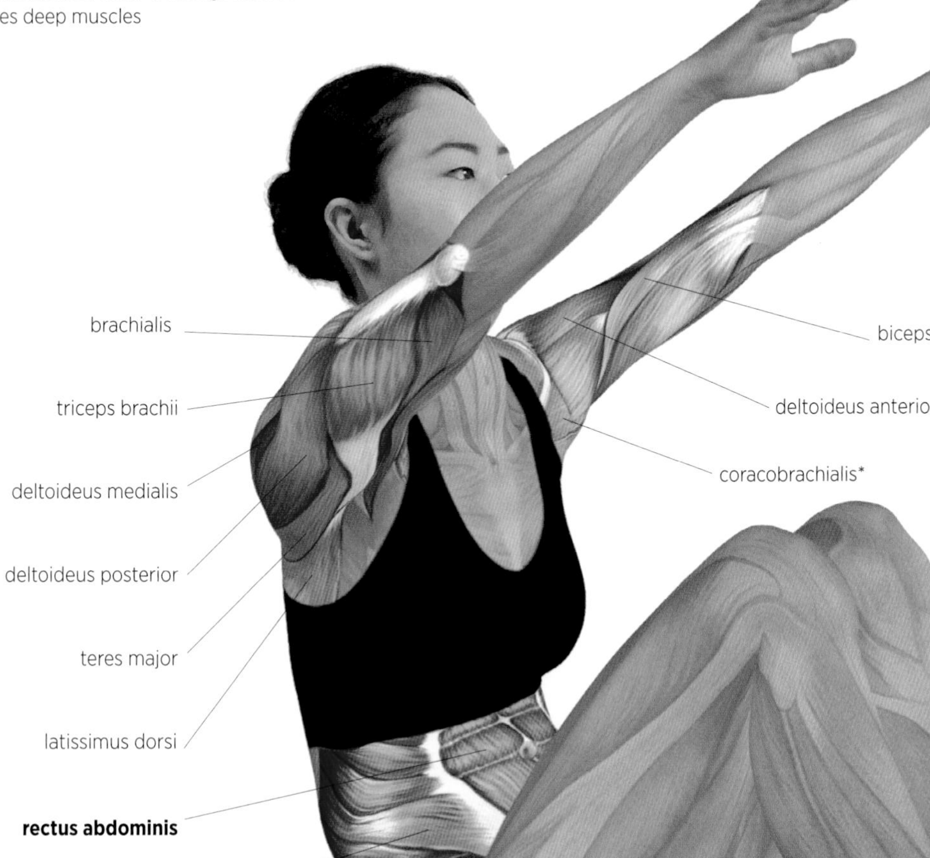

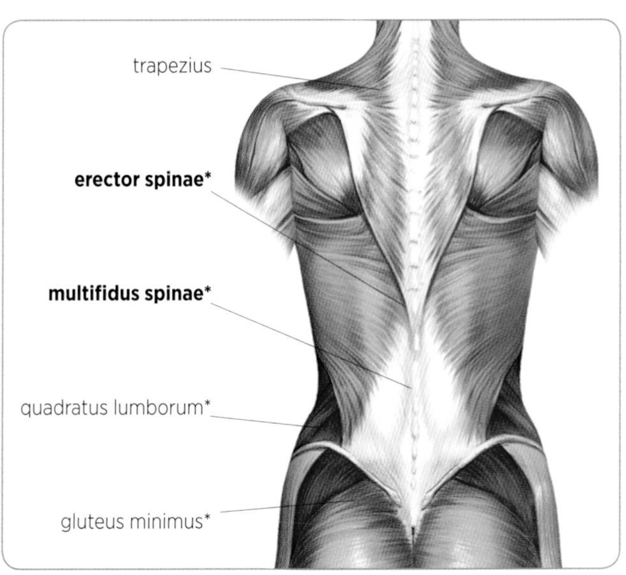

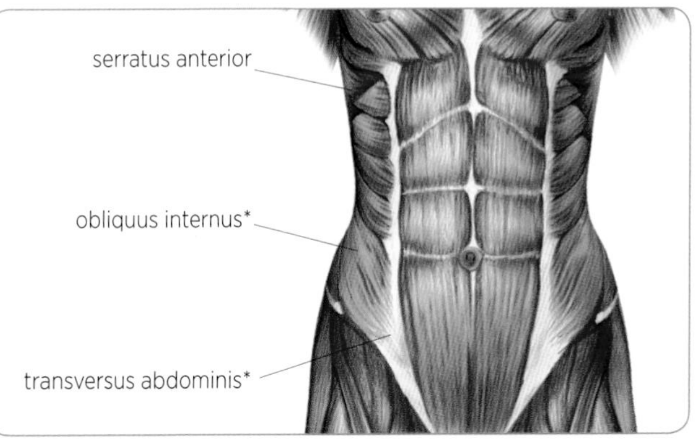

Swiss Ball Jackknife

The Swiss Ball Jackknife builds strength, primarily in your core and hip flexors. It targets both the front and back core muscles—especially your rectus abdominis and spinal erectors. For proper performance, you need excellent coordination, timing, accuracy, and strength.

HOW TO DO IT

- Begin in a high plank position with your arms shoulder-width apart and your shins resting on a Swiss ball.
- Bend your knees to roll the ball in toward your chest until your buttocks touch your heels.
- Slowly extend your legs, rolling the ball back to the starting position. Repeat for the recommended repetitions.

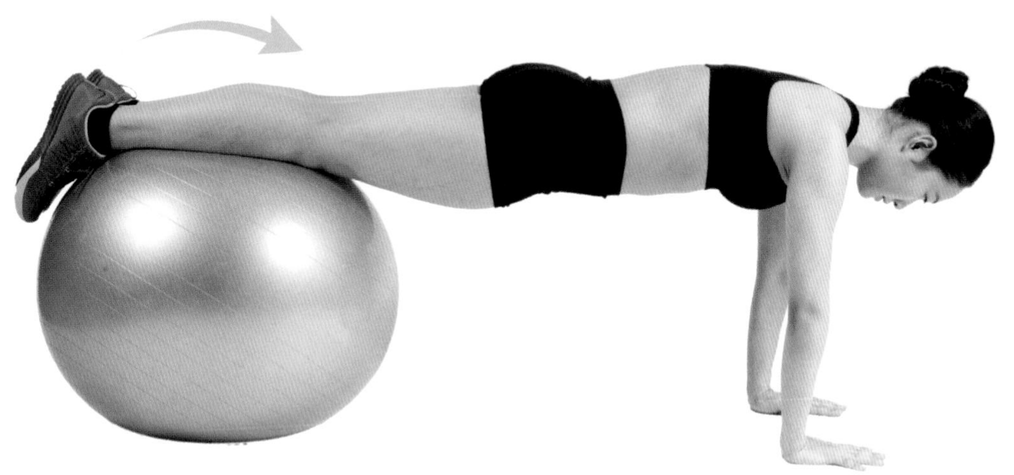

DO IT RIGHT

- Keep your abdominals contracted and tight.
- Keep both hands anchored to the floor.
- Keep your gaze directed toward the floor.
- Avoid rounding your back.
- Avoid straining your neck by trying to look forward.

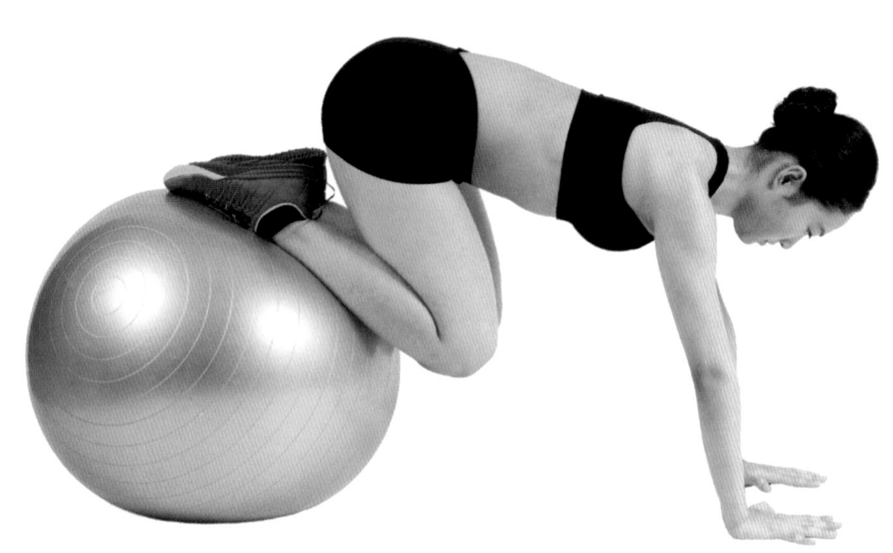

serratus anterior
rectus abdominis
iliopsoas*
sartorius

trapezius
subscapularis*
rhomboideus*

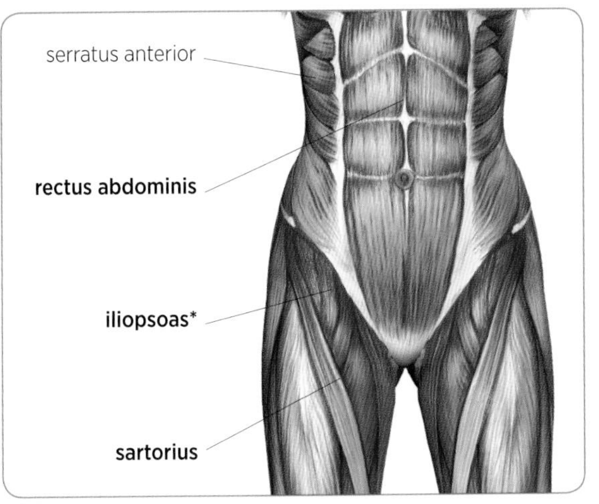

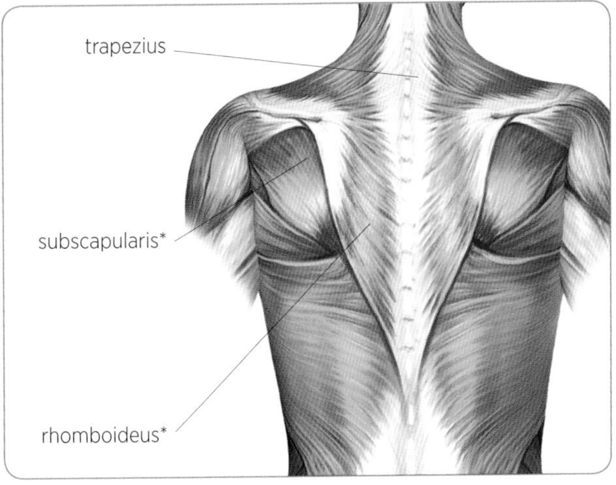

FACT FILE

TARGETS
- Abdominals
- Hip flexors

EQUIPMENT
- Swiss ball

BENEFITS
- Stabilizes core
- Strengthens abdominal and hip flexors

CAUTIONS
- Lower-back issues
- Shoulder issues
- Neck issues

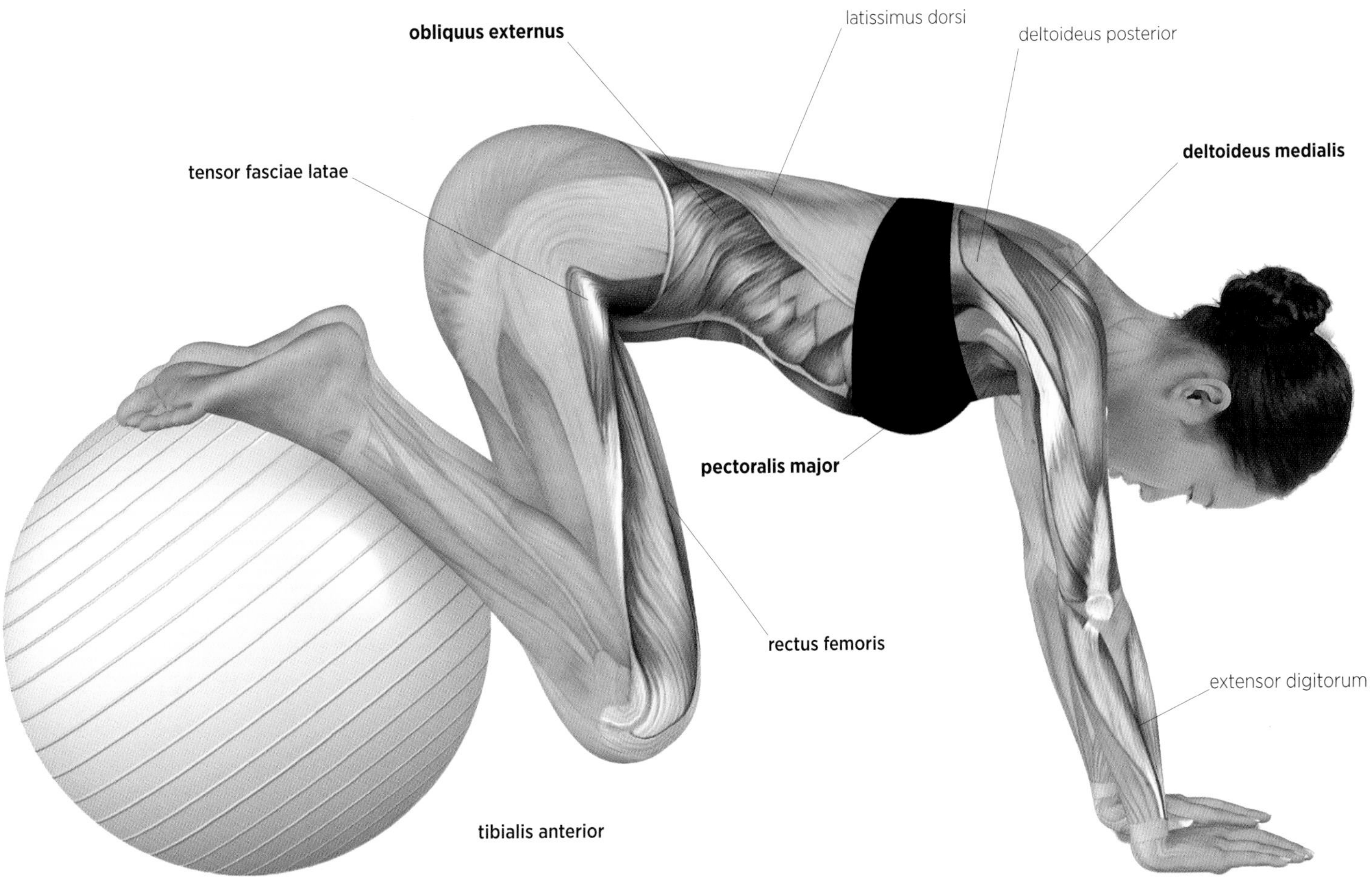

obliquus externus
latissimus dorsi
deltoideus posterior
tensor fasciae latae
deltoideus medialis
pectoralis major
rectus femoris
extensor digitorum
tibialis anterior

Annotation Key

Bold text indicates target muscles
Light text indicates other working muscles
* indicates deep muscles

Medicine Ball Pike-Up

The Medicine Ball Pike-Up is especially good for building core strength and stability. In addition to targeting your core muscles, it works glutes, hamstrings, and calves.

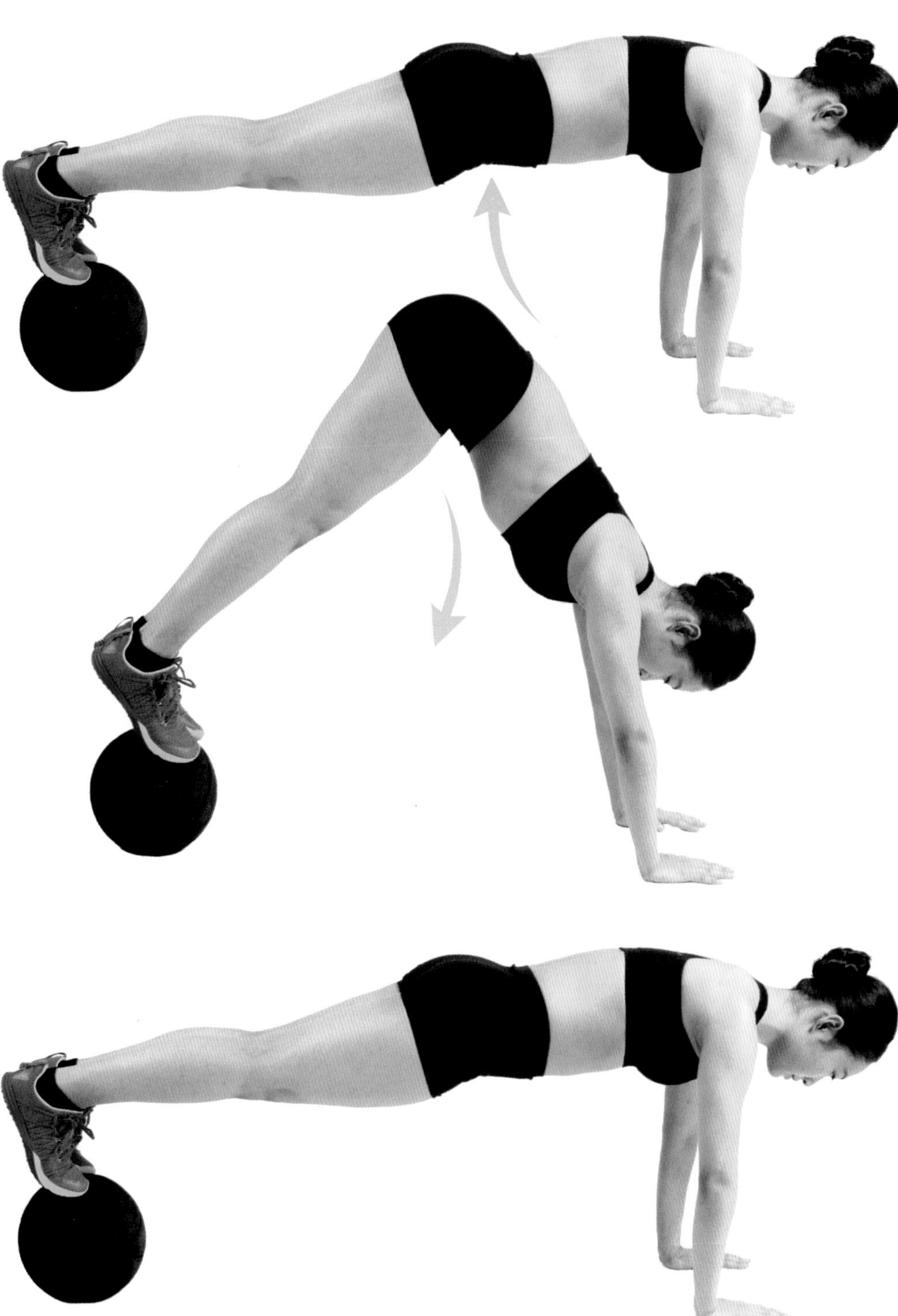

HOW TO DO IT

- Begin in a high plank position with your arms shoulder-width apart and your toes planted on a medicine ball.
- Raise your hips to the ceiling, rolling the medicine ball toward your hands as you do so.
- Reverse the movement, lowering yourself back down to the starting position. Repeat for the recommended repetitions.

DO IT RIGHT

- Keep your abdominals contracted and tight.
- Keep both hands anchored to the floor.
- Keep your gaze directed toward the floor.
- Keep your legs locked.
- Avoid lowering your torso farther than parallel to the floor.

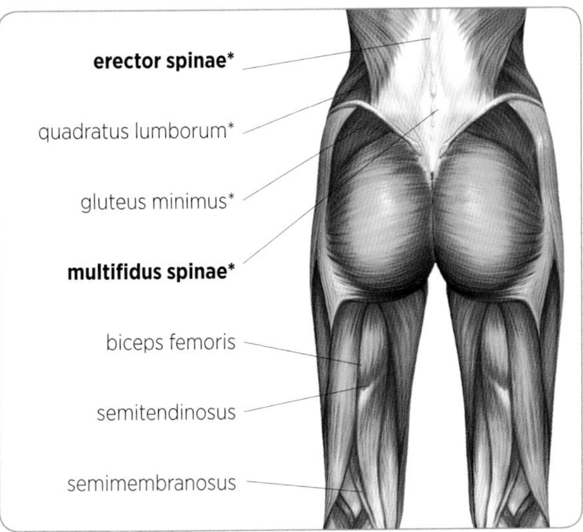

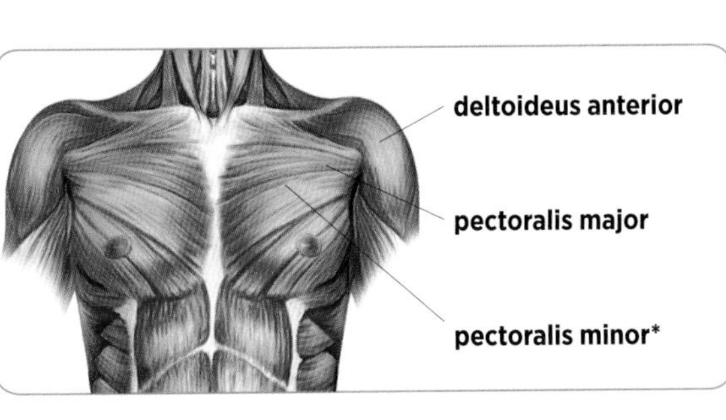

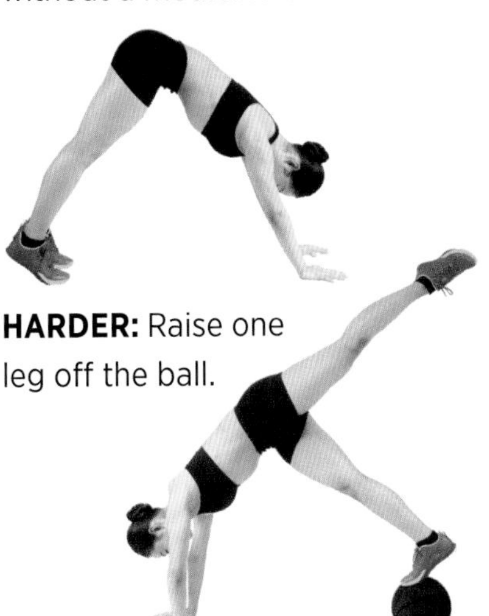

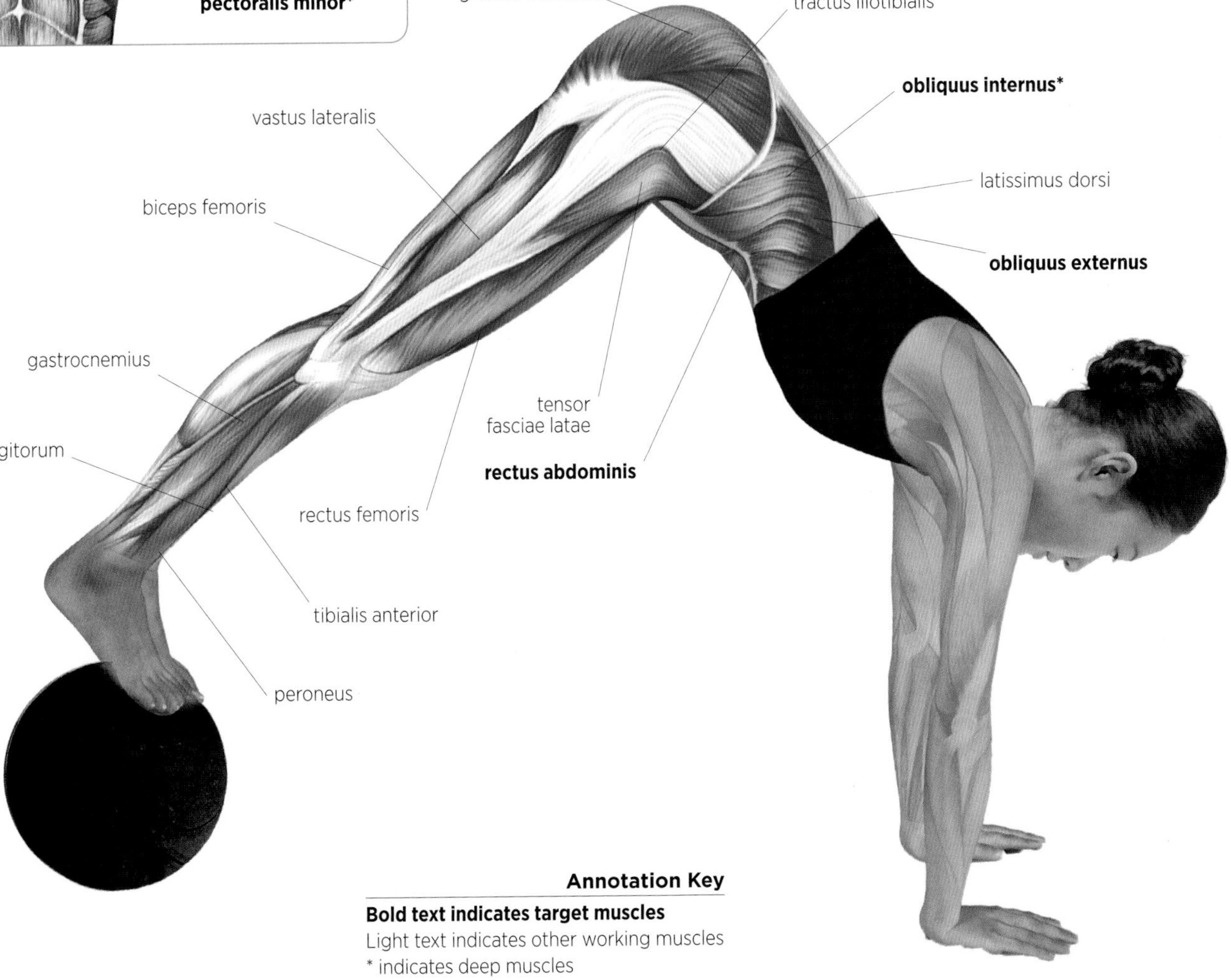

FACT FILE

TARGETS
- Abdominals
- Hip flexors
- Shoulders

EQUIPMENT
- Medicine ball

BENEFITS
- Stabilizes core
- Strengthens abdominals and hip flexors

CAUTIONS
- Lower-back issues
- Shoulder issues
- Neck issues

erector spinae*
quadratus lumborum*
gluteus minimus*
multifidus spinae*
biceps femoris
semitendinosus
semimembranosus

deltoideus anterior
pectoralis major
pectoralis minor*

MODIFICATIONS

EASIER: Perform the exercise without a medicine ball.

HARDER: Raise one leg off the ball.

gluteus maximus
tractus iliotibialis
obliquus internus*
vastus lateralis
latissimus dorsi
biceps femoris
obliquus externus
gastrocnemius
tensor fasciae latae
extensor digitorum
rectus abdominis
rectus femoris
tibialis anterior
peroneus

Annotation Key

Bold text indicates target muscles

Light text indicates other working muscles

* indicates deep muscles

Swiss Ball Rollout

The Swiss Ball Rollout stabilizes your cores muscles, which prepares them for many everyday movements. When performing this exercise, you more effectively activate the rectus abdominis and obliques than when performing sit-ups and crunches.

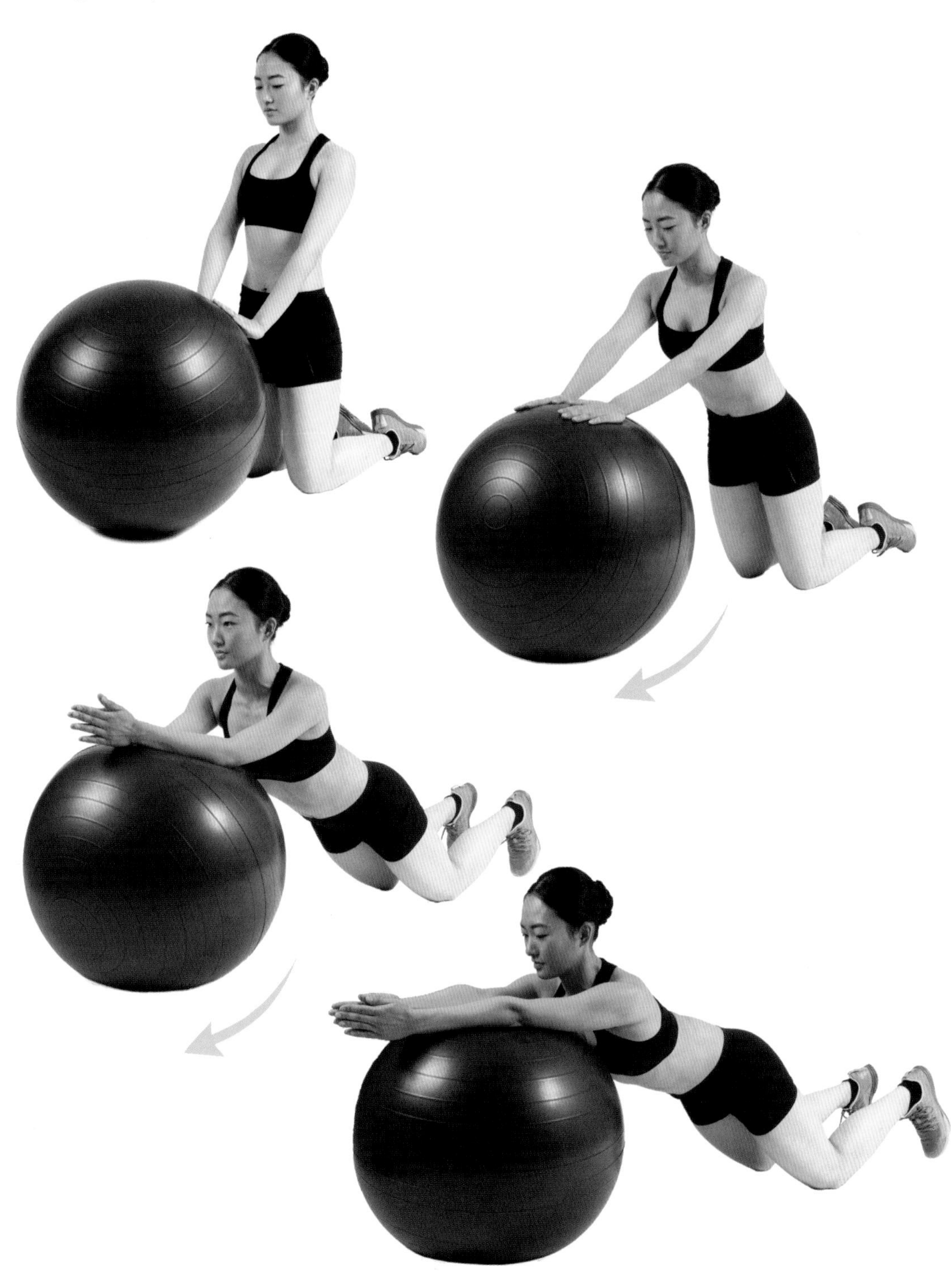

HOW TO DO IT

- Kneel in front of a Swiss ball, and place your hands on it at about hip height.
- Slowly roll the ball forward, extending your body as you go.
- While keeping a flat back and remaining anchored on your knees, continue to roll forward until you are completely stretched out.
- To return to the starting position, engage your abdominal and lower-back muscles and roll back to the starting position. Repeat for the recommended repetitions.

DO IT RIGHT

- Keep your abdominals contracted and tight.
- Keep your body elongated throughout the movement.
- Avoid bridging your back.
- Avoid allowing your hips or lower back to sag.

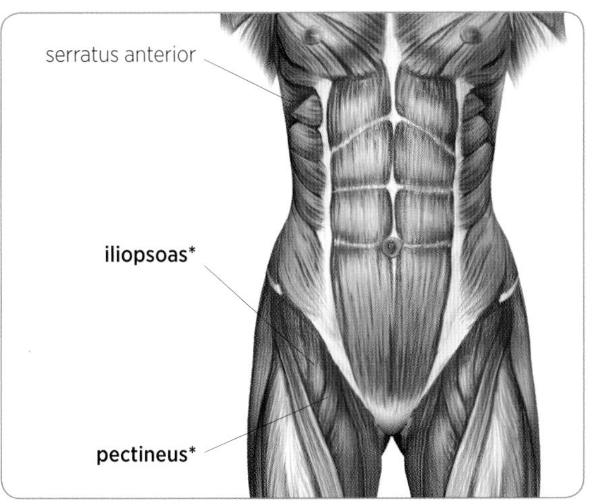

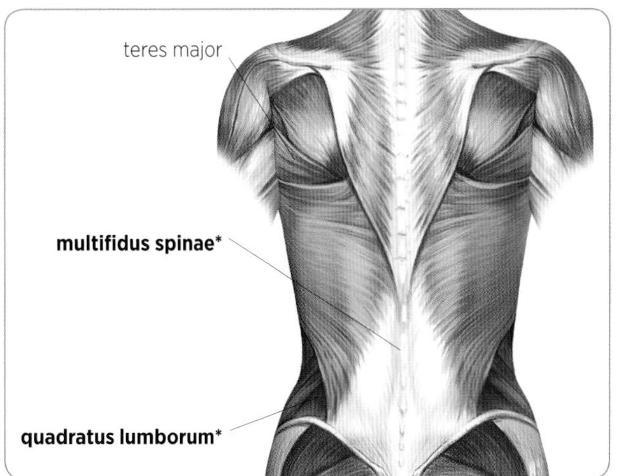

FACT FILE

TARGETS
- Abdominals
- Obliques
- Lower back

EQUIPMENT
- Swiss ball

BENEFITS
- Stabilizes core
- Strengthens abdominals, obliques, and back

CAUTIONS
- Shoulder issues
- Knee issues

serratus anterior
iliopsoas*
pectineus*

teres major
multifidus spinae*
quadratus lumborum*

Annotation Key

Bold text indicates target muscles
Light text indicates other working muscles
* indicates deep muscles

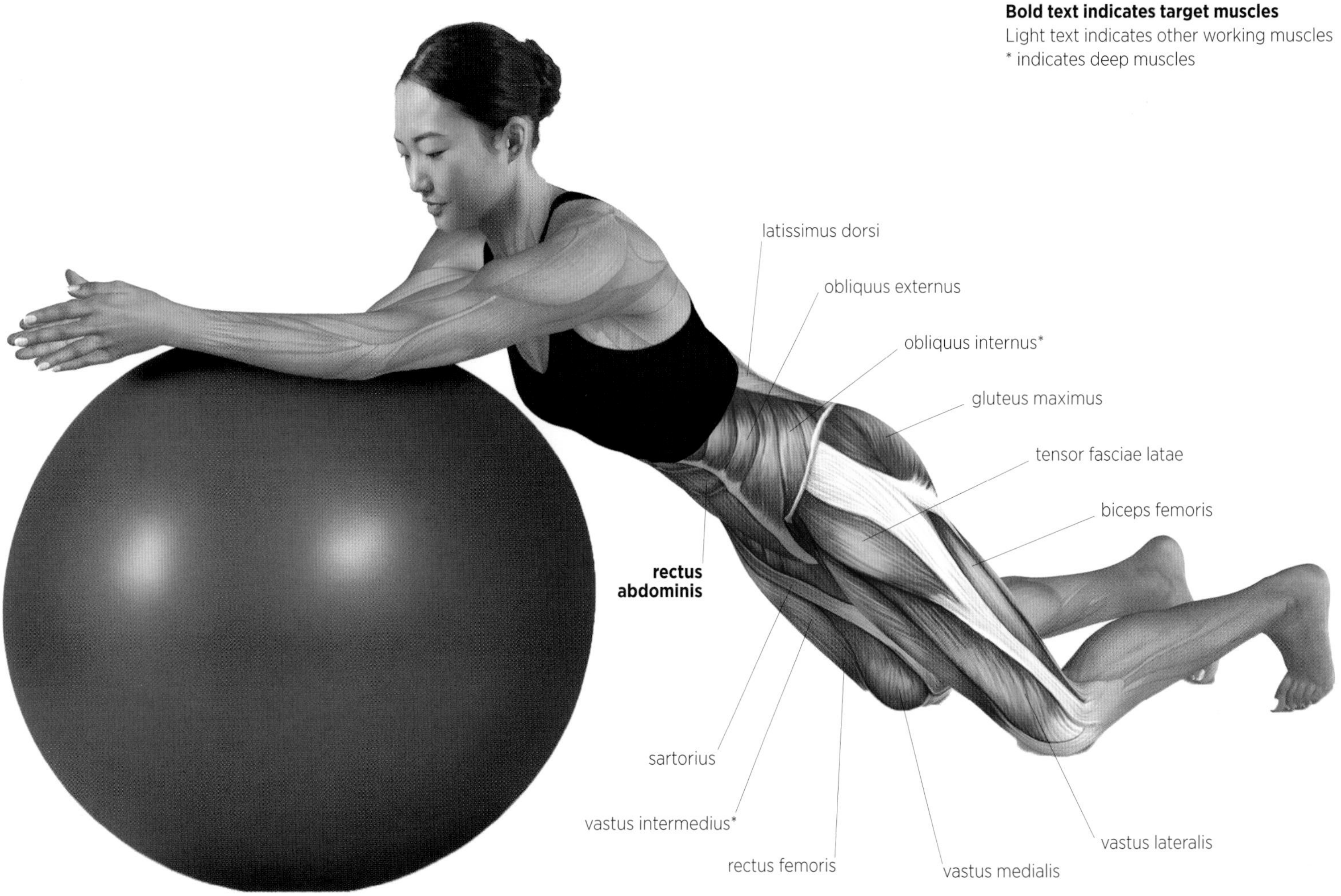

latissimus dorsi
obliquus externus
obliquus internus*
gluteus maximus
tensor fasciae latae
biceps femoris
rectus abdominis
sartorius
vastus intermedius*
rectus femoris
vastus medialis
vastus lateralis

Barbell Squat

This weight-training classic is one of the most effective strengthening exercises you perform. The Barbell Squat is fantastic for working your lower body and core, and revs up your metabolism.

HOW TO DO IT

- To begin, set a bar on a squat rack just below shoulder level. Load the bar with the proper weights, step under the bar, and position the bar high on the back of your shoulders and grasp barbell to sides. Dismount the bar from the rack, and carefully take a step back to stand with your feet shoulder-width apart and your knees slightly bent.

- Keeping your back straight, slowly bend your knees until your thighs and calves form an angle of slightly less than 90 degrees.

- Pushing down into your heels, begin to raise the bar by straightening your legs back to the upright starting position. Repeat for the recommended repetitions.

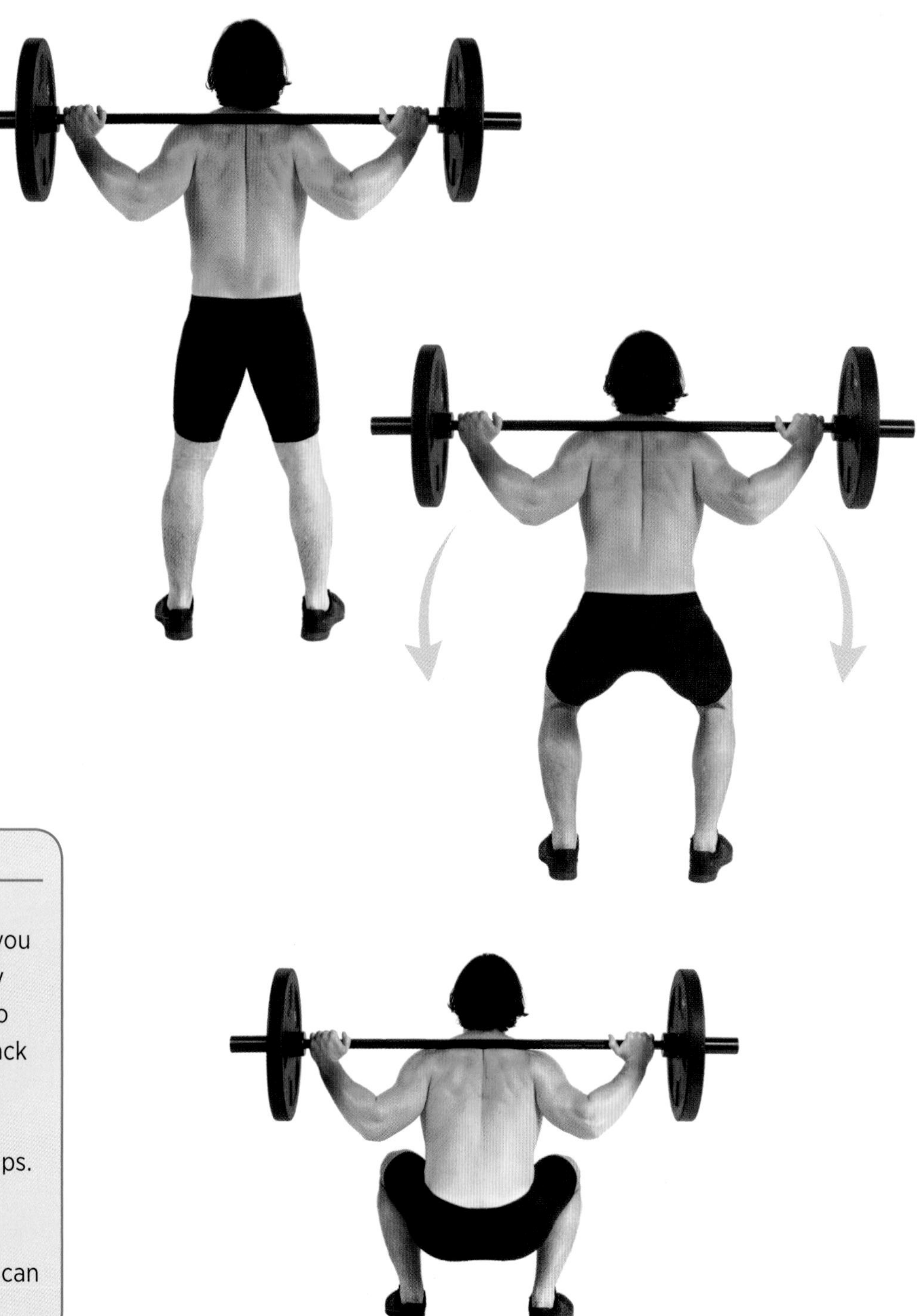

DO IT RIGHT

- This exercise is safest while being performed within a squat rack. When you are finished with this exercise, carefully step forward, aligning the bar back into the rack. Secure the weight onto the rack by bending your knees slightly.
- Keep the bar straight and balanced.
- Keep your spine stable from head to hips.
- Avoid rolling your shoulders or upper back forward.
- Avoid using a heavier weight than you can safely handle.

FACT FILE

TARGETS
- Quadriceps
- Glutes

EQUIPMENT
- Barbell
- Squat rack

BENEFITS
- Strengthens lower body

CAUTIONS
- Shoulder issues
- Back issues

Annotation Key

Bold text indicates target muscles
Light text indicates other working muscles
* indicates deep muscles

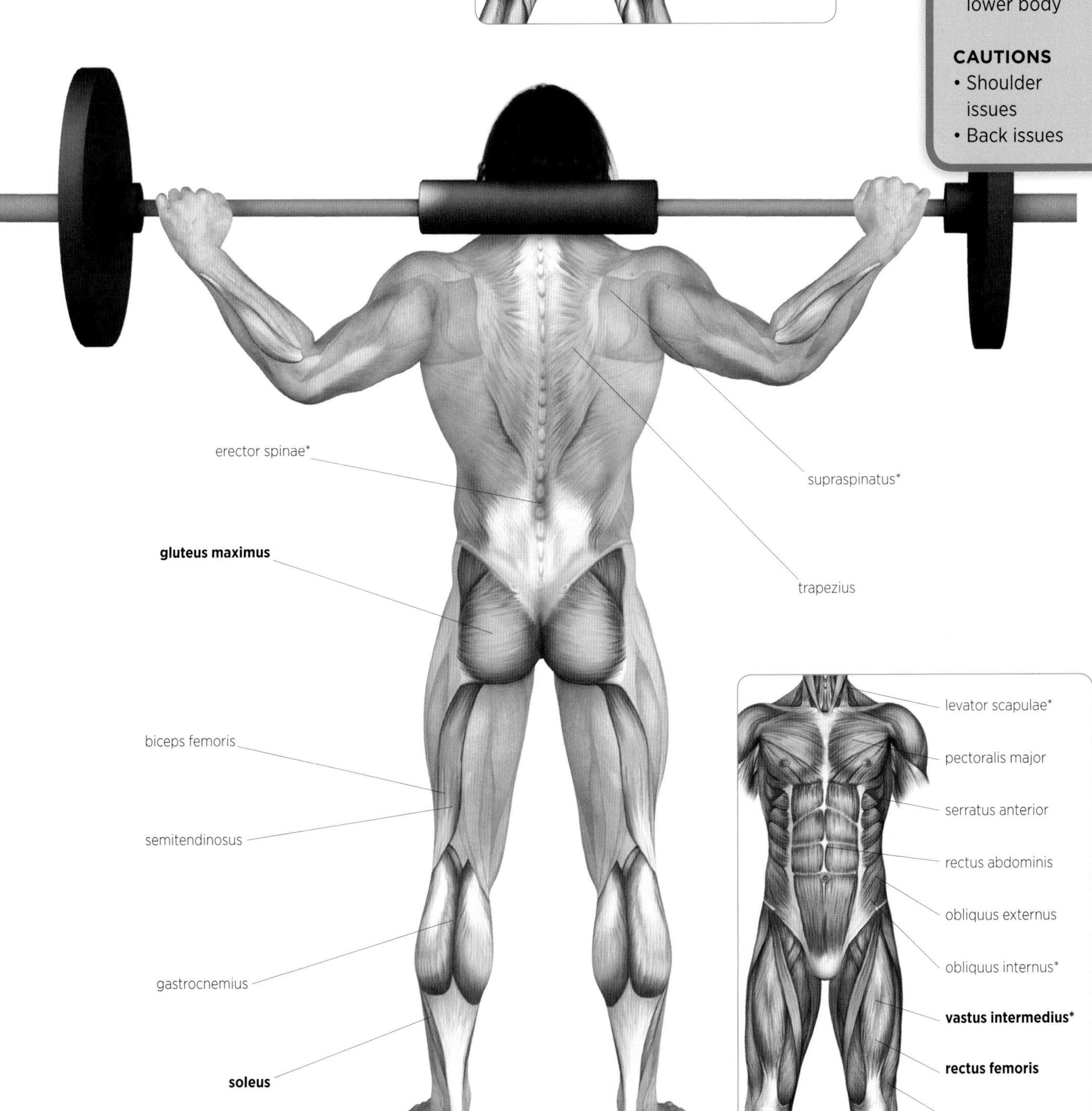

Power Squat

The Power Squat effectively targets your thighs and glutes. It improves balance and helps to stabilize your pelvis, trunk, and knees. It also boosts general movement strength.

HOW TO DO IT

- Stand holding a medicine ball in front of your torso.
- Shift your weight to your left foot, and bend your right knee, lifting your right foot toward your buttocks. Bend your elbows to draw the ball toward the outside of your right ear.
- Maintaining a neutral spine, bend your hips and left knee. Lower your torso toward to the left, bringing the ball toward your left ankle.
- Press into your left leg as you straighten your knee and torso to return to the starting position.
- Repeat for the recommended repetitions, and then repeat all steps, moving in the opposite direction.

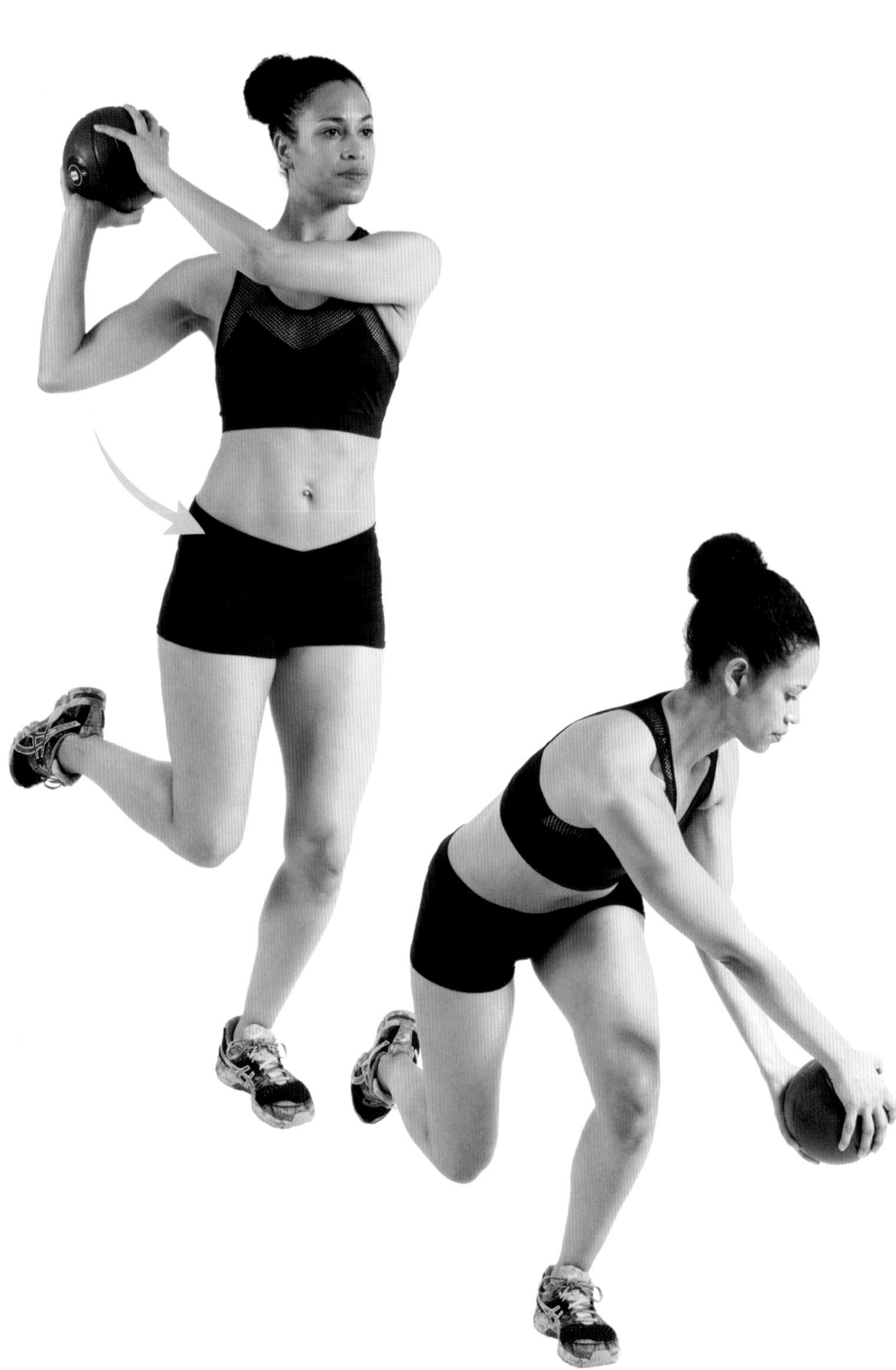

DO IT RIGHT

- Create a smooth arc in the air with the ball.
- Keep the hips and knees of both legs aligned.
- Keep your shoulders and neck relaxed.
- Avoid allowing your knee to extend beyond your toes as you bend and rotate.
- Keep your standing foot firmly anchored to the floor.
- Avoid flexing your spine.

FACT FILE

TARGETS
- Quadriceps
- Glutes

EQUIPMENT
- Medicine ball

BENEFITS
- Strengthens lower body
- Improves balance
- Stabilizes pelvis, trunk, and knees
- Promotes stronger movement patterns

CAUTIONS
- Knee pain
- Lower-back issues
- Shoulder issues

piriformis*
adductor magnus
biceps femoris
semitendinosus
semimembranosus

trapezius
infraspinatus*
supraspinatus*
teres minor
subscapularis*
rhomboideus*

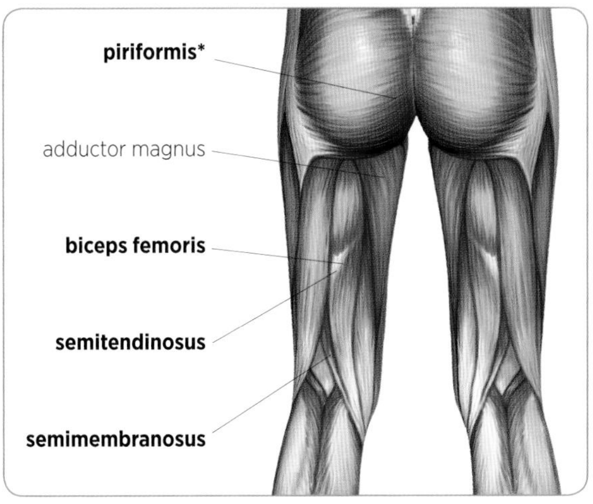

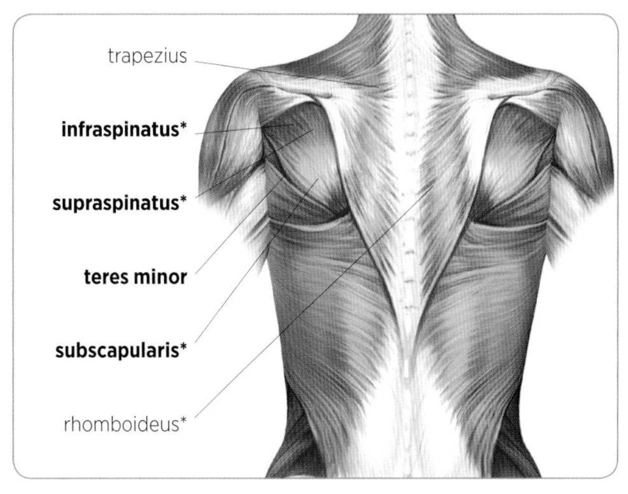

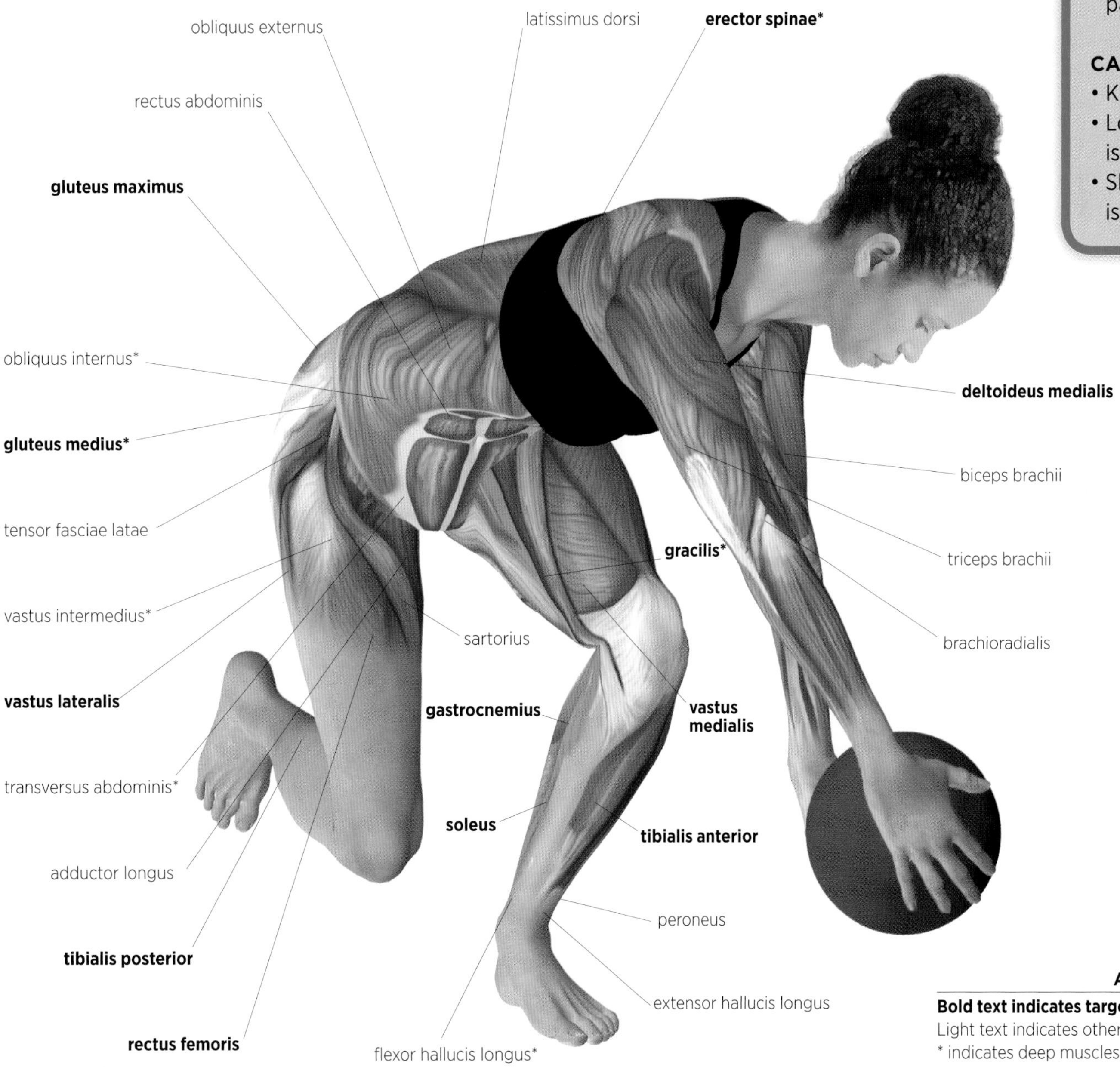

obliquus externus
latissimus dorsi
erector spinae*
rectus abdominis
gluteus maximus
obliquus internus*
deltoideus medialis
gluteus medius*
biceps brachii
tensor fasciae latae
gracilis*
triceps brachii
vastus intermedius*
sartorius
brachioradialis
vastus lateralis
gastrocnemius
vastus medialis
transversus abdominis*
soleus
tibialis anterior
adductor longus
peroneus
tibialis posterior
extensor hallucis longus
rectus femoris
flexor hallucis longus*

Annotation Key

Bold text indicates target muscles
Light text indicates other working muscles
* indicates deep muscles

Swiss Ball Hamstrings Curl

The Swiss Ball Hamstrings Curl is a challenging exercise that targets your hamstrings and glutes. Choose a ball size that you are comfortable with, keeping in mind that the larger the ball the greater the muscle contraction.

HOW TO DO IT

- Lie on your back with your arms along your sides, angled slightly away from your body. Extend your legs, and rest your lower legs and ankles on top of a Swiss ball.

- Pressing downward with your feet, bend your knees as you roll the ball toward you. Curl your pelvis, and raise your lower body off the floor. Hold for a few moments.

- With control, return to the starting position. Repeat for the recommended repetitions.

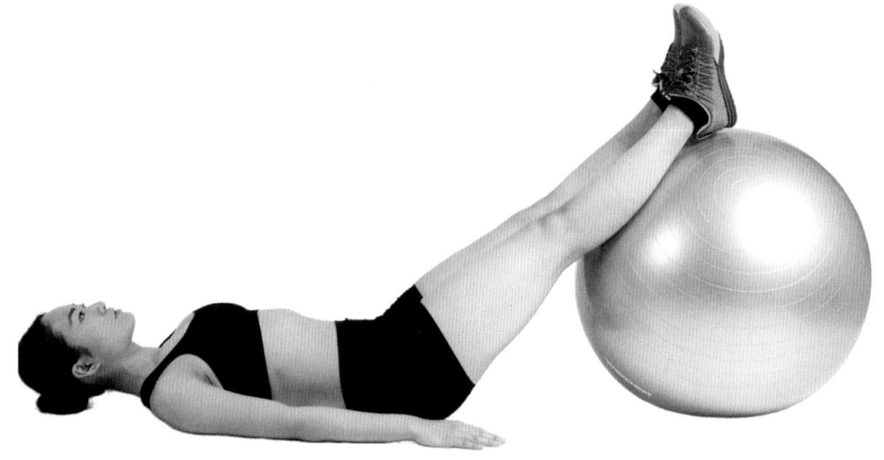

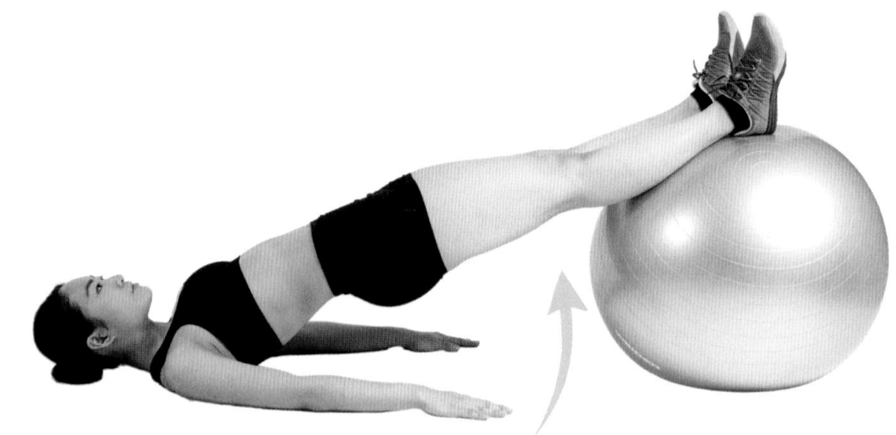

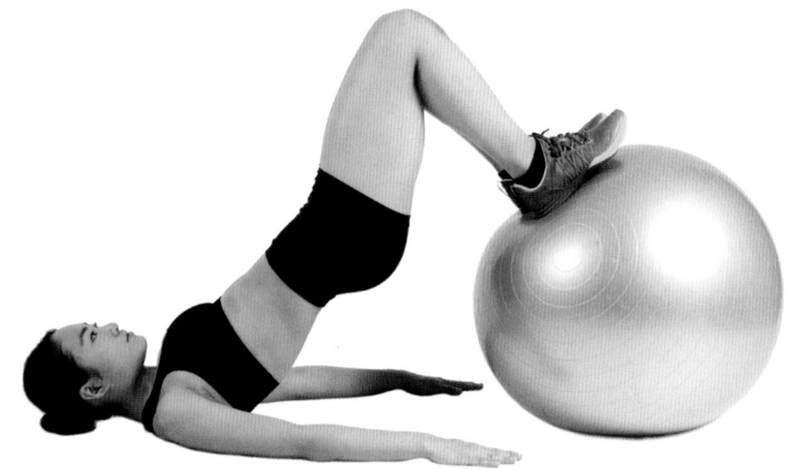

DO IT RIGHT

- Position your legs on the ball to form a 45-degree angle with the rest of your body before you curl.
- Move smoothly, maintaining control of the ball.
- Keep your arms anchored to the floor.
- Engage your abdominals, and squeeze your glutes.
- Avoid rushing through the movement.
- Avoid arching your back in the curl position.

FACT FILE

TARGETS
- Glutes
- Hamstrings

EQUIPMENT
- Swiss ball

BENEFITS
- Strengthens glutes and hamstrings
- Stretches chest and spine

CAUTIONS
- Lower-back issues
- Neck issues
- Shoulder issues

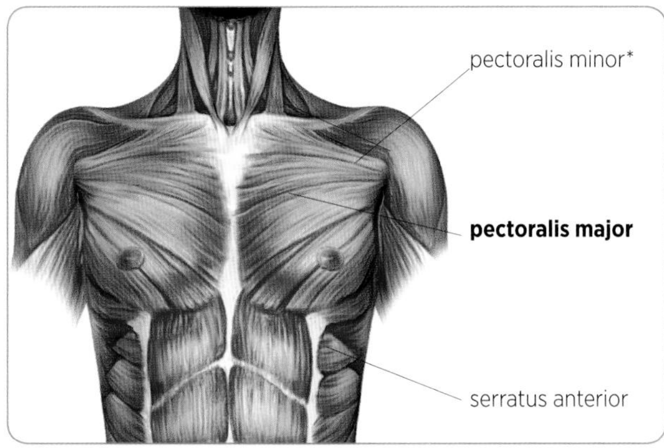

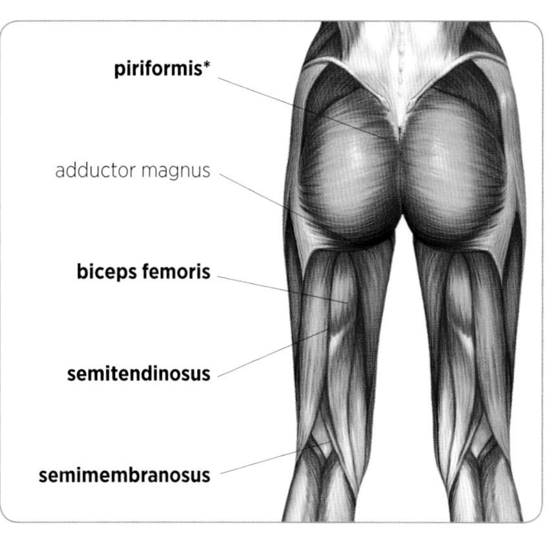

Annotation Key

Bold text indicates target muscles
Light text indicates other working muscles
* indicates deep muscles

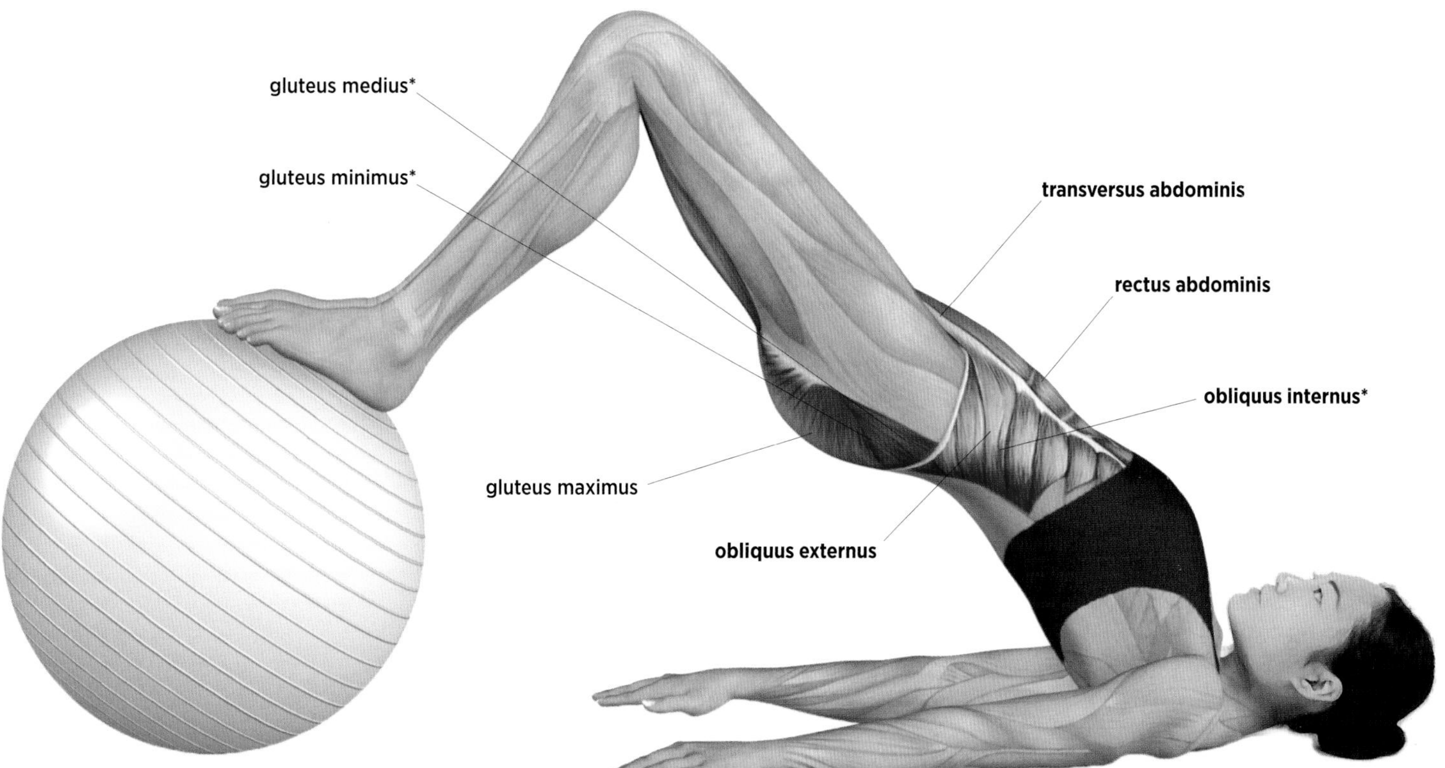

Hamstring Pull-In

The Hamstring Pull-In is a challenging exercise. The difficulty lies in controlling the range of motion of the foam roller. Master the move, however, and you will give your hamstrings and glutes a great workout, increasing the strength and endurance in both. It also helps to strengthen your pelvic stabilizers.

HOW TO DO IT

- Lie faceup with your knees bent and a roller under your feet.
- Bridge up, lifting your hips so that they align with your shoulders in a neutral position.
- Squeezing your glutes, pull your calves in and out as you roll the roller under your feet. Repeat for the recommended repetitions.

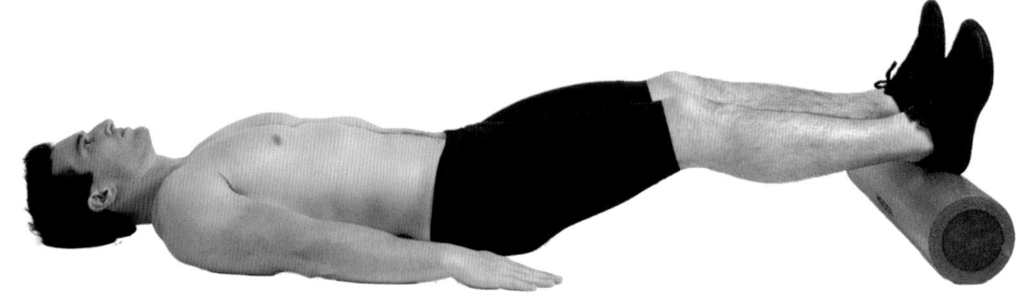

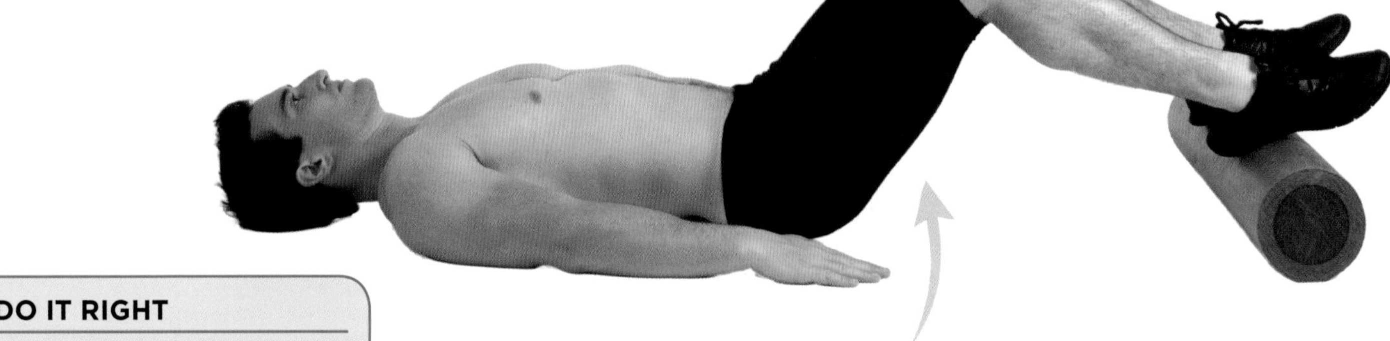

DO IT RIGHT

- Keep your shoulders relaxed.
- Align your body from shoulder to knee.
- Avoid allowing your hips and lower back to drop.
- Avoid arching your back.

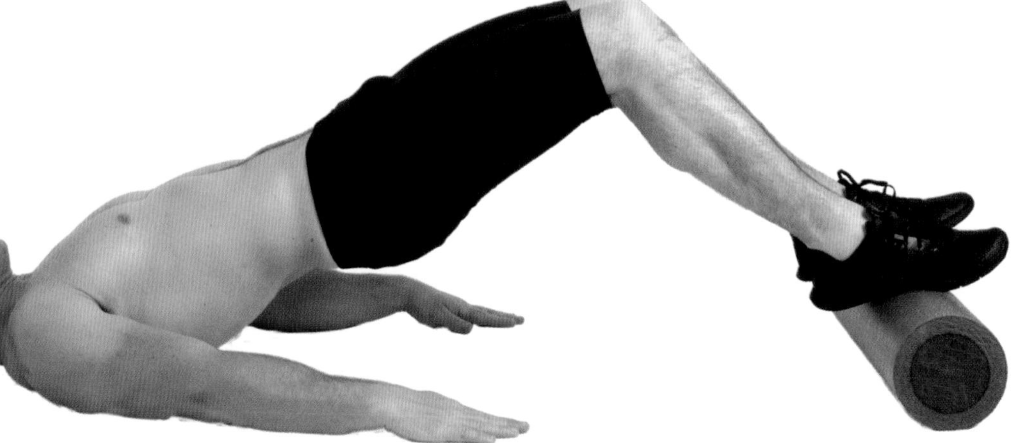

FACT FILE

TARGETS
- Hamstrings
- Glutes
- Pelvic stabilizers

EQUIPMENT
- Foam roller

BENEFITS
- Strengthens hamstrings, glutes, and pelvic stabilizers
- Increases lower-body endurance

CAUTIONS
- Hamstring injury
- Lower-back pain
- Ankle pain
- Neck issues

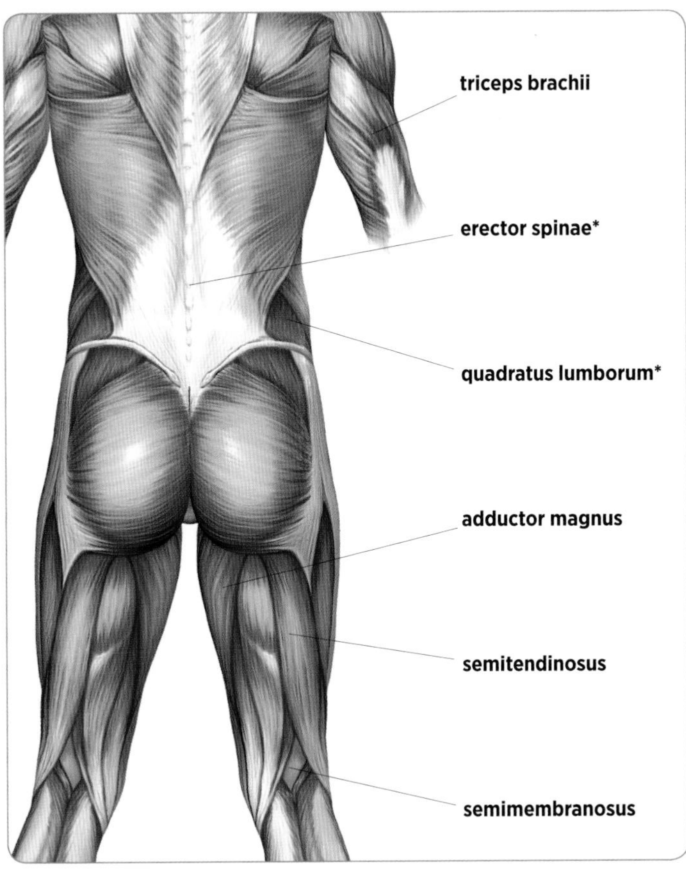

Annotation Key

Bold text indicates target muscles
Light text indicates other working muscles
* indicates deep muscles

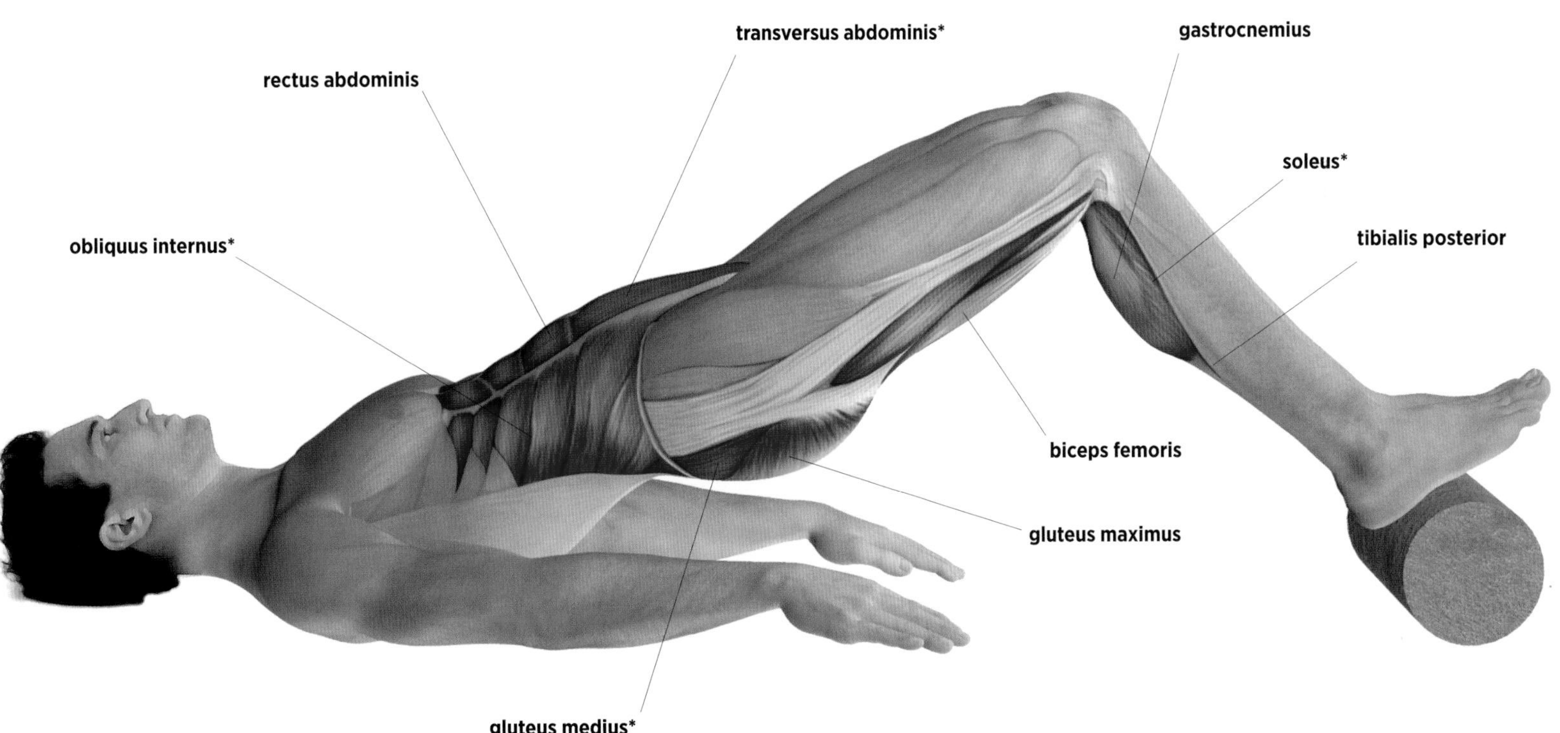

Reach-and-Twist Walking Lunge

The Reach-and-Twist Walking Lunge does a lot of work, building both lower-body and core strength. The deep lunge combined with the torso rotation engages the quads, glutes, and core while improving balance.

HOW TO DO IT

- Stand with feet hip-width apart and holding a medicine ball in both hands in front of your chest.
- Lunge your left foot forward, bending both knees and lowering your entire body into the lunge. At the same time, raise the medicine ball over your right shoulder.
- In a single motion, rise up to stand, bring the ball back to center, and then perform the lunge and reach in the other direction.
- Continue to lunge and move the ball from side to side as you walk forward. Repeat for the recommended repetitions, time, or distance.

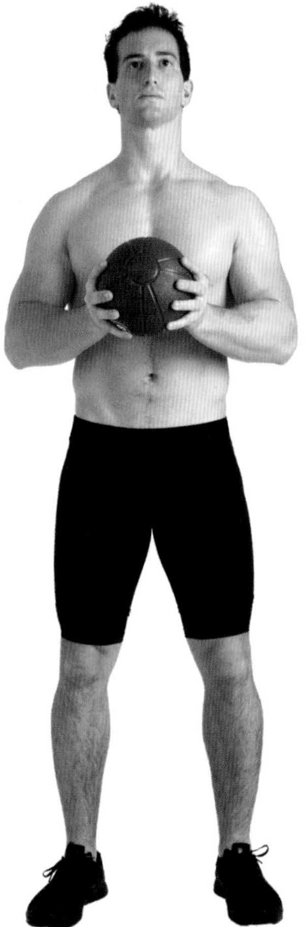

DO IT RIGHT

- Keep your torso facing forward.
- Keep your abdominals contracted and tight.
- Move smoothly and with control; avoid rushing through the exercise.
- Keep the weight of the ball balanced between both hands.
- Avoid hunching your shoulders.
- Avoid arching your back.
- Avoid turning your neck in either direction.
- Avoid letting your abdominals bulge outward.

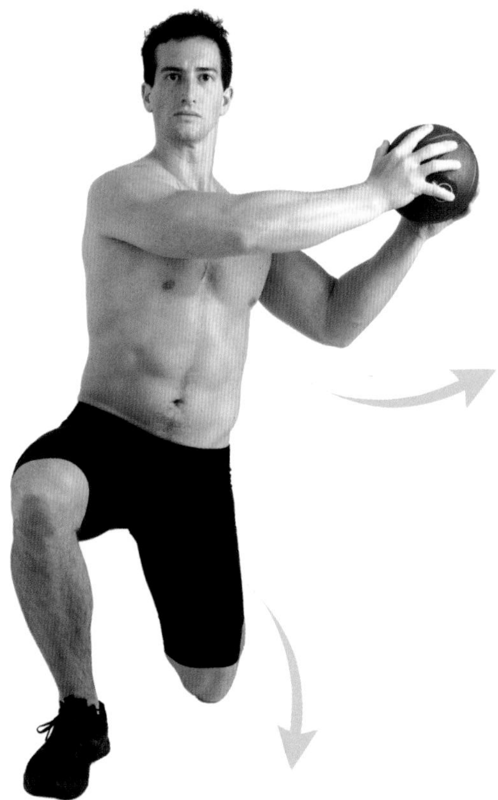

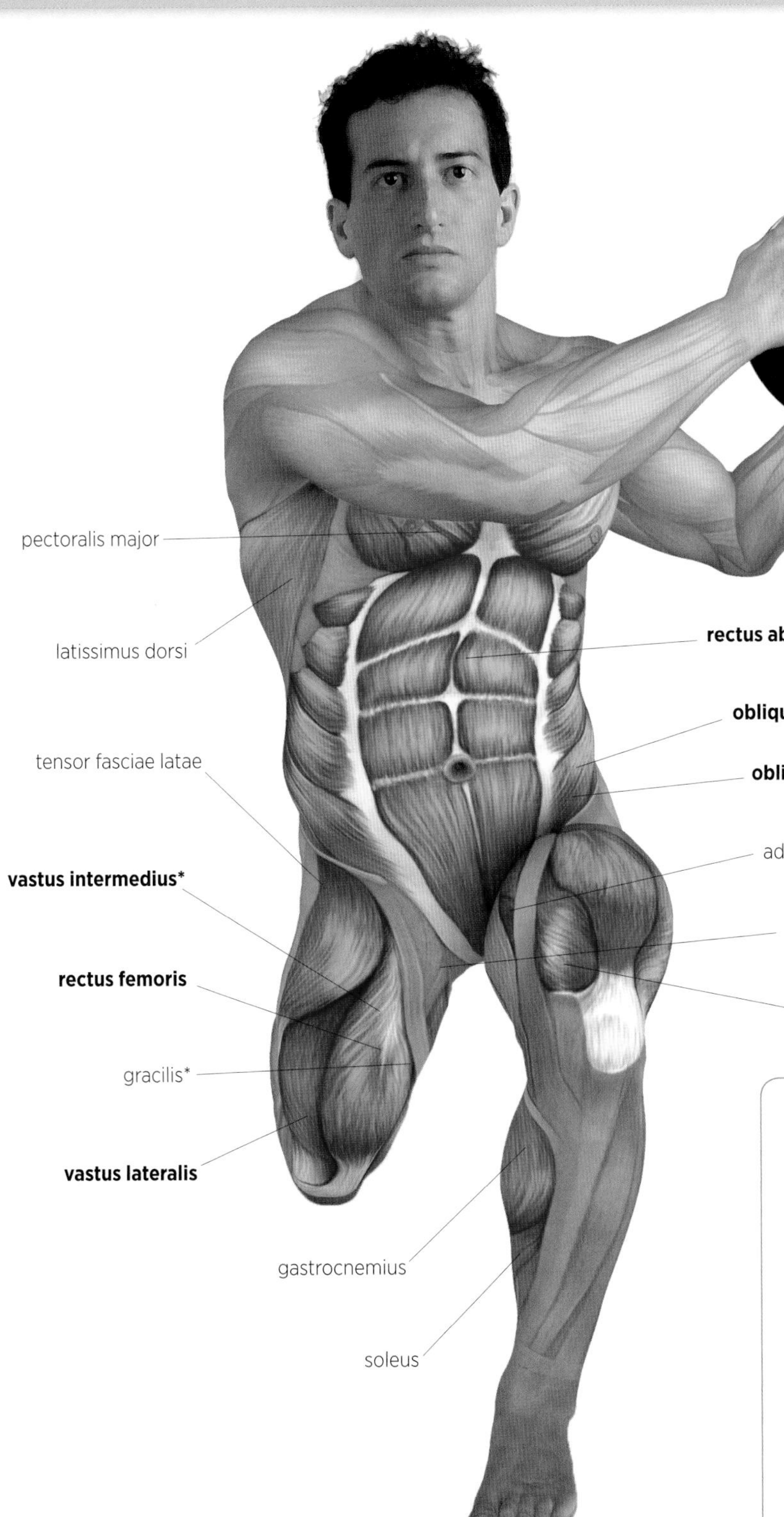

FACT FILE

TARGETS
- Quadriceps
- Hip flexors
- Hamstrings
- Abdominals
- Glutes

EQUIPMENT
- Medicine ball

BENEFITS
- Improves endurance and coordination
- Strengthens lower body and core

CAUTIONS
- Shoulder issues
- Knee issues

Annotation Key

Bold text indicates target muscles
Light text indicates other working muscles
* indicates deep muscles

Front Rack Barbell Lunge

The high demand of the Front Rack Barbell Lunge will have you on your knees. This exercise offers all the benefits of a basic lunge and then adds a resistance load that will force you to use your back, core, glutes, and quads more than ever before.

HOW TO DO IT

- Stand with your feet hip-width apart, the barbell in the front rack position, placed on your shoulders, with your hands grasping the bar just outside shoulder-width apart, and your elbows pointing forward and up.
- Keeping your core engaged, step your right foot forward to perform a lunge, bending both knees and dropping your left knee toward the floor.
- To return to the starting position, press through your glutes and legs and extend your knees to power off your right leg until both legs are straight before bringing your feet together.
- Repeat on the opposite side. Continue alternating sides for the recommended repetitions.

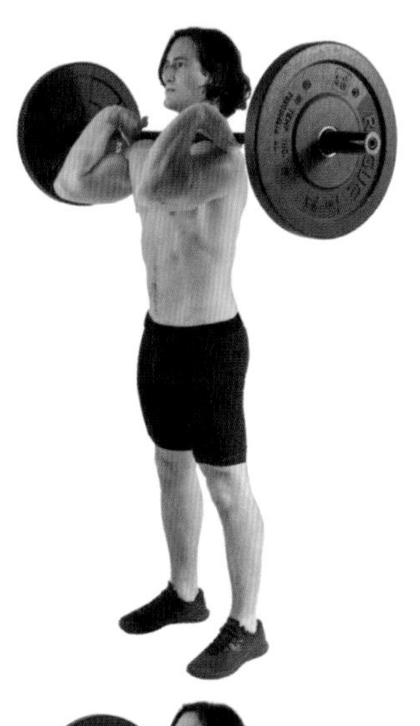

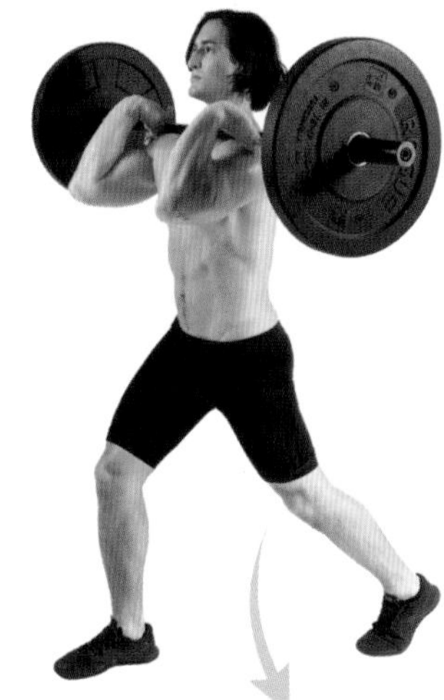

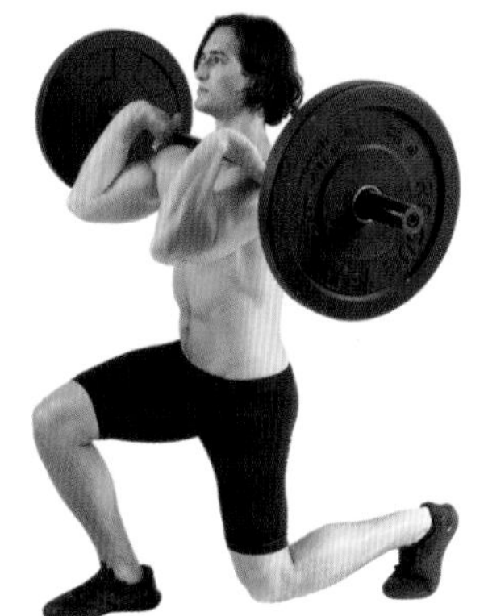

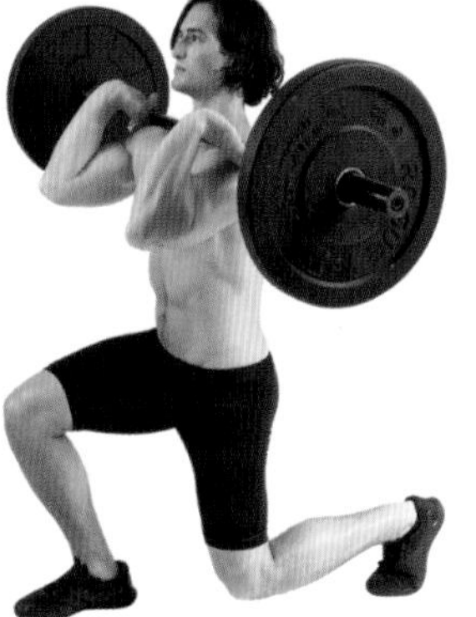

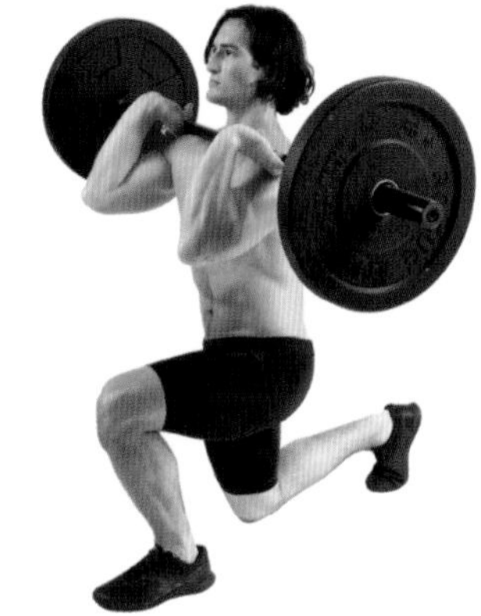

DO IT RIGHT

- Keep your back straight.
- Keep your elbows pointing forward and up.
- Track your knees over your toes.

Annotation Key
Bold text indicates target muscles
Light text indicates other working muscles
* indicates deep muscles

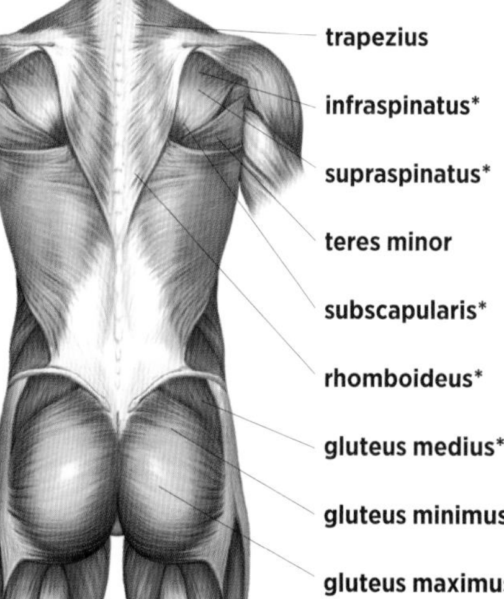

rectus abdominis
obliquus internus*
obliquus externus
transversus abdominis*
vastus intermedius*
rectus femoris
vastus lateralis
vastus medialis

FACT FILE

TARGETS
- Quadriceps
- Glutes
- Back
- Abdominals

EQUIPMENT
- Barbell

BENEFITS
- Strengthens and tones legs, back, and abdominals
- Improves balance

CAUTIONS
- Knee issues
- Shoulder/rotator cuff issues
- Wrist issues

Overhead Squat

The Overhead Squat, although focused on the lower extremities, works just about all of your body. This exercise will build strength from the bottom up, requiring a fair amount of mobility, strength, and stability in both your upper and lower body, as well as your core.

FACT FILE

TARGETS
- Quadriceps
- Glutes
- Triceps
- Deltoids
- Abdominals
- Back

EQUIPMENT
- Barbell

BENEFITS
- Strengthens and tones legs, abdominals, back, chest, and arms
- Improves coordination

CAUTIONS
- Shoulder/ rotator cuff issues
- Knee issues
- Back issues
- Wrist issues

HOW TO DO IT

- Stand with your feet hip-width apart, holding a barbell with an overhand grip, your hands placed wider than shoulder-width apart close to the weight plates. Keeping your arms straight and your core engaged, press the bar overhead. This is your starting position.

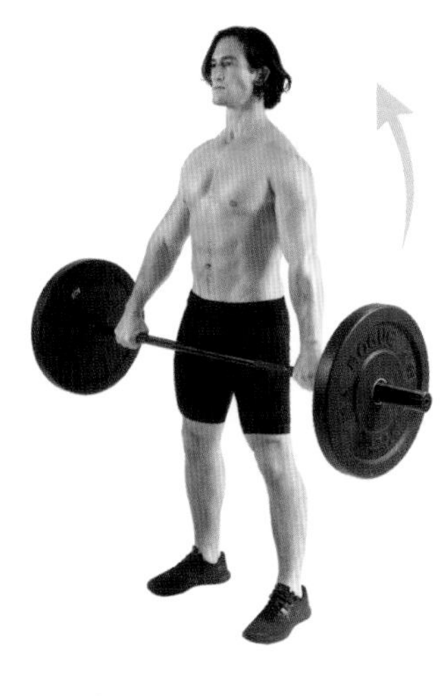

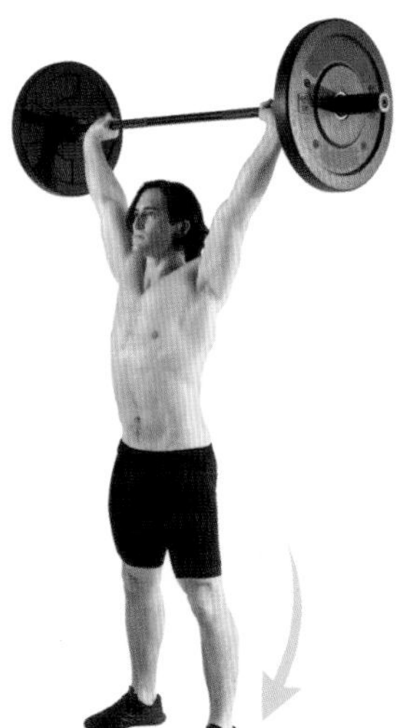

- Keeping your torso as upright as possible and the bar pressed overhead, drop down into a squat, shifting your hips backward, bending at the hips, knees, and ankles, until the tops of your thighs are parallel to the floor.

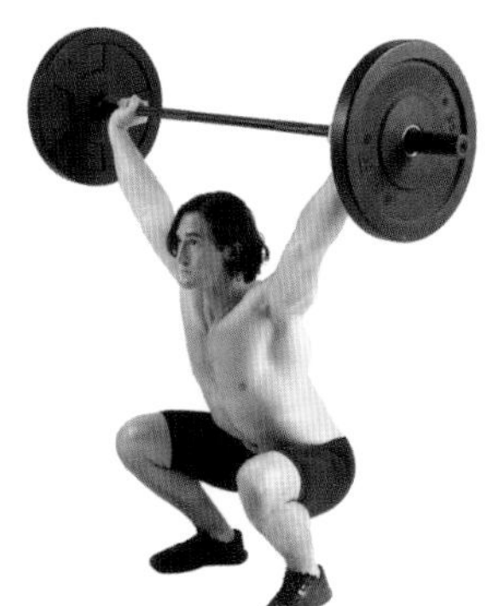

- To return to the starting position, extend your hips and legs, powering through your heels, until both legs are straight. Repeat for the recommended repetitions.

DO IT RIGHT

- Keep your back in a neutral position.
- Keep weight shifted back and through your heels.
- Avoid excessive trunk or shoulder movement.
- Avoid using a heavier weight than you can safely handle.

Annotation Key

Bold text indicates target muscles

Light text indicates other working muscles

* indicates deep muscles

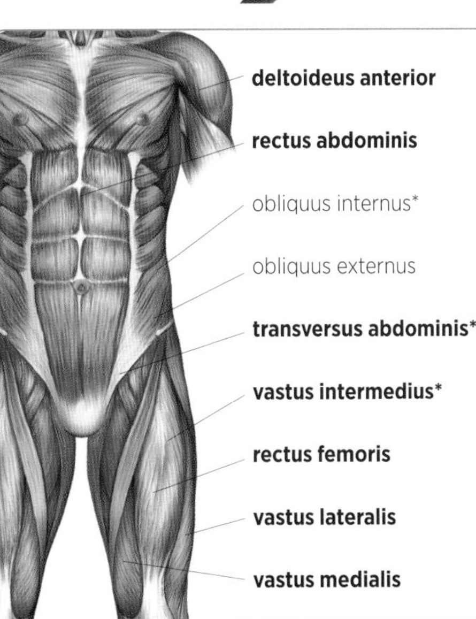

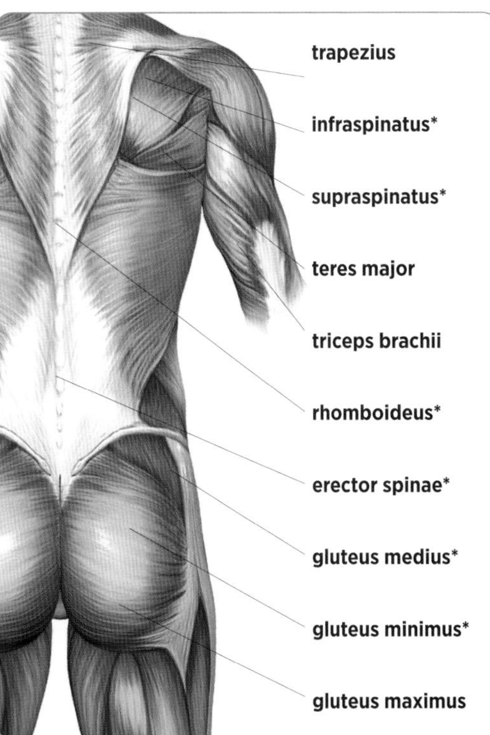

Jump Rope

Channel your inner child and perform this school-yard favorite. Jump Rope, also called Skip Rope, is a great cardio and strength exercise. This calorie burner works mainly on your calf muscles, while strengthening your bones and improving your balance and coordination. Perform as a rest between other exercise sets to recover your heart rate.

HOW TO DO IT

- Stand holding a rope in your hands, letting it hang behind your feet.

- Swing the rope around your body and jump over it. Keep your arms as straight as you can during the movement, and land with both feet together on the floor. Perform for recommended time.

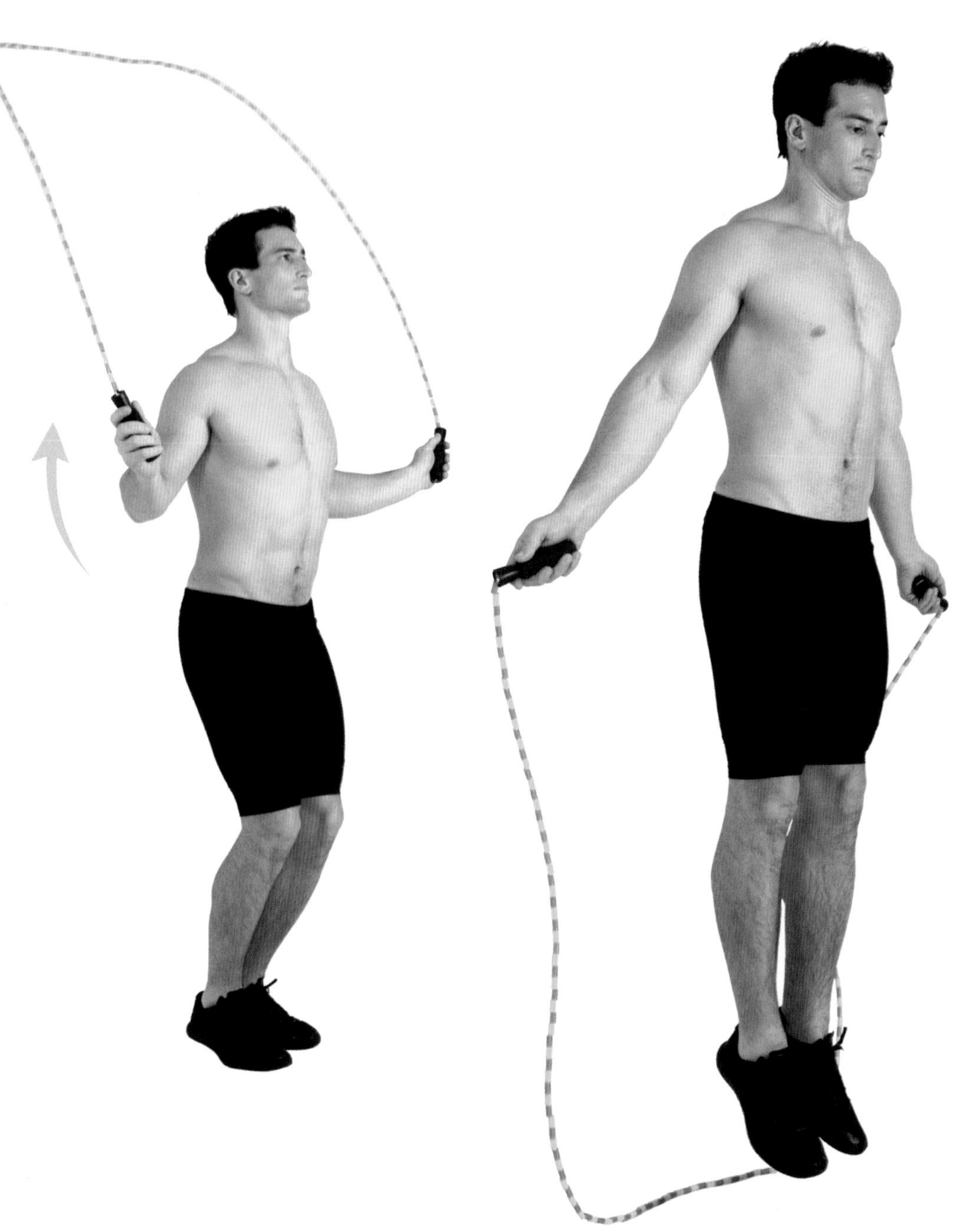

DO IT RIGHT

- Land on the balls of your feet; landing flat on your feet can compact your knees.
- To check if a jump rope is the right size for you, place one foot in the center of the rope, and then lift the handles—they shouldn't reach higher than your armpits.

FACT FILE

TARGETS
- Legs
- Arms
- Shoulders
- Back

EQUIPMENT
- Jump rope

BENEFITS
- Strengthens arms, legs, back, and shoulders
- Increases cardiovascular endurance

CAUTIONS
- Wrist issues
- Ankle issues
- Knee pain

deltoideus posterior
triceps brachii

biceps femoris
semitendinosus
semimembranosus

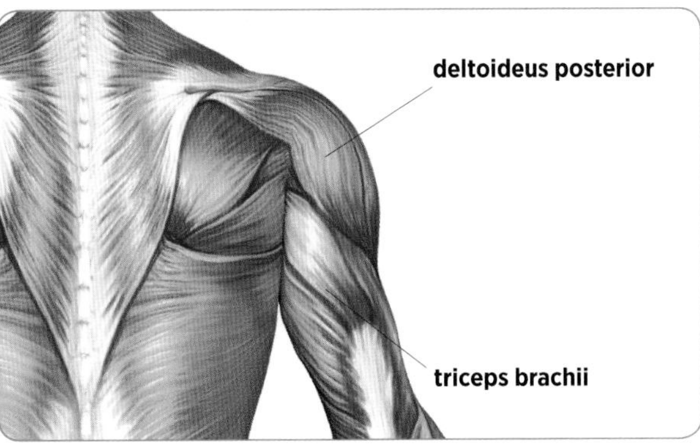

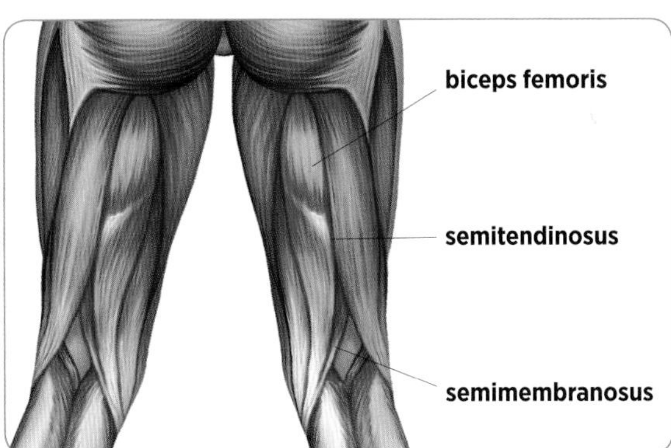

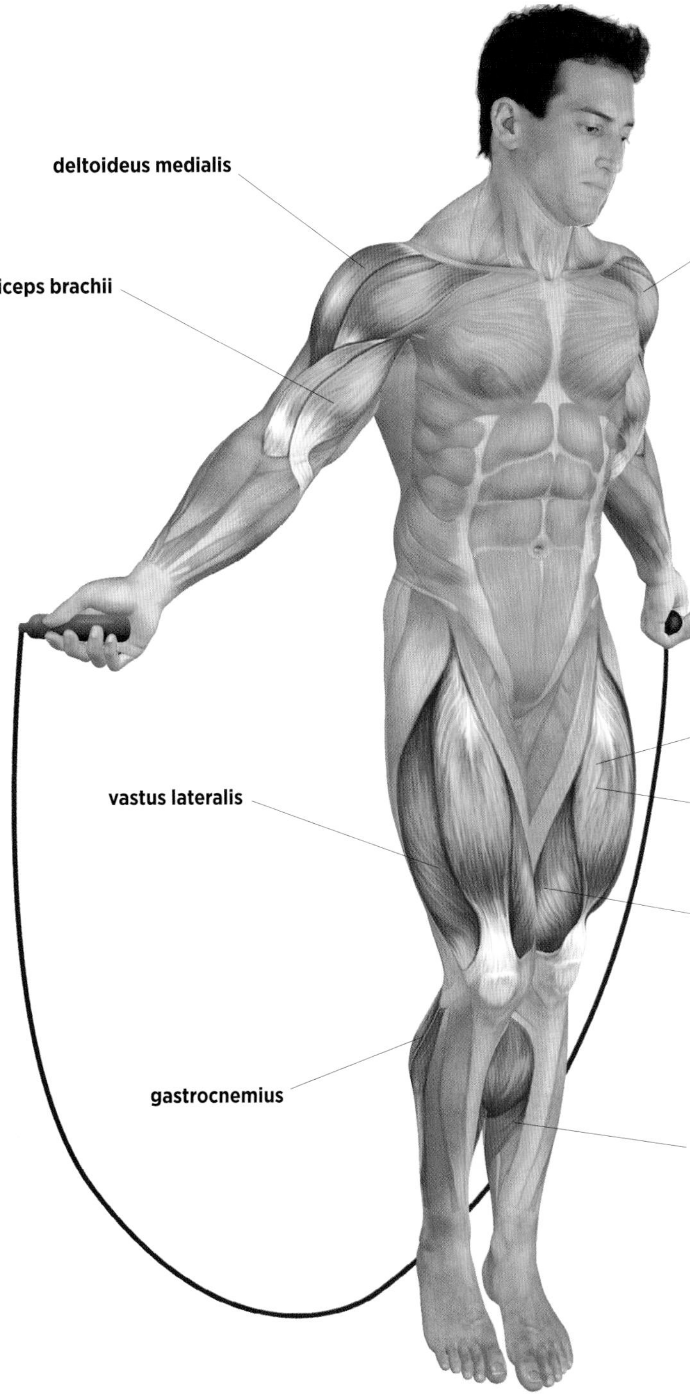

deltoideus medialis
deltoideus anterior
biceps brachii
vastus intermedius*
vastus lateralis
rectus femoris
vastus medialis
gastrocnemius
soleus

Annotation Key

Bold text indicates target muscles

Light text indicates other working muscles

* indicates deep muscles

Chin-Up with Hanging Leg Raise

The Chin-Up with Hanging Leg Raise adds a core challenge to the basic back and arm exercise. The leg-raising motion will work like a midair crunch to target your abdominals and lower body.

HOW TO DO IT

- Standing in front of a pull-up bar, either reach up or step on a stool. Place your hands shoulder-width apart, and take a close, underhand grip on the bar, and hang until your arms are straight.
- Pull yourself up until your chin is as close to the bar as possible.
- With your abdominal muscles strongly engaged, raise your knees. Hold for as long as possible.
- Slowly straighten your legs, and then, with control, lower yourself to the hanging position. Repeat for the recommended repetitions.

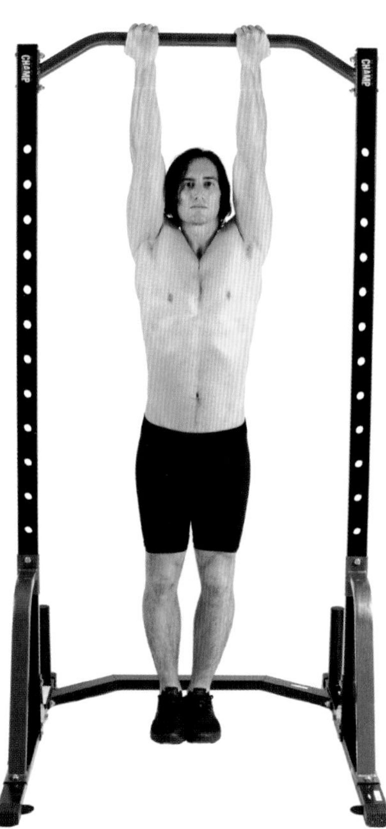

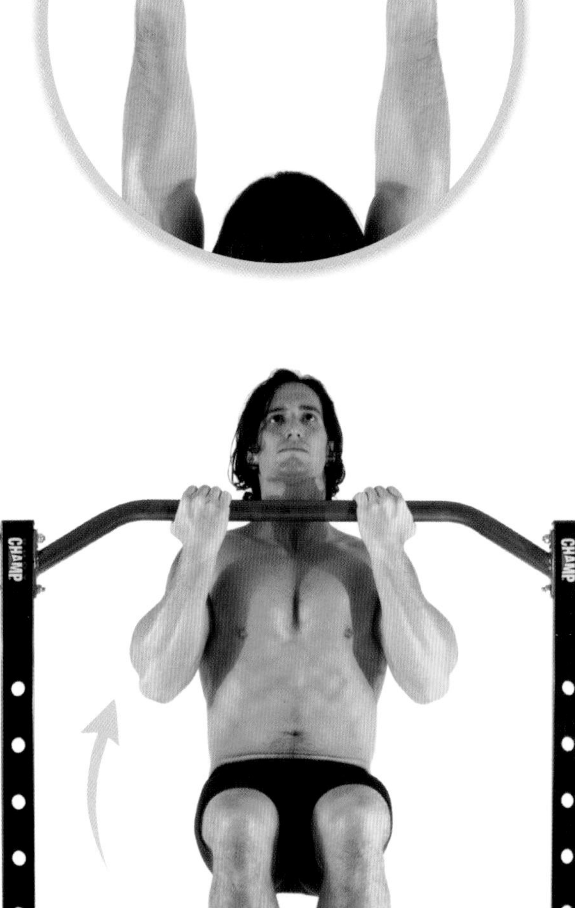

DO IT RIGHT

- Keep your feet together as you raise your knees.
- Move smoothly and with control; avoid rushing through the exercise.
- Keep your abdominals contracted and tight.
- Avoid arching your back.
- Avoid tensing your neck.
- Avoid suddenly dropping your body weight.
- Avoid swinging, or kipping, your body—a swinging movement can injure your rotator cuffs.

FACT FILE

TARGETS
- Back
- Arms
- Abdominals

EQUIPMENT
- Pull-up bar

BENEFITS
- Strengthens back, arms, and core

CAUTIONS
- Shoulder issues
- Wrist issues

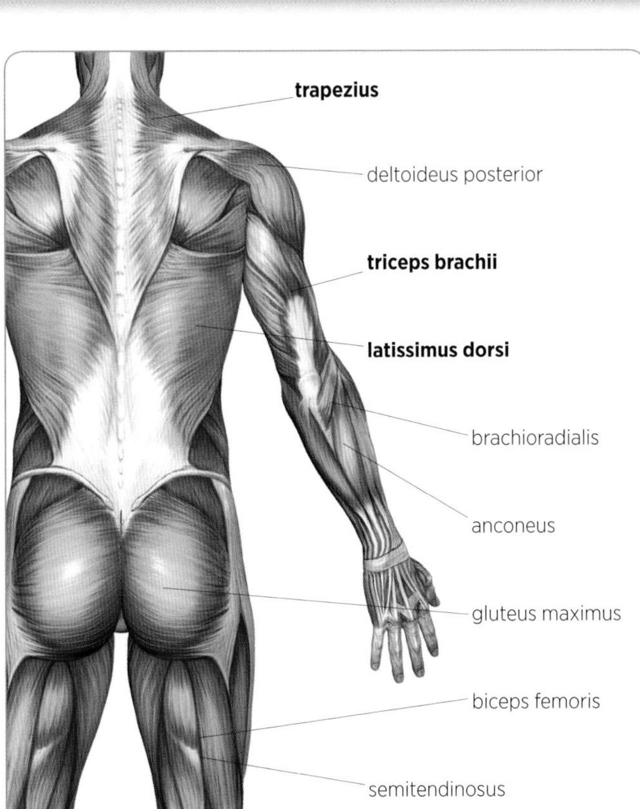

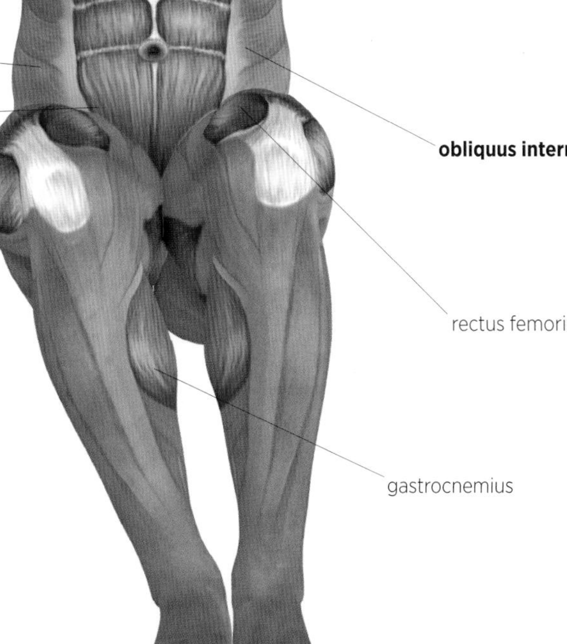

Annotation Key

Bold text indicates target muscles

Light text indicates other working muscles

* indicates deep muscles

Barbell Power Clean and Jerk

The Barbell Power Clean and Jerk boosts power and mass in your shoulders and upper back, especially your deltoids and triceps. It also benefits the thighs, glutes, hamstrings, and core.

HOW TO DO IT

- Stand with your feet parallel and shoulder-width apart, your knees slightly bent and your midfoot under the bar. Squat down to grab the bar with your hands about shoulder-width apart in a wide overhand grip.
- As you return to a standing position, flip the barbell until it is nearly touching your upper chest. This is a Power Clean.
- Push the barbell overhead with your arms fully extended to complete the clean and jerk movement.
- Lower the barbell back to your upper chest, reverse the flip, and return it to the floor. Repeat for the recommended repetitions.

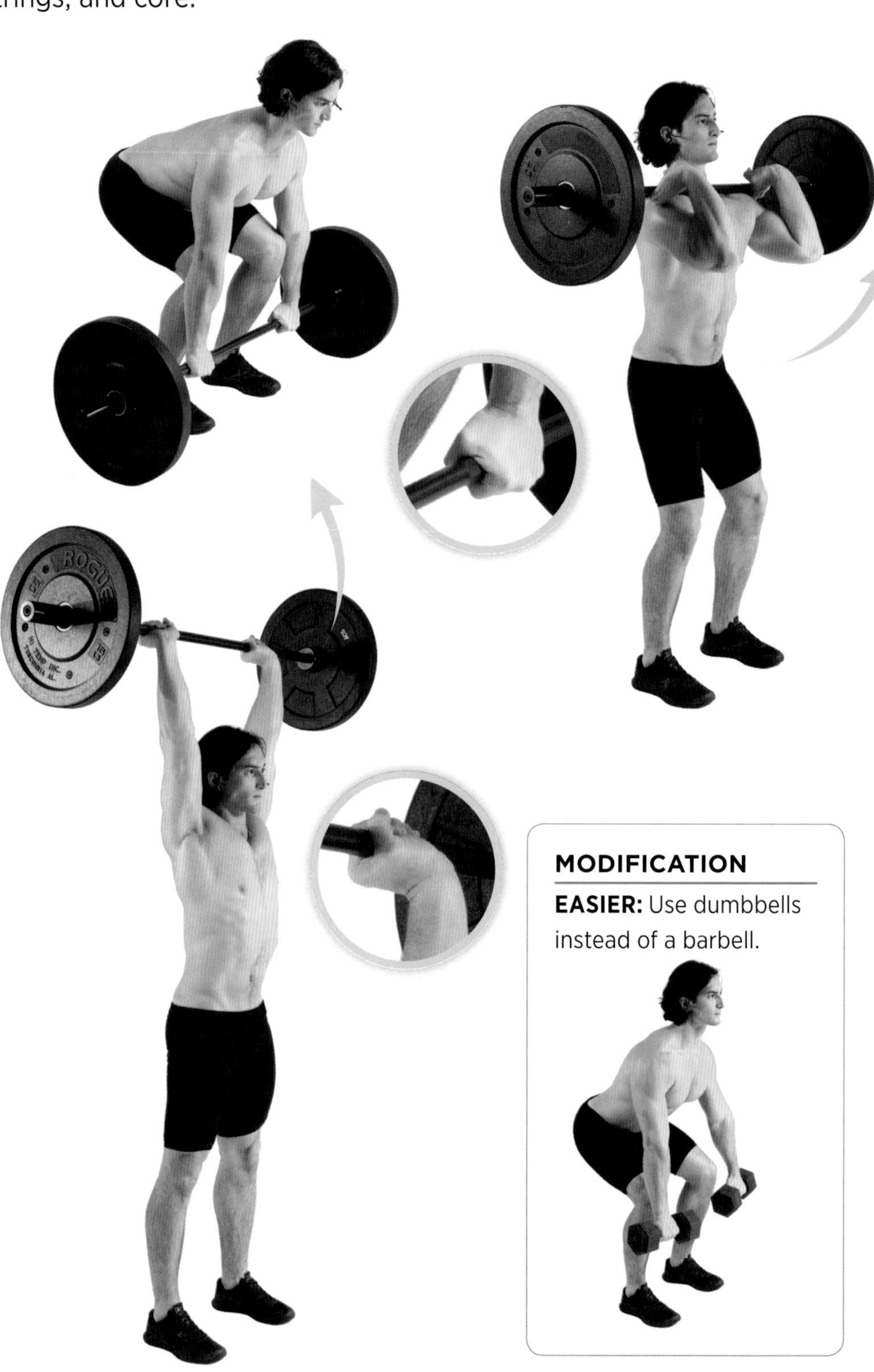

DO IT RIGHT

- Use your legs to help with the start of the movement.
- Avoid overarching your back.
- Avoid using a heavier weight than you can safely handle.

MODIFICATION

EASIER: Use dumbbells instead of a barbell.

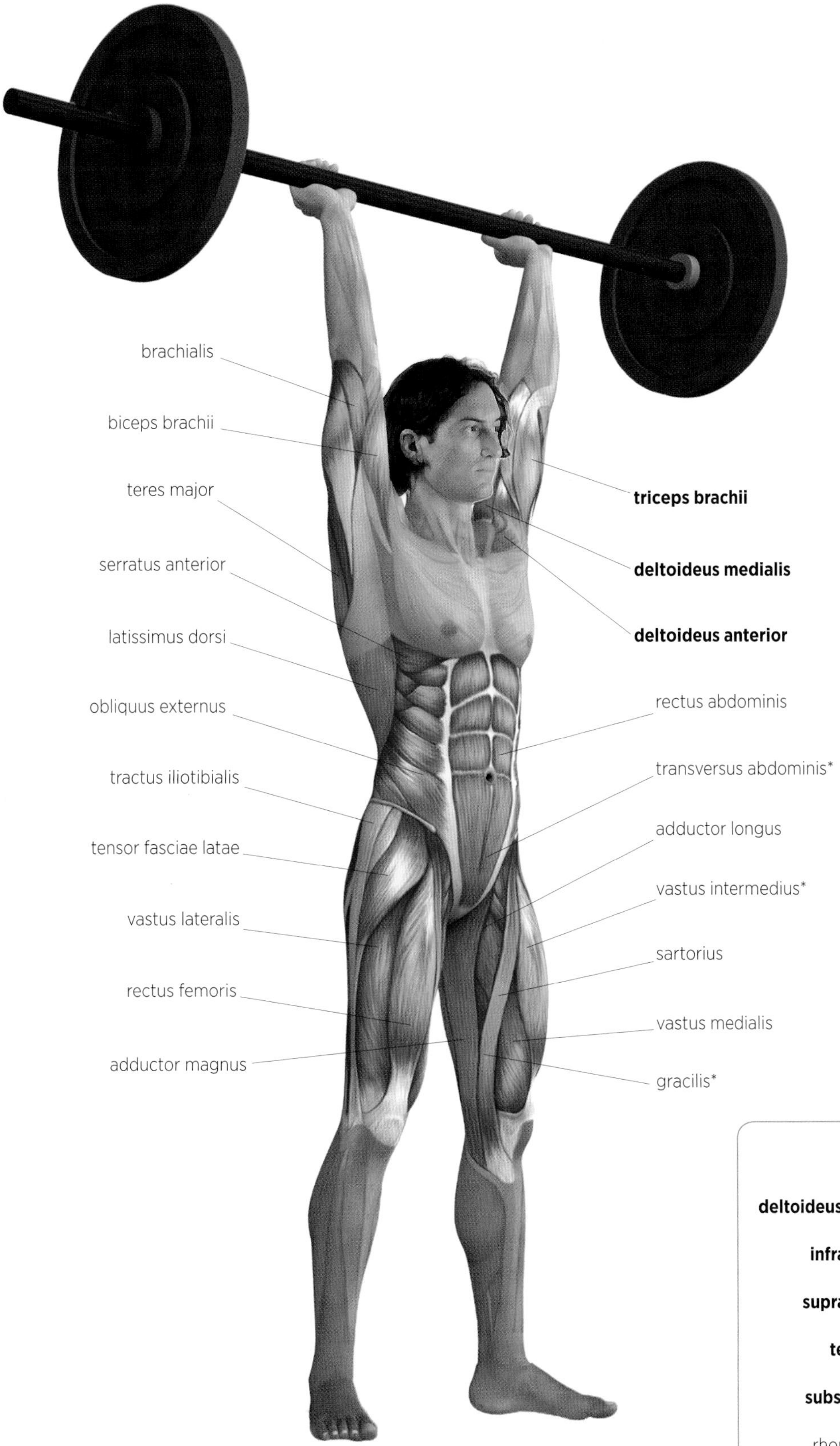

brachialis
biceps brachii
teres major
serratus anterior
latissimus dorsi
obliquus externus
tractus iliotibialis
tensor fasciae latae
vastus lateralis
rectus femoris
adductor magnus
triceps brachii
deltoideus medialis
deltoideus anterior
rectus abdominis
transversus abdominis*
adductor longus
vastus intermedius*
sartorius
vastus medialis
gracilis*

FACT FILE

TARGETS
- Deltoids
- Upper back
- Triceps
- Thighs
- Glutes
- Hamstrings
- Core

EQUIPMENT
- Barbell

BENEFITS
- Strengthens upper and lower body
- Increases shoulder and upper-body power and mass

CAUTIONS
- Shoulder issues
- Wrist issues

Annotation Key

Bold text indicates target muscles
Light text indicates other working muscles
* indicates deep muscles

trapezius
deltoideus posterior
infraspinatus*
supraspinatus*
teres minor
subscapularis*
rhomboideus*
erector spinae*

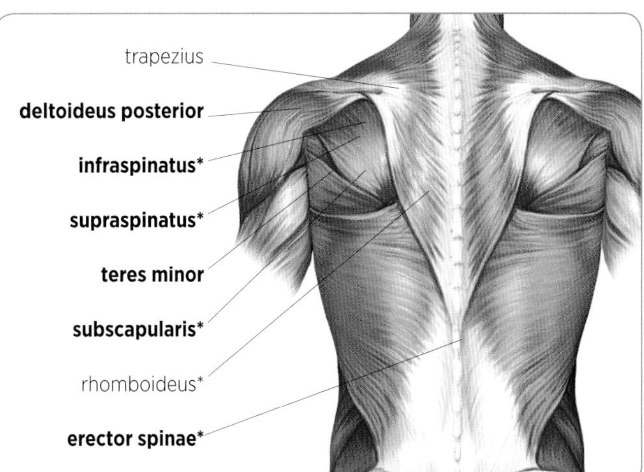

Barbell Squat Snatch

The Barbell Squat Snatch targets your deltoids and glutes, while also working your upper back, core, and hamstrings. Perform to increase power and mass in your shoulders and thighs.

HOW TO DO IT

- Stand with your feet parallel and shoulder-width apart, your knees slightly bent and your midfoot under the bar. Squat down to grab the bar with a wide overhand grip. Make sure your knees are close to the bar.
- As you return to a standing position, flip the barbell directly overhead with your arms locked.
- Carefully lower the barbell to the floor. Repeat for the recommended repetitions.

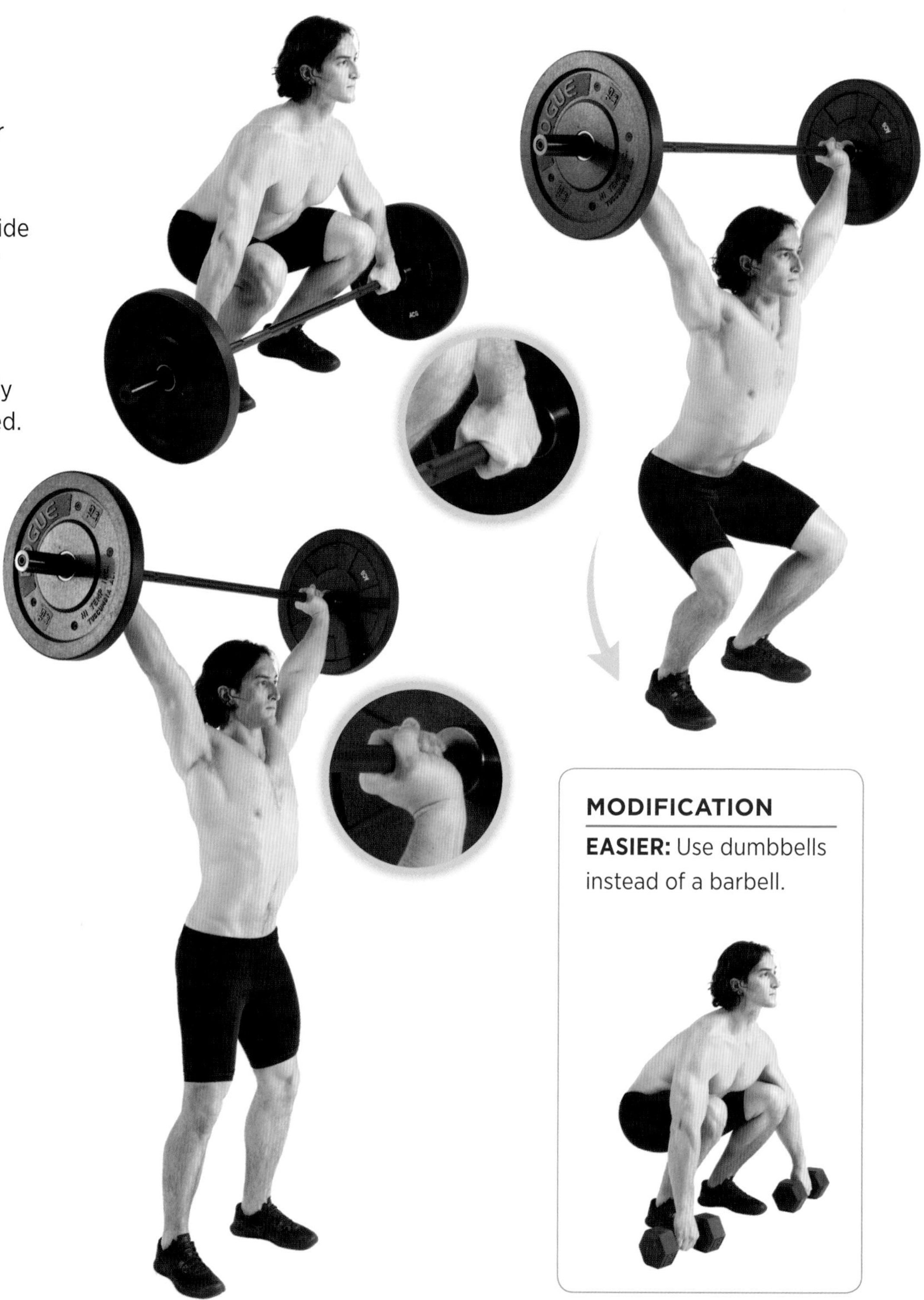

DO IT RIGHT

- Use your legs to help with the start of the movement.
- Avoid overarching your back.
- Avoid using a heavier weight than you can safely handle.

MODIFICATION

EASIER: Use dumbbells instead of a barbell.

FACT FILE

TARGETS
- Deltoids
- Thighs
- Glutes
- Upper back
- Core
- Triceps
- Hamstrings

EQUIPMENT
- Barbell

BENEFITS
- Strengthens upper and lower body
- Increases shoulder and thigh power and mass

CAUTIONS
- Shoulder issues
- Wrist issues

Annotation Key
Bold text indicates target muscles
Light text indicates other working muscles
* indicates deep muscles

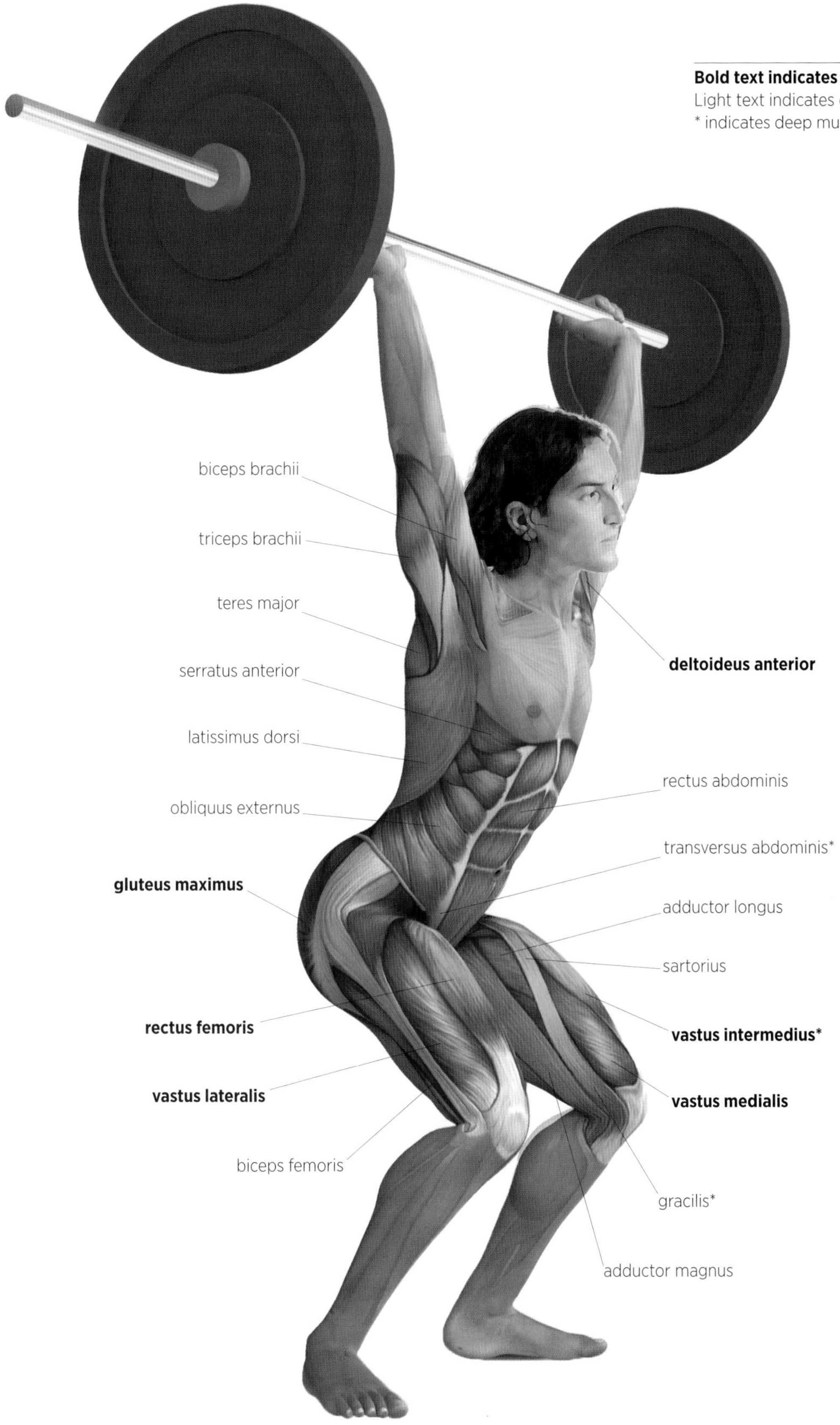

biceps brachii
triceps brachii
teres major
serratus anterior
latissimus dorsi
obliquus externus
gluteus maximus
rectus femoris
vastus lateralis
biceps femoris
deltoideus anterior
rectus abdominis
transversus abdominis*
adductor longus
sartorius
vastus intermedius*
vastus medialis
gracilis*
adductor magnus

trapezius
deltoideus medialis
deltoideus posterior
erector spinae*
multifidus spinae*
gluteus medius*
gluteus minimus*

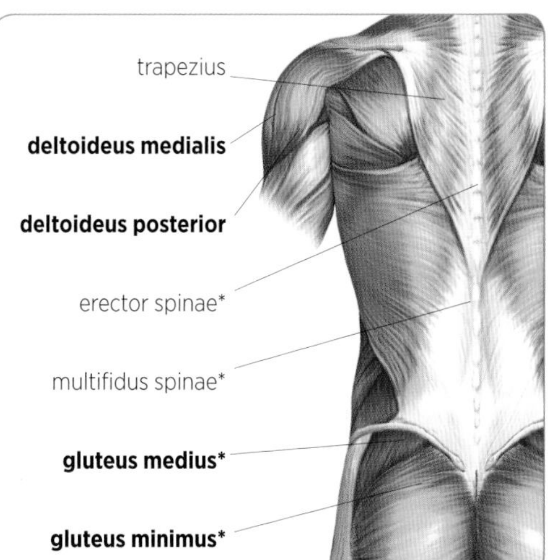

Medicine Ball Slam

The Medicine Ball Slam is all about explosive power. It is a simple move, but offers numerous benefits. It is a calorie burner that builds abdominal, shoulder, leg, glute, and back strength, while improving cardiovascular endurance and hand-eye coordination.

HOW TO DO IT

- Stand with your feet shoulder-width apart with your knees slightly bent, holding a medicine ball above your head with your arms outstretched.
- Keeping your back straight, lean forward at the waist and forcefully throw the ball onto the floor.
- Pick up the ball, and repeat for the recommended repetitions.

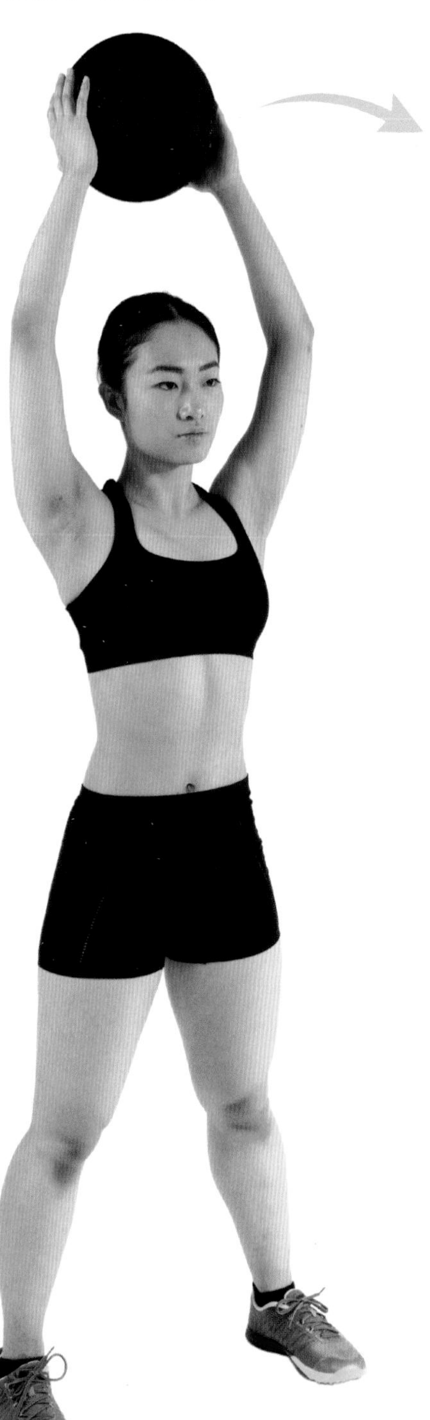

DO IT RIGHT

- Keep your torso straight on throughout the movement.
- Keep your heels on the floor.
- Keep your abdominals contracted and tight.
- Avoid rounding your back.
- Aggressively perform the slam.

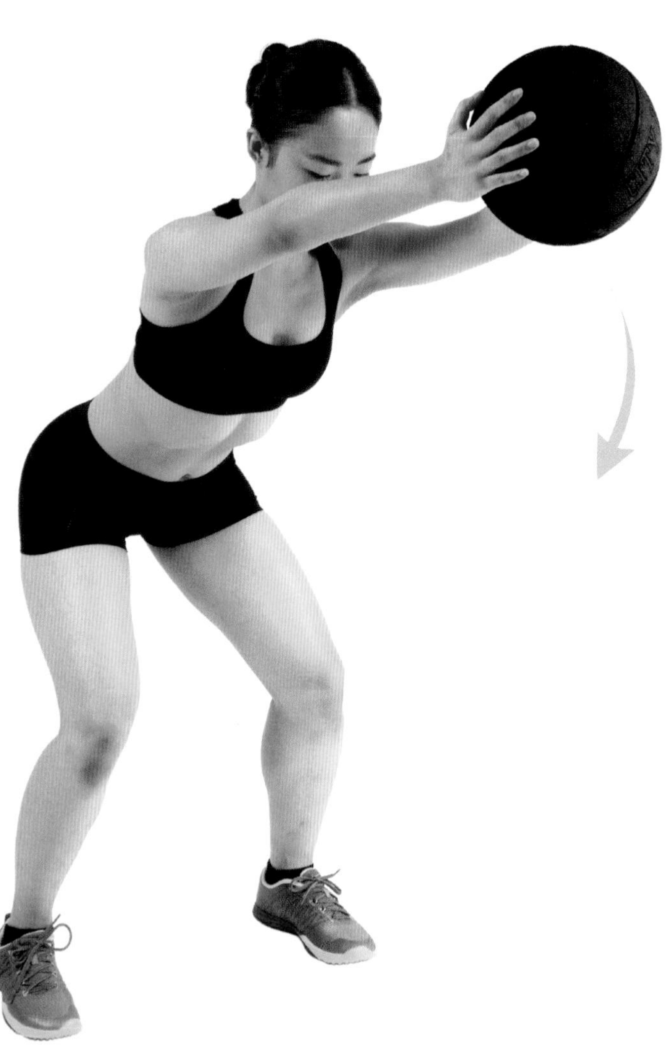

Annotation Key

Bold text indicates target muscles
Light text indicates other working muscles
* indicates deep muscles

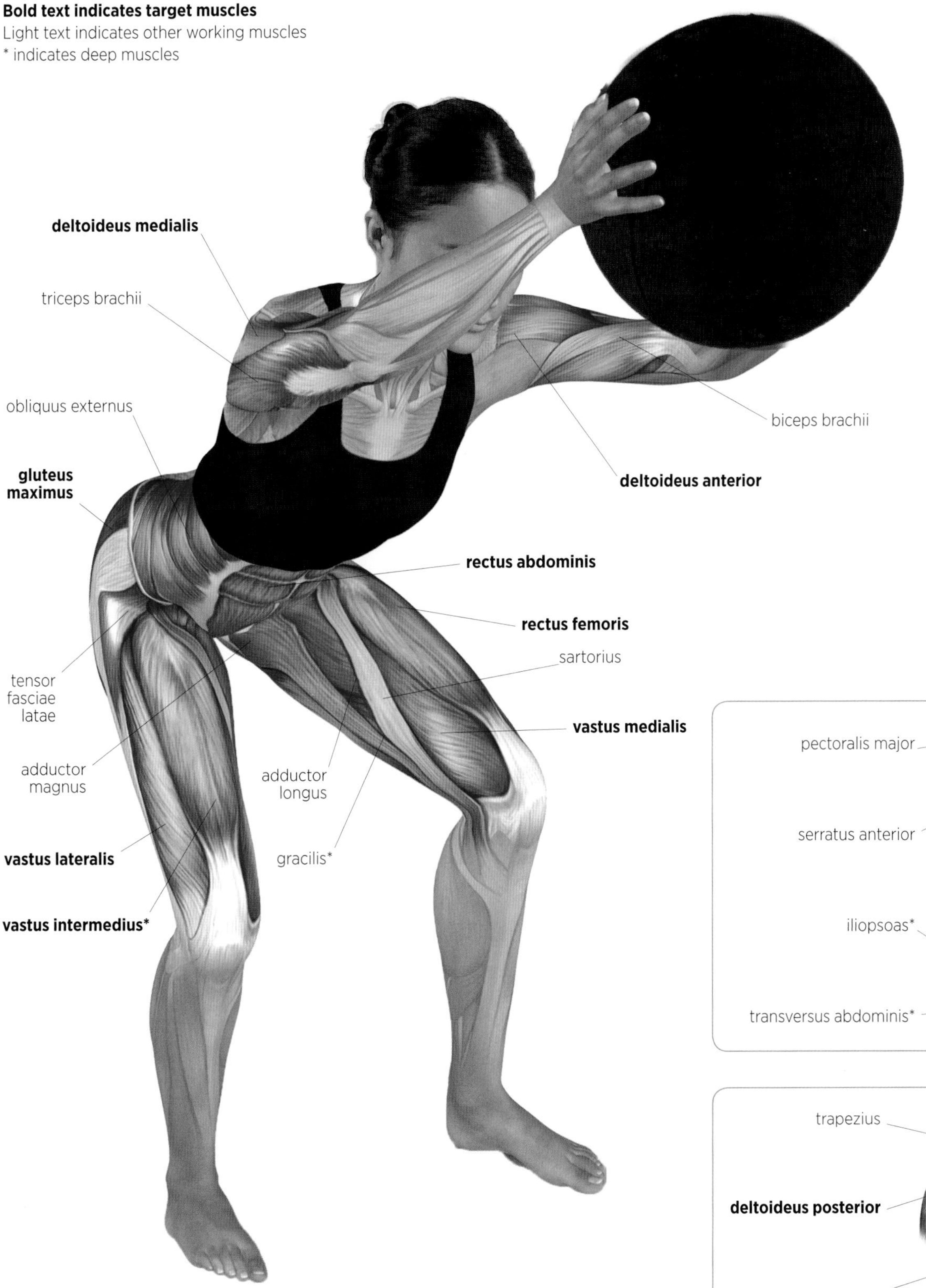

deltoideus medialis
triceps brachii
obliquus externus
gluteus maximus
tensor fasciae latae
adductor magnus
vastus lateralis
vastus intermedius*
biceps brachii
deltoideus anterior
rectus abdominis
rectus femoris
sartorius
vastus medialis
adductor longus
gracilis*

pectoralis major
serratus anterior
iliopsoas*
transversus abdominis*

trapezius
deltoideus posterior
rhomboideus*
latissimus dorsi

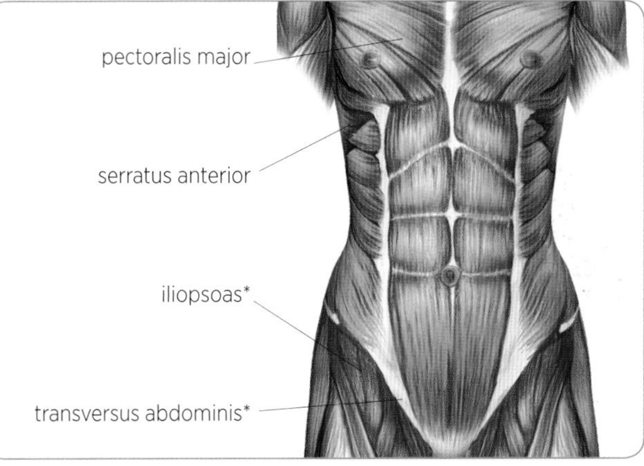

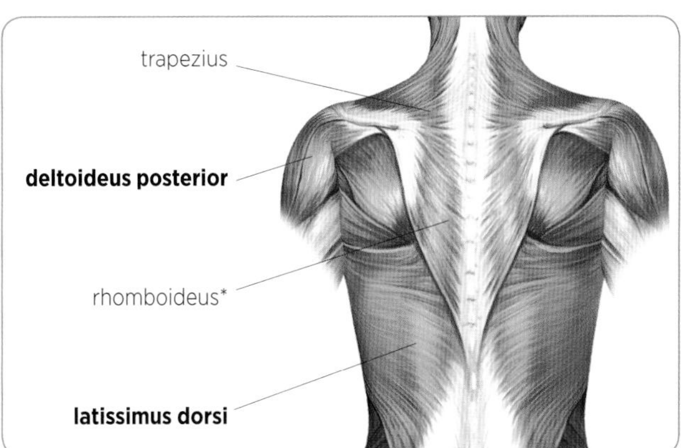

FACT FILE

TARGETS
- Abdominals
- Shoulders
- Legs
- Glutes
- Back

EQUIPMENT
- Medicine ball

BENEFITS
- Strengthens core, back, glutes, and arms
- Improves coordination
- Increases cardiovascular endurance
- Develops power, speed, and strength

CAUTIONS
- Shoulder issues
- Wrist issues

Wall Ball Shot

You will often see Wall Ball Shots listed as a component of grueling cross-training regimens. Try them for a sweat-producing, calorie-burning workout that targets your upper and lower body.

HOW TO DO IT

- Stand with your feet shoulder-width apart facing a wall and holding a large medicine ball in front of your chest.
- Pull your shoulders back and keep your chest up high as you descend into a squat, dropping as low as possible while keeping the medicine ball at your chest.
- As soon as you reach a full squat, drive through your heels to explosively rise up. At the same time, throw the ball up at the wall, aiming for a height of about 10 feet.
- Catch the ball on the rebound, squat again, and repeat for the recommended repetitions.

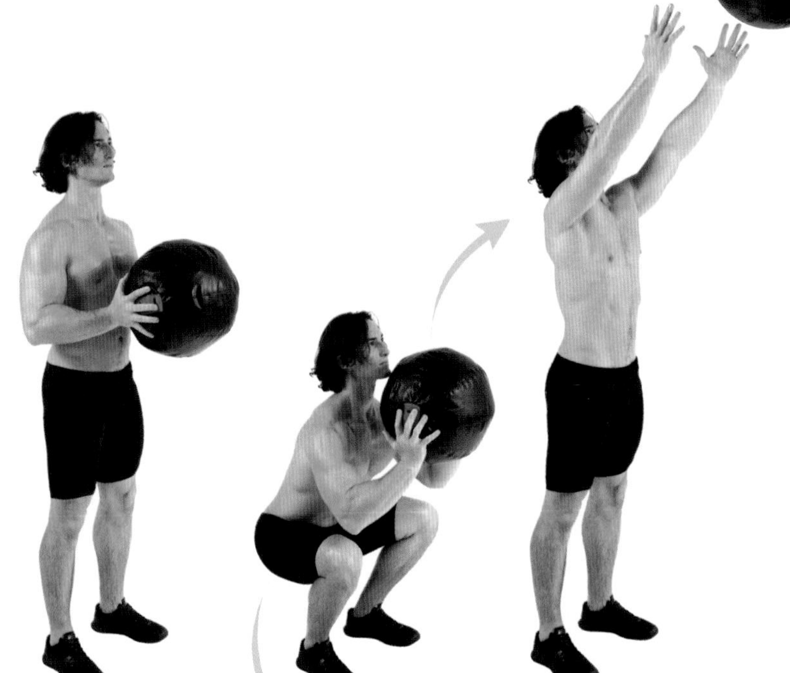

DO IT RIGHT

- Keep a proper distance from the wall to throw and catch efficiently.
- Drop as low as you can into the squat.
- Avoid holding your breath.

Annotation Key
Bold text indicates target muscles
Light text indicates other working muscles
* indicates deep muscles

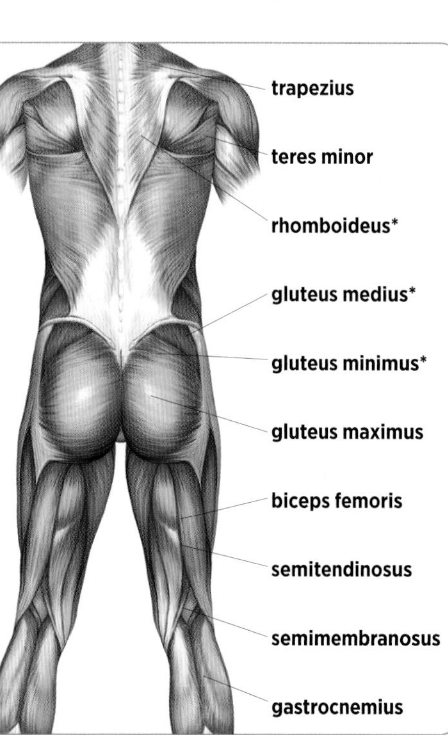

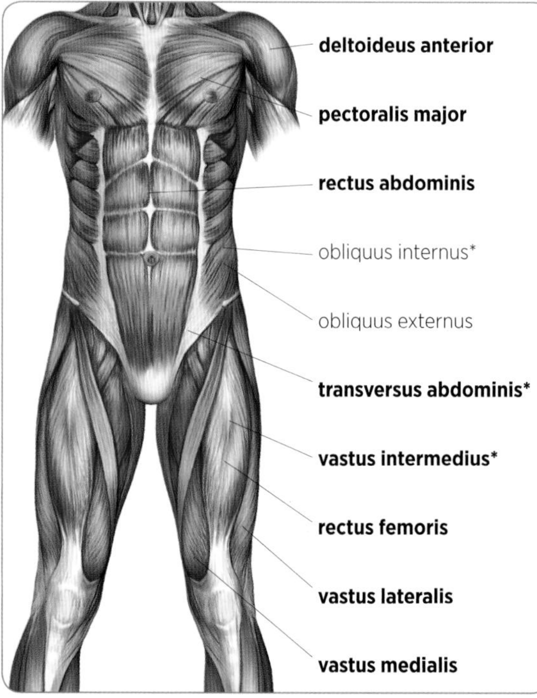

FACT FILE

TARGETS
- Chest
- Back
- Abdominals
- Arms
- Glutes
- Legs

EQUIPMENT
- Medicine ball

BENEFITS
- Strengthens entire body
- Increases endurance
- Increases overall power and explosiveness

CAUTIONS
- Knee issues
- Shoulder issues

Barbell Shoulder Press

Don't let its name fool you. The Barbell Shoulder Press is a multipurpose exercise that targets more than your shoulders. It will work your back, abdominals, and arms as it helps stabilize your core.

FACT FILE

TARGETS
- Shoulders
- Back
- Chest
- Abdominals
- Spine

EQUIPMENT
- Barbell

BENEFITS
- Strengthens shoulders and upper body
- Stabilizes core and lower back

CAUTIONS
- Shoulder issues
- Wrist issues

HOW TO DO IT

- Stand with your feet shoulder-width apart, grasping a barbell with your hands placed slightly wider than shoulder-width using an overhand grip. Position the bar near your upper chest.
- Press the bar upward until your arms are extended overhead.
- Lower the bar to your upper chest to return to the starting position. Repeat for the recommended repetitions.

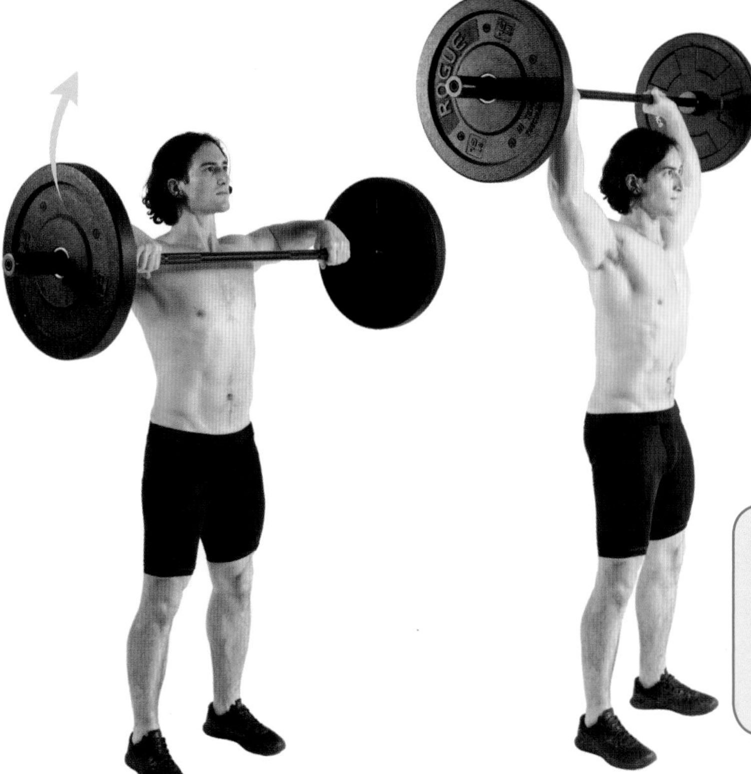

DO IT RIGHT
- Avoid arching your back.
- Avoid using a heavier weight than you can safely handle.

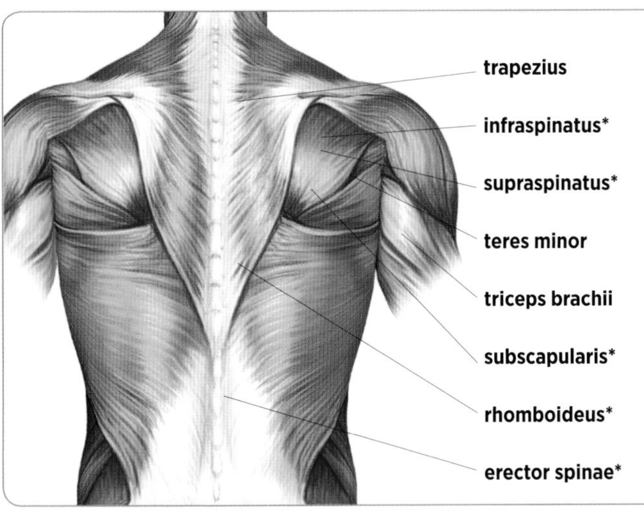

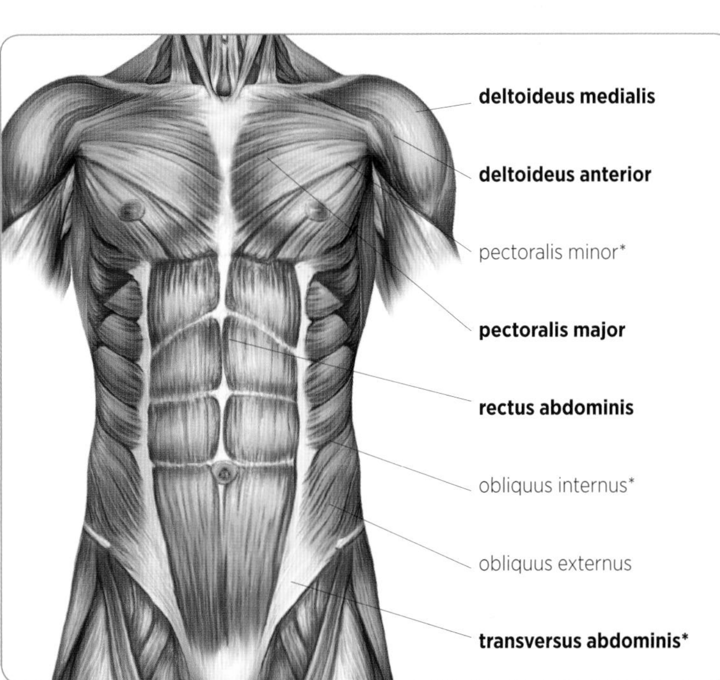

Annotation Key
Bold text indicates target muscles
Light text indicates other working muscles
* indicates deep muscles

Bear Complex

The Bear Complex is a total-body movement that leaves no muscle unscathed, requiring strength, perseverance, and will. This movement sequence is a combination of a variety of power and strength exercises; practice them individually before attempting this sequence.

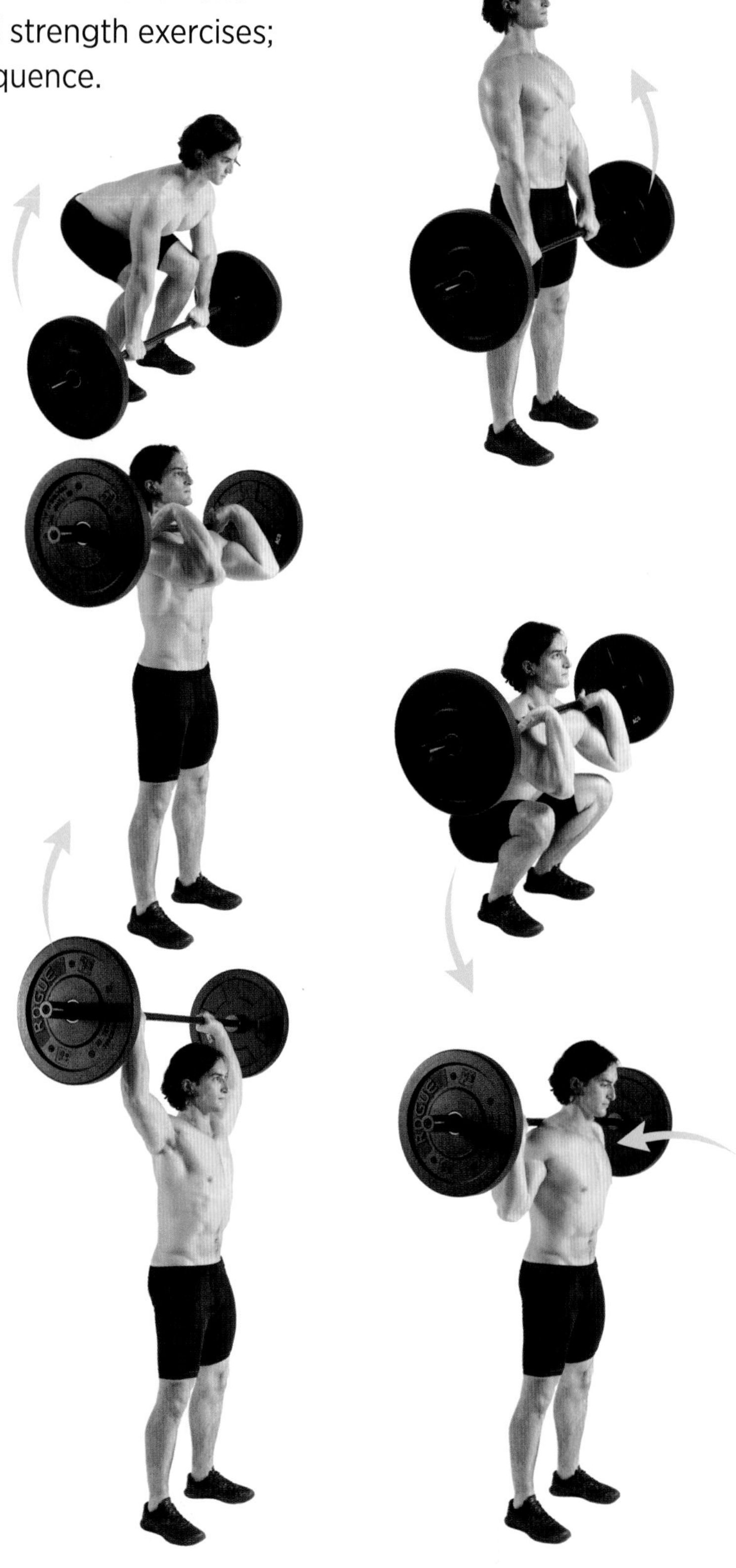

HOW TO DO IT

- Place a barbell at your feet, and stand with your feet shoulder-width apart. Squat down to grasp the weight with your hands positioned just outside shoulder-width apart with your palms facing inward.
- Perform a Barbell Deadlift (pages 240–241), lifting the bar up and away from the floor, powering through your heels until you are standing with your legs straight and the barbell lifted to thigh height.
- With an explosive motion, perform a Barbell Power Clean and Jerk (pages 314–315), shrugging your shoulders and drawing your elbows up to pull the bar to shoulder level. Catch the bar on your shoulders with your elbows pointed forward in the front rack position.
- Perform a squat while keeping your torso as upright as possible and the bar positioned on your shoulders in front of you. Power through your heels until your legs are straight, to return to a standing position.
- Perform a Barbell Shoulder Press (page 321), driving the barbell overhead until your arms are fully extended.
- Lower the weight behind your head until it rests on your shoulders and upper back.
- Perform a Barbell Squat (pages 298–299), while keeping your torso as upright as possible and the bar positioned on your upper back. Power through your heels until your legs are straight, to return to a standing position.
- Finally, perform another Barbell Shoulder Press.
- Lower the weight down until it rests on the floor in front you. Repeat all steps for the recommended repetitions.

FACT FILE

TARGETS
- Arms
- Shoulders
- Abdominals
- Back
- Legs
- Glutes

EQUIPMENT
- Barbell

BENEFITS
- Strengthens and tones entire body
- Promotes total-body functional movement
- Improves coordination
- Increases cardiovascular endurance

CAUTIONS
- Wrist issues
- Knee issues
- Back issues
- Shoulder issues

rectus abdominis
transversus abdominis*
obliquus externus
vastus medialis
obliquus internus*
sartorius
vastus intermedius*
adductor magnus
vastus lateralis
rectus femoris

DO IT RIGHT
- Keep your back in a neutral position.
- Avoid using a heavier weight than you can safely handle.
- Keep your core engaged.
- Find a steady, maintainable pace; this compound exercise requires high energy expenditure.

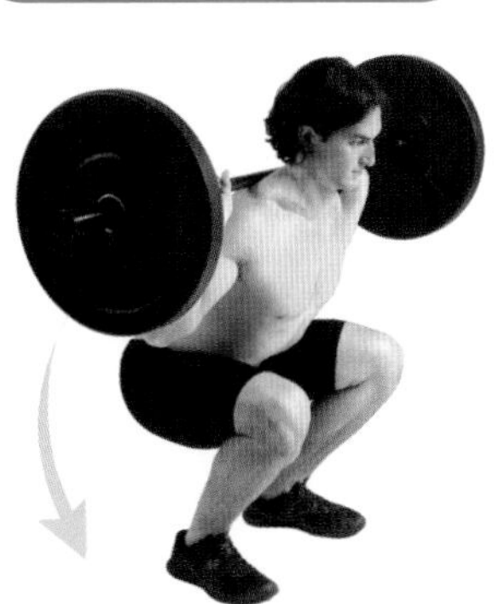

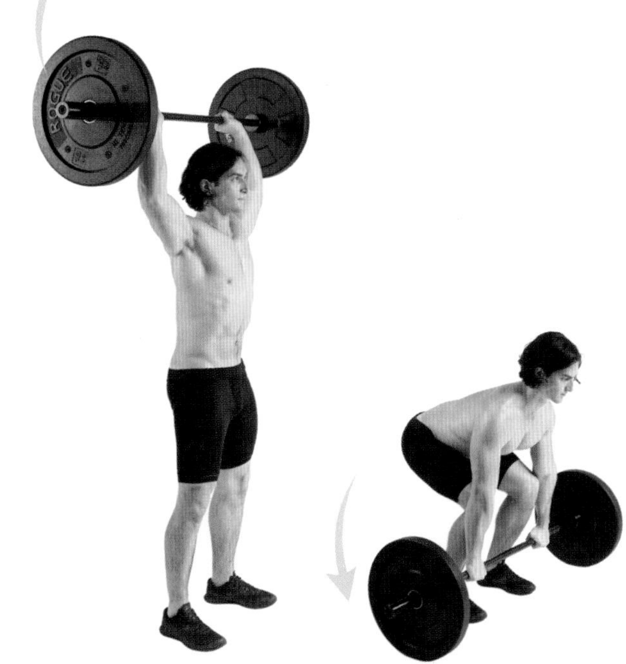

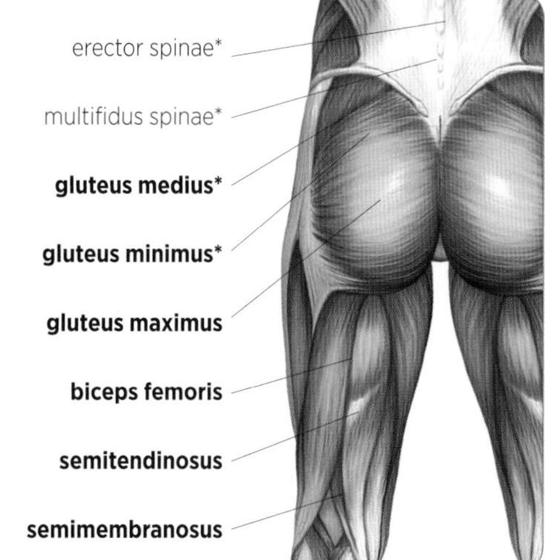

Annotation Key
Bold text indicates target muscles
Light text indicates other working muscles
* indicates deep muscles

CHAPTER FIVE

WORKOUT ROUTINES

Once you have gone through the exercises illustrated in this book, your next step is to put these moves together. The following routines are just samples of the many ways that you can combine exercises to create HIIT workouts. You'll find routines crafted for beginner, intermediate, and advanced practitioners, as well as a mix-and-match selection to inspire you to create your own routines geared to your individual objectives.

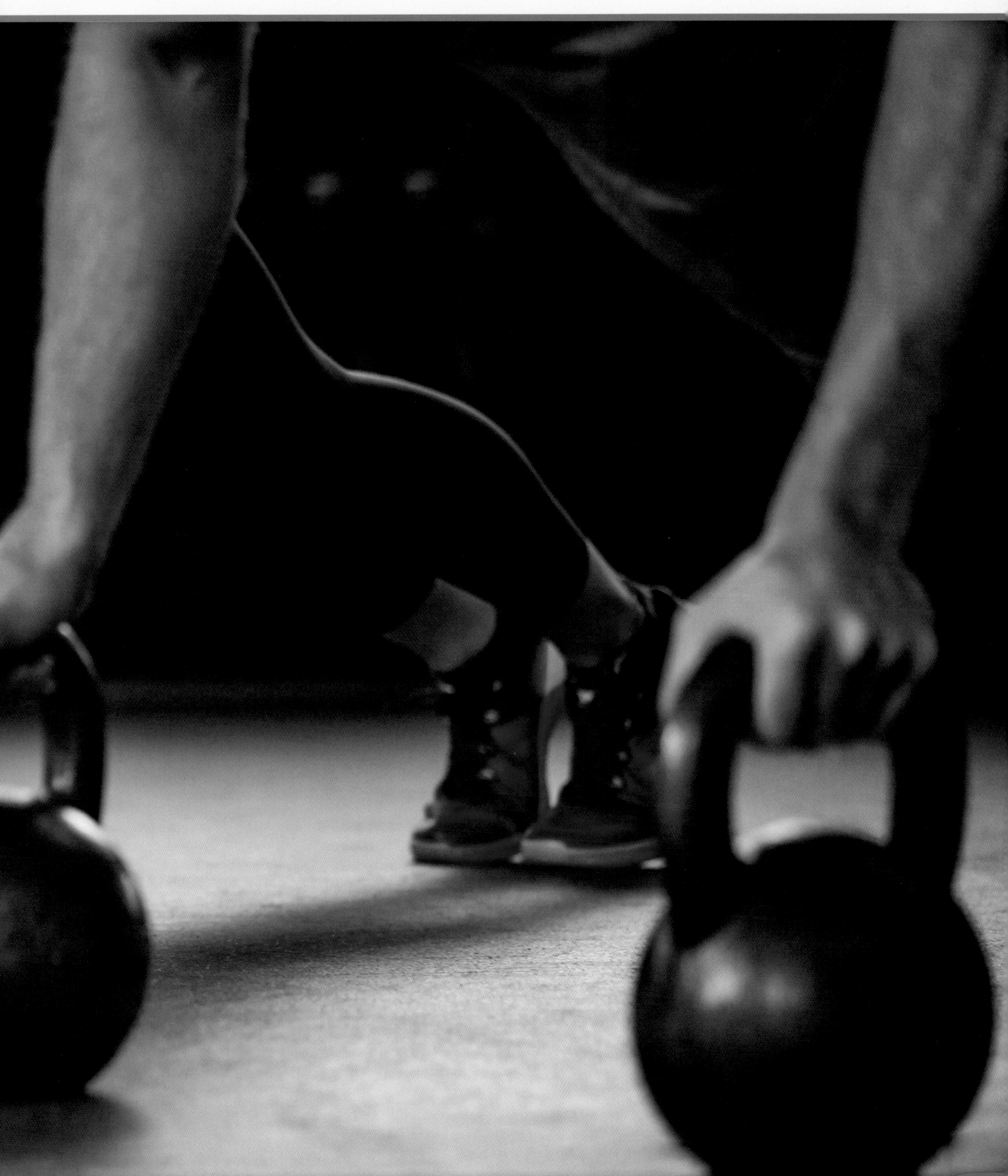

Before-and-After Routine

This routine, crafted for all levels of HIIT, takes you through movements that warm up your body and stretch your muscles to get you ready for any workout. Use them after to cooldown.

1 WARM-UP OBSTACLE COURSE

pages 32–33

- Perform for 60 seconds.
- Aim for as many repetitions as you can perform.

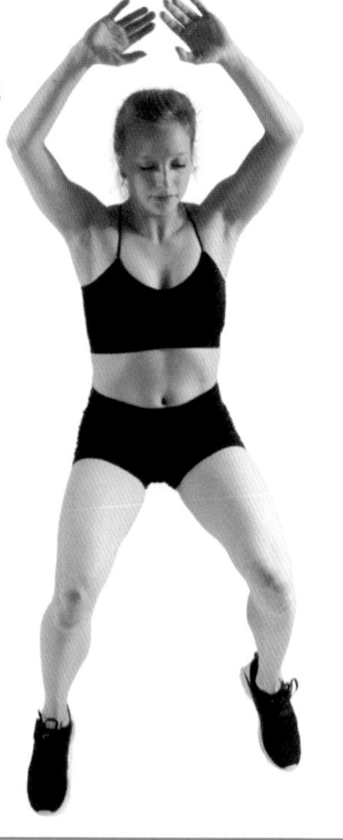

2 ADDUCTOR STRETCH

page 36

- Perform for 60 seconds.
- Aim for as many repetitions as you can perform.

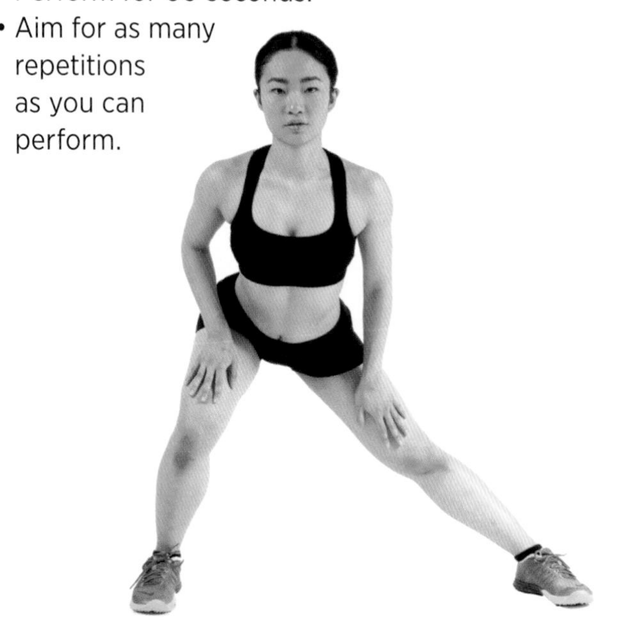

3 COBRA STRETCH

pages 40–41

- Perform for 60 seconds.
- Aim for as many repetitions as you can perform.

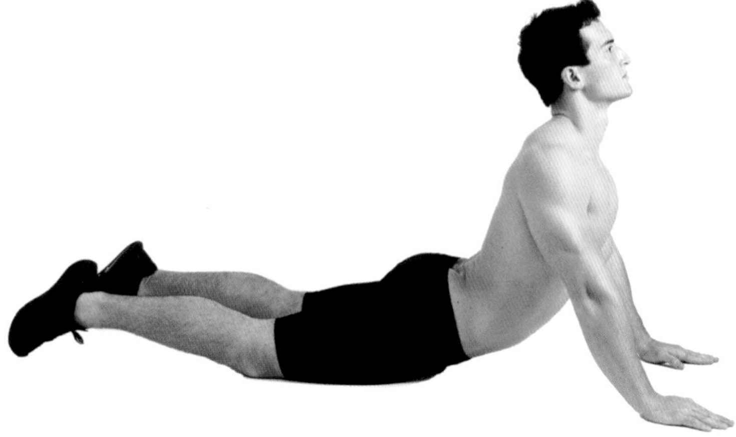

4 HIP FLEXOR STRETCH

page 37

- Perform for 60 seconds.
- Aim for as many repetitions as you can perform.

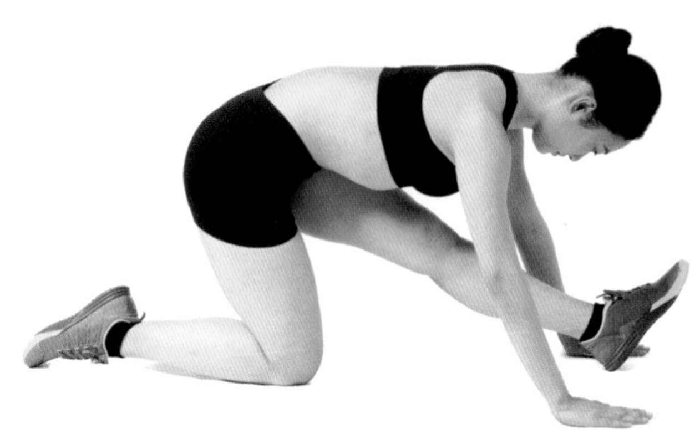

FACT FILE

LEVEL
- All levels

OBJECTIVE
- Extensibility of soft tissues

WORK/REST
- 60 seconds per exercise

TOTAL TIME
- 8 minutes

TOTAL COMPLETED CIRCUIT SETS
- 1 set

5 PIRIFORMIS BRIDGE

pages 30–31

- Perform for 60 seconds.
- Aim for as many repetitions as you can perform.

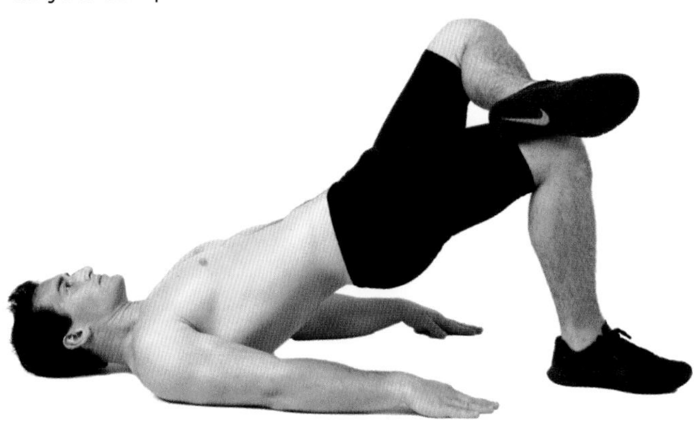

6 HIGH LUNGE

pages 38–39

- Perform for 60 seconds.
- Aim for as many repetitions as you can perform.

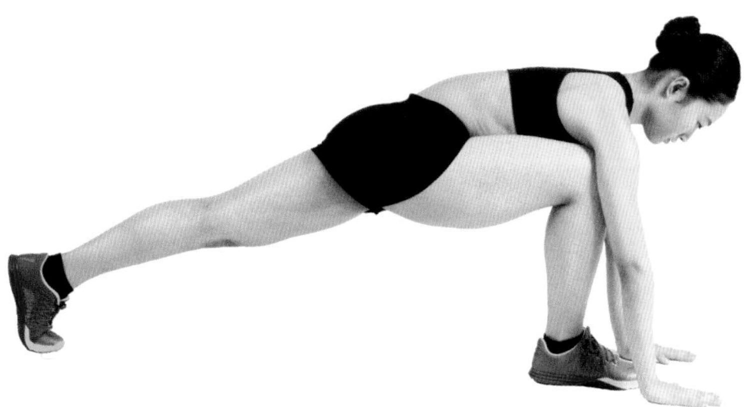

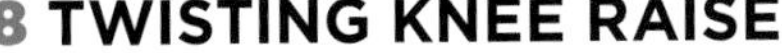

7 SINGLE-LEG CROSSOVER

pages 34–35

- Perform for 60 seconds.
- Aim for as many repetitions as you can perform.

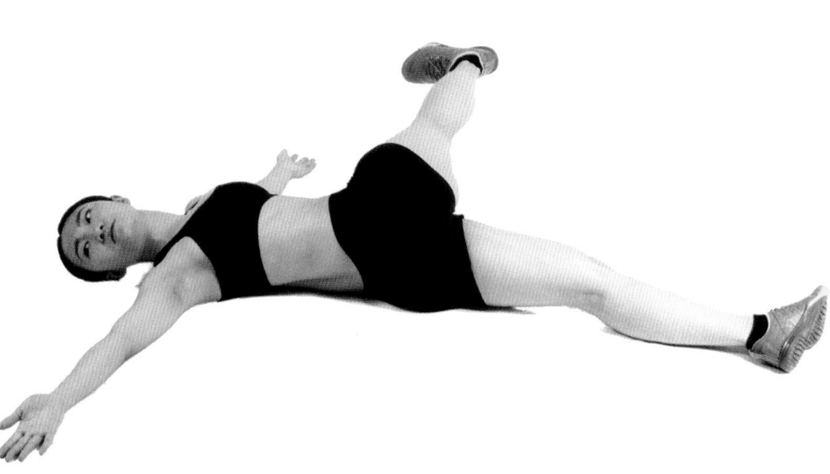

8 TWISTING KNEE RAISE

pages 28–29

- Perform for 60 seconds.
- Aim for as many repetitions as you can perform.

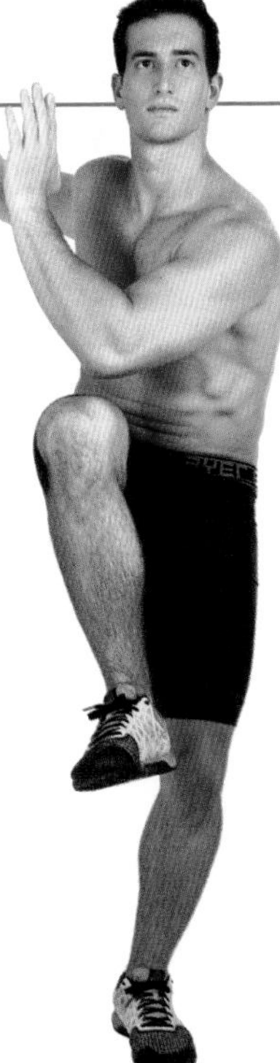

Body-Weight Routine I

This body-weight routine takes you through movements that work out your upper and lower body without added resistance.

1 GOOD MORNING

page 60

- Perform for 30 seconds.
- Aim for 15+ repetitions.

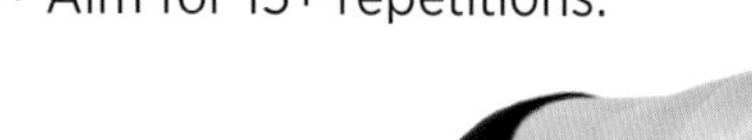

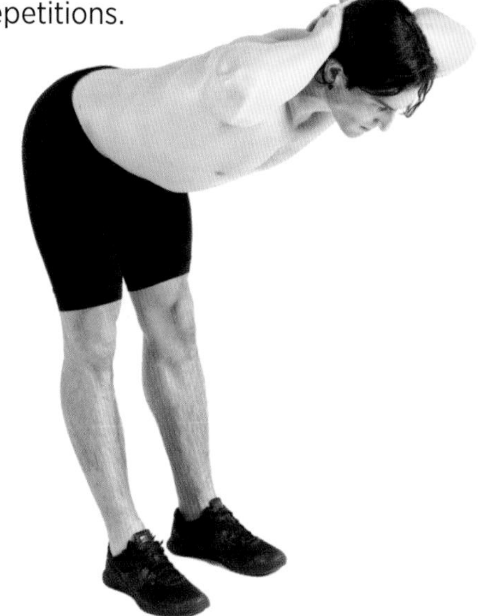

2 HIGH LUNGE WITH TWIST

pages 114–115

- Perform for 30 seconds.
- Aim for 15+ repetitions.

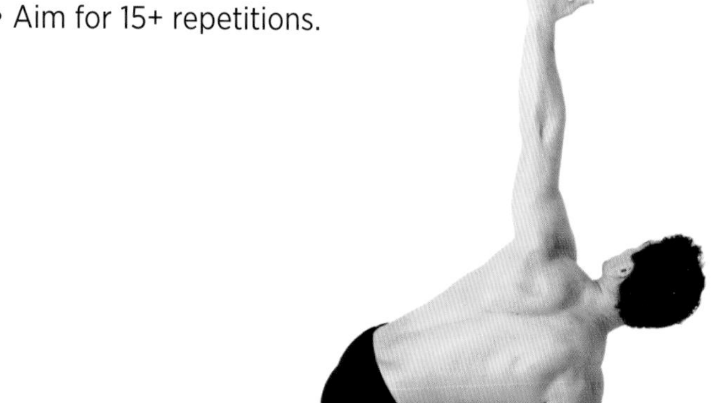

3 BUTT KICK

pages 108–109

- Perform for 30 seconds.
- Aim for 15+ repetitions.

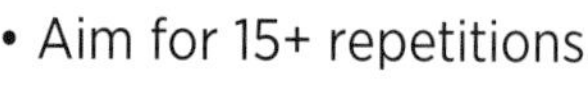

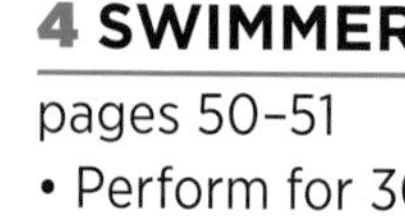

4 SWIMMER

pages 50–51

- Perform for 30 seconds.
- Aim for 15+ repetitions.

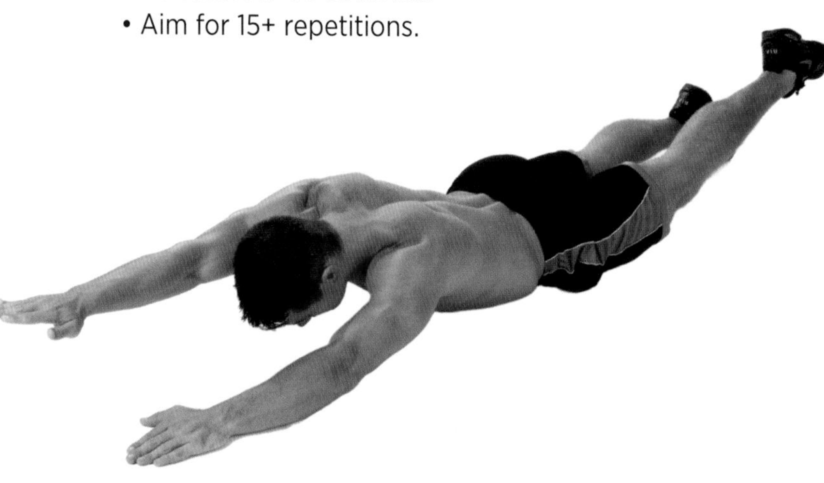

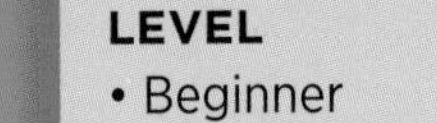

FACT FILE

LEVEL
- Beginner

OBJECTIVE
- Full-body endurance

WORK/REST
- 1:3 (30 seconds per exercise/90 seconds rest)

TOTAL TIME
- 48 minutes

TOTAL COMPLETED CIRCUIT SETS
- 3 sets

5 HIGH KNEES

pages 94–95
- Perform for 30 seconds.
- Aim for 15+ repetitions.

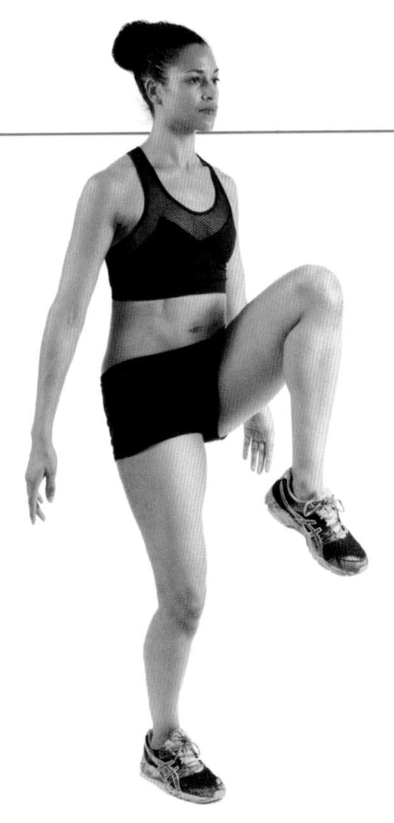

6 ABDOMINAL KICK

pages 100–101
- Perform for 30 seconds.
- Aim for 15+ repetitions.

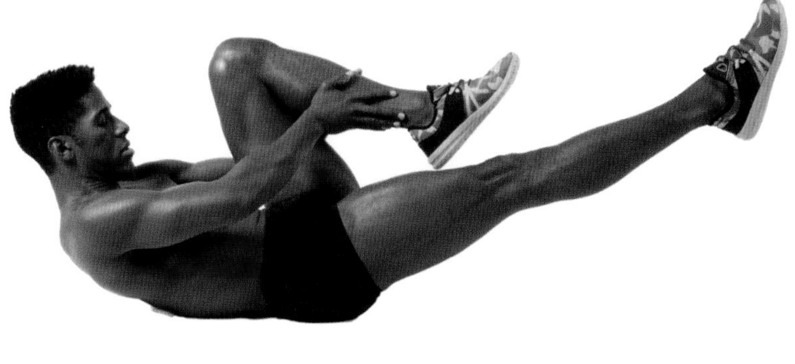

7 SQUAT

pages 106–107
- Perform for 30 seconds.
- Aim for 15+ repetitions.

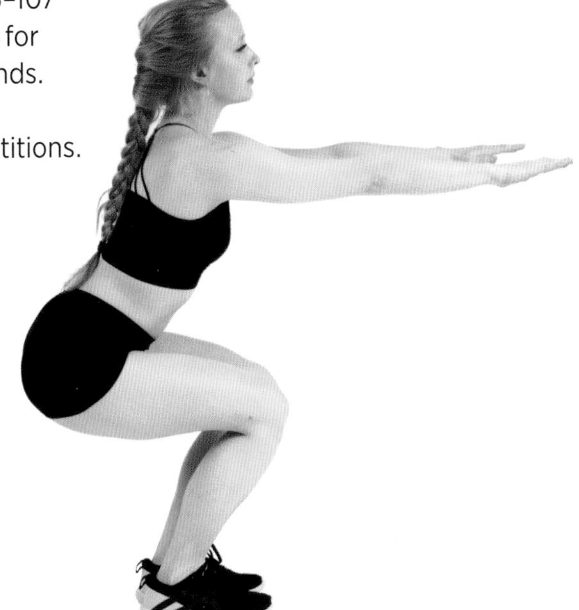

8 PUSH-UP

pages 76–77
- Perform for 30 seconds.
- Aim for 15+ repetitions.

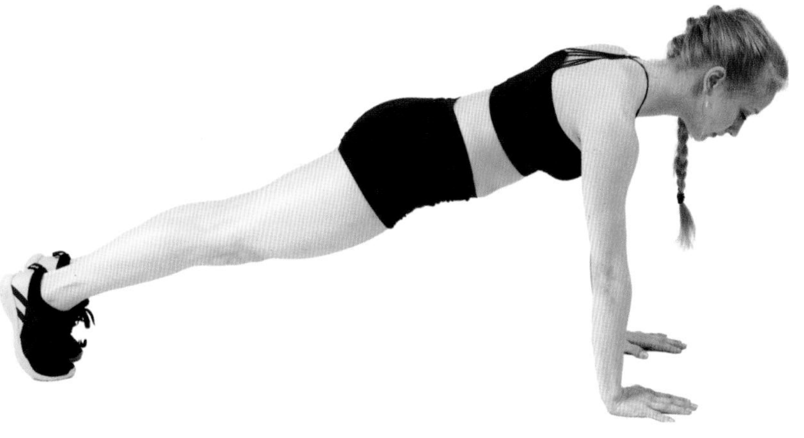

Body-Weight Routine II

Another take on a body-weight routine takes you through movements that will challenge your entire body.

1 SQUAT

pages 106–107

- Perform for 30 seconds.
- Aim for 15+ repetitions.

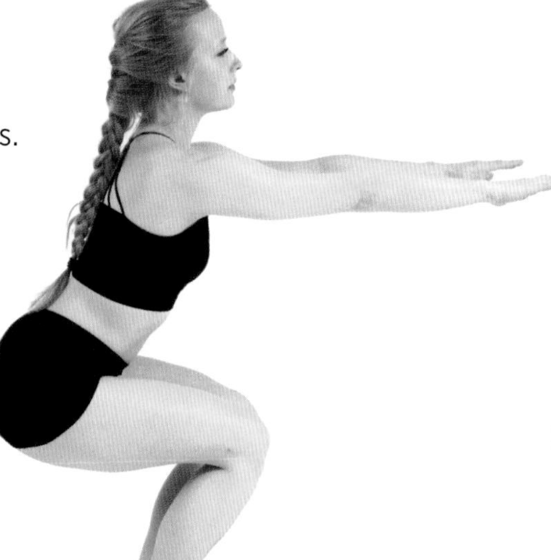

2 TRICEPS PUSH-UP

pages 64–65

- Perform for 30 seconds.
- Aim for 15+ repetitions.

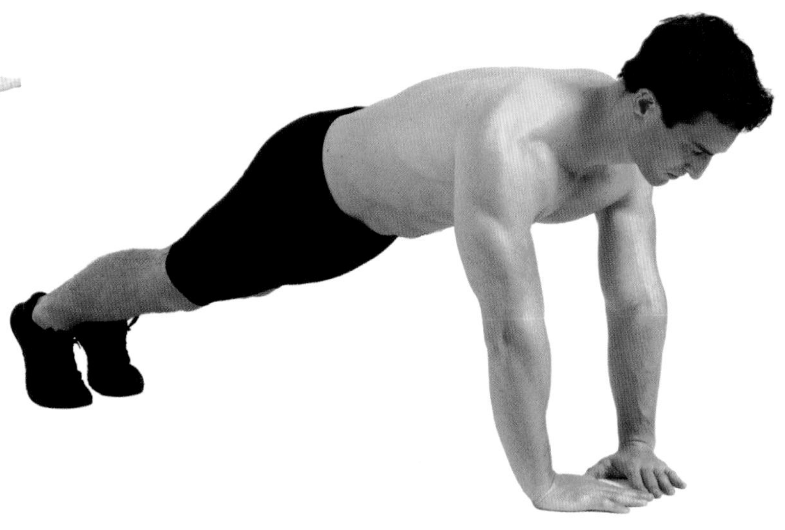

3 ARM HAULER

pages 48–49

- Perform for 30 seconds.
- Aim for 15+ repetitions.

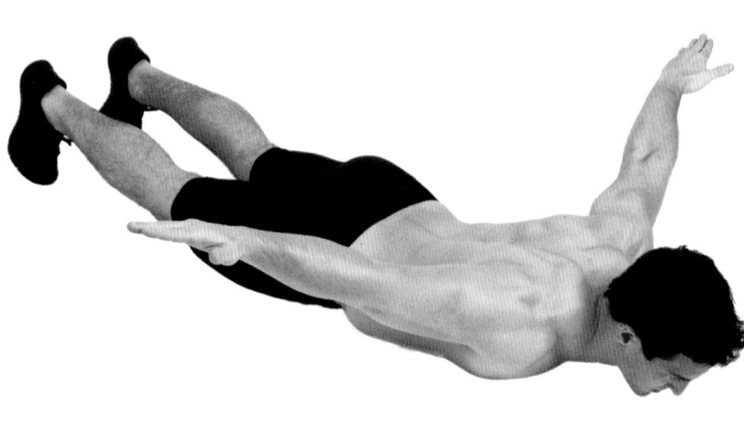

4 BENCH DIP

pages 62–163

- Perform for 30 seconds.
- Aim for 15+ repetitions.

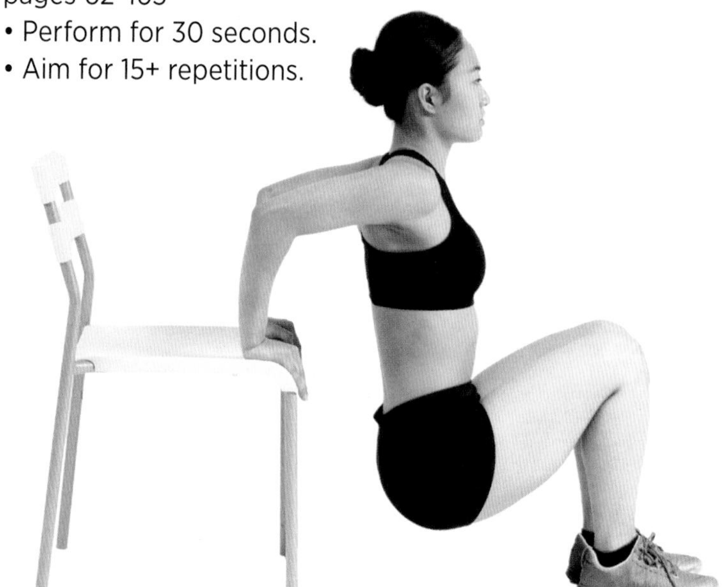

FACT FILE

LEVEL
- Beginner

OBJECTIVE
- Full-body endurance

WORK/REST
- 1:3 (30 seconds per exercise/90 seconds rest)

TOTAL TIME
- 48 minutes

TOTAL COMPLETED CIRCUIT SETS
- 3 sets

5 BENT-KNEE SIT-UP

pages 90–91
- Perform for 30 seconds.
- Aim for 15+ repetitions.

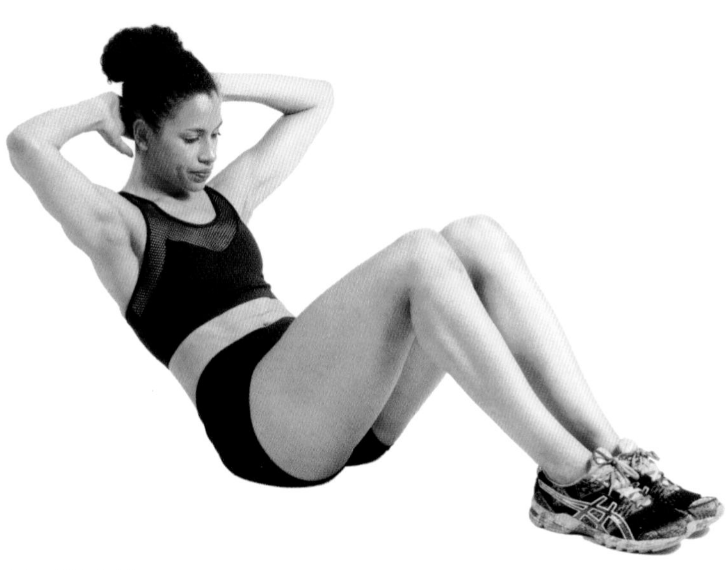

6 BRIDGE WITH LEG LIFT

pages 120–121
- Perform for 30 seconds.
- Aim for 15+ repetitions.

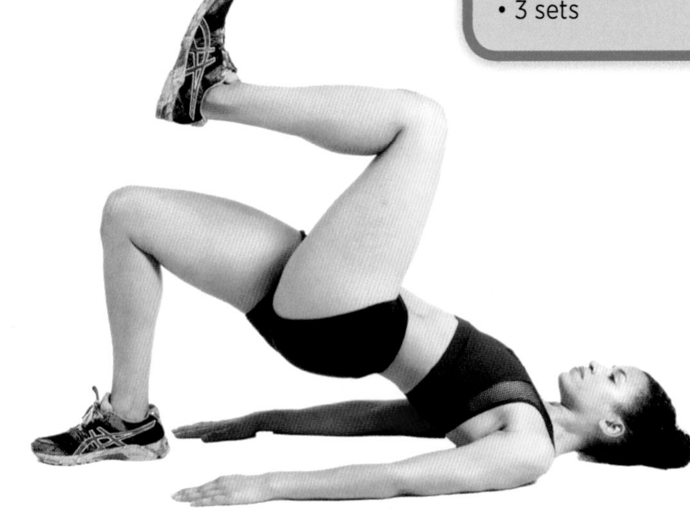

7 THE Y

page 53
- Perform for 30 seconds.
- Aim for 15+ repetitions.

8 BICYCLE CRUNCH

pages 92–93
- Perform for 30 seconds.
- Aim for 15+ repetitions.

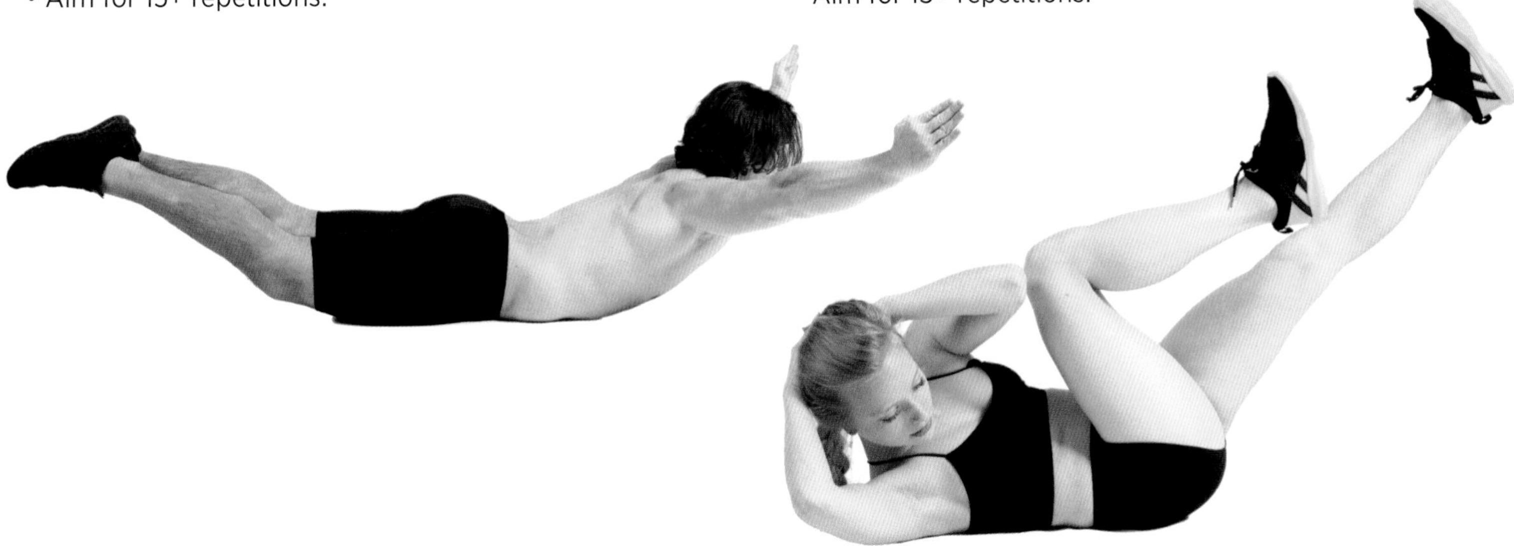

Dumbbell Routine

This routine takes you through movements that will condition your entire body with the use of dumbbells.

1 SUMO SQUAT WITH DUMBBELL

pages 216–217

- Perform for 30 seconds.
- Aim for 15+ repetitions.

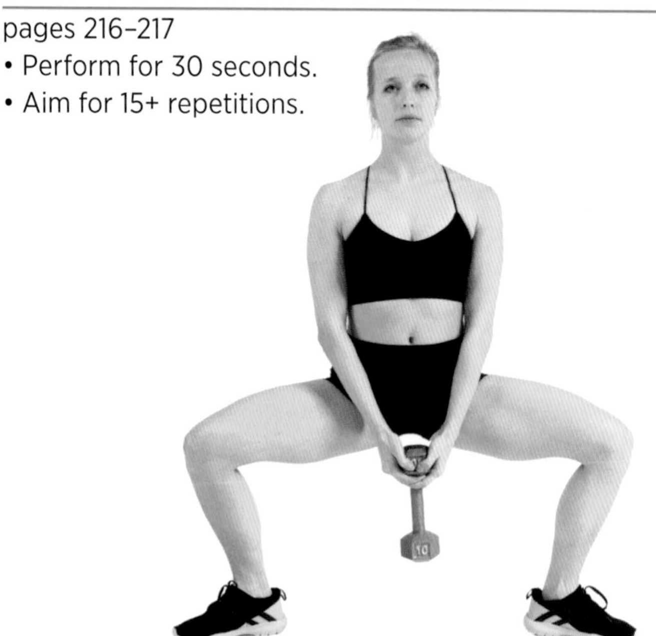

2 DUMBBELL DEADLIFT

pages 150–151

- Perform for 30 seconds.
- Aim for 15+ repetitions.

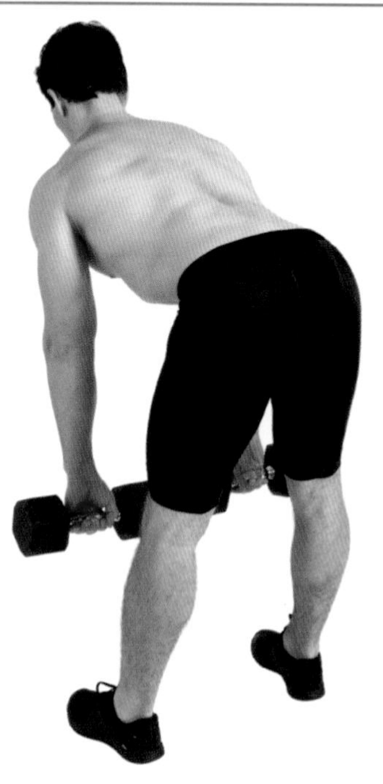

3 ALTERNATING DUMBBELL BICEPS CURL

page 166

- Perform for 30 seconds.
- Aim for 15+ repetitions.

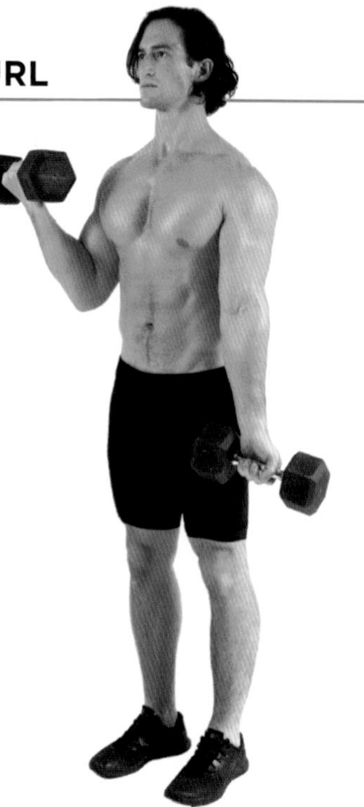

4 TRICEPS KICKBACK

page 180

- Perform for 30 seconds.
- Aim for 15+ repetitions.

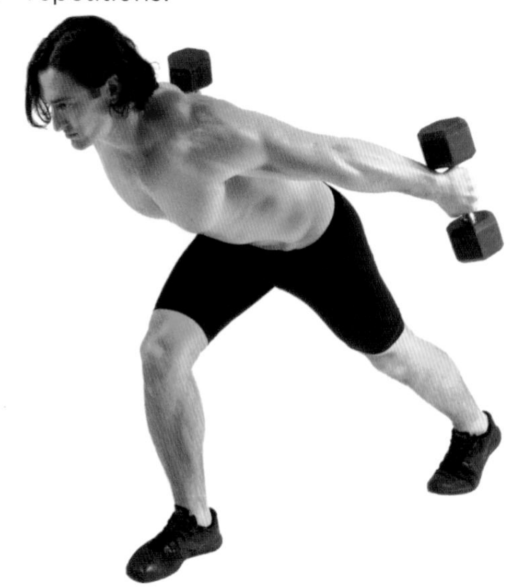

FACT FILE

LEVEL
- Beginner

OBJECTIVE
- Full-body endurance

WORK/REST
- 1:3 (30 seconds per exercise/90 seconds rest)

TOTAL TIME
- 48 minutes

TOTAL COMPLETED CIRCUIT SETS
- 3 sets

5 SEATED DUMBBELL RUSSIAN TWIST

pages 198–199

- Perform for 30 seconds.
- Aim for 15+ repetitions.

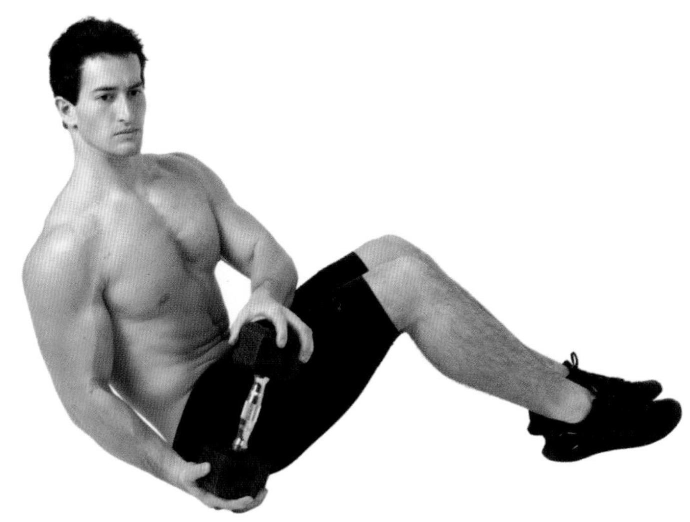

6 MOUNTAIN CLIMBER

pages 138–139

- Perform for 30 seconds.
- Aim for 15+ repetitions.

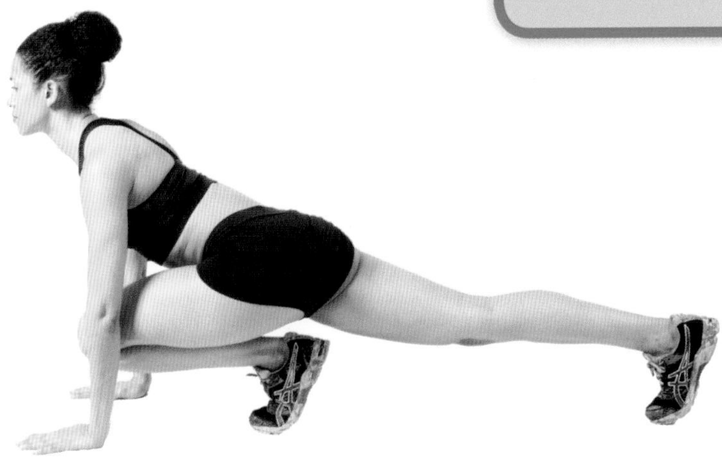

7 DUMBBELL ROW

page 154–155

- Perform for 30 seconds.
- Aim for 15+ repetitions.

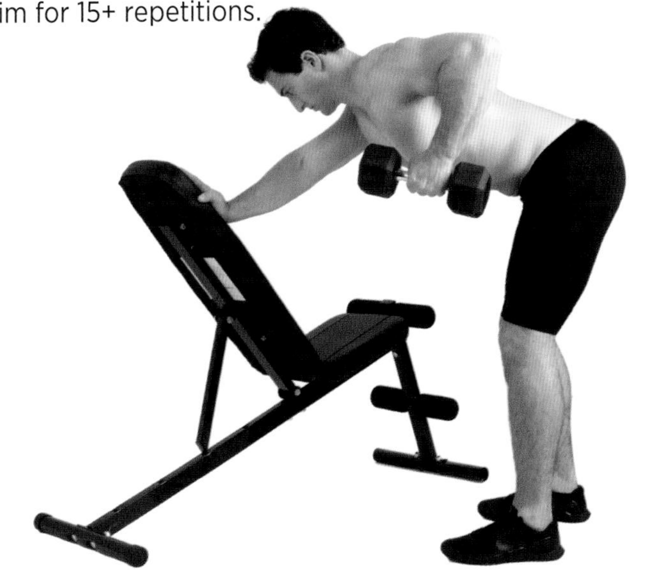

8 SINGLE-ARM DUMBBELL PRESS

page 182

- Perform for 30 seconds.
- Aim for 15+ repetitions.

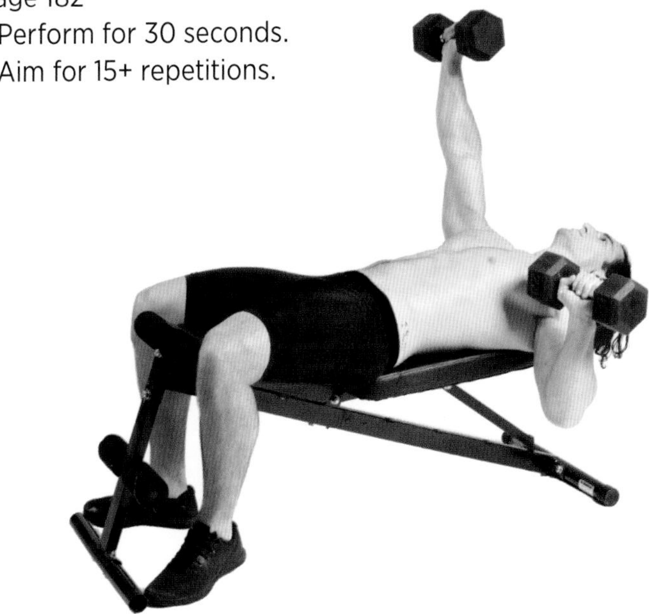

Barbell and Bench Routine

This routine takes you through movements that tone and engage your entire body with the use of a barbell, a bench, and your own body weight.

1 BARBELL DEADLIFT

pages 240–241

- Perform for 20 seconds.
- Aim for 15+ repetitions.

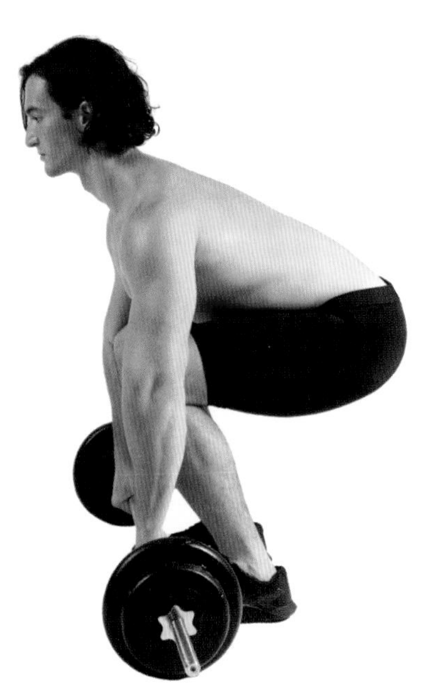

2 BARBELL BENCH PRESS

pages 270–271

- Perform for 20 seconds.
- Aim for 15+ repetitions.

3 V-UP

pages 96–97

- Perform for 20 seconds.
- Aim for 15+ repetitions.

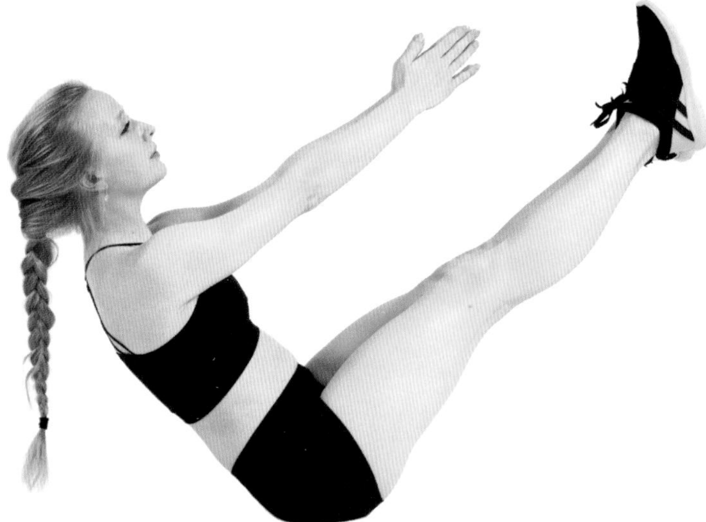

4 BARBELL CURL

pages 254–255

- Perform for 20 seconds.
- Aim for 15+ repetitions.

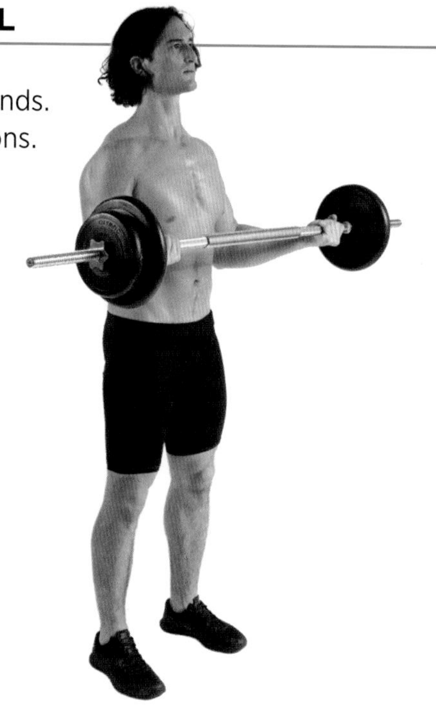

FACT FILE

LEVEL
- Beginner

OBJECTIVE
- Full-body endurance

WORK/REST
- 1:4 (20 seconds per exercise/80 seconds rest)

TOTAL TIME
- 40 minutes

TOTAL COMPLETED CIRCUIT SETS
- 3 sets

5 SKULL CRUSHER

pages 260–261

- Perform for 20 seconds.
- Aim for 15+ repetitions.

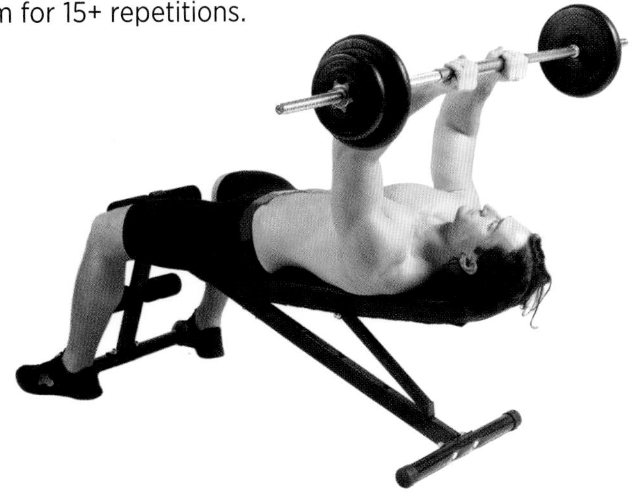

6 BARBELL UPRIGHT ROW

pages 248–249

- Perform for 20 seconds.
- Aim for 15+ repetitions.

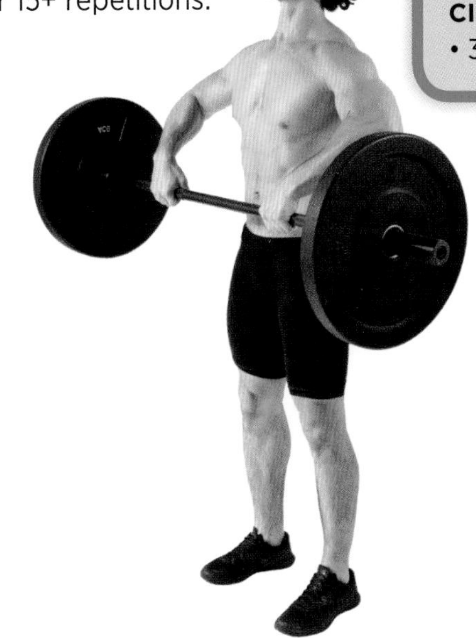

7 KNEES TO CHEST

pages 98–99

- Perform for 20 seconds.
- Aim for 15+ repetitions.

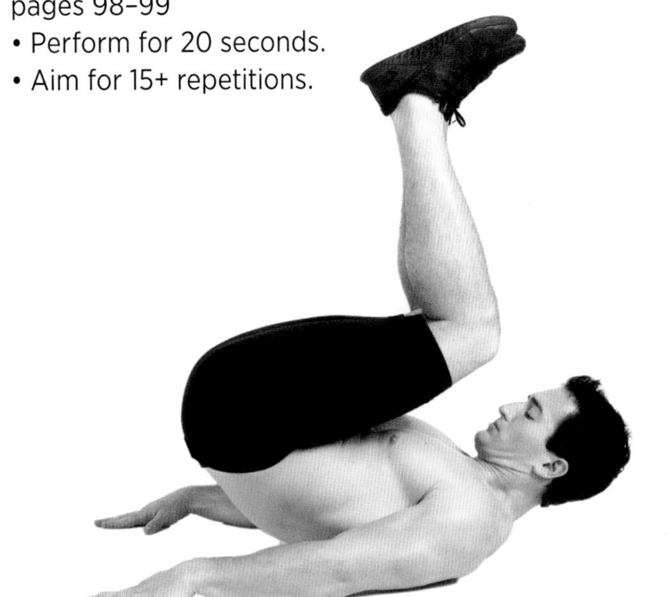

8 BARBELL SQUAT

pages 298–299

- Perform for 20 seconds.
- Aim for 15+ repetitions.

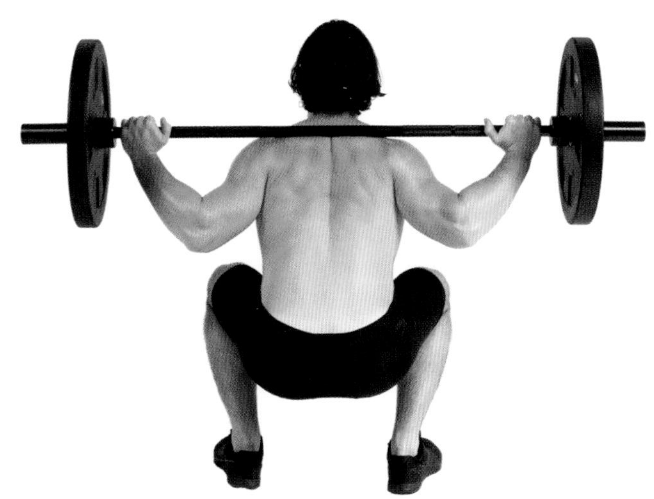

Party-Bag Routine

This routine takes you through movements utilizing a variety of different equipment to challenge your conditioning and keep your body guessing.

1 JUMP ROPE

pages 310–311

- Perform for 20 seconds.
- Aim for 15+ repetitions.

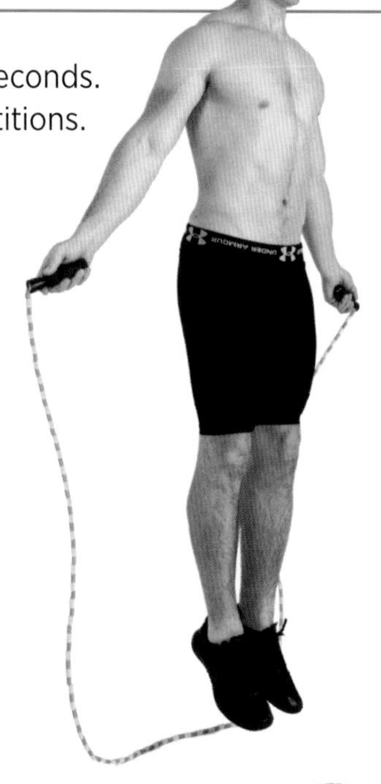

2 GOBLET SQUAT

page 213

- Perform for 20 seconds.
- Aim for 15+ repetitions.

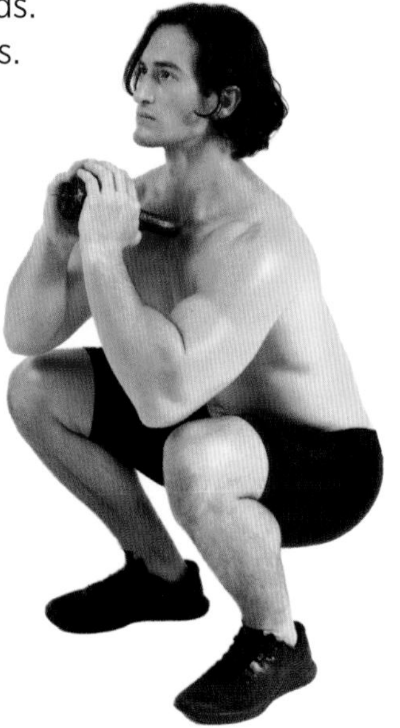

3 PLATE CURL

pages 256–257

- Perform for 20 seconds.
- aim for 15+ repetitions.

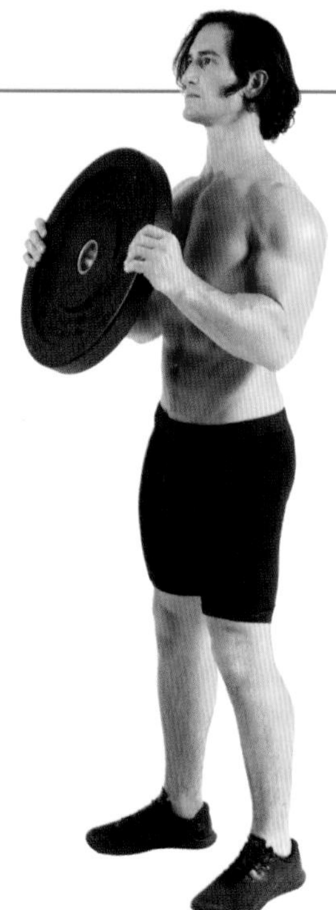

4 TOWEL HAMSTRINGS PULL

page 124

- Perform for 20 seconds.
- Aim for 15+ repetitions.

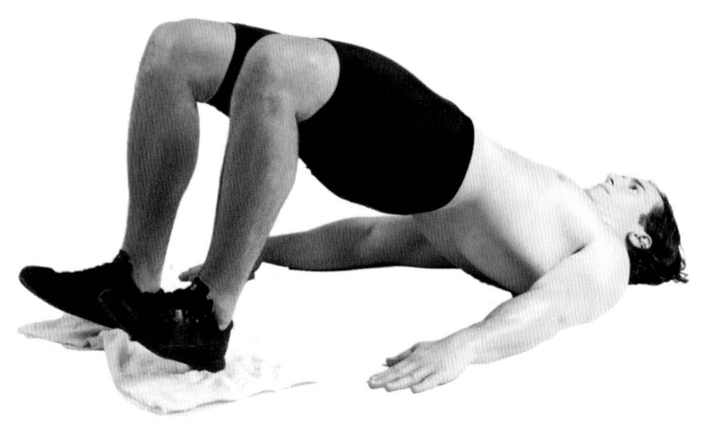

FACT FILE

LEVEL
• Beginner

OBJECTIVE
• Full-body endurance

WORK/REST
• 1:4 (20 seconds per exercise/80 seconds rest)

TOTAL TIME
• 40 minutes

TOTAL COMPLETED CIRCUIT SETS
• 3 sets

5 FRONT PLATE RAISE

pages 258–259

- Perform for 20 seconds.
- Aim for 15+ repetitions.

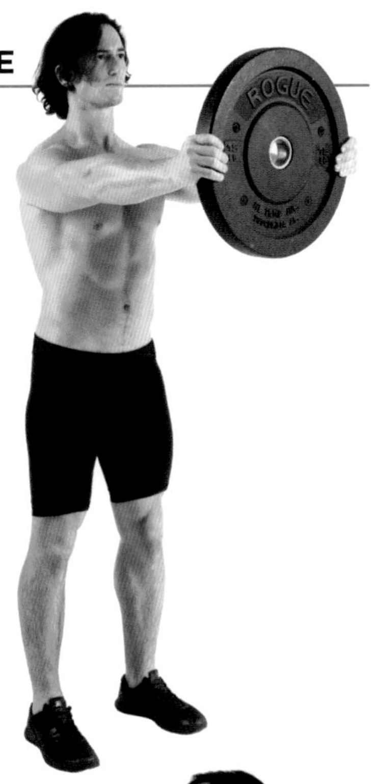

6 STIFF-LEGGED BARBELL DEADLIFT

pages 242–243

- Perform for 20 seconds.
- Aim for 15+ repetitions.

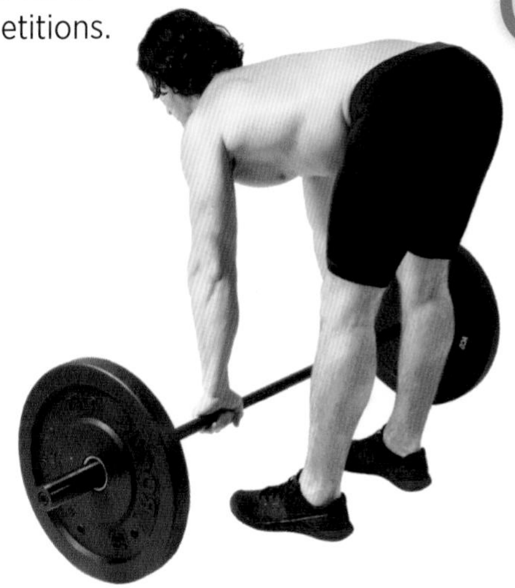

7 MEDICINE BALL CORE TWIST

page 283

- Perform for 20 seconds.
- Aim for 15+ repetitions.

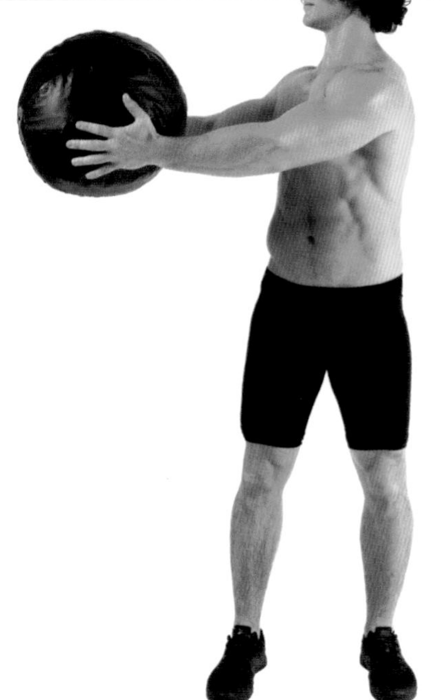

8 FARMER'S WALK

pages 202–203

- Perform for 20 seconds.
- Aim for 15+ repetitions.

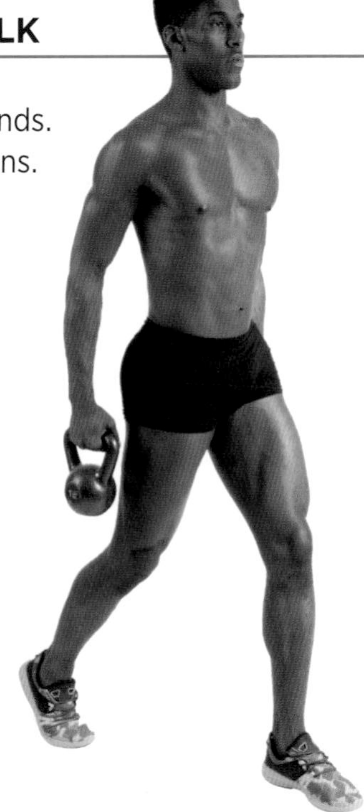

Back Routine

This routine takes you through body-weight movements and utilizes various equipment. It is designed to condition a number muscle groups that support your back.

1 DUMBBELL PULLOVER

pages 162–163

- Perform for 30 seconds.
- Aim for 8–12 repetitions.

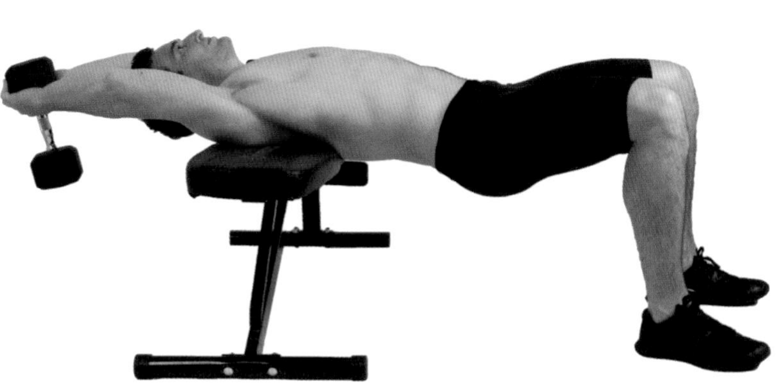

2 BARBELL GOOD MORNING

pages 244–245

- Perform for 30 seconds.
- Aim for 8–12 repetitions.

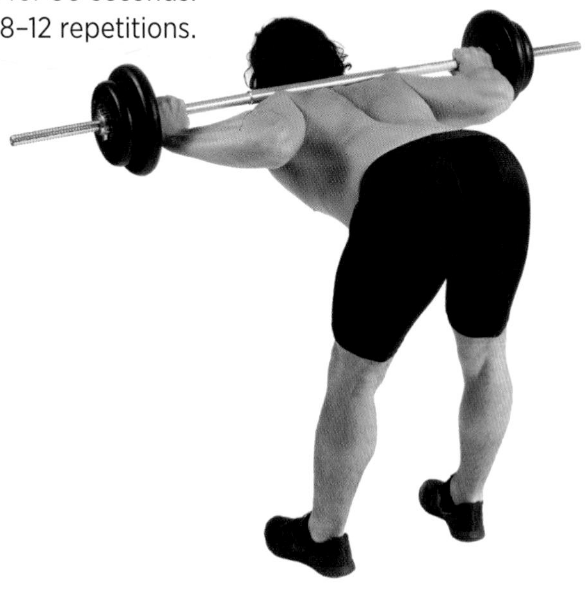

3 PULL-UP

pages 44–45

- Perform for 30 seconds.
- Aim for 8–12 repetitions.

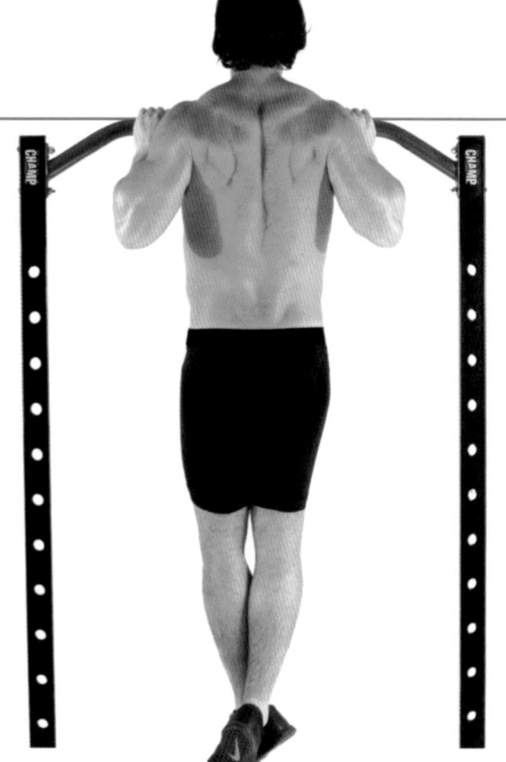

4 ROTATED BACK EXTENSION

pages 58–59

- Perform for 30 seconds.
- Aim for 8–12 repetitions.

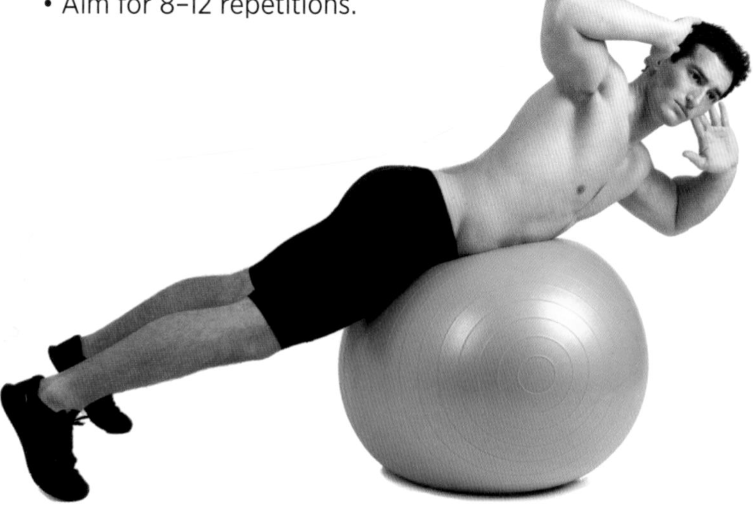

FACT FILE

LEVEL
- Intermediate

OBJECTIVE
- Back-muscle hypertrophy

WORK/REST
- 1:2 (30 seconds per exercise/60 seconds rest)

TOTAL TIME
- 60 minutes

TOTAL COMPLETED CIRCUIT SETS
- 5 sets

5 MEDICINE BALL SLAM

pages 318–319
- Perform for 30 seconds.
- Aim for 8–12 repetitions.

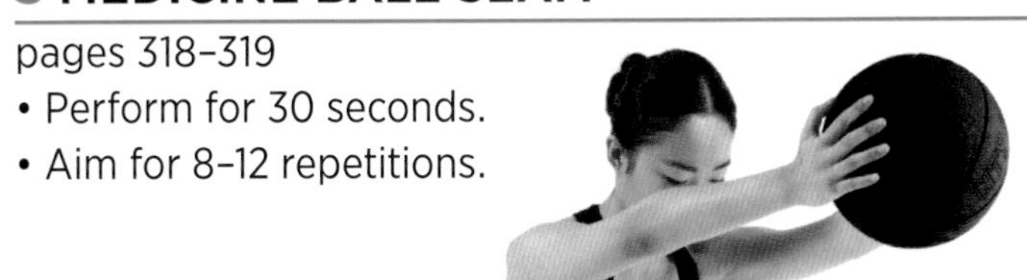

6 SINGLE-ARM T-ROW

page 152–153
- Perform for 30 seconds.
- Aim for 8–12 repetitions.

7 SWISS BALL HYPEREXTENSION

pages 56–57
- Perform for 30 seconds.
- Aim for 8–12 repetitions.

8 MEDICINE BALL PULLOVER ON SWISS BALL

pages 252–253
- Perform for 30 seconds.
- Aim for 8–12 repetitions.

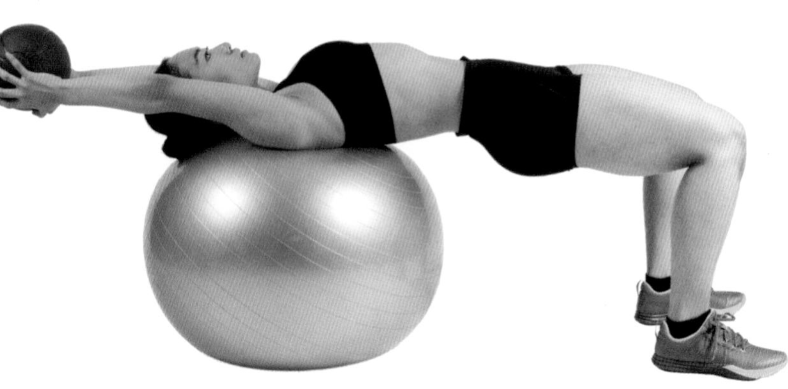

Arm Routine

This routine takes you through both equipment and body-weight movement to condition and tone your arms, alternating through resistance and power motions.

1 MEDICINE BALL THROW

pages 268–269

- Perform for 30 seconds.
- Aim for 8–12 repetitions.

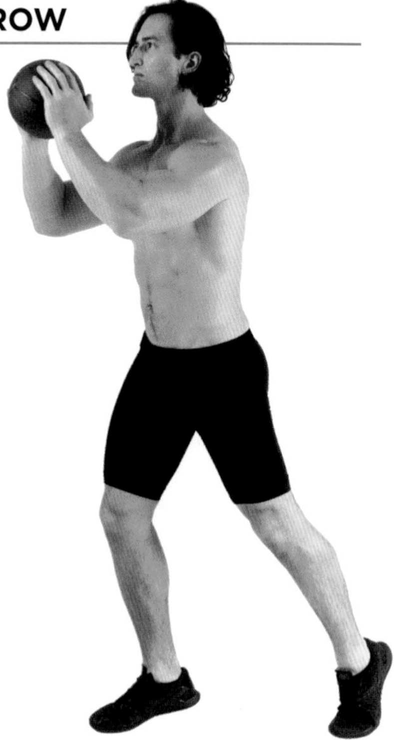

2 4-COUNT OVERHEAD

pages 174–175

- Perform for 30 seconds.
- Aim for 8–12 repetitions.

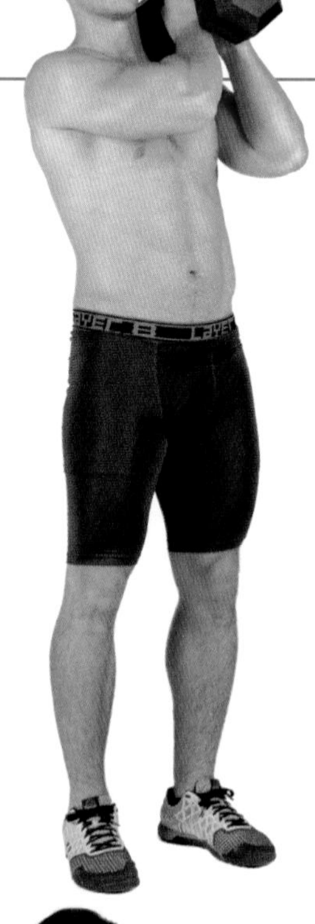

3 REAR LATERAL RAISE

pages 160–161

- Perform for 30 seconds.
- Aim for 8–12 repetitions.

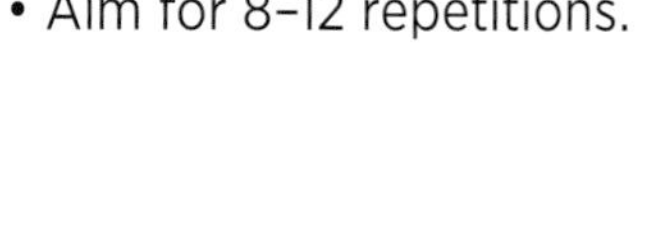

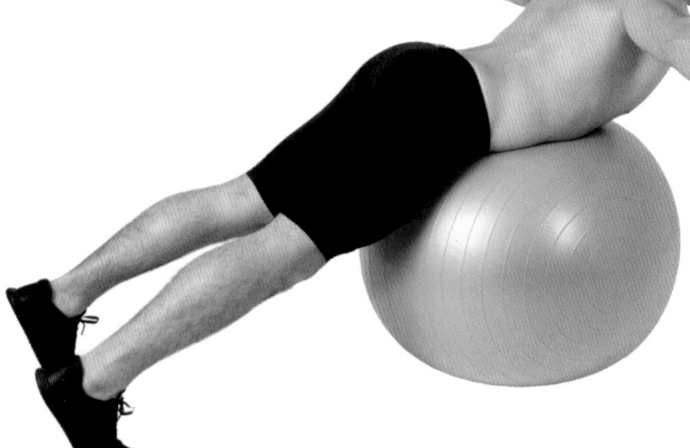

4 POWER PUNCH

pages 70–71

- Perform for 30 seconds.
- Aim for 8–12 repetitions.

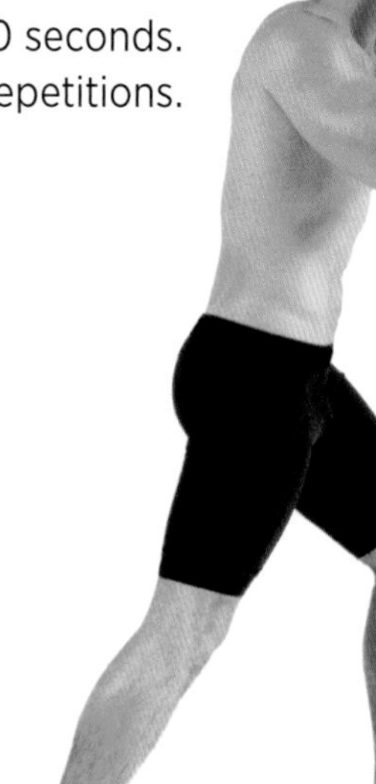

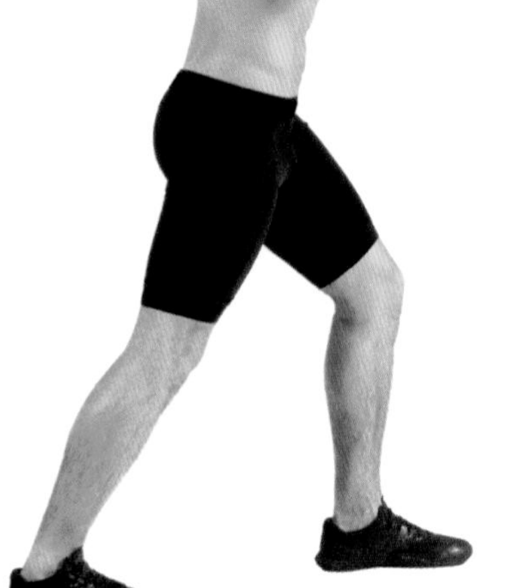

FACT FILE

LEVEL
- Intermediate

OBJECTIVE
- Arm and shoulder hypertrophy

WORK/REST
- 1:2 (30 seconds per exercise/60 seconds rest)

TOTAL TIME
- 60 minutes

TOTAL COMPLETED CIRCUIT SETS
- 5 sets

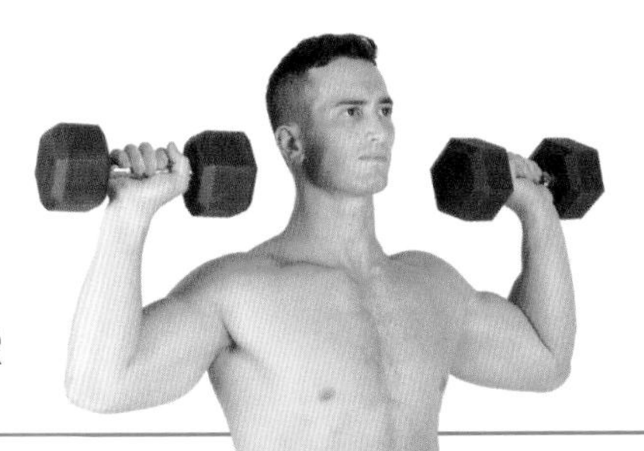

5 SHOULDER CRUSHER

pages 176–177
- Perform for 30 seconds.
- Aim for 8–12 repetitions.

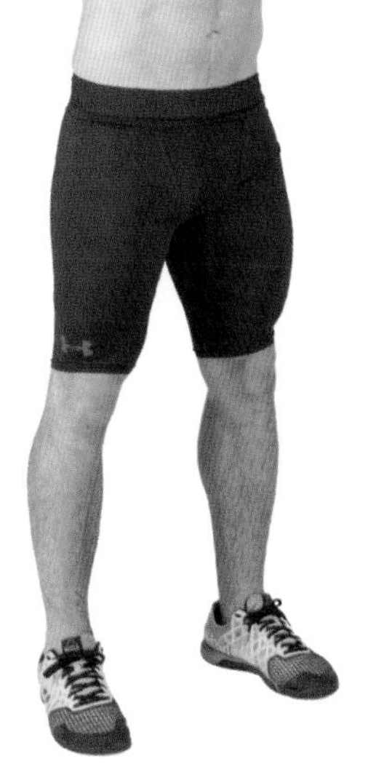

6 WALL BALL SHOT

page 320
- Perform for 30 seconds.
- Aim for 8–12 repetitions.

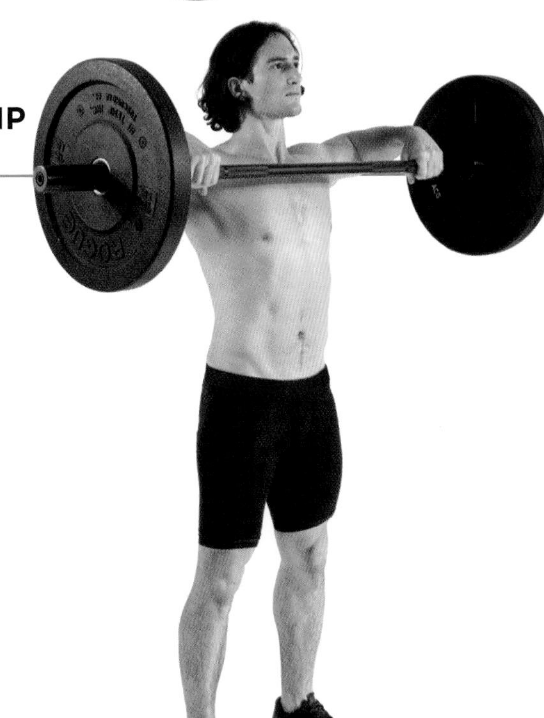

7 WIDE-GRIP HIGH PULL

pages 250–251
- Perform for 30 seconds.
- Aim for 8–12 repetitions.

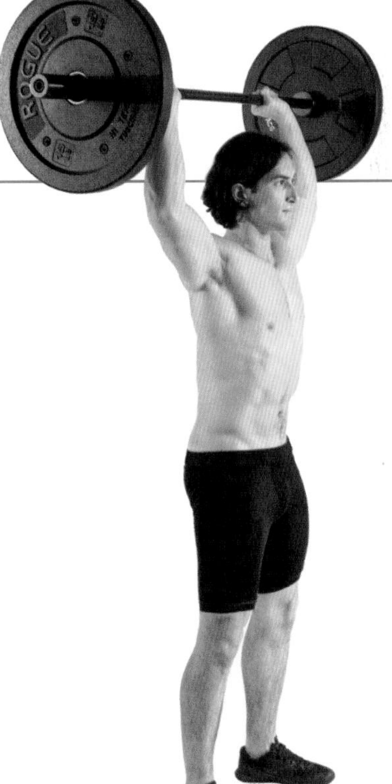

8 BARBELL SHOULDER PRESS

page 321
- Perform for 30 seconds.
- Aim for 8–12 repetitions.

Chest Routine

This routine utilizes body weight and resistance to condition your chest throughout its entire range of motion.

1 DUMBBELL FLY

pages 188–189

- Perform for 30 seconds.
- Aim for 8–12 repetitions.

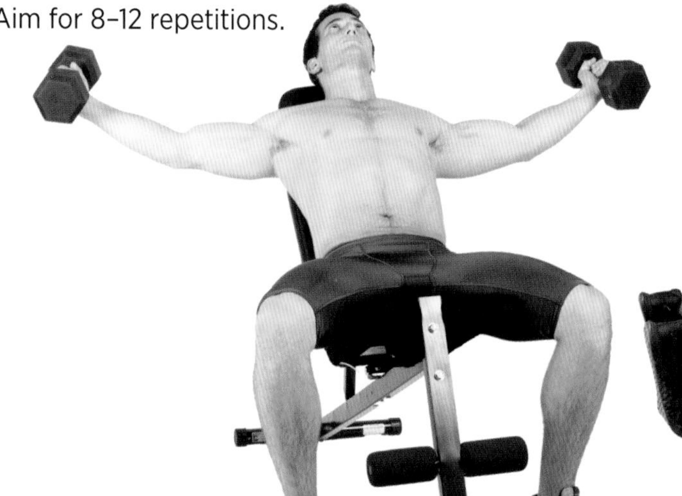

2 PLATE PUSH-UP

pages 276–277

- Perform for 30 seconds.
- Aim for 8–12 repetitions.

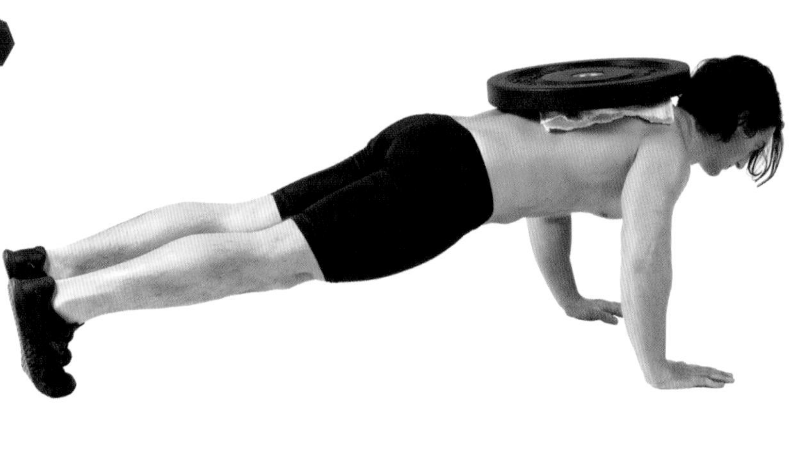

3 PUSH-UP WALKOUT

pages 26–27

- Perform for 30 seconds.
- Aim for 8–12 repetitions.

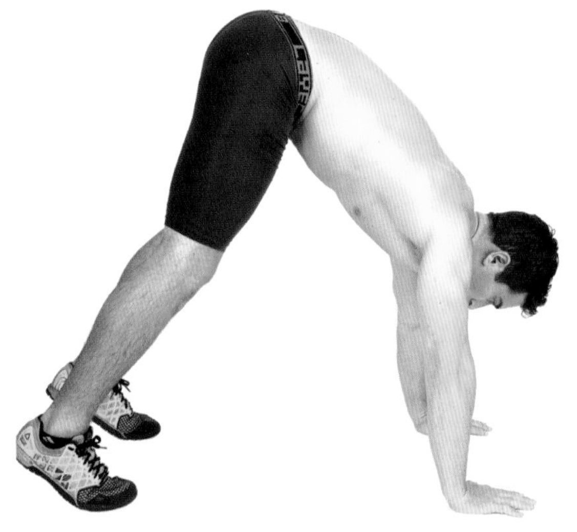

4 HAMMER-GRIP PRESS

pages 186–187

- Perform for 30 seconds.
- Aim for 8–12 repetitions.

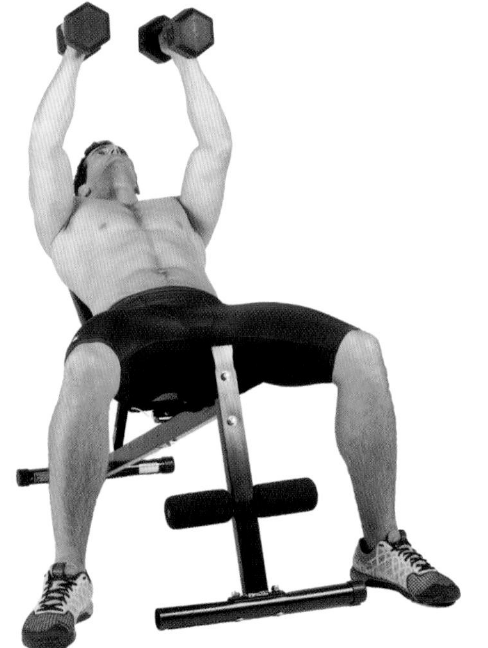

FACT FILE

LEVEL
- Intermediate

OBJECTIVE
- Pectoral hypertrophy

WORK/REST
- 1:2 (30 seconds per exercise/60 seconds rest)

TOTAL TIME
- 60 minutes

TOTAL COMPLETED CIRCUIT SETS
- 5 sets

5 PUSH-UP HAND WALK-OVER

pages 272–273

- Perform for 30 seconds.
- Aim for 8–12 repetitions.

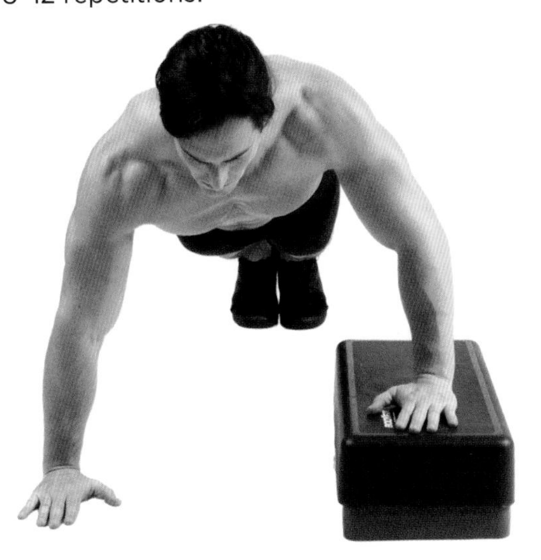

6 SPHINX PUSH-UP

page 88

- Perform for 30 seconds.
- Aim for 8-12 repetitions.

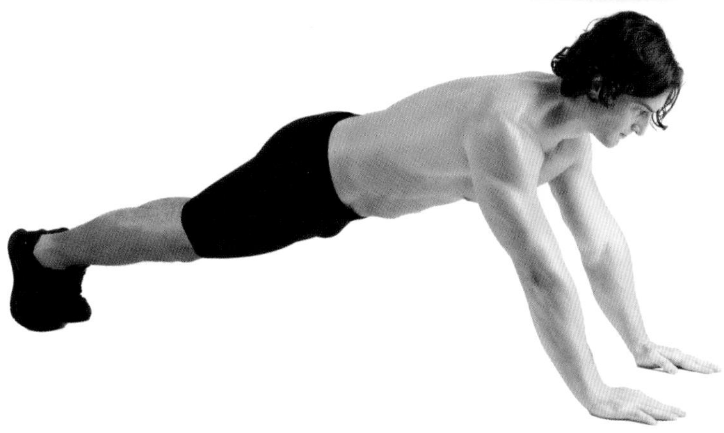

7 SWISS BALL INCLINE DUMBBELL PRESS

page 183

- Perform for 30 seconds.
- Aim for 8–12 repetitions.

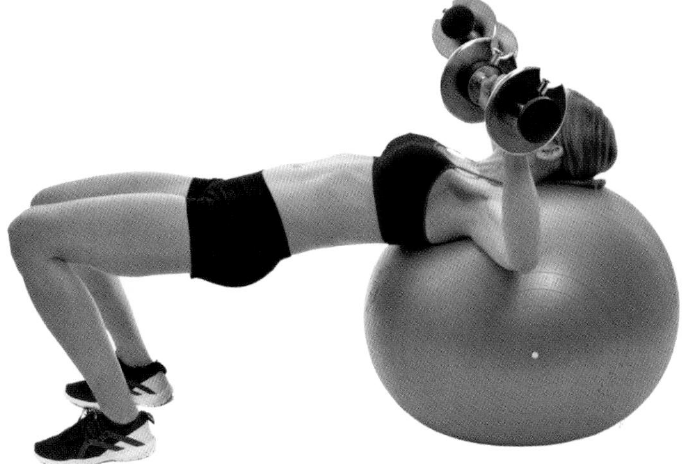

8 TRIANGLE PUSH-UP WITH MEDICINE BALL

page 281

- Perform for 30 seconds.
- Aim for 8–12 repetitions.

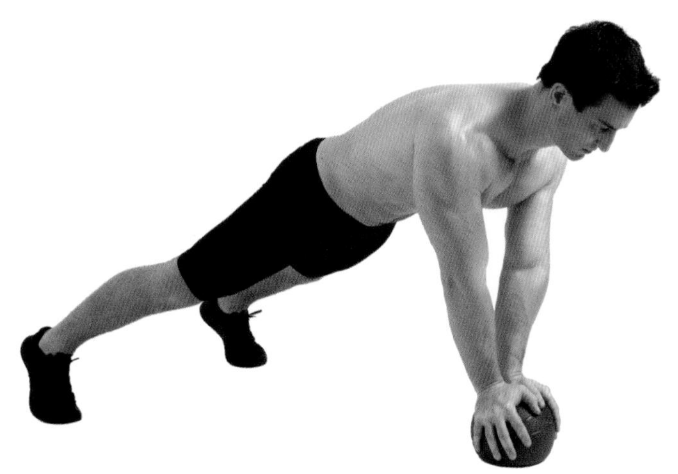

Core Routine

This routine takes you through an hour-long workout utilizing equipment and body weight to tone and define the multitude of muscle groups that make up your abdominal core.

1 MEDICINE BALL PIKE-UP

pages 294–295

- Perform for 30 seconds.
- Aim for 8–12 repetitions.

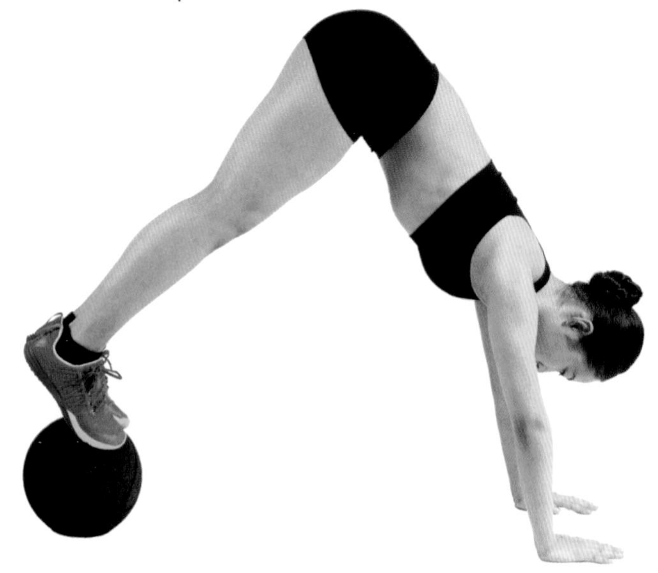

2 BATTLE ROPE SIDE-TO-SIDE SWING

pages 266–267

- Perform for 30 seconds.
- Aim for 8–12 repetitions.

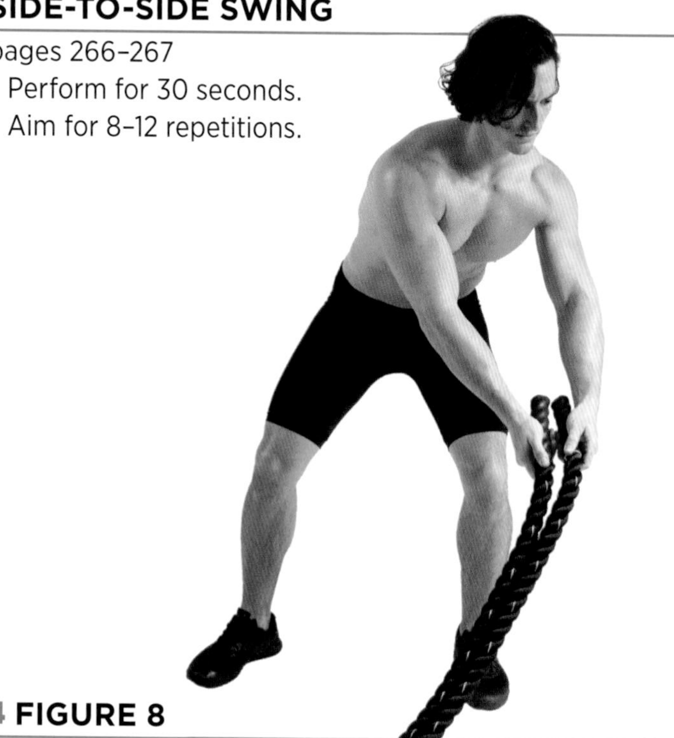

3 SWISS BALL JACKKNIFE

pages 292–293

- Perform for 30 seconds.
- Aim for 8–12 repetitions.

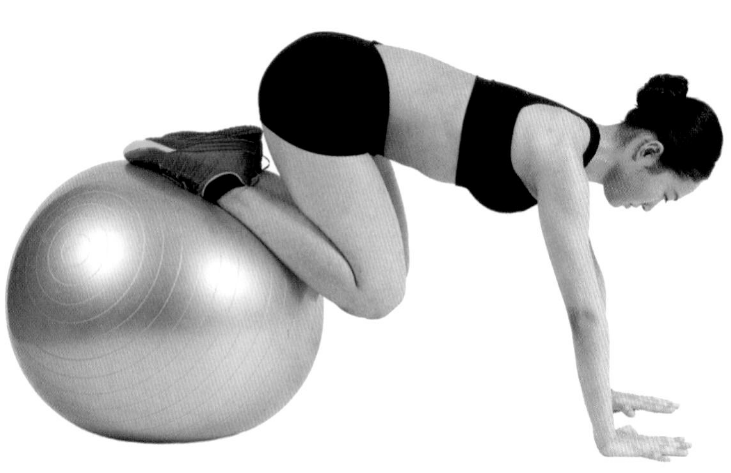

4 FIGURE 8

pages 286–287

- Perform for 30 seconds.
- Aim for 8–12 repetitions.

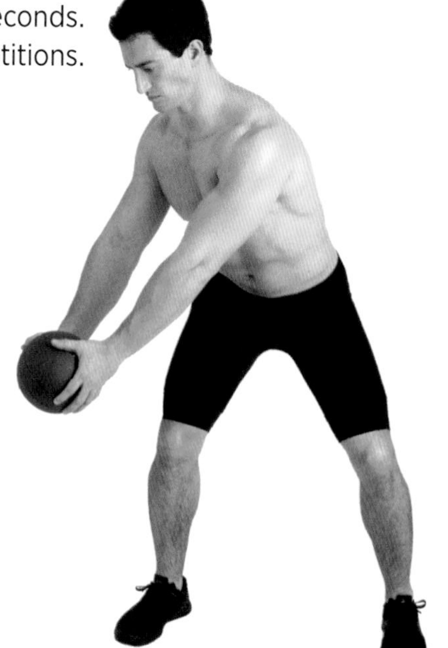

FACT FILE

LEVEL
- Intermediate

OBJECTIVE
- Abdominal and oblique hypertrophy

WORK/REST
- 1:2 (30 seconds per exercise/60 seconds rest)

TOTAL TIME
- 60 minutes

TOTAL COMPLETED CIRCUIT SETS
- 5 sets

5 ROPE PULL-DOWN

pages 284–285
- Perform for 30 seconds.
- Aim for 8–12 repetitions.

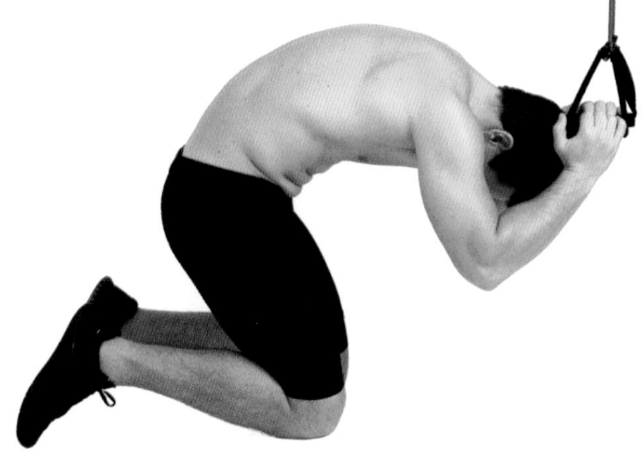

6 KETTLEBELL TOE TOUCHER

page 205
- Perform for 30 seconds.
- Aim for 8–12 repetitions.

7 TWISTING KNEE RAISE

pages 28–29
- Perform for 30 seconds.
- Aim for 8–12 repetitions.

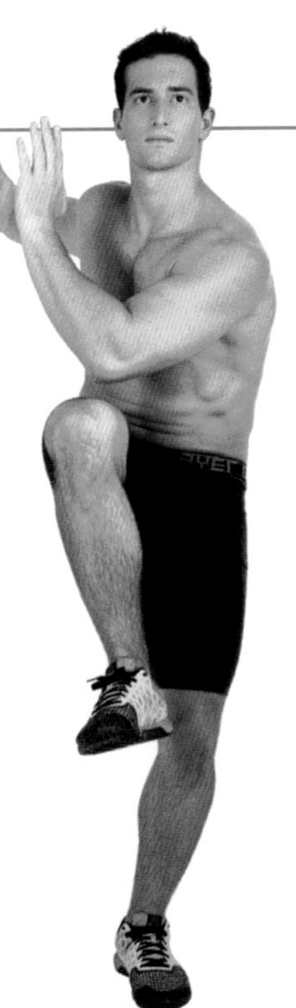

8 PULLOVER PASS

pages 290–291
- Perform for 30 seconds.
- Aim for 8–12 repetitions.

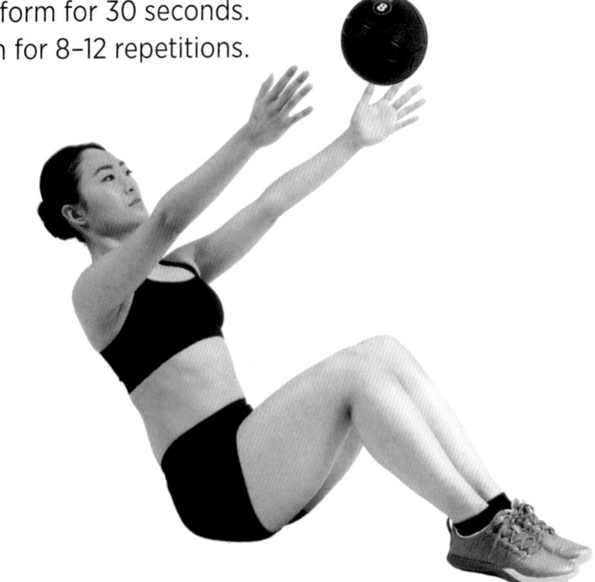

Body-Weight Legs

This routine takes you through movements using just your own body weight to condition your lower body.

1 LATERAL LUNGE WITH SQUAT

pages 112–113

- Perform for 30 seconds.
- Aim for 8–12 repetitions.

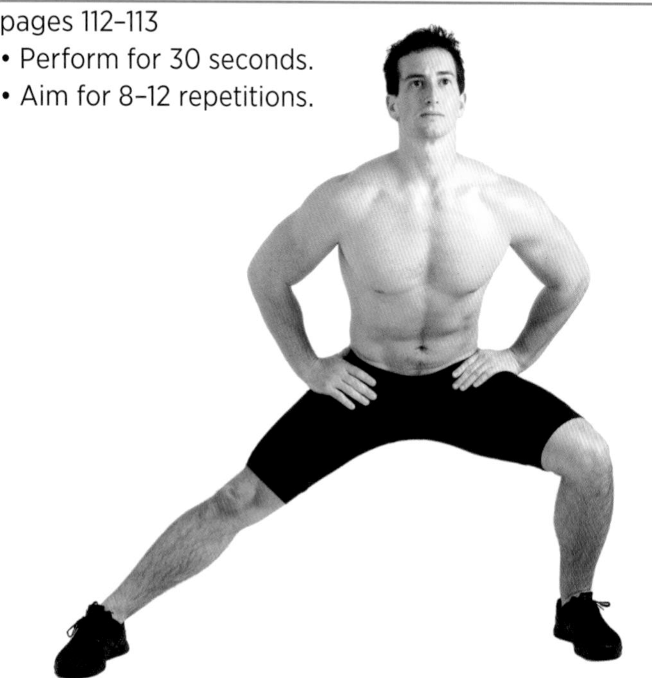

2 POWER SQUAT

pages 300–301

- Perform for 30 seconds.
- Aim for 8–12 repetitions.

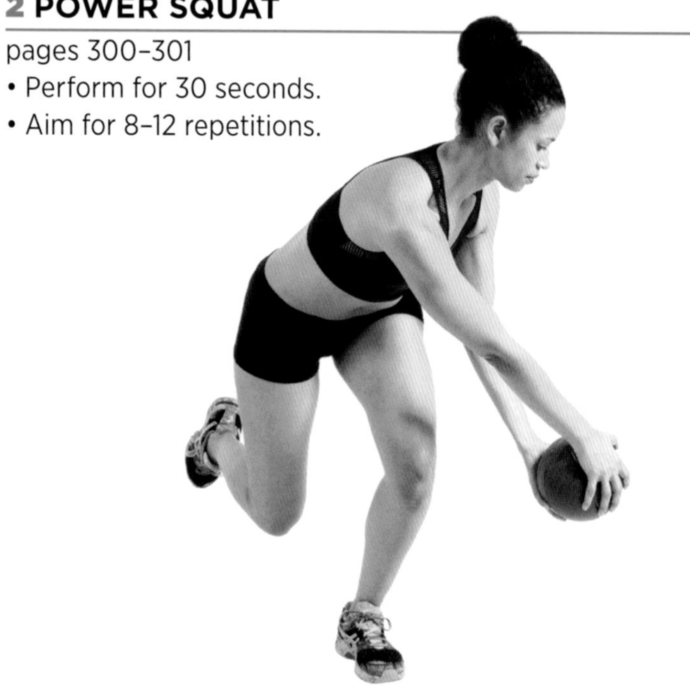

3 SLALOM SKIER

pages 136–137

- Perform for 30 seconds.
- Aim for 8–12 repetitions.

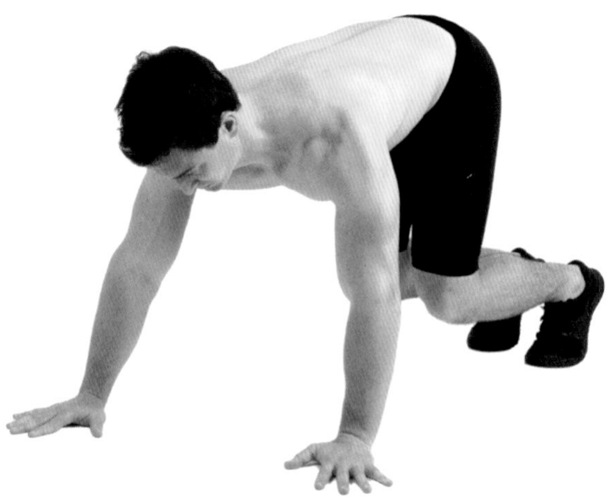

4 SINGLE-LEG CROSSOVER

pages 34–35

- Perform for 30 seconds.
- Aim for 8–12 repetitions.

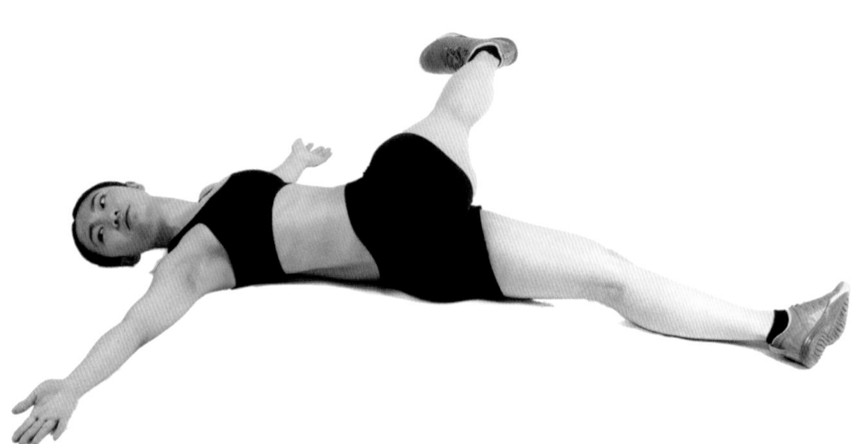

FACT FILE

LEVEL

- Intermediate

OBJECTIVE

- Lower-extremity hypertrophy

WORK/REST

- 1:2 (30 seconds per exercise/60 seconds rest)

TOTAL TIME

- 60 minutes

TOTAL COMPLETED CIRCUIT SETS

- 5 sets

5 REACH-AND-TWIST WALKING LUNGE

pages 306–307

- Perform for 30 seconds.
- Aim for 8–12 repetitions.

6 SPEED SKATER

pages 118–119

- Perform for 30 seconds.
- Aim for 8–12 repetitions.

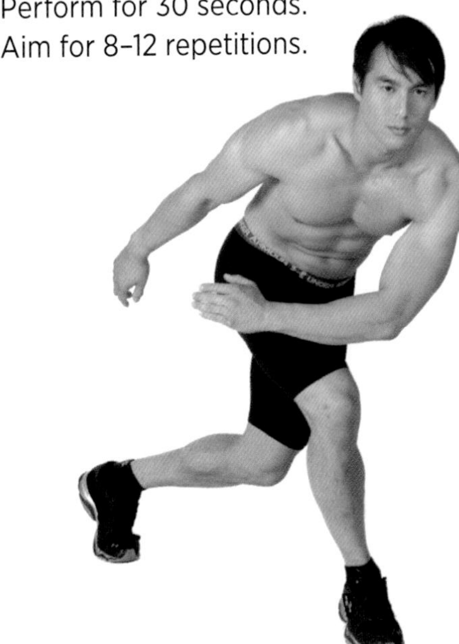

7 STAR JUMP

pages 130–131

- Perform for 30 seconds.
- Aim for 8–12 repetitions.

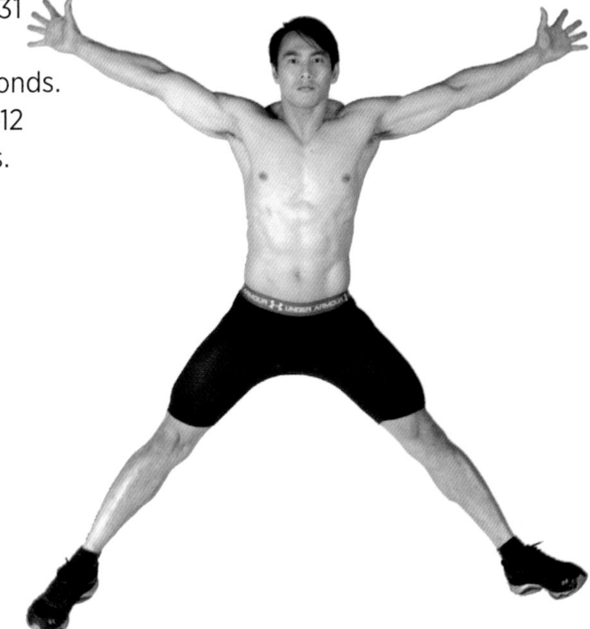

8 SWITCH LUNGE

pages 110–111

- Perform for 30 seconds.
- Aim for 8–12 repetitions.

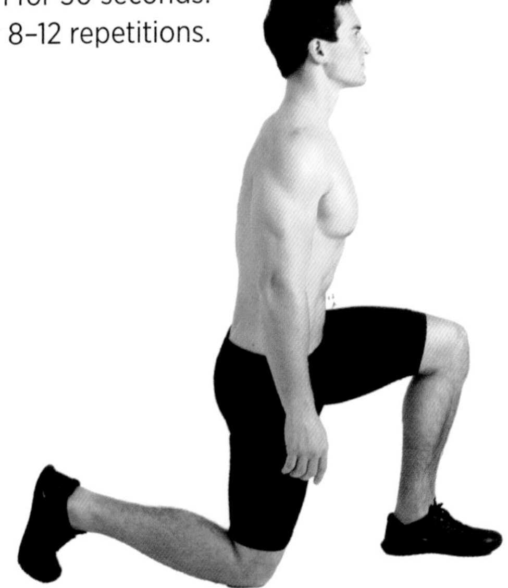

Resisted Legs

This routine takes you through movements that use a variety of resistance tools to condition your lower body.

1 DUMBBELL LUNGE

pages 210–211

- Perform for 30 seconds.
- Aim for 8–12 repetitions.

2 KETTLEBELL FIGURE 8

pages 218–219

- Perform for 30 seconds.
- Aim for 8–12 repetitions.

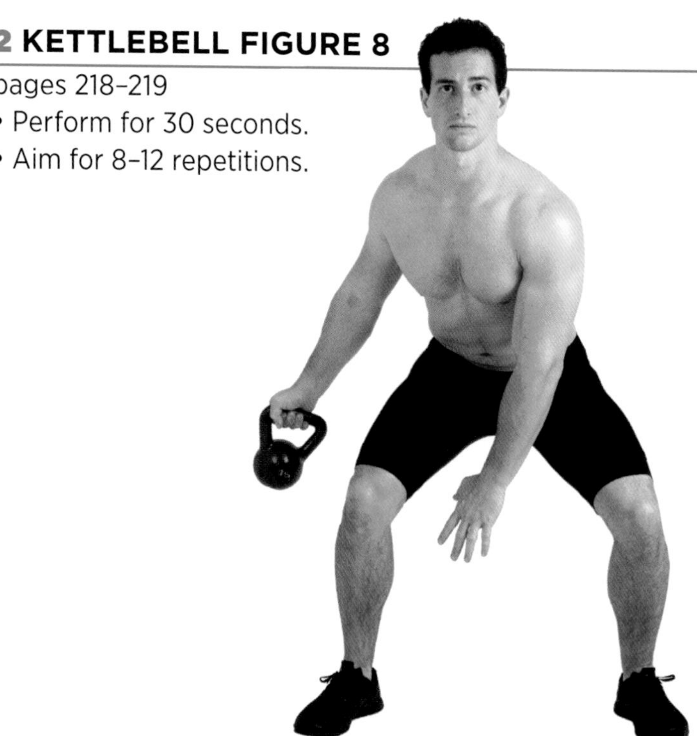

3 FRONT RACK BARBELL LUNGE

page 308

- Perform for 30 seconds.
- Aim for 8–12 repetitions.

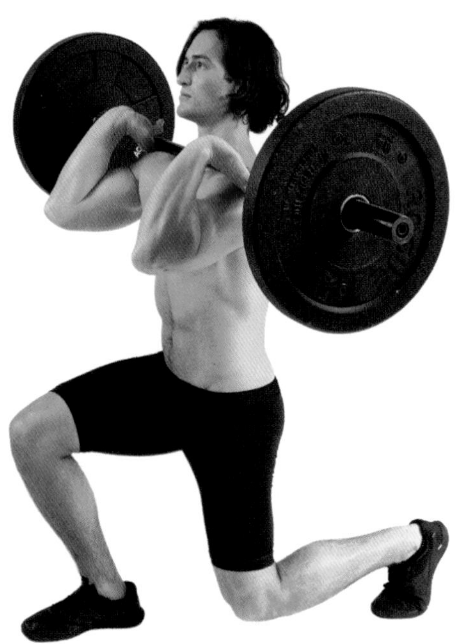

4 FLAT BENCH DUMBBELL SQUAT

pages 206–207

- Perform for 30 seconds.
- Aim for 8–12 repetitions.

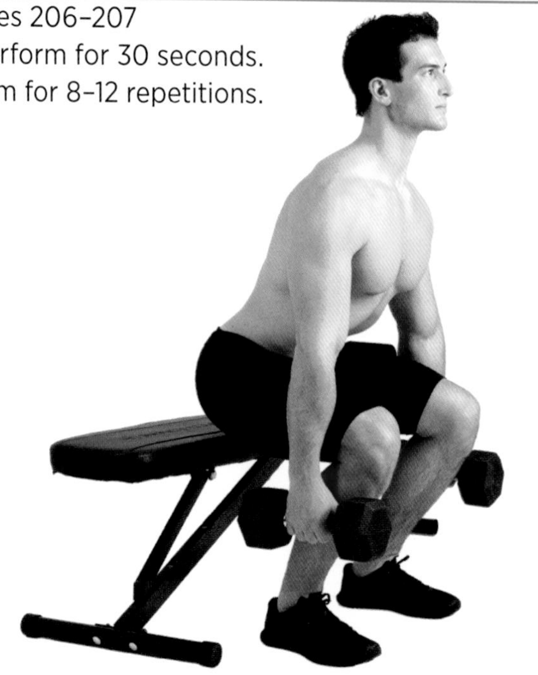

FACT FILE

LEVEL
- Intermediate

OBJECTIVE
- Lower-extremity hypertrophy

WORK/REST
- 1:2 (30 seconds per exercise/60 seconds rest)

TOTAL TIME
- 60 minutes

TOTAL COMPLETED CIRCUIT SETS
- 5 sets

5 SWISS BALL HAMSTRINGS CURL

pages 302–303

- Perform for 30 seconds.
- Aim for 8–12 repetitions.

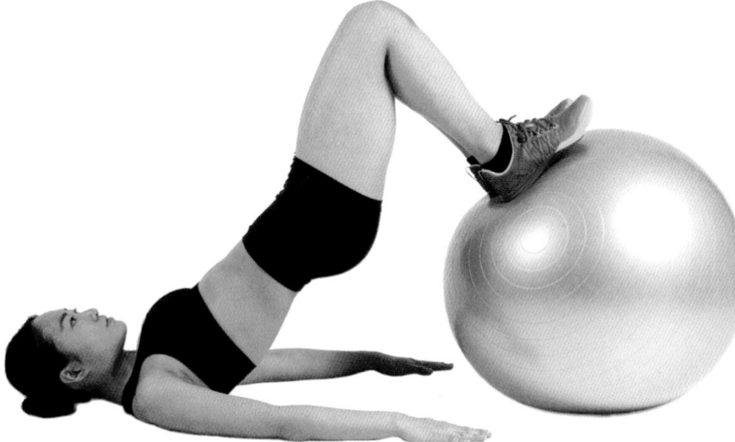

6 KETTLEBELL SINGLE-LEG RUSSIAN DEADLIFT

page 212

- Perform for 30 seconds.
- Aim for 8–12 repetitions.

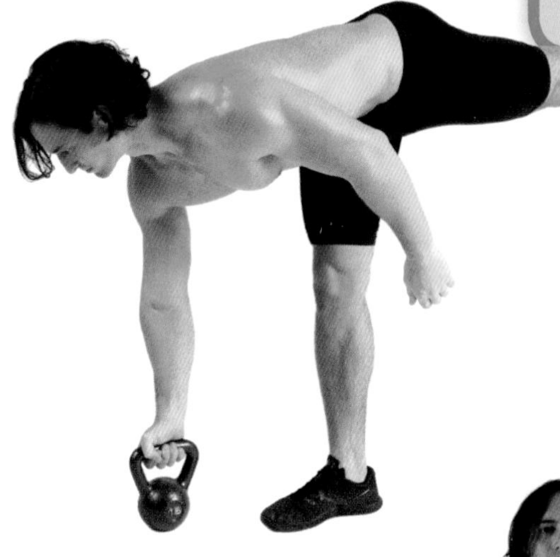

7 SPLIT SQUAT WITH OVERHEAD PRESS

pages 228–229

- Perform for 30 seconds.
- Aim for 8–12 repetitions.

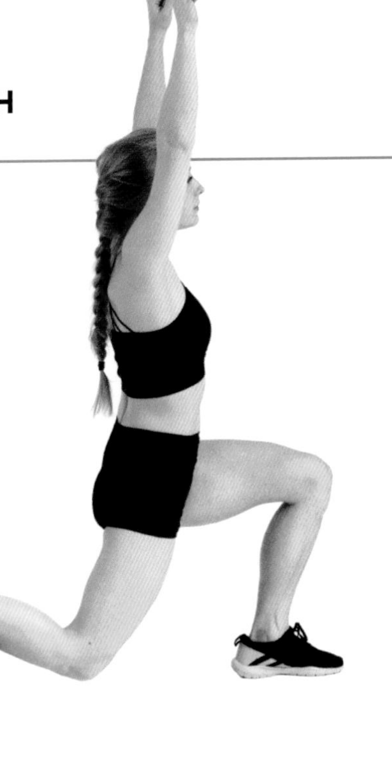

8 TOWEL ABDUCTION AND ADDUCTION

page 125

- Perform for 30 seconds.
- Aim for 8–12 repetitions.

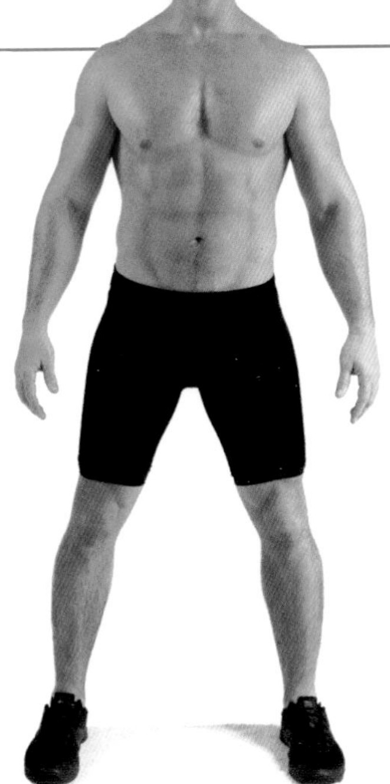

Push Circuit I

This routine takes you through an hour-long circuit of pushing exercises to tone and define a majority of the muscle groups that make up your ventral aspect.

1 SINGLE-ARM KETTLEBELL PRESS-UP

page 204

- Perform for 30 seconds.
- Aim for 8–12 repetitions.

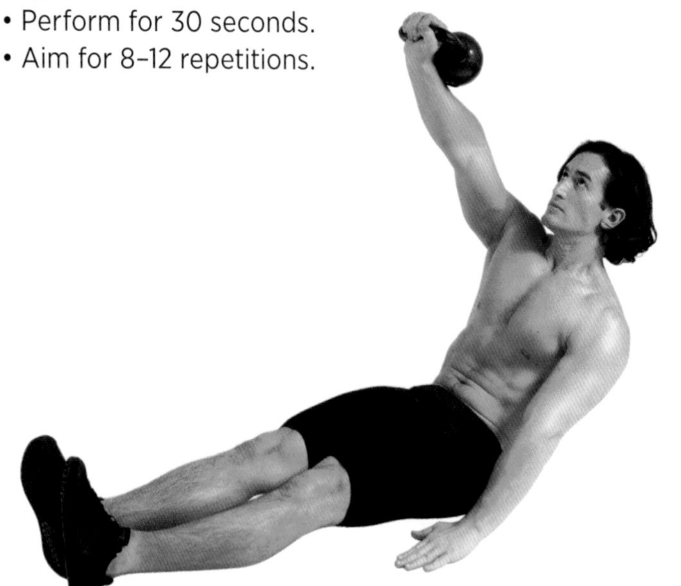

2 SHOULDER RAISE AND PULL

pages 170–171

- Perform for 30 seconds.
- Aim for 8–12 repetitions.

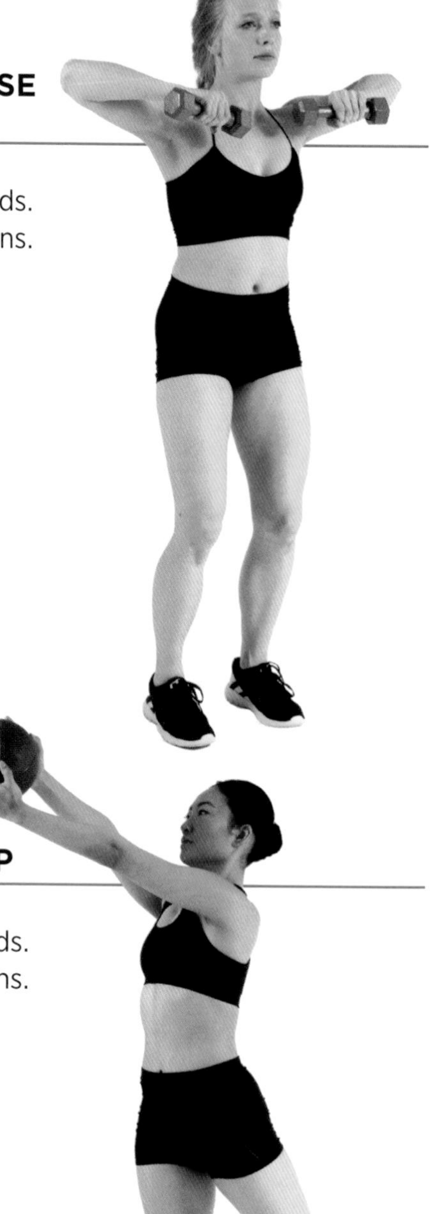

3 PLYO POWER STAND PUSH-UP

pages 190–191

- Perform for 30 seconds.
- Aim for 8–12 repetitions.

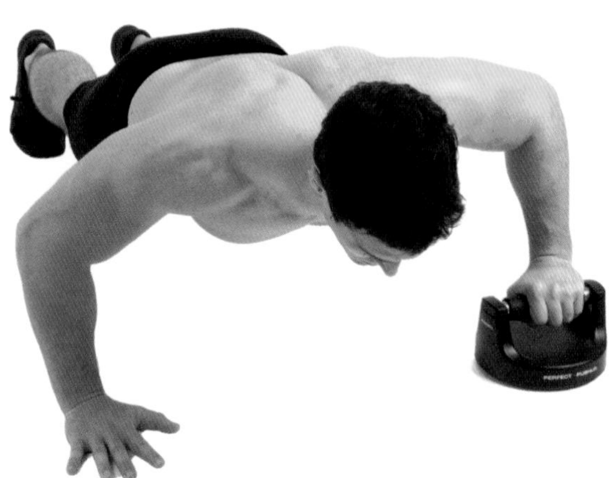

4 MEDICINE BALL WOODCHOP

pages 288–289

- Perform for 30 seconds.
- Aim for 8–12 repetitions.

FACT FILE

LEVEL
- Intermediate

OBJECTIVE
- Chest, abdominal, leg, shoulder, and arm hypertrophy

WORK/REST
- 1:2 (30 seconds per exercise/60 seconds rest)

TOTAL TIME
- 60 minutes

TOTAL COMPLETED CIRCUIT SETS
- 5 sets

5 PLANK-UP

pages 68–69

- Perform for 30 seconds.
- Aim for 8–12 repetitions.

6 BEAR CRAWL

page 132-133

- Perform for 30 seconds.
- Aim for 8–12 repetitions.

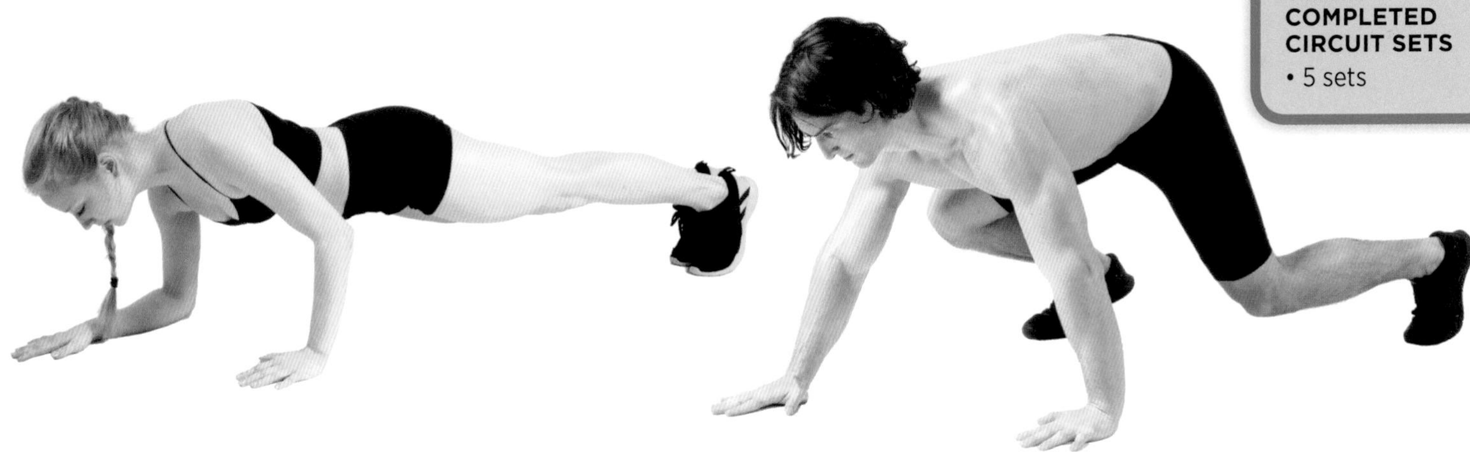

7 BOX JUMP

pages 116–117

- Perform for 30 seconds.
- Aim for 8–12 repetitions.

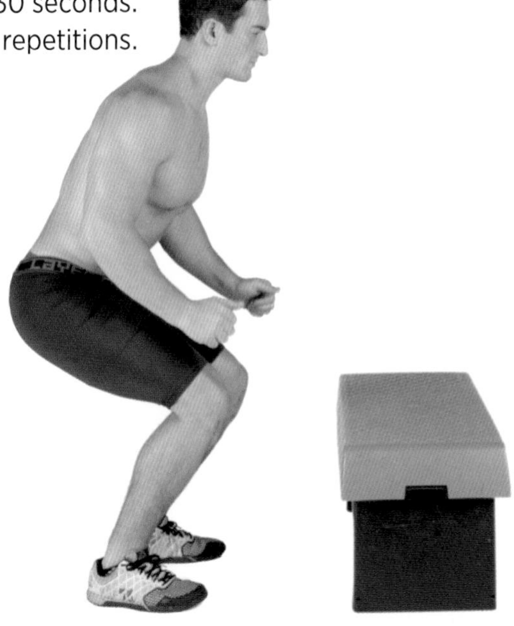

8 TOWEL FLY

pages 84–85

- Perform for 30 seconds.
- Aim for 8–12 repetitions.

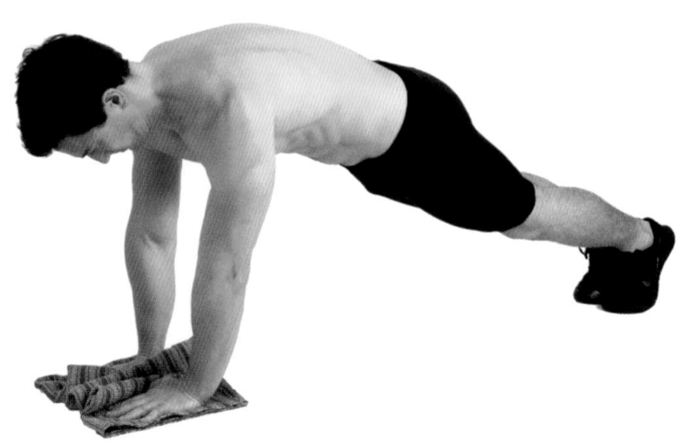

Pull Circuit I

This routine takes you through various equipment movements to tone and condition all of your pulling muscles.

1 CHIN-UP

pages 46–47

- Perform for 30 seconds.
- Aim for 8–12 repetitions.

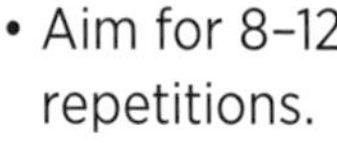

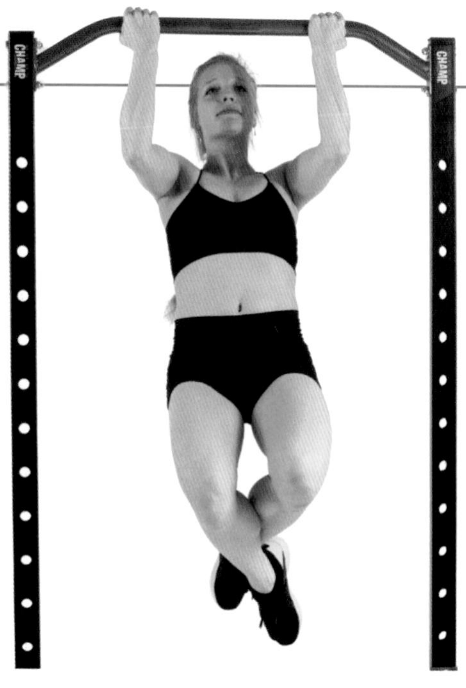

2 ADVANCED SUPERMAN

page 52

- Perform for 30 seconds.
- Aim for 8–12 repetitions.

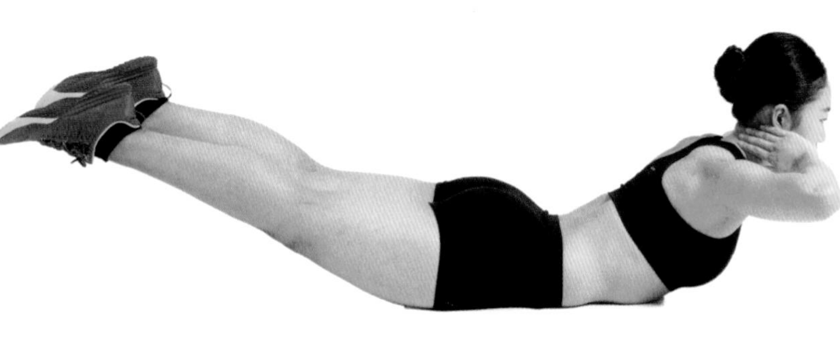

3 DUMBBELL UPRIGHT ROW

page 148

- Perform for 30 seconds.
- Aim for 8–12 repetitions.

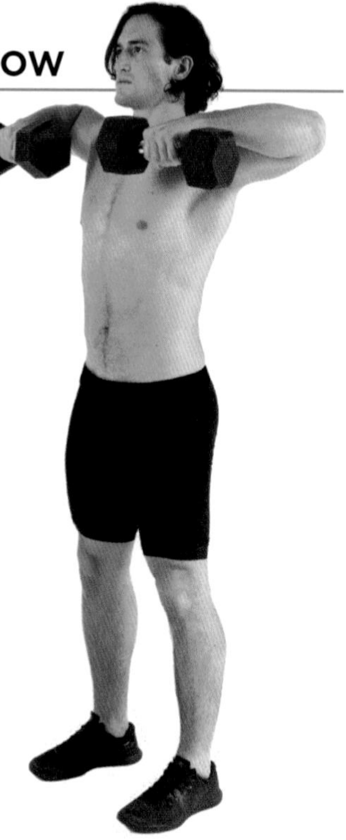

4 SUPINE REVERSE-GRIP BACK ROW

page 72

- Perform for 30 seconds.
- Aim for 8–12 repetitions.

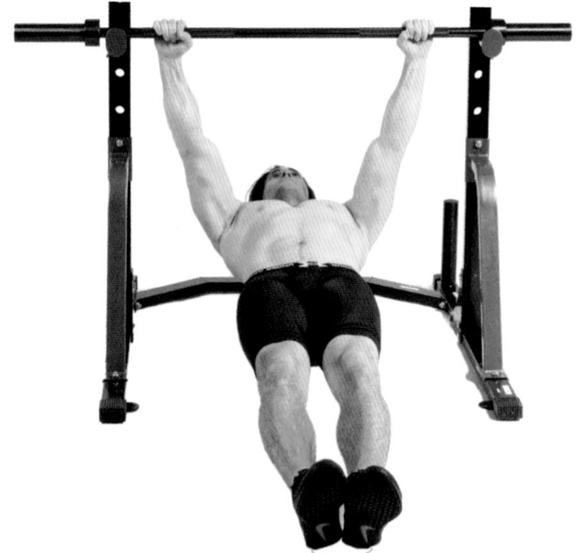

FACT FILE

LEVEL
- Intermediate

OBJECTIVE
- Arm, back, and rear shoulder hypertrophy

WORK/REST
- 1:2 (30 seconds per exercise/60 seconds rest)

TOTAL TIME
- 60 minutes

TOTAL COMPLETED CIRCUIT SETS
- 5 sets

5 HAMSTRINGS PULL-IN

pages 304–305
- Perform for 30 seconds.
- Aim for 8–12 repetitions.

6 BARBELL BENT-OVER ROW

pages 246–247
- Perform for 30 seconds.
- Aim for 8–12 repetitions.

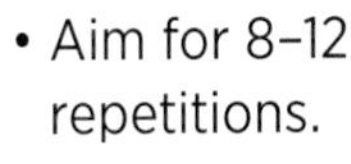

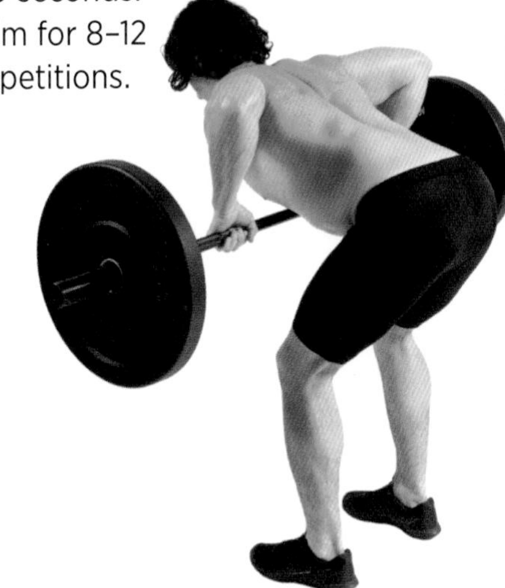

7 ROLL-UP

page 142
- Perform for 30 seconds.
- Aim for 8–12 repetitions.

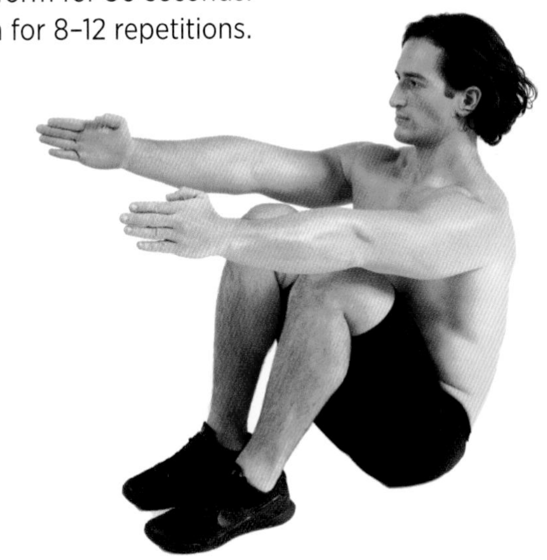

8 BARBELL HANG CLEAN

pages 264–265
- Perform for 30 seconds.
- Aim for 8–12 repetitions.

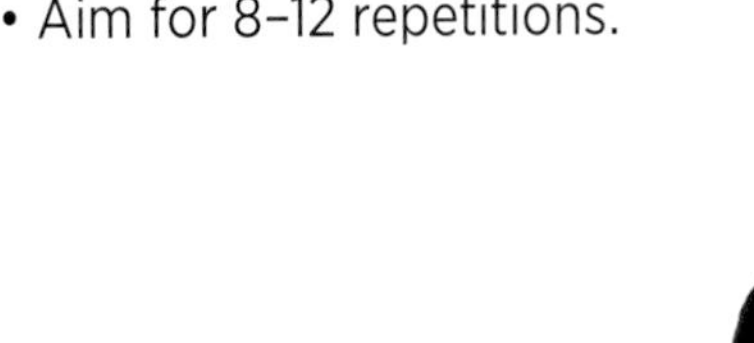

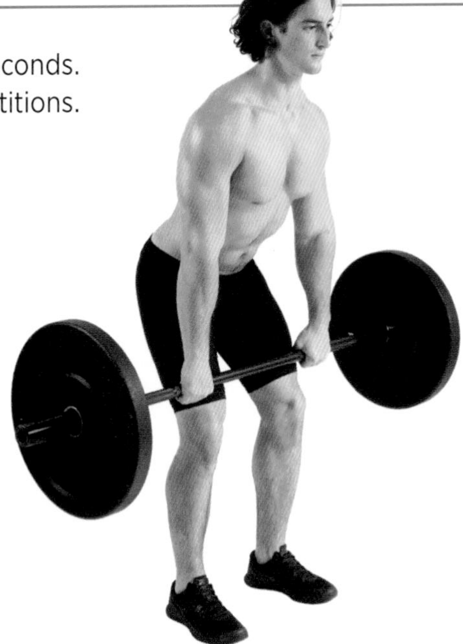

Push Circuit II

In this circuit, rather than a rest interval, you will have a sub-max interval, performing another exercise at less intensity. You'll challenge your body without reprieve, getting the ultimate workout.

1 PLYO GOBLET SQUAT

pages 214–215

- Perform for 60 seconds.
- Aim for as many repetitions as you can perform.

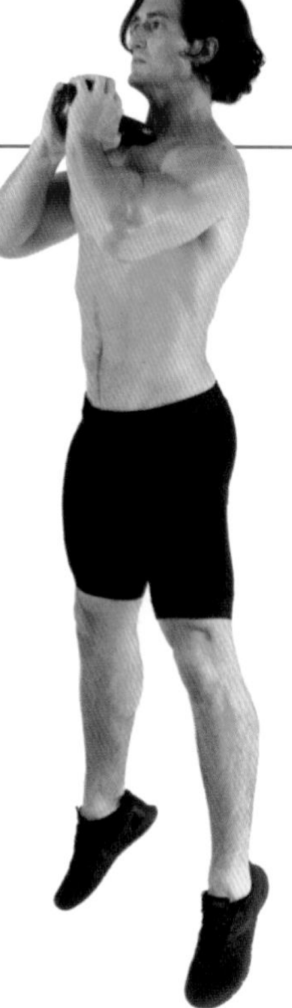

2 ROLLING DUMBBELL FLY

page 193

- Perform for 60 seconds, sub-max.
- Aim for 4–6 repetitions.

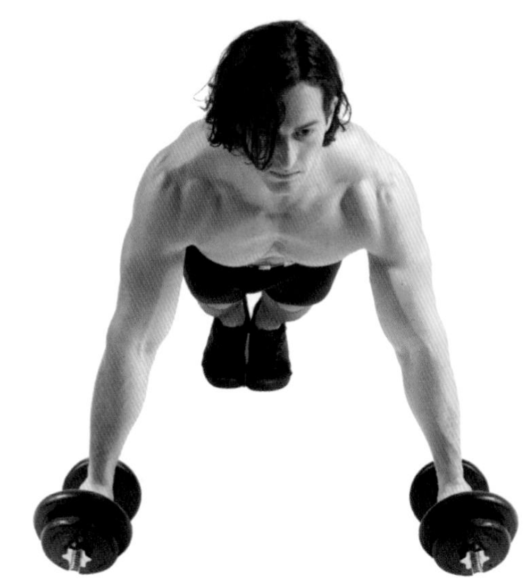

3 HANDSTAND PUSH-UP

pages 74–75

- Perform for 60 seconds.
- Aim for as many repetitions as you can perform.

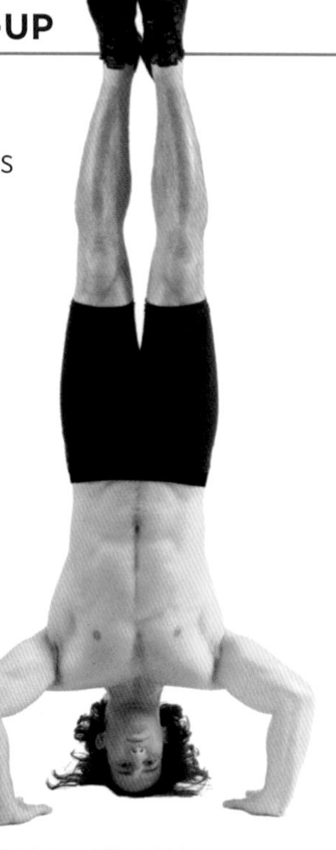

4 SPRAWL PUSH-UP

pages 86–87

- Perform for 60 seconds, sub-max.
- Aim for 4–6 repetitions.

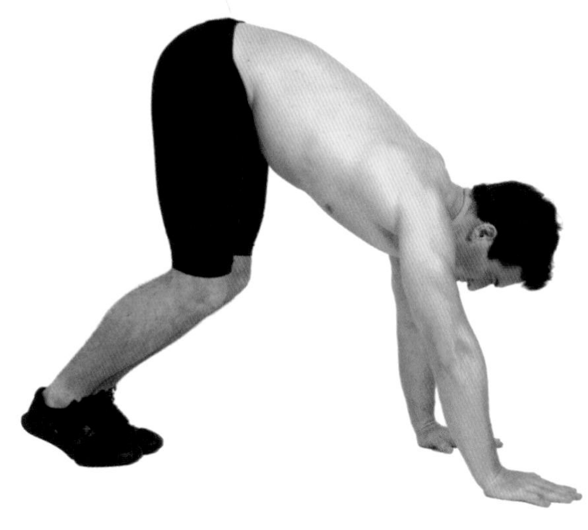

5 TWO-LEVEL PUSH-UP

pages 278–279

- Perform for 60 seconds.
- Aim for as many repetitions as you can perform.

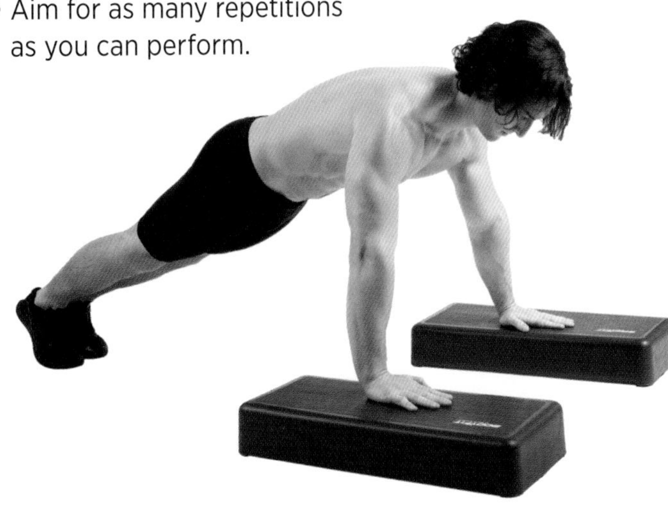

6 ALTERNATING SINGLE-ARM PUSH-UP

pages 80–81

- Perform for 60 seconds, sub-max.
- Aim for 4–6 repetitions.

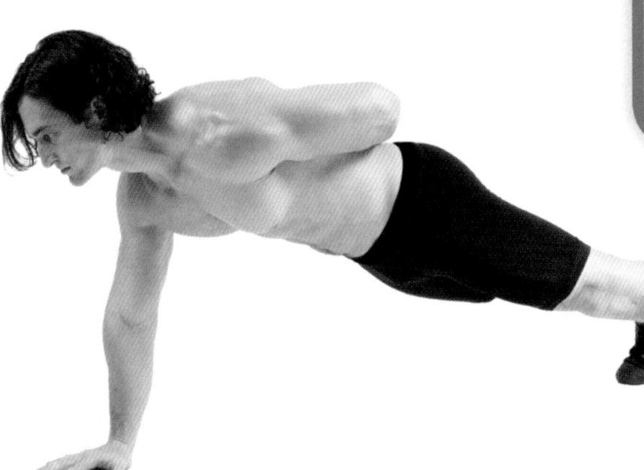

7 BARBELL POWER CLEAN AND JERK

pages 314–315

- Perform for 60 seconds.
- Aim for as many repetitions as you can perform.

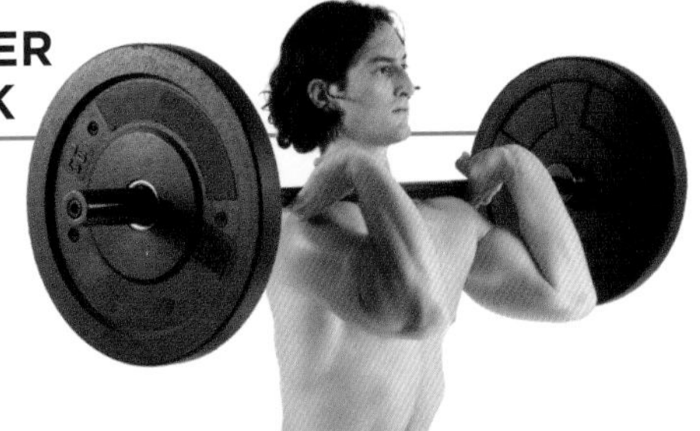

8 LAYOUT PUSH-UP

page 61

- Perform for 60 seconds, sub-max.
- Aim for 4–6 repetitions.

FACT FILE

LEVEL
- Advanced

OBJECTIVE
- Total-body strength

WORK/SUB-MAX WORK
- 1:1 (60 seconds per exercise/60 seconds per sub-max exercise)

TOTAL TIME
- 40 minutes

TOTAL COMPLETED CIRCUIT SETS
- 5 sets

Pull Circuit II

This routine focuses mainly on pulling movements driven by your posterior chain. With body-weight and resistance exercises intertwined, this circuit calls for you to bring your best.

1 CHIN-UP WITH HANGING LEG RAISE

pages 312–313

- Perform for 30 seconds.
- Aim for 4–6 repetitions.

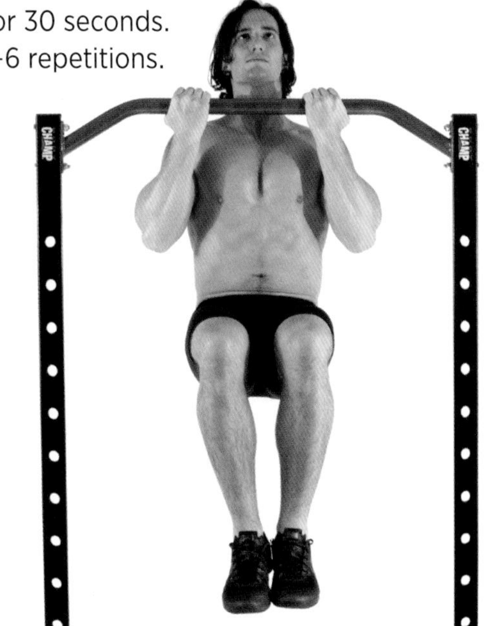

2 KETTLEBELL WINDMILL

pages 200–201

- Perform for 30 seconds.
- Aim for 4–6 repetitions.

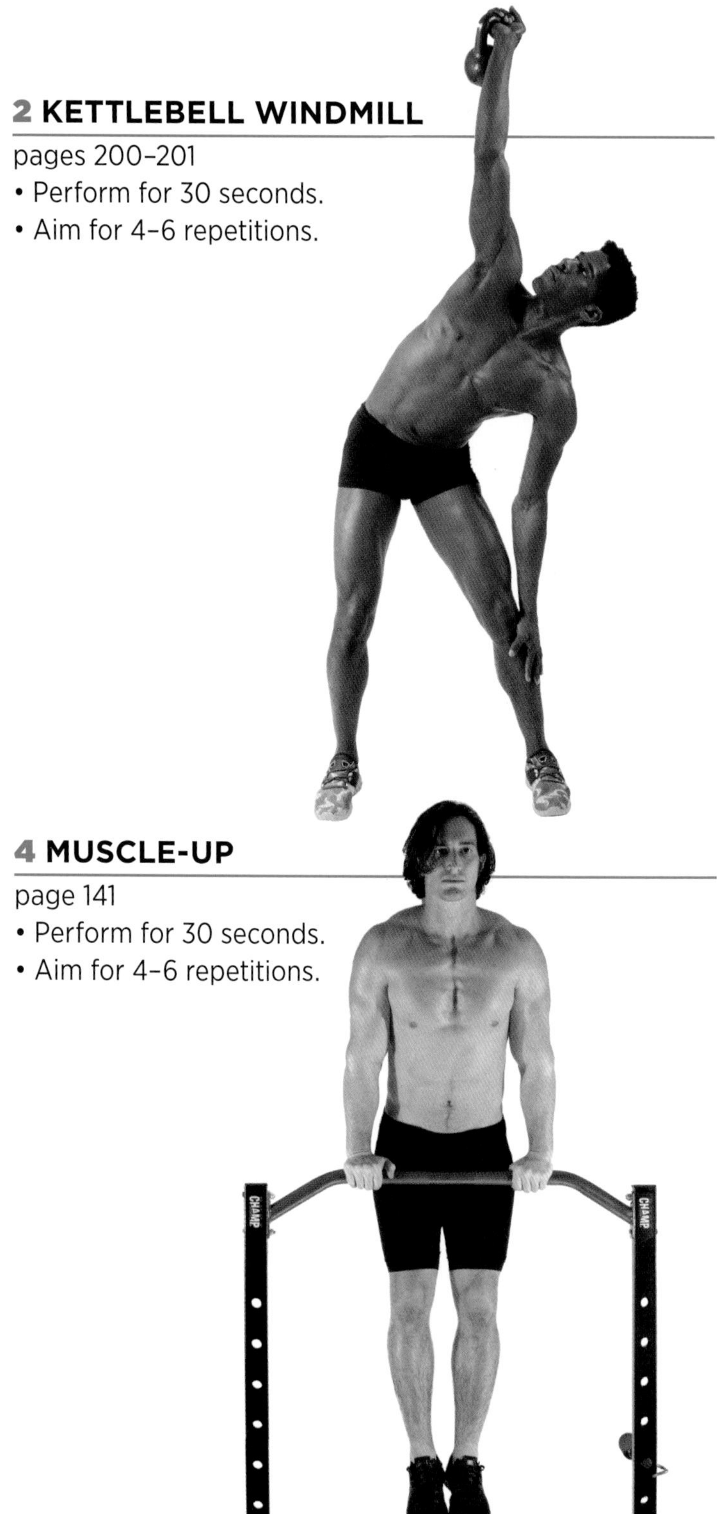

3 ALTERNATING RENEGADE ROW

pages 158–159

- Perform for 30 seconds.
- Aim for 4–6 repetitions.

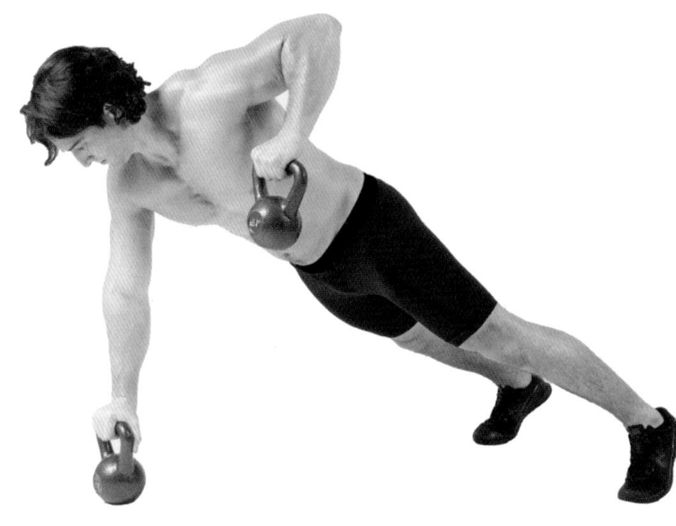

4 MUSCLE-UP

page 141

- Perform for 30 seconds.
- Aim for 4–6 repetitions.

FACT FILE

LEVEL
- Advanced

OBJECTIVE
- Total-body strength

WORK/REST
- 1:1 (30 seconds per exercise/30 seconds rest)

TOTAL TIME
- 40 minutes

TOTAL COMPLETED CIRCUIT SETS
- 5 sets

5 SWISS BALL ROLLOUT

pages 296–297
- Perform for 30 seconds.
- Aim for 4–6 repetitions.

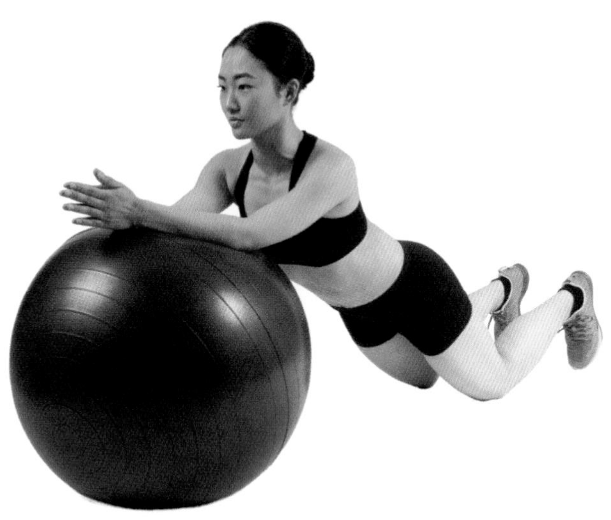

6 DUMBBELL POWER CLEAN AND PRESS

page 233
- Perform for 30 seconds.
- Aim for 4–6 repetitions.

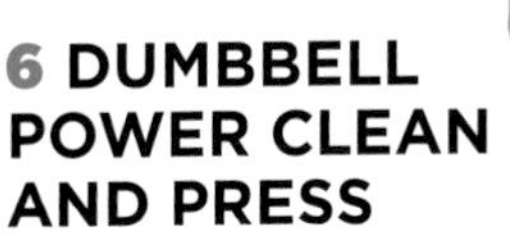

7 DOUBLE KETTLEBELL SNATCH

pages 222–223
- Perform for 30 seconds.
- Aim for 4–6 repetitions.

8 LUNGE WITH DUMBBELL UPRIGHT ROW

pages 230–231
- Perform for 30 seconds.
- Aim for 4–6 repetitions.

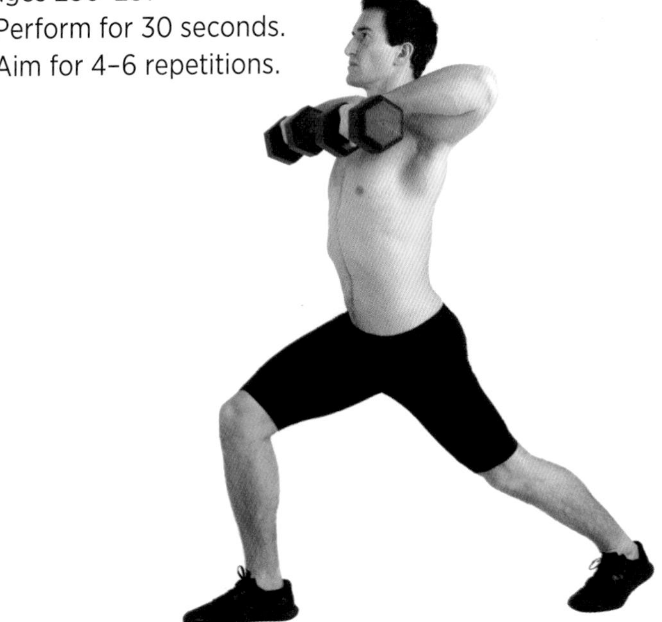

Functional Circuit

This routine uses functional movements to create a circuit that will give you an intense full-body workout that hits every part of you.

1 SINGLE-ARM MEDICINE BALL PUSH-UP

page 280

- Perform for 60 seconds.
- Aim for 4–6 repetitions.

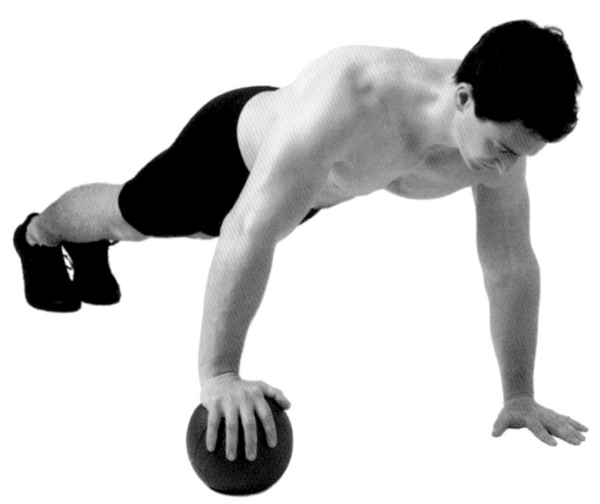

2 OVERHEAD SQUAT

page 309

- Perform for 60 seconds.
- Aim for 4–6 repetitions.

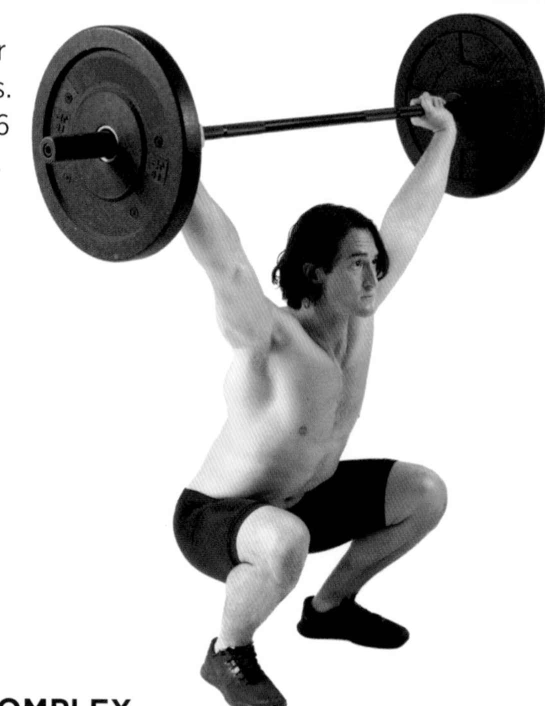

3 BARBELL DEADLIFT

pages 240–241

- Perform for 60 seconds.
- Aim for 4–6 repetitions.

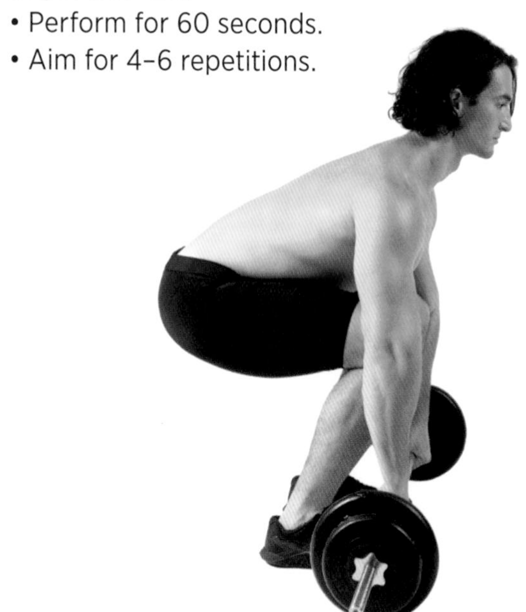

4 BEAR COMPLEX

pages 322–323

- Perform for 60 seconds.
- Aim for 4–6 repetitions.

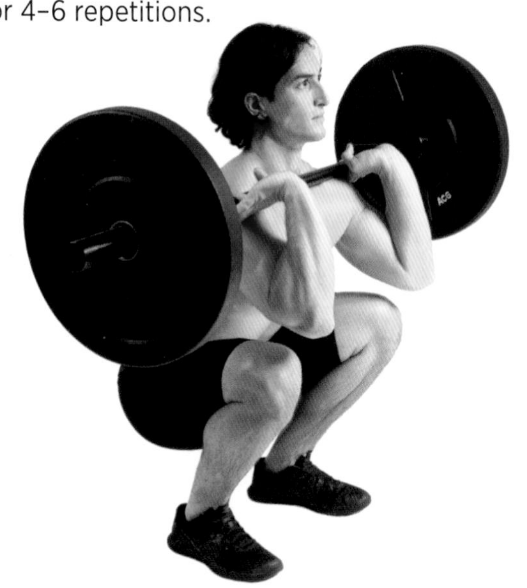

5 BARBELL SQUAT SNATCH

pages 316–317

- Perform for 60 seconds.
- Aim for 4–6 repetitions.

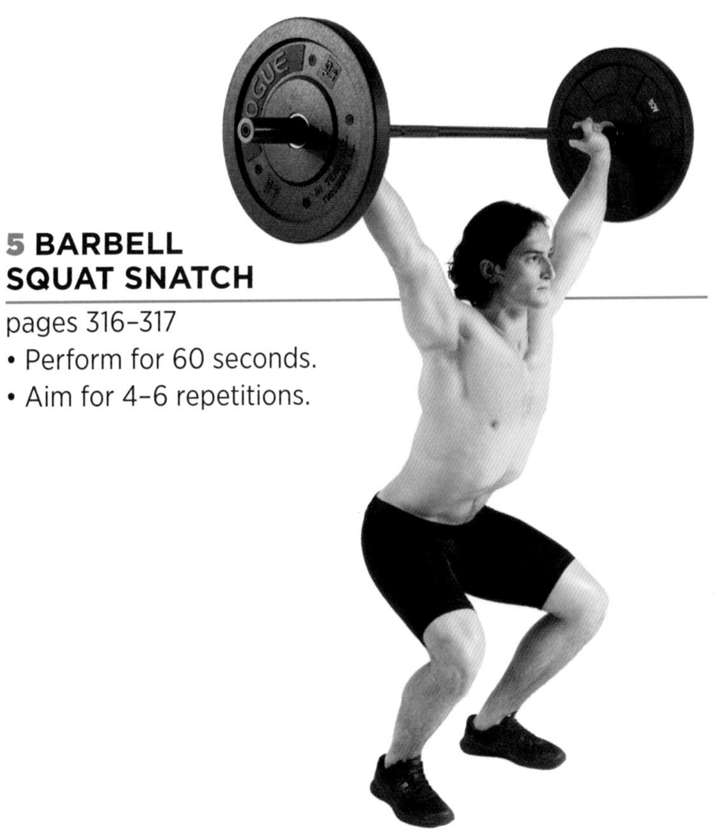

6 BURPEE

pages 128-129

- Perform for 60 seconds.
- Aim for 4–6 repetitions.

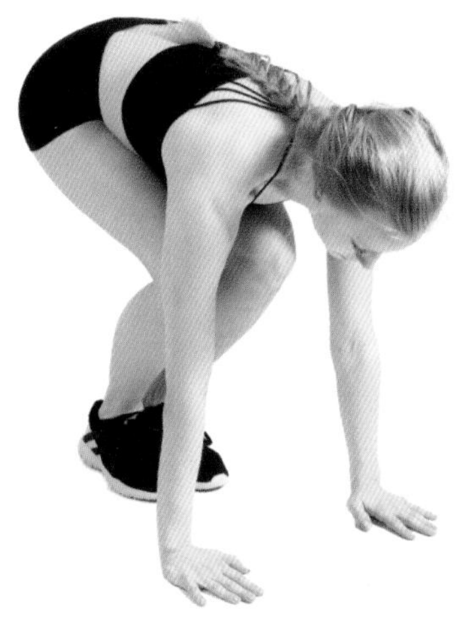

FACT FILE

LEVEL

- Advanced

OBJECTIVE

- Total-body strength

WORK/REST

- 1:1 (30 seconds per exercise/30 seconds rest)

TOTAL TIME

- 40 minutes

TOTAL COMPLETED CIRCUIT SETS

- 5 sets

7 V-SIT KETTLEBELL HOLD WITH LEG LIFT

page 197

- Perform for 60 seconds.
- Aim for 4–6 repetitions.

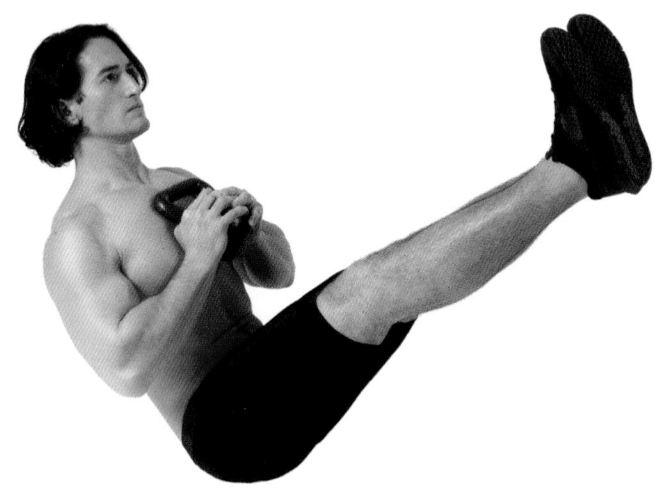

8 ALTERNATING KETTLEBELL SWING

pages 224–225

- Perform for 60 seconds.
- Aim for 4–6 repetitions.

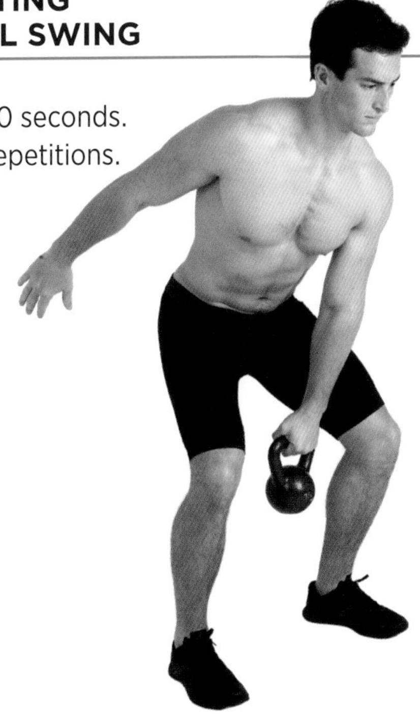

High-Energy Circuit

This routine uses high-energy movements that include jumping, crawling, rolling, and squatting to give yourself a full-body workout.

1 PISTOL

page 123

- Perform for 60 seconds.
- Aim for 4–6 repetitions.

2 STAR PUSH-UP

page 89

- Perform for 60 seconds.
- Aim for 4–6 repetitions.

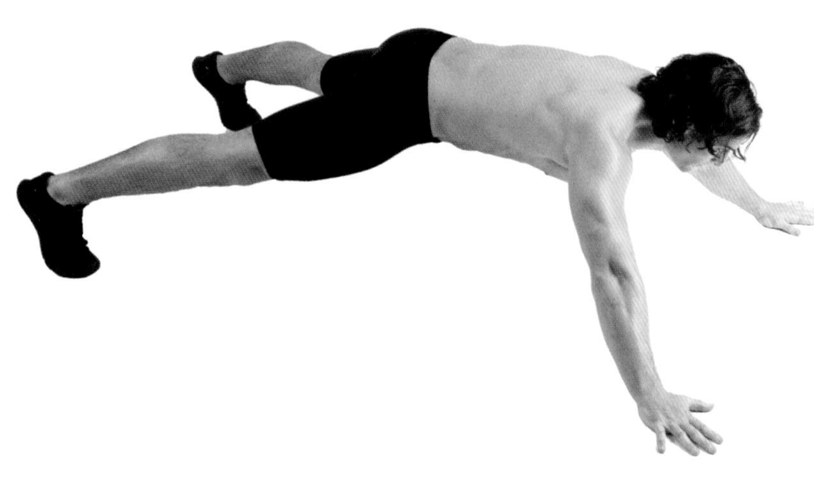

3 HANDSTAND WALK

page 140

- Perform for 60 seconds.
- Aim for 4–6 repetition.

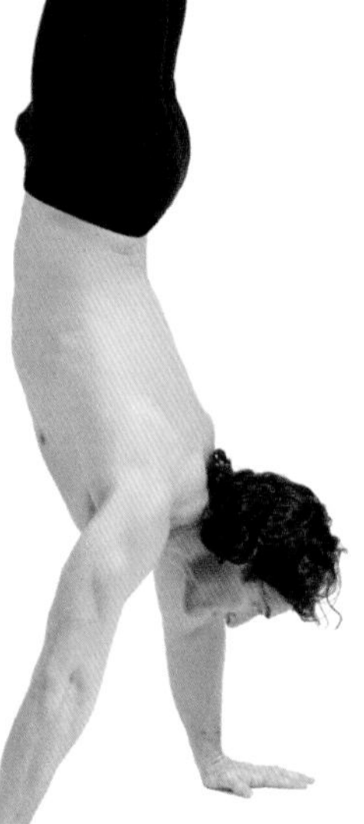

4 HOLLOW HOLD TO SUPERMAN

page 105

- Perform for 60 seconds.
- Aim for 4–6 repetitions.

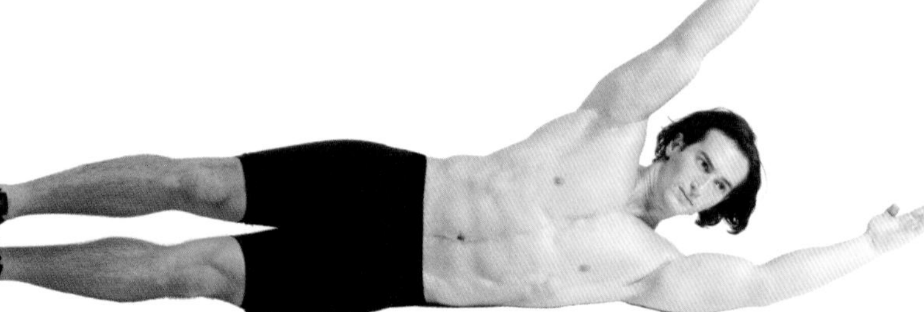

FACT FILE

LEVEL
• Advanced

OBJECTIVE
• Total-body strength

WORK/REST
• 1:1 (30 seconds per exercise/30 seconds rest)

TOTAL TIME
• 40 minutes

TOTAL COMPLETED CIRCUIT SETS
• 5 sets

5 KNEELING SQUAT JUMP

page 127

• Perform for 60 seconds.
• Aim for 4–6 repetitions.

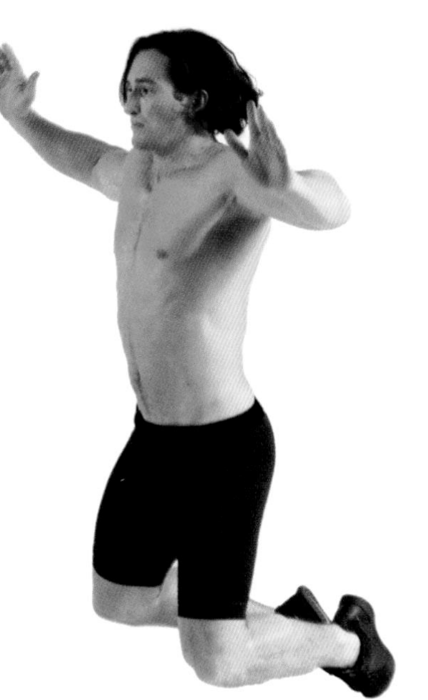

6 ALLIGATOR CRAWL

pages 134-135

• Perform for 60 seconds.
• Aim for 4–6 repetitions.

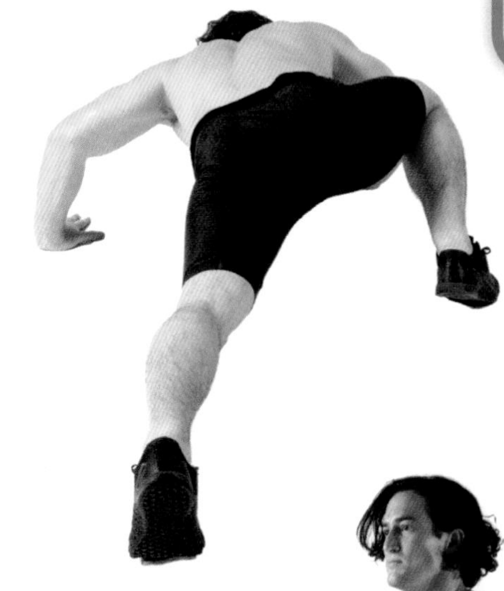

7 KITCHEN SINK

pages 234–235

• Perform for 60 seconds.
• Aim for 4–6 repetitions.

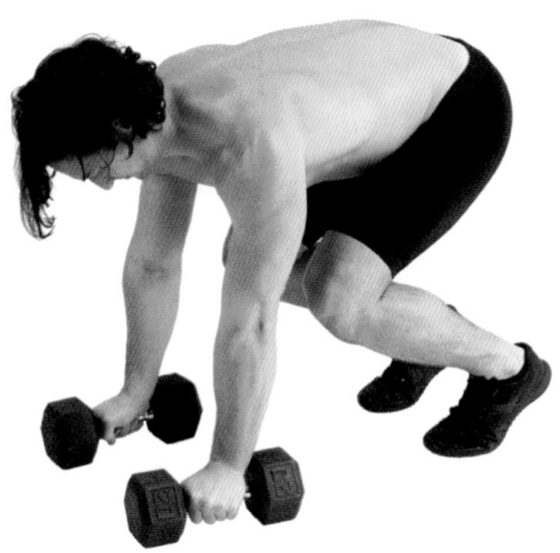

8 PLYO KNEE DRIVE

page 122

• Perform for 60 seconds.
• Aim for 4–6 repetitions.

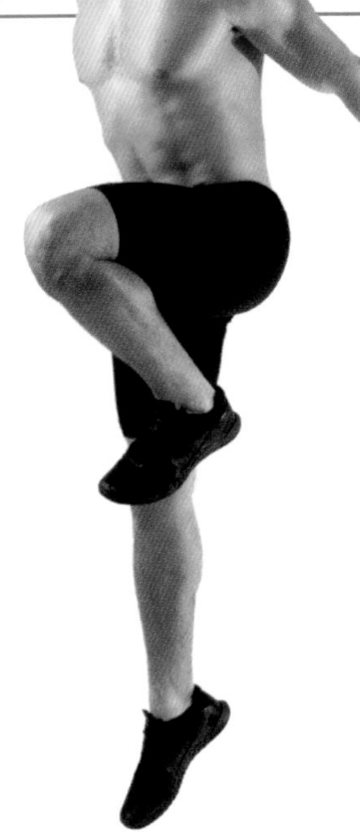

Mix-and-Match Circuits

Once you have become familiar with the fundamentals of HIIT, you will be ready to start formulating your own workouts to suit your unique fitness goals and level of ability. The following pages feature sample circuits that will inspire you to create HIIT routines that work for you. Refer to Chart A on page 15 to determine the number of repetitions to aim for, depending on your goal.

Back Circuit

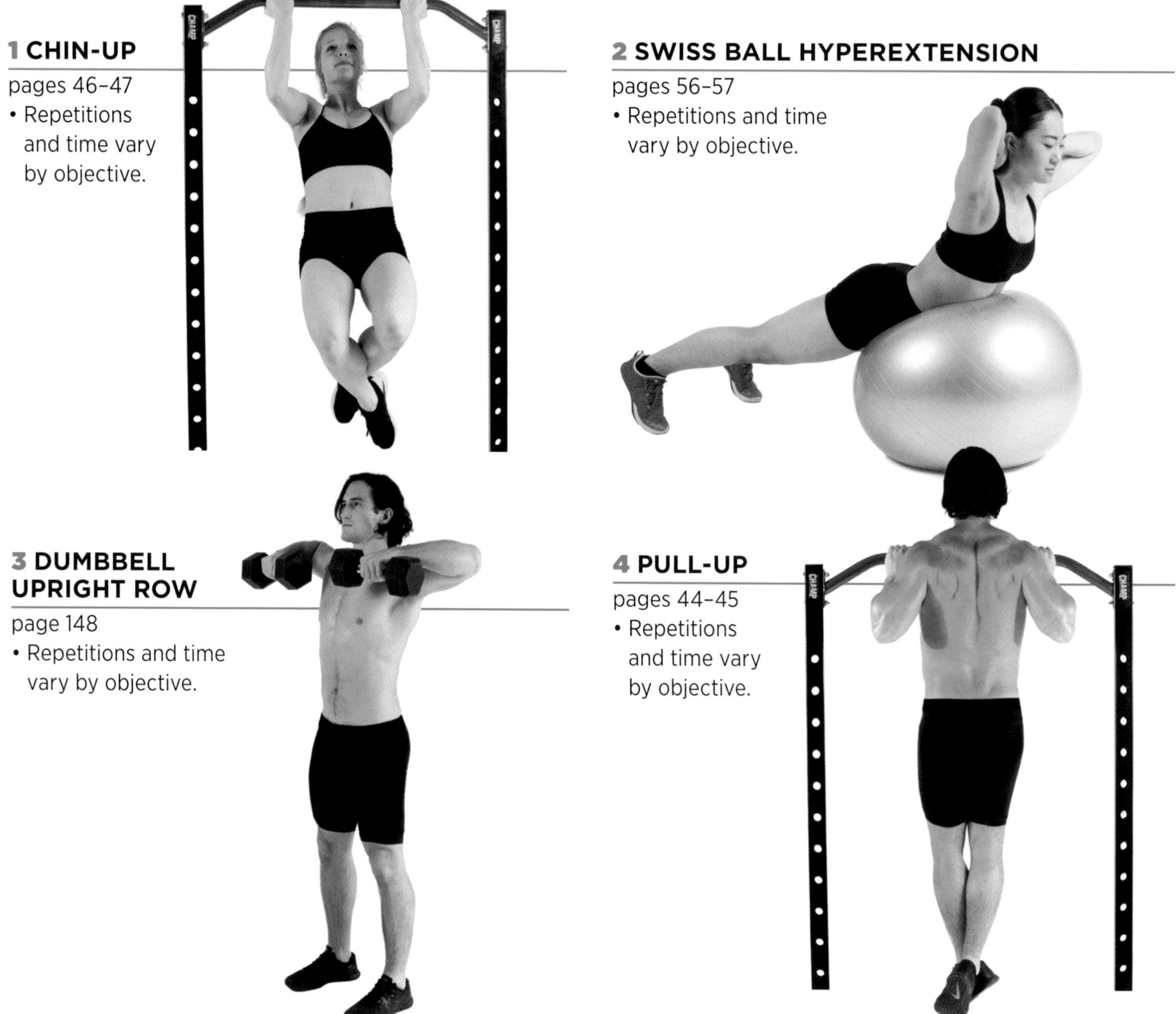

1 CHIN-UP
pages 46–47
- Repetitions and time vary by objective.

2 SWISS BALL HYPEREXTENSION
pages 56–57
- Repetitions and time vary by objective.

3 DUMBBELL UPRIGHT ROW
page 148
- Repetitions and time vary by objective.

4 PULL-UP
pages 44–45
- Repetitions and time vary by objective.

Arm Circuit

FACT FILE

LEVEL
- All levels

OBJECTIVE
- Varies

WORK/REST
- Varies by objective

TOTAL TIME
- Varies by objective

TOTAL COMPLETED CIRCUIT SETS
- Varies by objective

1 SINGLE-ARM TRICEPS KICKBACK

page 181
- Repetitions and time vary by objective.

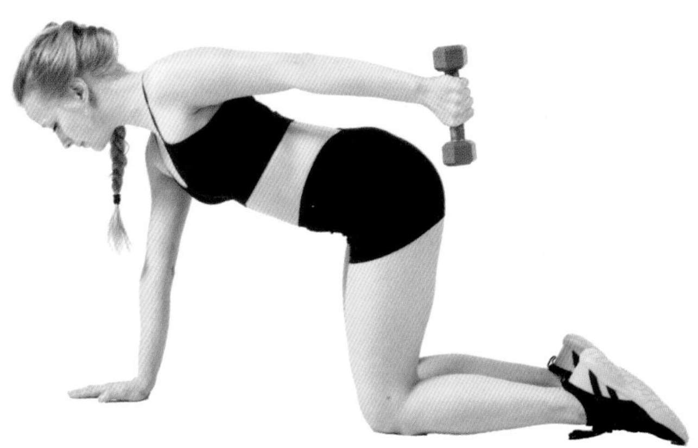

2 INCHWORM

pages 66–67
- Repetitions and time vary by objective.

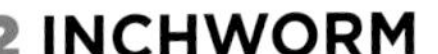

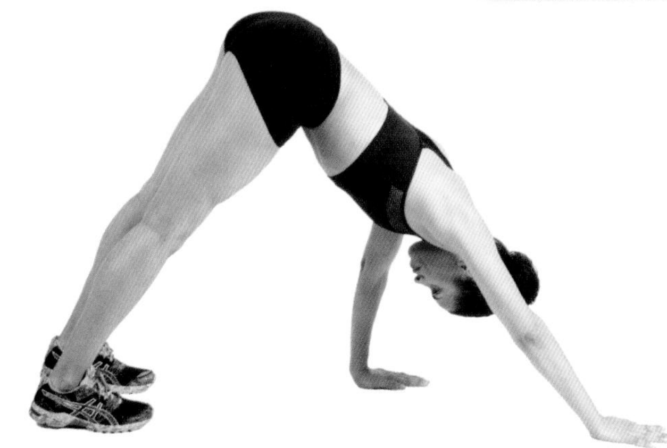

3 ARNOLD PRESS

page 167
- Repetitions and time vary by objective.

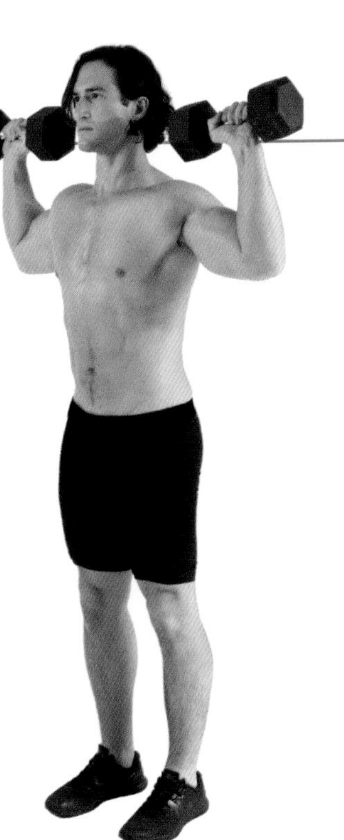

4 BAR DIP

page 73
- Repetitions and time vary by objective.

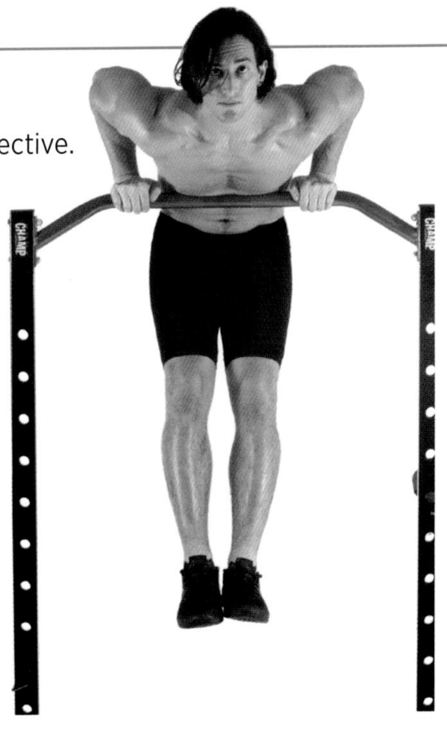

Chest Circuit

1 SHOULDER-TAP PUSH-UP

pages 78–79

- Repetitions and time vary by objective.

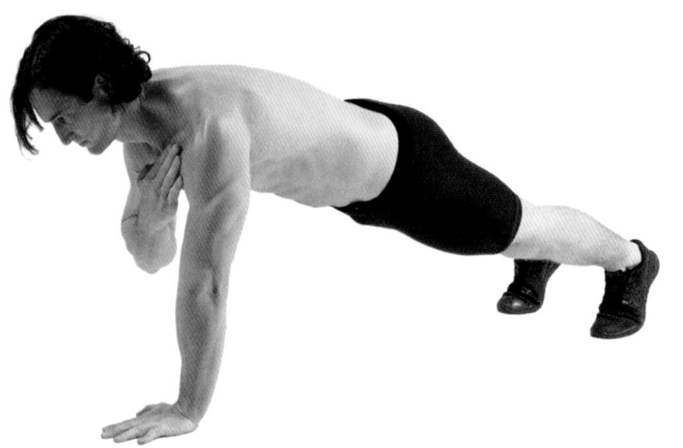

2 SINGLE DUMBBELL PUSH-UP

page 192

- Repetitions and time vary by objective.

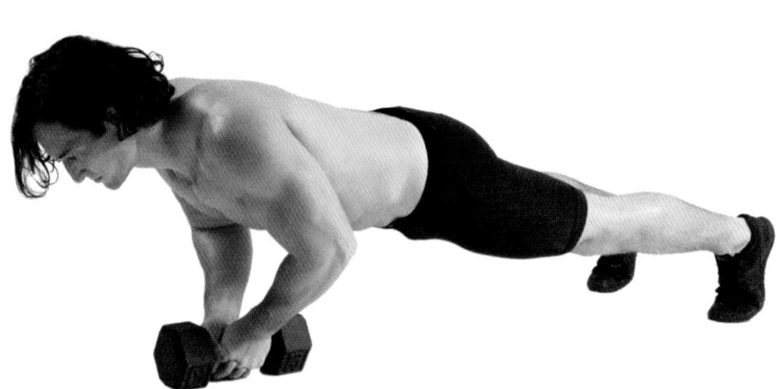

3 DIVE-BOMBER PUSH-UP

pages 82–83

- Repetitions and time vary by objective.

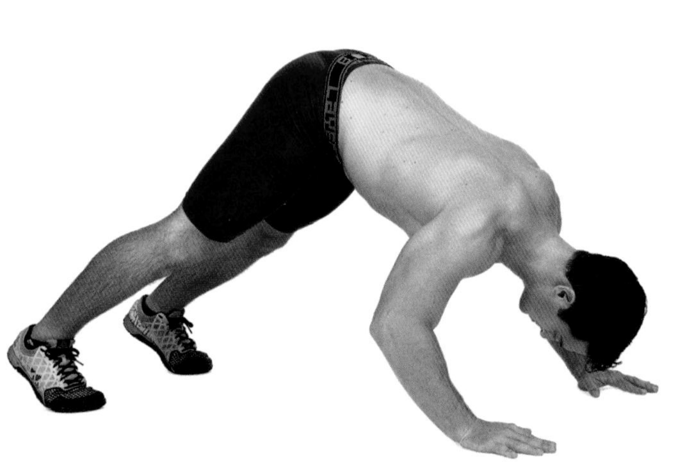

4 ROLLER PUSH-UP

pages 274–275

- Repetitions and time vary by objective.

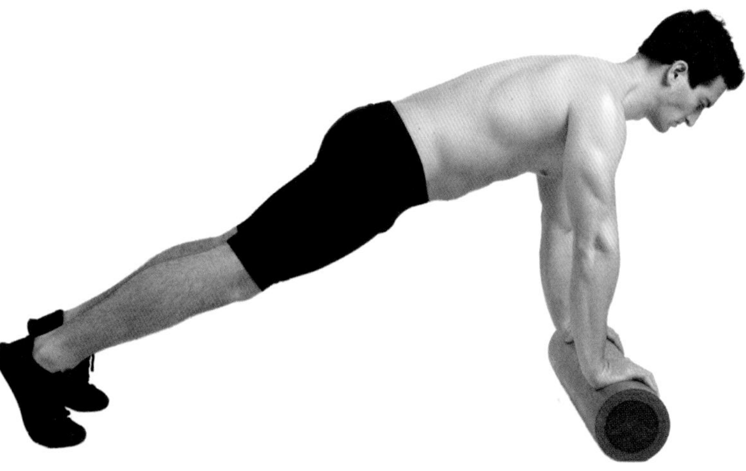

Core Circuit

FACT FILE

LEVEL
- All levels

OBJECTIVE
- Varies

WORK/REST
- Varies by objective

TOTAL TIME
- Varies by objective

TOTAL COMPLETED CIRCUIT SETS
- Varies by objective

1 METRONOME

page 104
- Repetitions and time vary by objective.

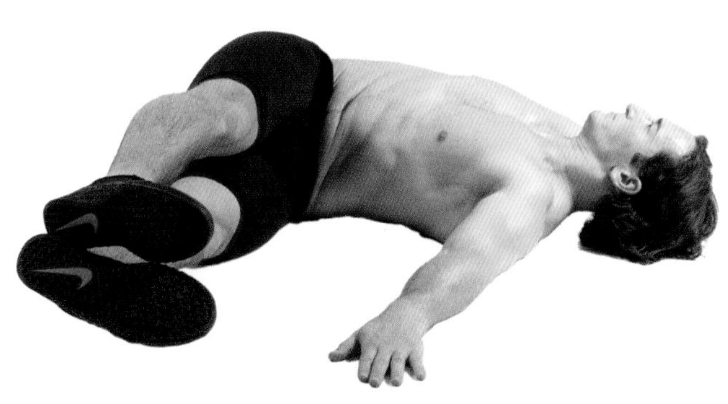

2 HIGH PLANK KICK-THROUGH

page 143
- Repetitions and time vary by objective.

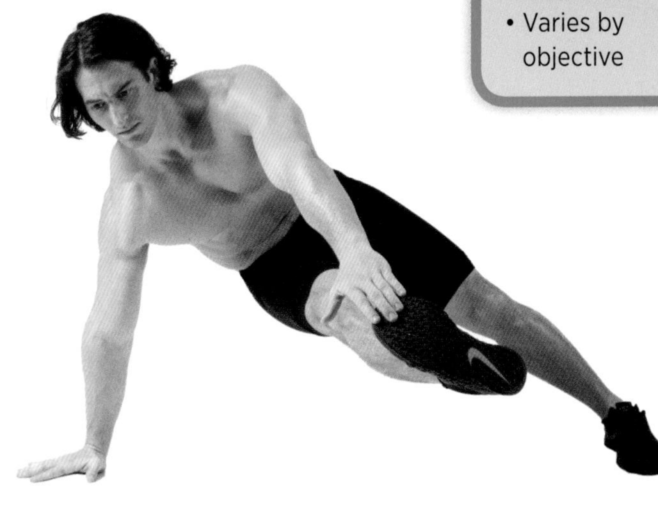

3 SCISSORS OVER DUMBBELLS

pages 194–195
- Repetitions and time vary by objective.

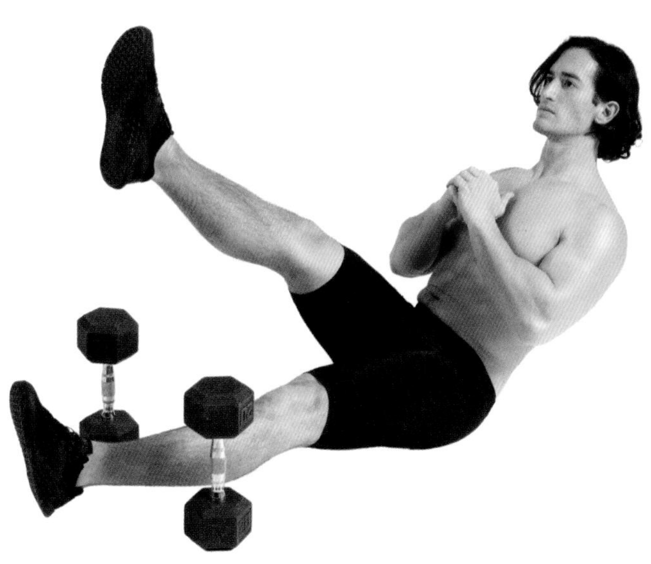

4 FLOOR WIPER

page 282
- Repetitions and time vary by objective.

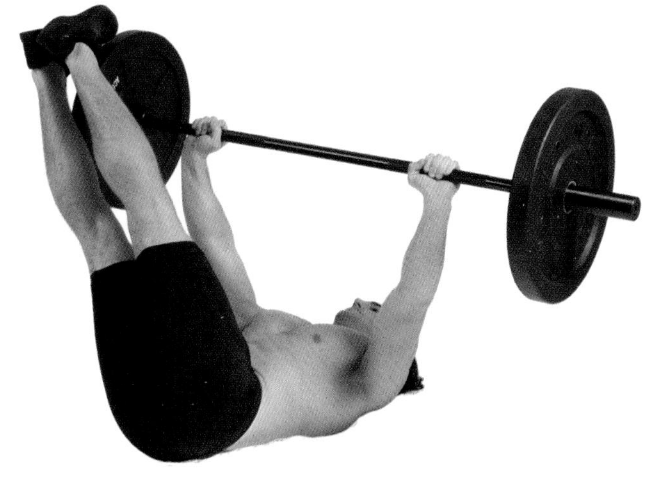

Mixed Circuit

1 TURKISH GET-UP

pages 144–145

• Repetitions and time vary by objective.

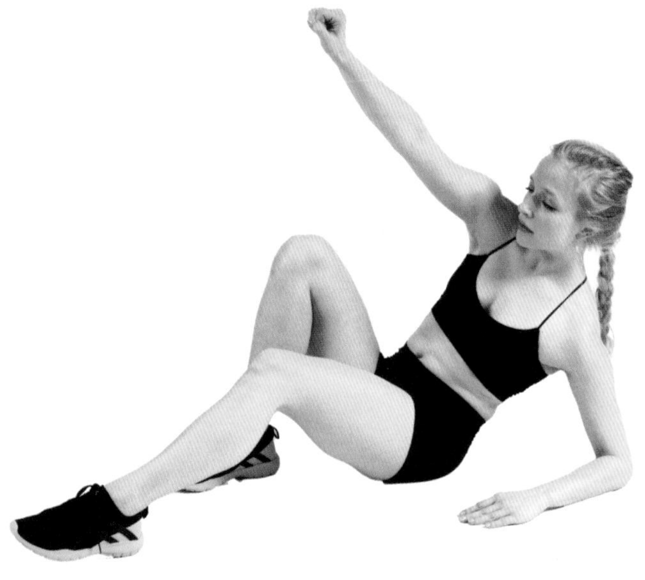

2 BARBELL HANG CLEAN

pages 264–265

• Repetitions and time vary by objective.

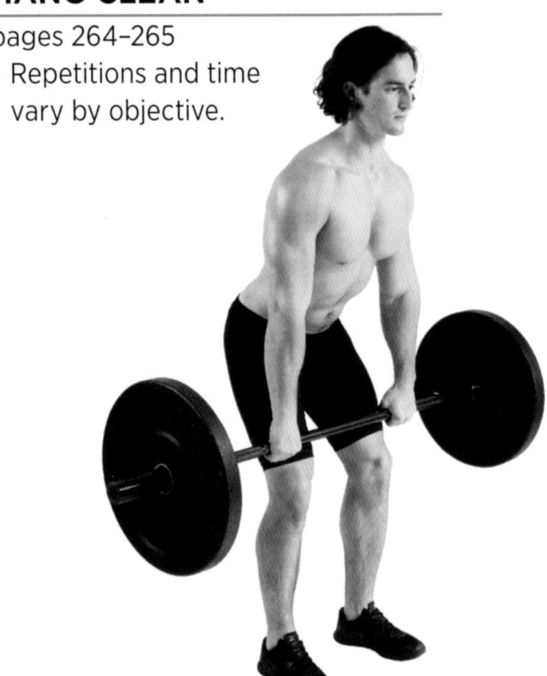

3 12-COUNT BODY BUILDER

pages 226–227

• Repetitions and time vary by objective.

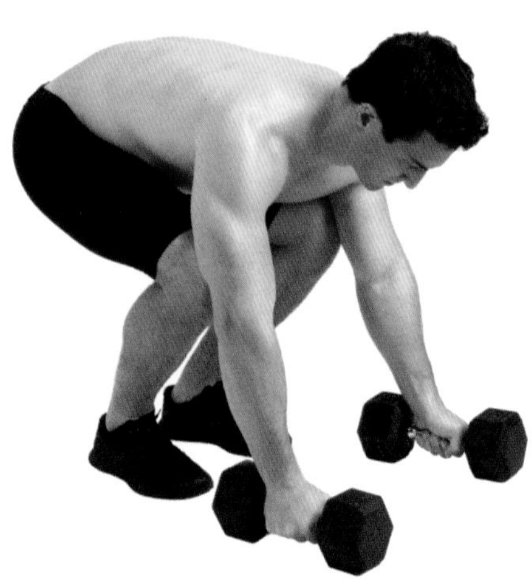

4 MOUNTAIN CLIMBER

pages 138–139

• Repetitions and time vary by objective.

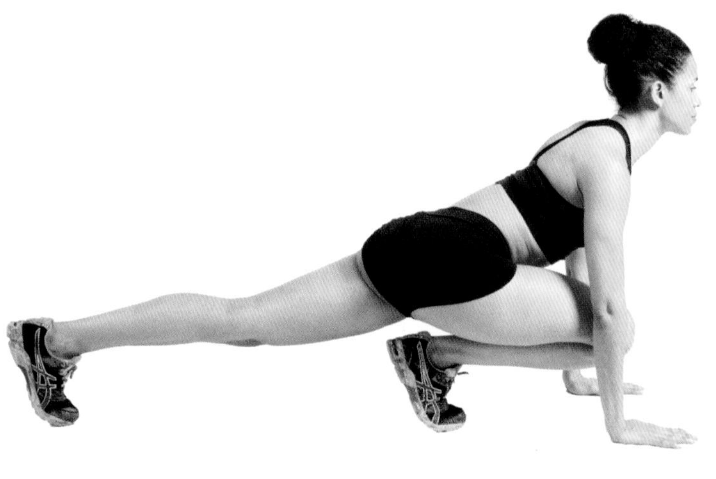

Resistance Circuit

FACT FILE

LEVEL
- All levels

OBJECTIVE
- Varies

WORK/REST
- Varies by objective

TOTAL TIME
- Varies by objective

TOTAL COMPLETED CIRCUIT SETS
- Varies by objective

1 V-SIT KETTLEBELL HOLD WITH LEG LIFT

page 197

- Repetitions and time vary by objective.

2 SWISS BALL FLAT DUMBBELL PRESS

pages 184–185

- Repetitions and time vary by objective.

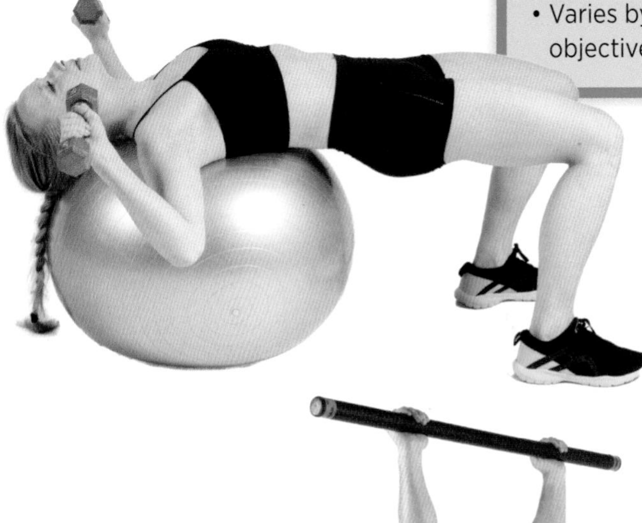

3 ALTERNATING KETTLEBELL ROW

pages 156–157

- Repetitions and time vary by objective.

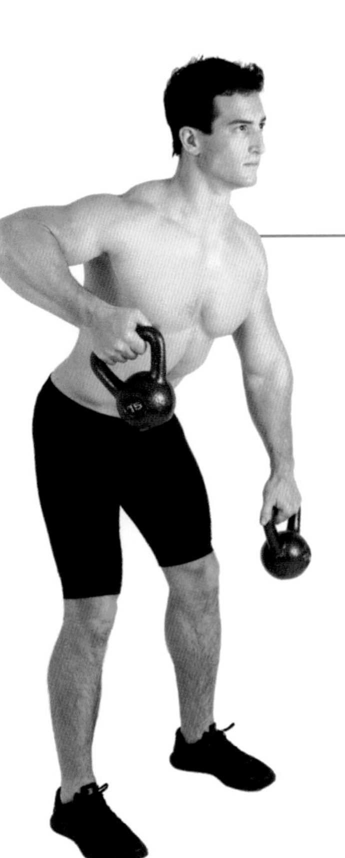

4 BARBELL FULL RAISE

pages 262–263

- Repetitions and time vary by objective.

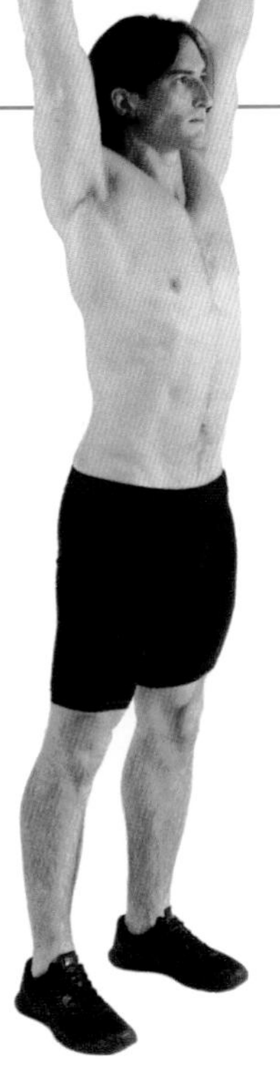

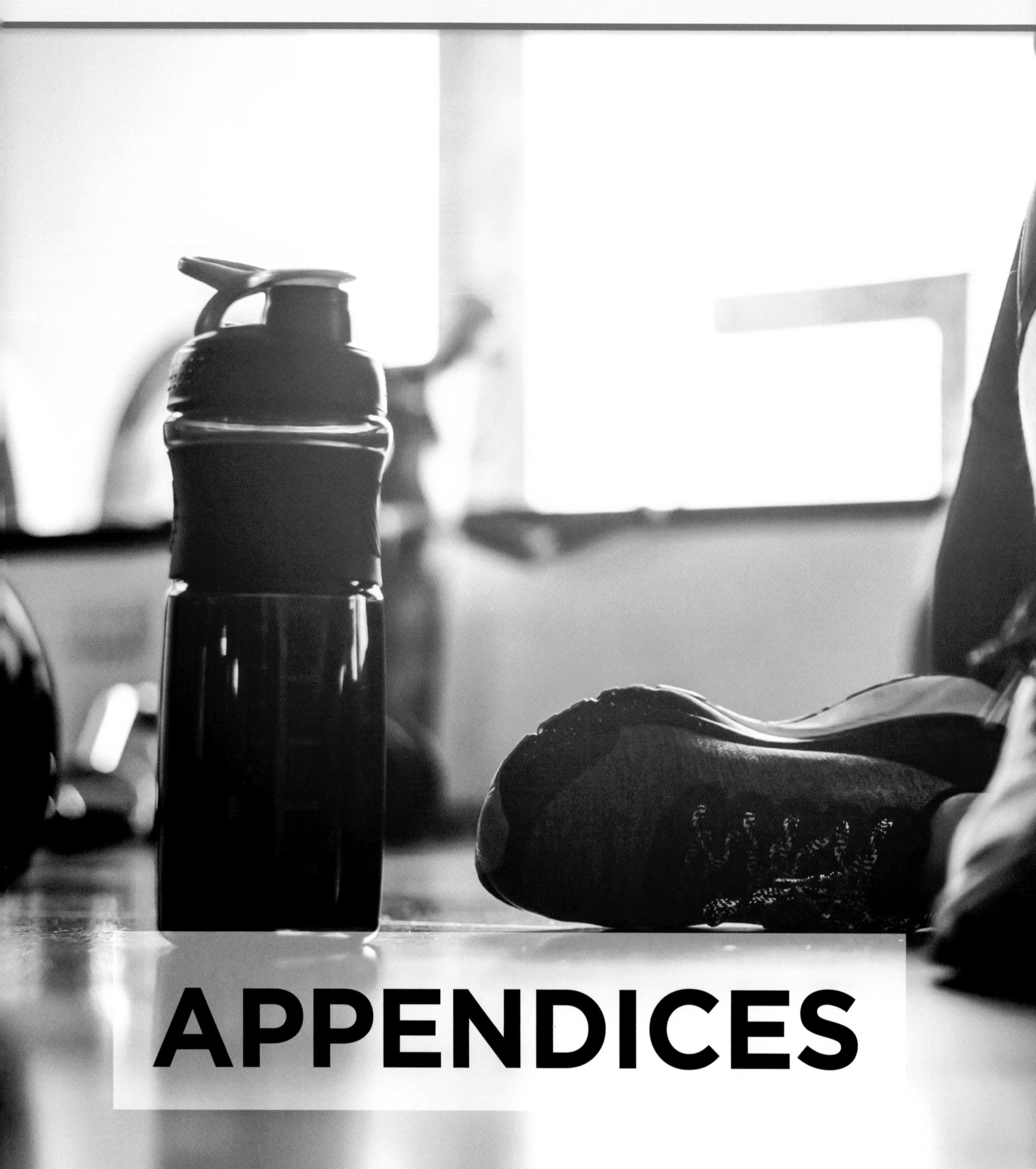

APPENDICES

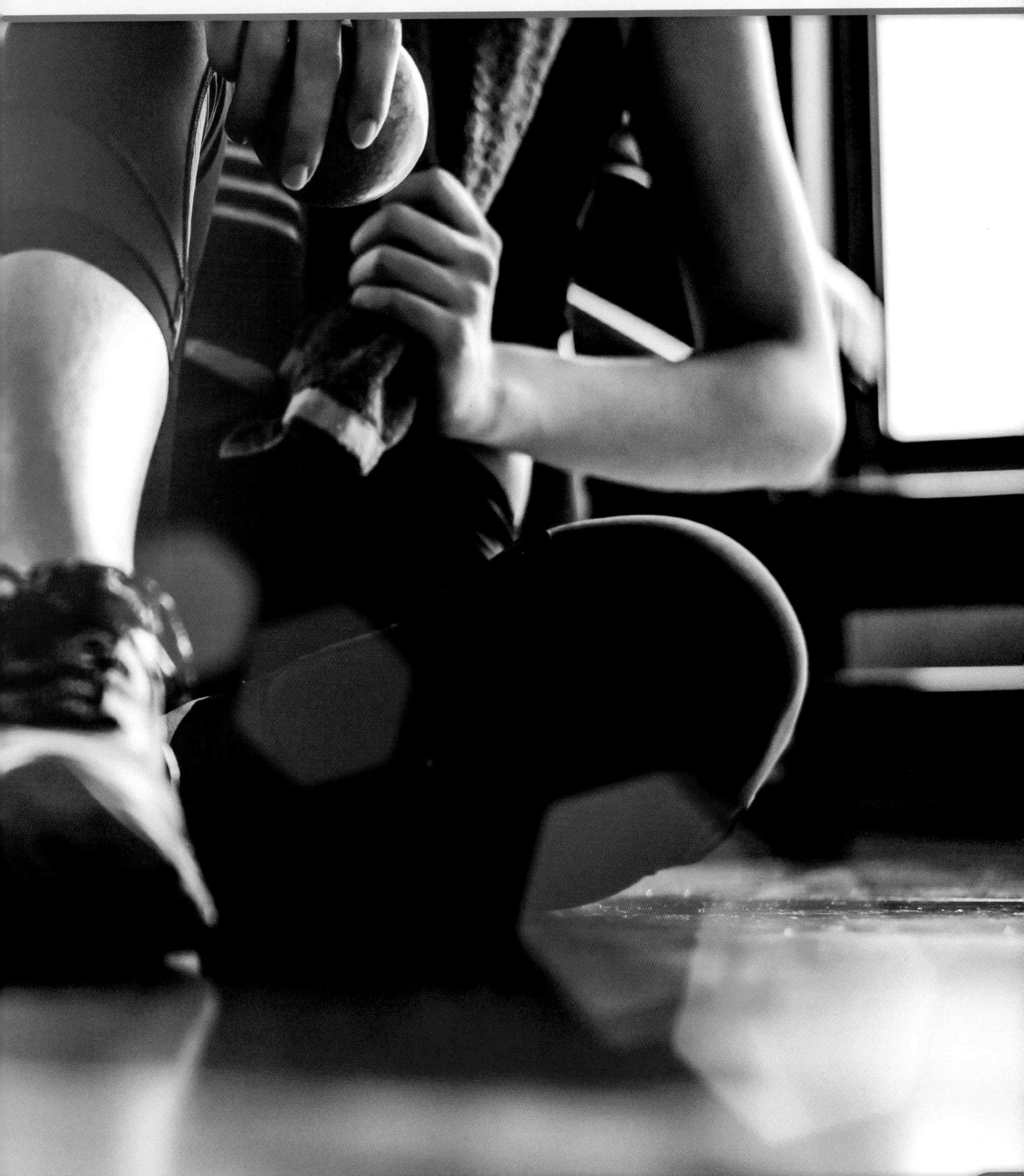

Glossary

GENERAL TERMS

abduction: Movement away from the body.

adduction: Movement toward the body.

aerobic exercise: An exercise form in which your body uses oxygen for energy.

aerobics step: A portable step or platform with adjustable risers designed for cardiovascular exercising

anaerobic exercise: An exercise form in which your muscles break down glucose sugar to use as energy.

anterior: Located in the front.

barbell: A long metal bar to which disks of varying weights are attached at each end.

battle rope: A rope of varying length and width that is anchored to a wall, or other secure object, and is used for strength, agility, and endurance training.

cardiovascular exercise: Any exercise that increases the heart rate, making oxygen and nutrient-rich blood available to working muscles.

circuit: A selection of exercises grouped together to be performed in order, with minimal rest in between each exercise.

clean: Lifting a weight from the floor into a front-racked squat to standing.

clean and jerk: A clean lift followed by powerfully moving the weight overhead in one smooth and powerful motion.

compound exercise: A move that incorporates multiple muscle groups, such as lunges, deadlifts, and squats. Also refers to two moves strung together, such as a power clean and press.

cooldown: An exercise performed at the end of the workout session that works to cool and relax the body.

core: Refers to the deep muscle layers that lie close to the spine and provide structural support for the entire body. The core is divided into two groups: the major and the minor. The major muscles reside on the trunk and include the stomach area and the middle and lower back. This area encompasses the pelvic floor muscles (levator ani, pubococcygeus, iliococcygeus, puborectalis, and coccygeus); the abdominals (rectus abdominis, transversus abdominis, obliquus externus, and obliquus internus); the spinal extensors (multifidus spinae, erector spinae, splenius, longissimus thoracis, and semispinalis); and the diaphragm. The minor core muscles include the latissimus dorsi, gluteus maximus and trapezius. Minor core muscles assist the major muscles when the body engages in activities or movements that require added stability.

core stabilizer: An exercise that calls for resisting motion at the lumbar spine though activation of the abdominal muscles and deep stabilizers; improves core strength and endurance.

core strengthener: An exercise that allows for motion in the lumbar spine, while working the abdominal muscles and deep stabilizers.

crunch: A common abdominal exercise that calls for curling the shoulders toward the pelvis while lying supine with hands behind head and knees bent.

curl: An exercise movement, usually targeting the biceps brachii, that calls for a weight to be moved through an arc, in a "curling" motion.

deadlift: An exercise movement that calls for lifting a weight, such as a dumbbell, off the floor from a stabilized bent-over position.

dumbbell: A basic piece of equipment that consists of a short bar on which plates are secured. A person can use a dumbbell in one or both hands during an exercise. Most gyms offer dumbbells with the weight plates welded on and poundage indicated on the plates, but dumbbells intended for home use come with removable plates that allow you to adjust the weight.

extension: The act of straightening.

extensor muscle: A muscle serving to extend a body part away from the body.

flexion: The bending of a joint.

flexor muscle: A muscle that decreases the angle between two bones, as when bending the arm at the elbow or raising the thigh toward the stomach.

fly: An exercise movement in which the hand and arm move through an arc while the elbow is kept at a constant angle. A fly works the muscles of the upper body.

foam roller: A tube that comes in a variety of sizes, materials, and densities that can be used for stretching, strengthening, and balance training.

front rack position: A barbell hold in which the bar rests on your clavicles and flexed shoulders.

functional exercise: A group of exercises that help you move in everyday life, often mimicking everyday movements, such as a squat or deadlift.

hamstrings: The three muscles of the posterior thigh (the semitendinosus, semimembranosus and biceps femoris) that work to flex the knee and extend the hip.

hyperextension: An exercise that works the lower back as well as the middle back and upper back, specifically the erector spinae, which usually involves raising the torso and/or lower body from the floor while keeping the pelvis firmly anchored.

internal rotation: The act of moving a body part toward the center of the body.

interval: A period of activity or a period of rest.

isolation exercise: A movement that focuses on just one muscle or muscle group.

kettlebell: A bell-shaped weight of varying poundage used to build strength and endurance, improve cardiovascular health, and increase grip strength.

iliotibial band (ITB): A thick band of fibrous tissue that runs down the outside of the leg, beginning at the hip and extending to the outer side of the tibia just below the knee joint. The band functions in concert with several of the thigh muscles to provide stability to the outside of the knee joint.

lateral: Located on, or extending toward, the outside.

lunge: A group of lower-body exercises in which one leg is positioned forward with knee bent and foot flat on the ground while the other leg is positioned behind.

medial: Located on, or extending toward, the middle.

neutral position: A position in which the natural curve of the spine is maintained, typically adopted when lying on one's back with one or both feet on the mat.

neutral: Describes the position of the legs, pelvis, hips, or other parts of the body that are neither arched nor curved forward.

plate: A cast-iron weight placed on a dumbbell. The weight of plates generally start at about 10 pounds and range upward to 50 pounds and higher.

plyometrics: Explosive exercises that increase power, such as jumps.

posterior: Located behind.

posterior chain: The glutes, hamstrings, and back.

press: An exercise movement that calls for moving a weight or other resistance away from the body.

pulling muscles: The upper-body muscles involved in pushing movements. They primarily include the chest, shoulders, and triceps brachii.

push-up: A basic exercise that involves raising and lowering the body using the arms.

pushing muscles: The upper-body muscles involved in pulling movements. They primarily include back and biceps brachii.

quadriceps: A large muscle group (full name: quadriceps femoris) that includes the four prevailing muscles on the front of the thigh: the rectus femoris, vastus intermedius, vastus lateralis and vastus medialis. It is the great extensor muscle of the knee, forming a large fleshy mass that covers the front and sides of the femur muscle.

range of motion: The distance and direction a joint can move between the flexed and the extended positions.

resistance: How much weight your muscles are working against to complete a movement, whether your own body weight or added weight, such as dumbbells.

row: An exercise movement that imitates the movement of rowing a boat. It primarily targets the upper back.

rotator muscle: One of a group of muscles that assist the rotation of a joint, such as the hip or the shoulder.

scapula: The protrusion of bone on the middle back to upper back, also known as the shoulder blade.

set: Refers to how many times you repeat a given number of repetitions of an exercise.

snatch A total-body move that brings a weight, such as a kettlebell, from floor to overhead.

split squat: An assisted one-legged squat in which the nonlifting leg is rested on the floor a few steps behind the lifting leg, as if it were a static lunge.

squat: An exercise movement that calls for moving the hips back and bending the knees and hips to lower the torso and an accompanying weight, and then returning to the upright position. A squat primarily targets the muscles of the thighs, hips, buttocks, and hamstrings.

Swiss ball: A flexible, inflatable PVC ball measuring approximately 12 to 30 inches in circumference that is used for weight training, physical therapy, balance training, and many other exercise regimens. It is also called a balance ball, fitness ball, stability ball, exercise ball, gym ball, physioball, body ball, therapy ball, and many other names.

ventral aspect: The front of the body.

warm-up: Any form of light exercise of short duration that prepares the body for more intense exercises.

weight: Refers to the plates or weight stacks, or the actual poundage listed on the bar or dumbbell.

work/rest ratio: The comparison between how much time spent working and how much time spent resting.

LATIN TERMS

The following glossary explains the Latin scientific terminology used to describe the muscles of the human body. Certain words are derived from Greek, which is indicated in each instance.

ABDOMEN

obliquus (externus and internus): *obliquus*, "slanting"

rectus abdominis: *rego,* "straight, upright," and *abdomen,* "belly"

serratus anterior: *serra*, "saw," and *ante*, "before"

transversus abdominis: *transversus*, "athwart," and *abdomen*, "belly"

BACK

erector spinae: *erectus*, "straight," and *spina*, "thorn"

latissimus dorsi: *latus*, "wide," and *dorsum*, "back"

multifidus spinae: *multifid*, "to cut into divisions," and *spinae*, "spine"

quadratus lumborum: *quadratus*, "square, rectangular," and *lumbus*, "loin"

rhomboideus: Greek *rhembesthai*, "to spin"

trapezius: Greek *trapezion*, "small table"

CHEST

coracobrachialis: Greek *korakoeidés*, "ravenlike," and *brachium*, "arm"

pectoralis (major and minor): *pectus*, "breast"

HIPS

gemellus (inferior and superior): *geminus*, "twin"

gluteus maximus: Greek *gloutós*, "rump," and *maximus*, "largest"

gluteus medius: Greek *gloutós*, "rump" and *medialis*, "middle"

gluteus minimus: Greek *gloutós*, "rump" and *minimus*, "smallest"

iliopsoas: *ilium,* "groin," and Greek *psoa*, "groin muscle"

obturator externus: *obturare,* "to block" and *externus,* "outward"

obturator internus: *obturare*, "to block," and *internus*, "within"

pectineus: *pectin*, "comb"

piriformis: *pirum*, "pear," and *forma,* "shape"

quadratus femoris: *quadratus*, "square, rectangular," and *femur*, "thigh"

LOWER ARM

anconeus: Greek *anconad*, "elbow"

brachioradialis: *brachium*, "arm," and *radius*, "spoke"

extensor carpi radialis: *extendere*, "to extend," Greek *karpós*, "wrist" and *radius*, "spoke"

extensor digitorum: *extendere*, "to extend," and *digitus*, "finger, toe"

flexor carpi pollicis longus: *flectere*, "to bend," Greek *karpós*, "wrist," *pollicis*, "thumb" and *longus*, "long"

flexor carpi radialis: *flectere*, "to bend," Greek *karpós*, "wrist" and *radius*, "spoke"

flexor carpi ulnaris: *flectere*, "to bend," Greek *karpós*, "wrist" and *ulnaris*, "forearm"

flexor digitorum: *flectere*, "to bend," and *digitus*, "finger, toe"

palmaris longus: *palmaris*, "palm," and *longus*, "long"

pronator teres: *pronate*, "to rotate," and *teres*, "rounded"

LOWER LEG

adductor digiti minimi: *adducere*, "to contract," *digitus*, "finger, toe" and *minimum* "smallest"

adductor hallucis: *adducere*, "to contract," and *hallex*, "big toe"

extensor digitorum longus: *extendere*, "to extend," *digitus*, "finger, toe" and *longus*, "long"

extensor hallucis longus: *extendere*, "to extend," *hallex*, "big toe," and *longus*, "long"

flexor digitorum longus: *flectere*, "to bend," *digitus*, "finger, toe" and *longus*, "long"

flexor hallucis longus: *flectere*, "to bend," and *hallex*, "big toe" and *longus*, "long"

gastrocnemius: Greek *gastroknémía*, "calf [of the leg]"

peroneus: *peronei*, "of the fibula"

plantaris: *planta*, "the sole"

soleus: *solea*, "sandal"

tibialis (anterior and posterior): *tibia*, "reed pipe"

NECK

scalenus: Greek *skalénós*, "unequal"

semispinalis: *semi*, "half," and *spinae*, "spine"

splenius: Greek *splénion*, "plaster, patch"

sternocleidomastoideus: Greek *stérnon,* "chest," Greek *kleís*, "key" and Greek *mastoeidés*, "breastlike"

SHOULDERS

deltoideus (anterior, medialis and posterior): Greek *deltoeidés*, "delta-shaped"

infraspinatus: *infra*, "under," and *spina*, "thorn"

levator scapulae: *levare*, "to raise," and *scapulae*, "shoulder [blades]"

subscapularis: *sub*, "below," and *scapulae*, "shoulder [blades]"

supraspinatus: *supra,* "above," and *spina*, "thorn"

teres (major and minor): *teres*, "rounded"

UPPER ARM

biceps brachii: *biceps*, "two-headed," and *brachium*, "arm"

brachialis: *brachium*, "arm"

triceps brachii: *triceps*, "three-headed" and *brachium*, "arm"

UPPER LEG

adductor longus: *adducere*, "to contract," and *longus*, "long"

adductor magnus: *adducere*, "to contract," and *magnus*, "major"

biceps femoris: *biceps*, "two-headed," and *femur*, "thigh"

gracilis: *gracilis*, "slim, slender"

rectus femoris: *rego*, "straight, upright," and *femur*, "thigh"

sartorius: *sarcio*, "to patch" or "to repair"

semimembranosus: *semi*, "half," and *membrum*, "limb"

semitendinosus: *semi*, "half," and *tendo*, "tendon"

tensor fasciae latae: *tenere*, "to stretch," *fasciae*, "band," and *latae*, "laid down"

vastus intermedius: *vastus*, "immense, huge," and *intermedius*, "between"

vastus lateralis: *vastus*, "immense, huge," and lateralis, "side"

vastus medialis: *vastus*, "immense, huge," and *medialis*, "middle"

Icon Index

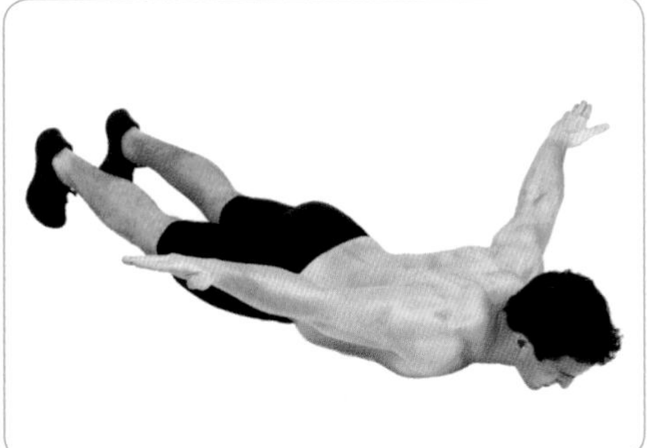

Arm Hauler
pages 48–49

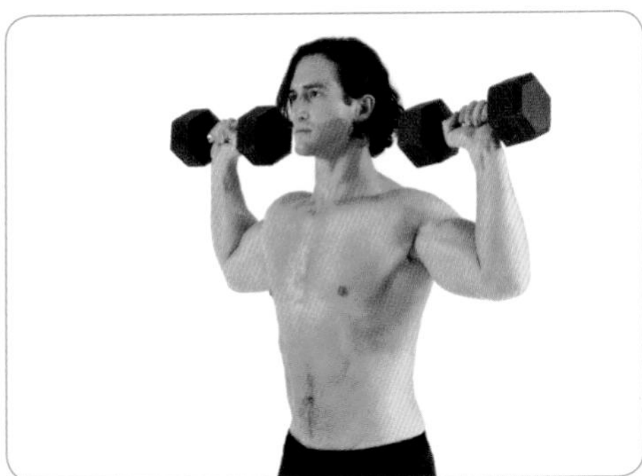

Arnold Press
page 167

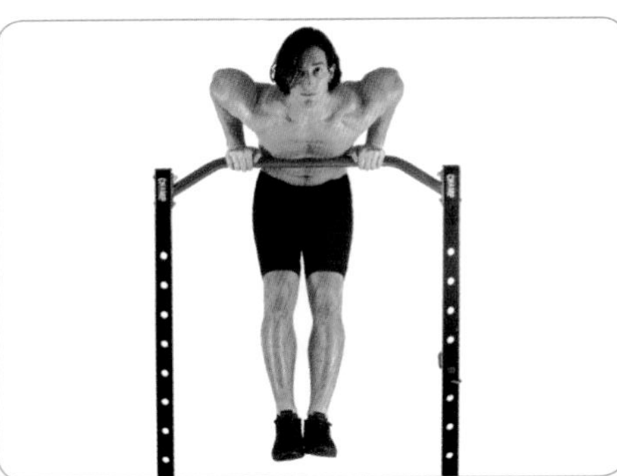

Bar Dip
page 73

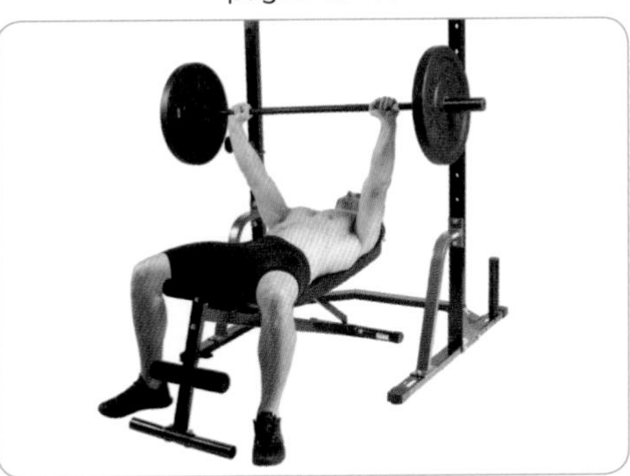

Barbell Bench Press
pages 270–271

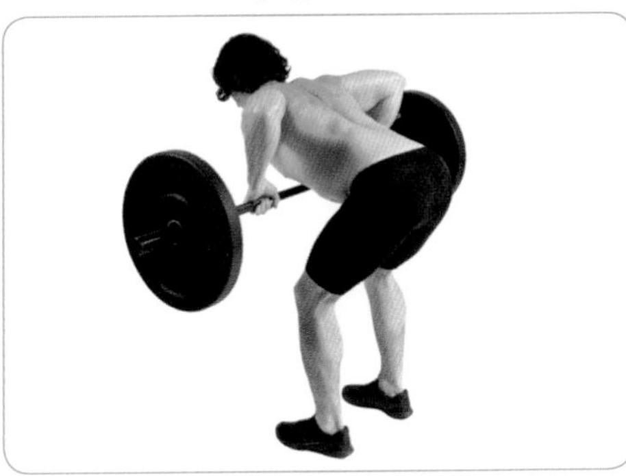

Barbell Bent-Over Row
pages 246–247

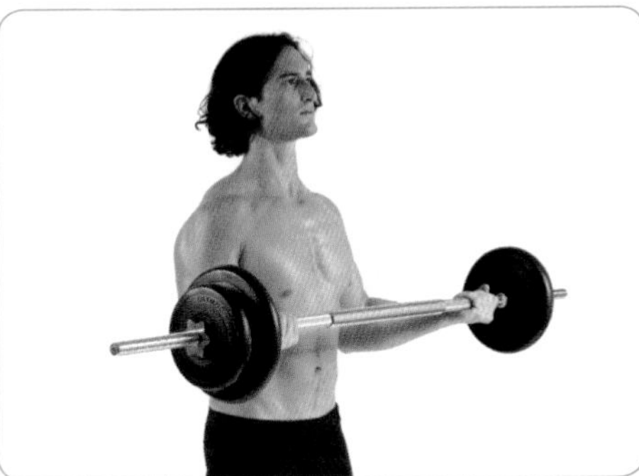

Barbell Curl
pages 254–255

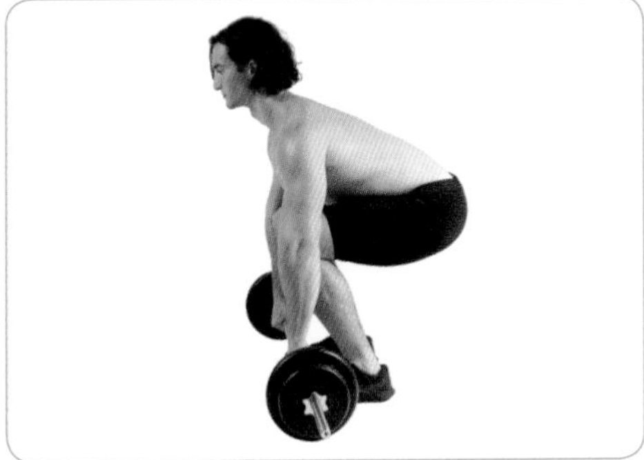

Barbell Deadlift
pages 240–241

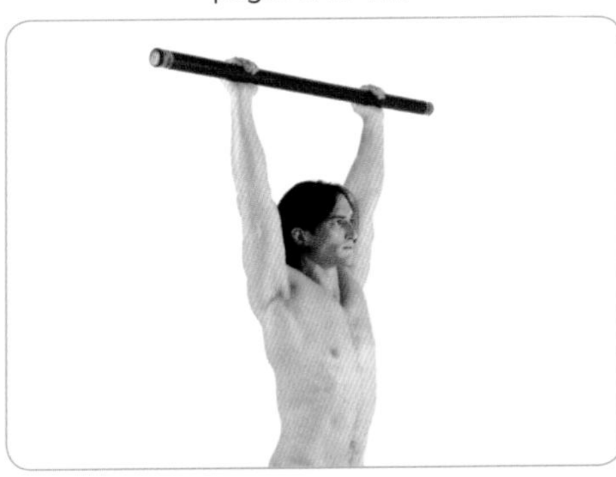

Barbell Full Raise
pages 262–263

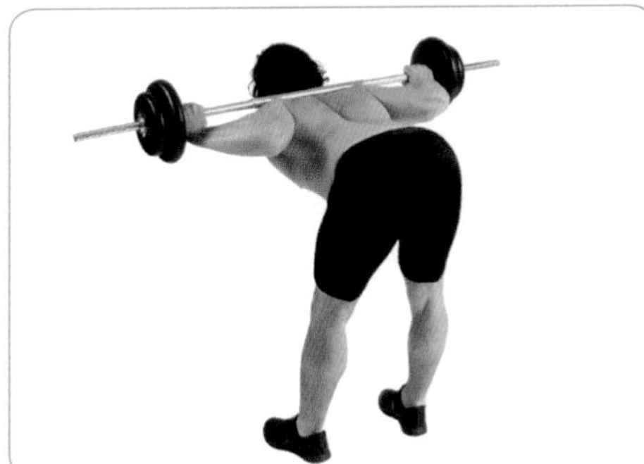

Barbell Good Morning
pages 244–245

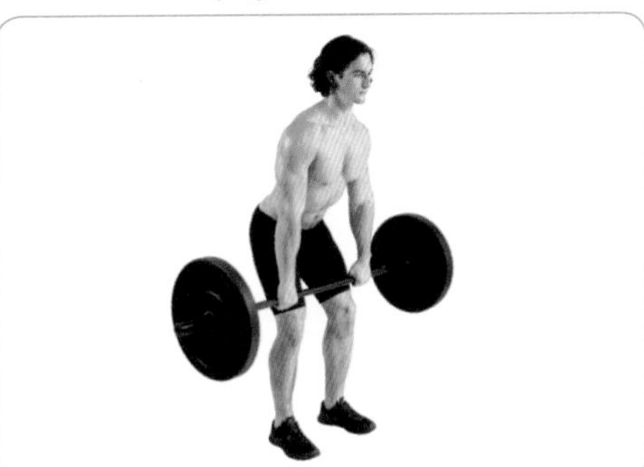

Barbell Hang Clean
pages 264–265

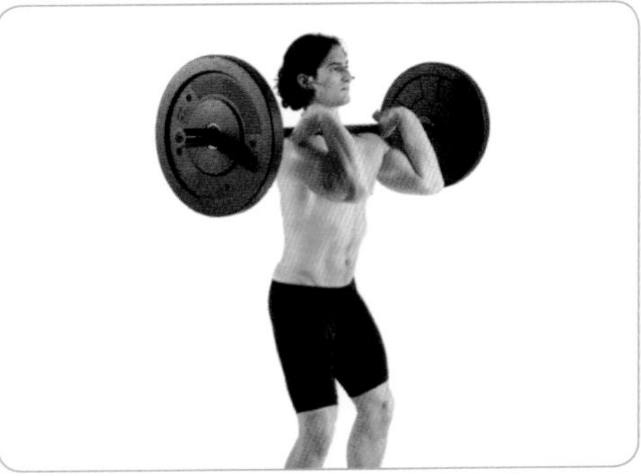

Barbell Power Clean and Jerk
pages 314–315

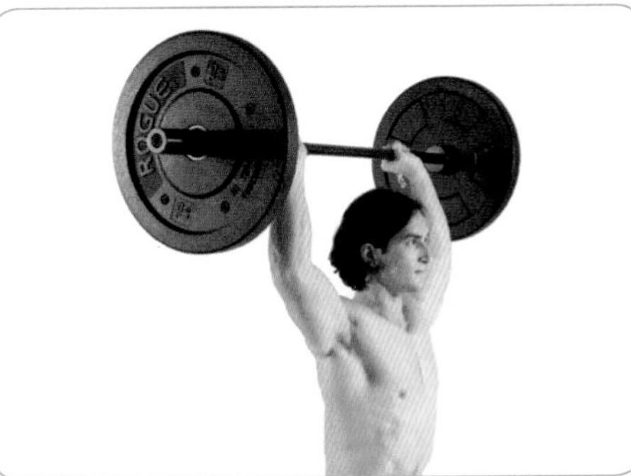

Barbell Shoulder Press
page 321

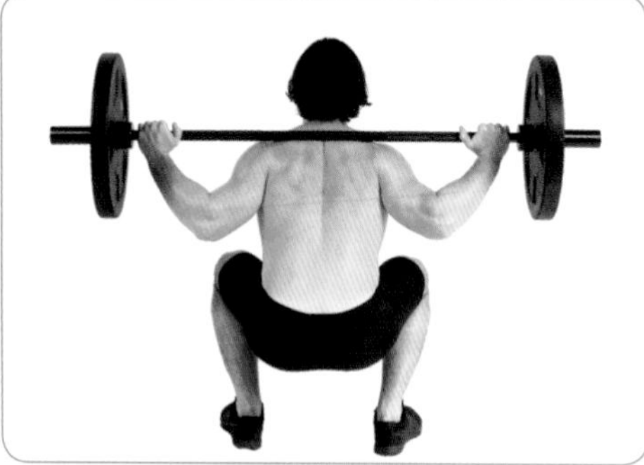
Barbell Squat
pages 298–299

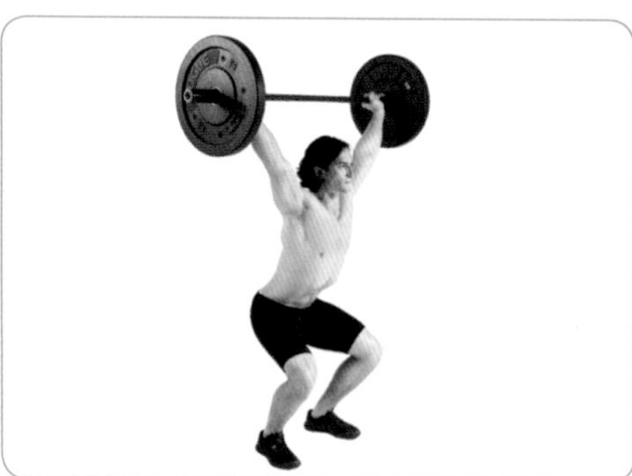
Barbell Squat Snatch
pages 316–317

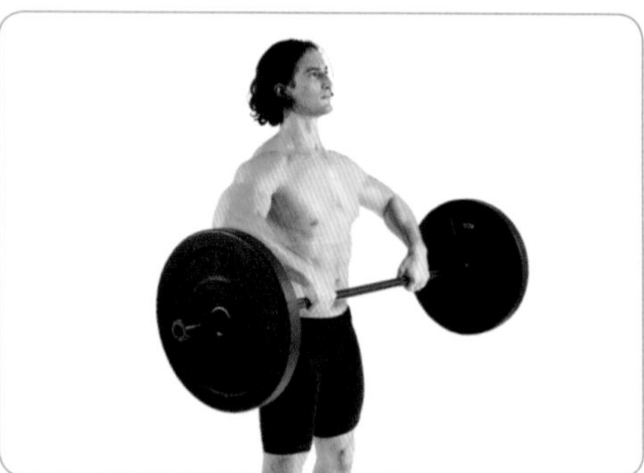
Barbell Upright Row
pages 248–249

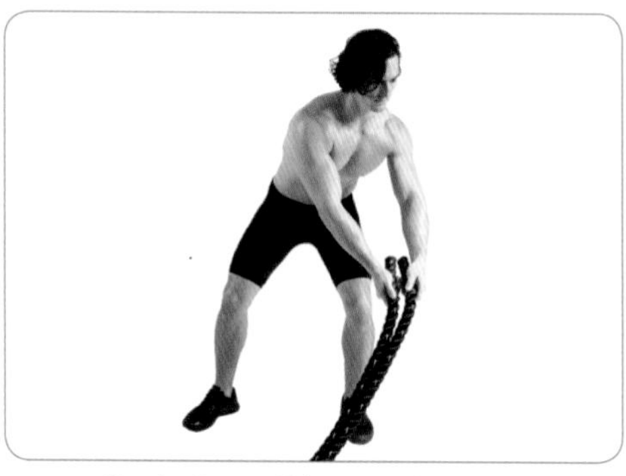
Battle Rope Side-to-Side Swing
pages 266–267

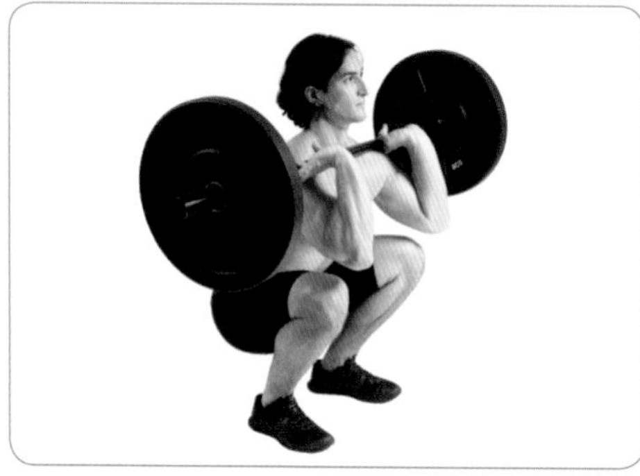
Bear Complex
pages 322–323

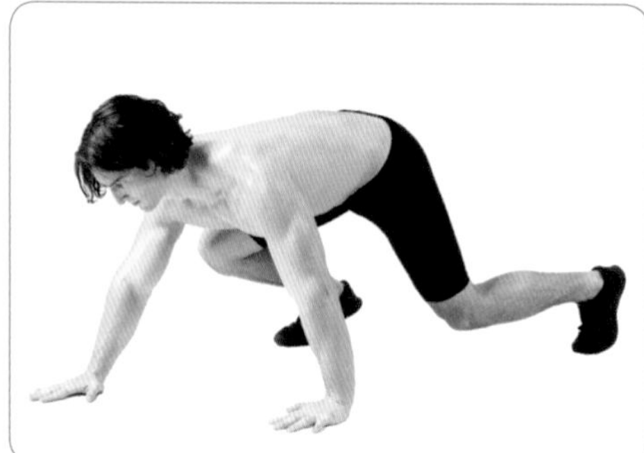
Bear Crawl
pages 132-133

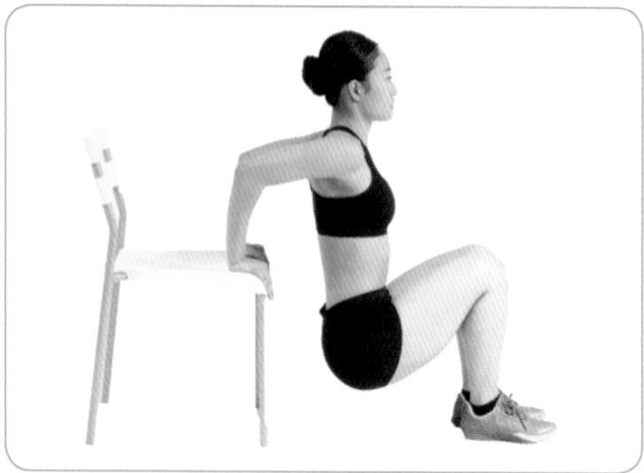
Bench Dip
pages 62–63

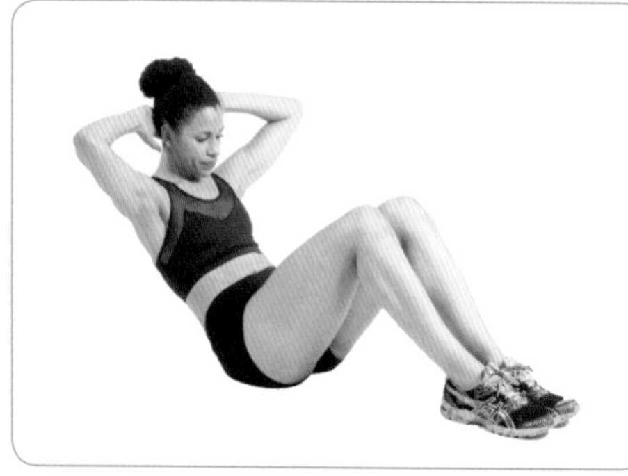
Bent-Knee Sit-Up
pages 90–91

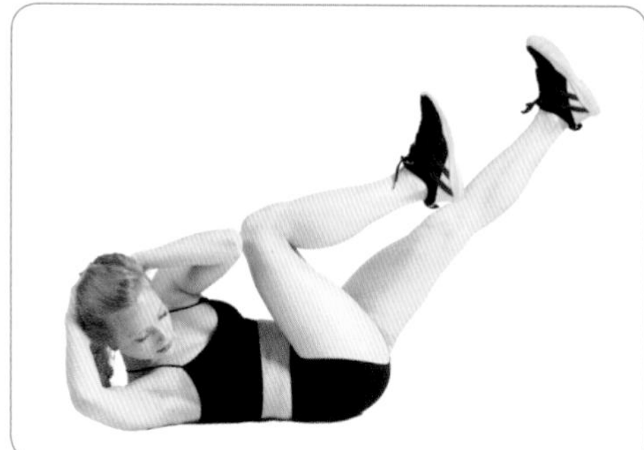
Bicycle Crunch
pages 92–93

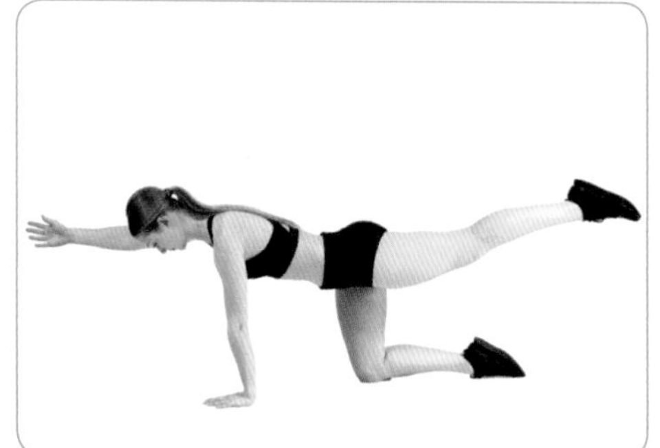
Bird-Dog
pages 54–55

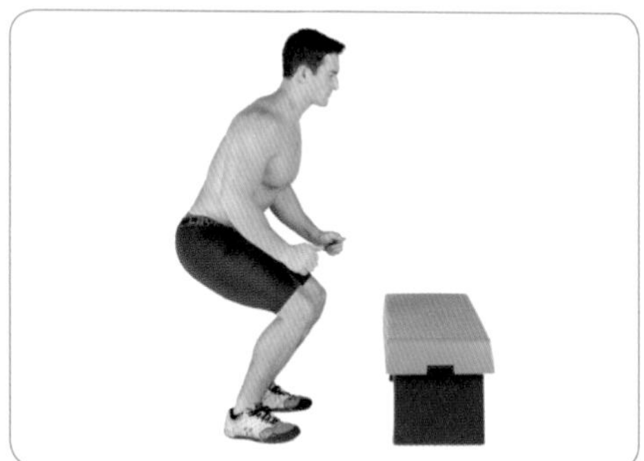
Box Jump
pages 116–117

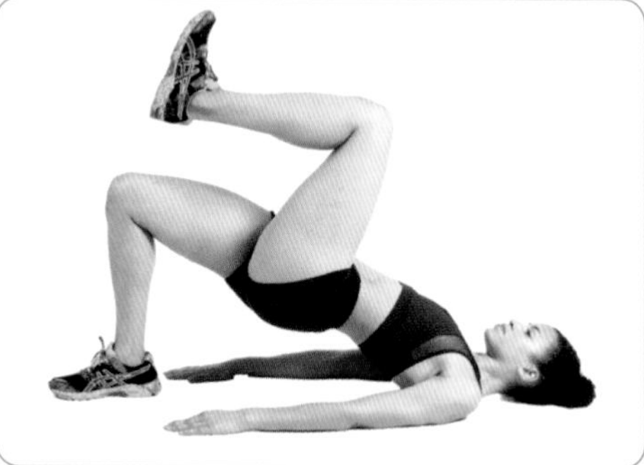
Bridge with Leg Lift
pages 120–121

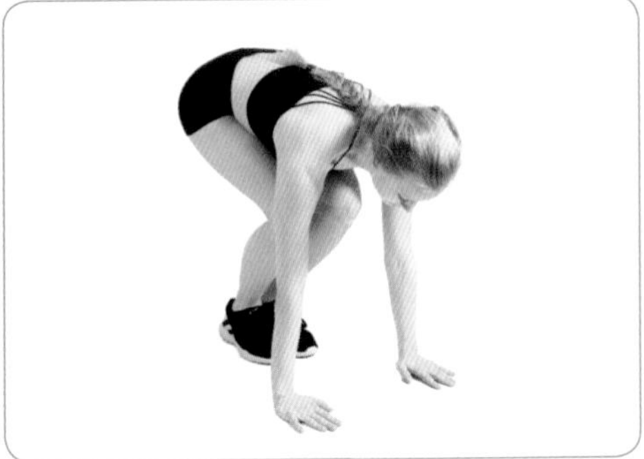
Burpee
pages 128–129

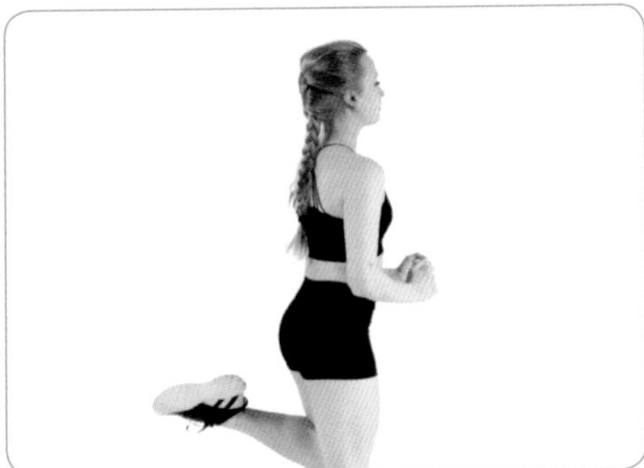
Butt Kick
pages 108–109

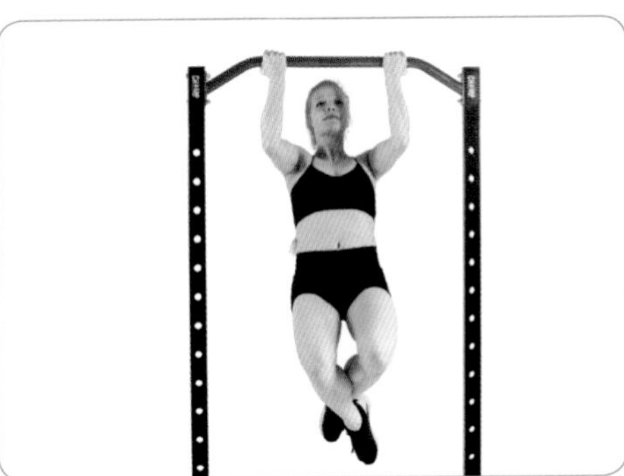
Chin-Up
pages 46–47

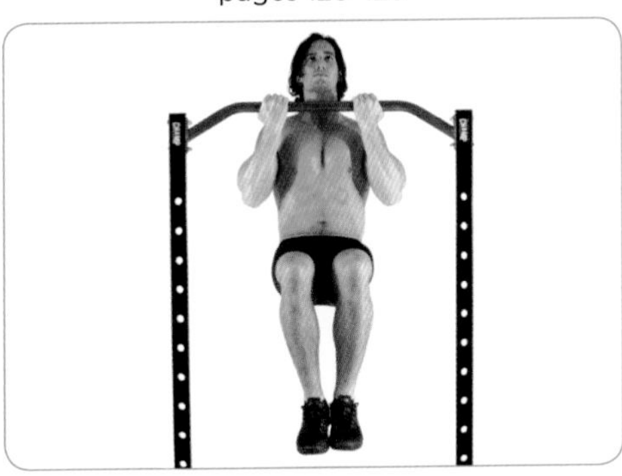
Chin-Up with Hanging Leg Raise
pages 312–313

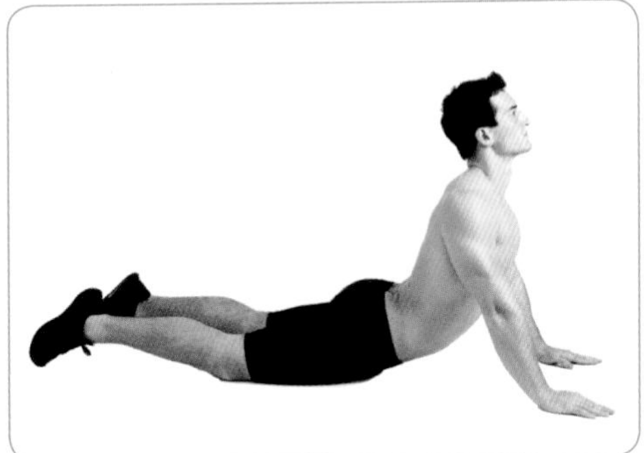
Cobra Stretch
pages 40–41

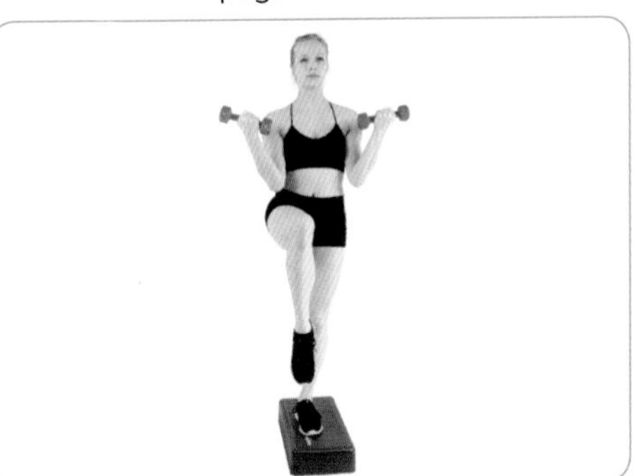
Curling Step and Raise
pages 168–169

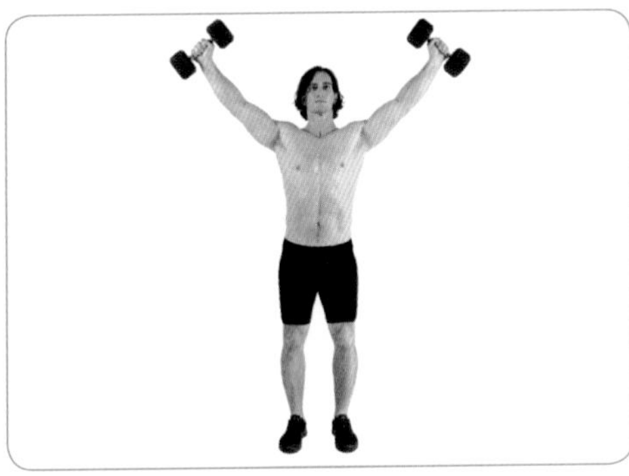
Da Vinci
pages 178–179

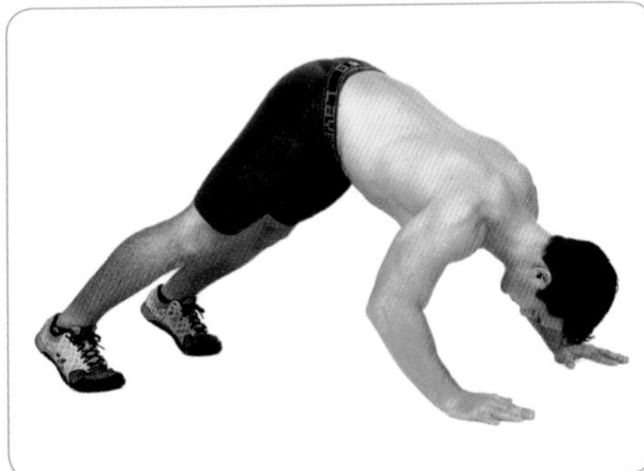
Dive-Bomber Push-Up
pages 82–83

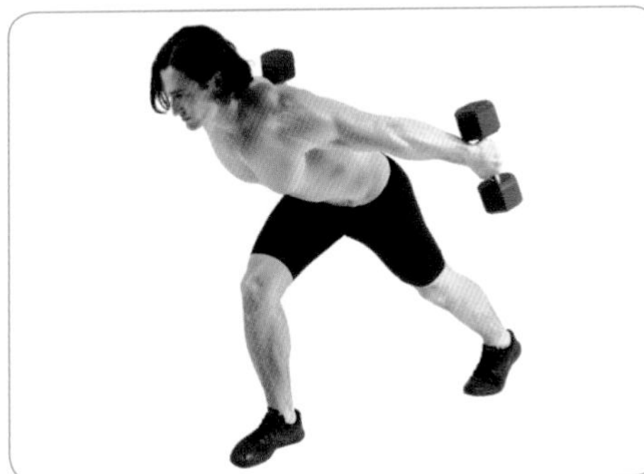
Double-Arm Triceps Kickback
page 180

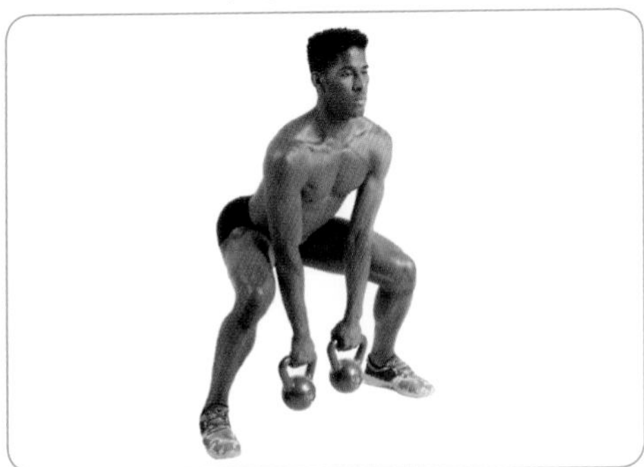
Double Kettlebell Snatch
pages 222–223

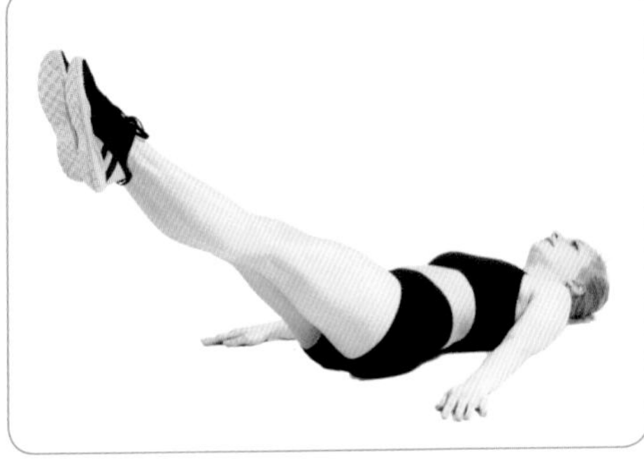
Double Leg Lift
pages 102–103

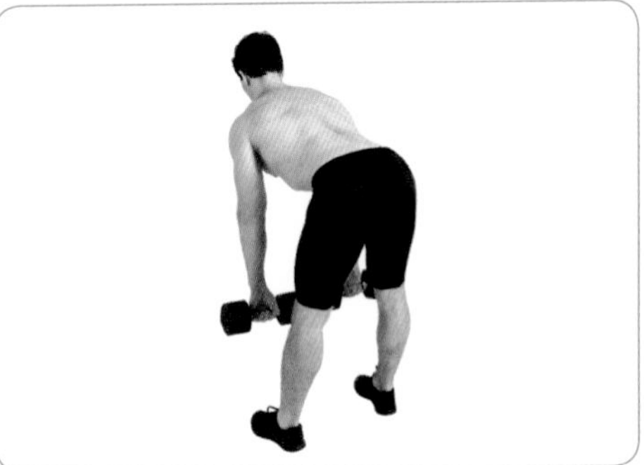
Dumbbell Deadlift
pages 150–151

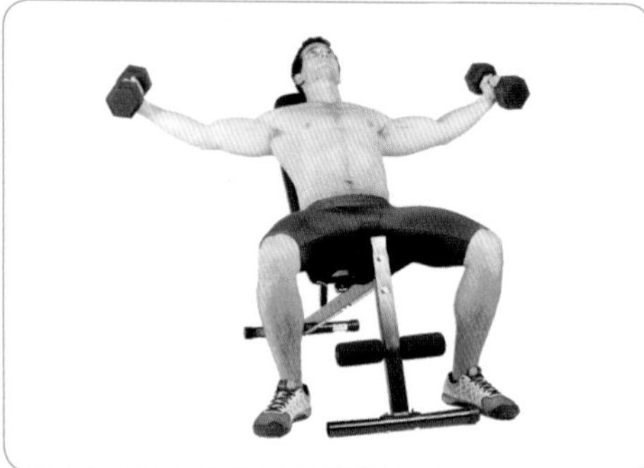
Dumbbell Fly
pages 188–189

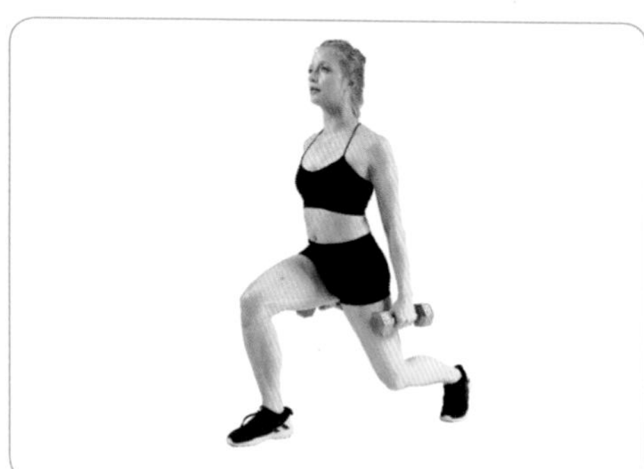
Dumbbell Lunge
pages 210–211

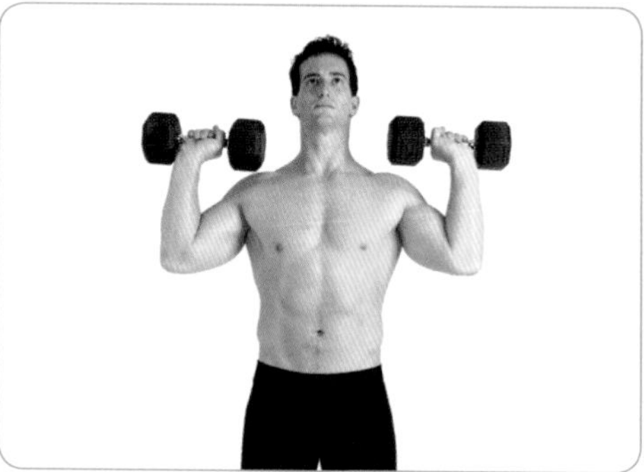
Dumbbell Power Clean
page 232

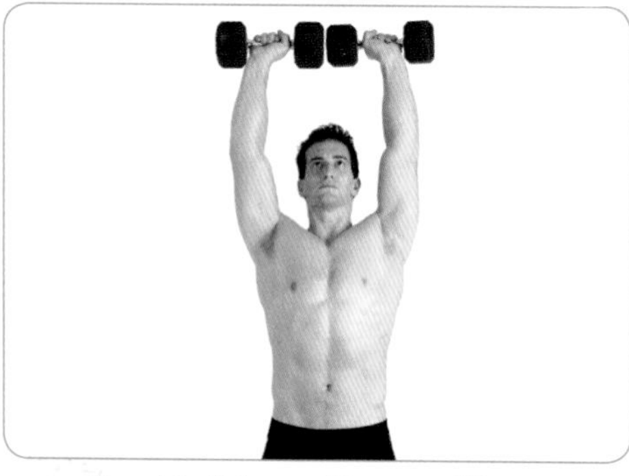
Dumbbell Power Clean and Press
page 233

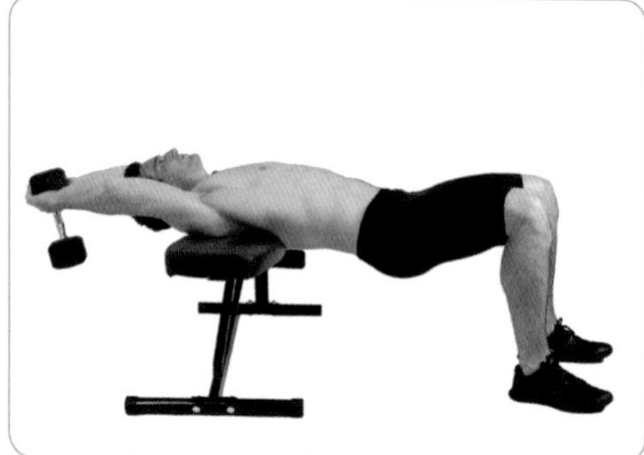
Dumbbell Pullover
pages 162–163

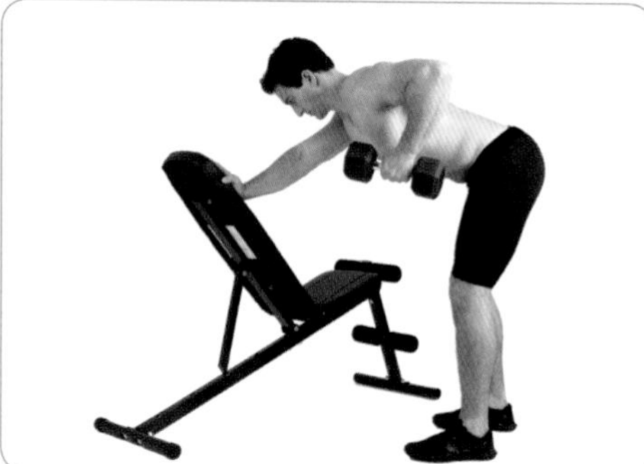
Dumbbell Row
page 154–155

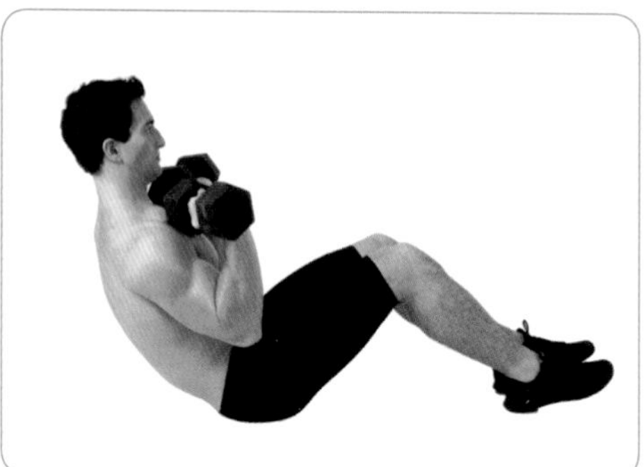
Dumbbell Sit-Up
page 196

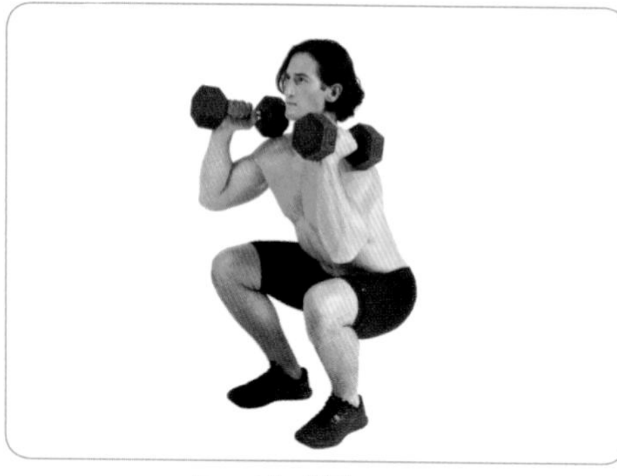
Dumbbell Thruster
pages 236–237

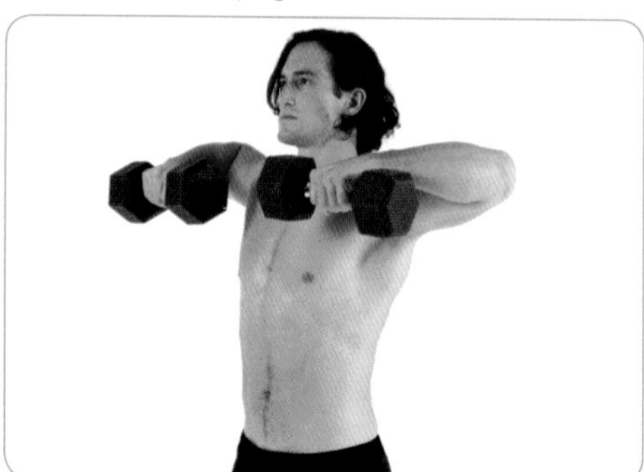
Dumbbell Upright Row
page 148

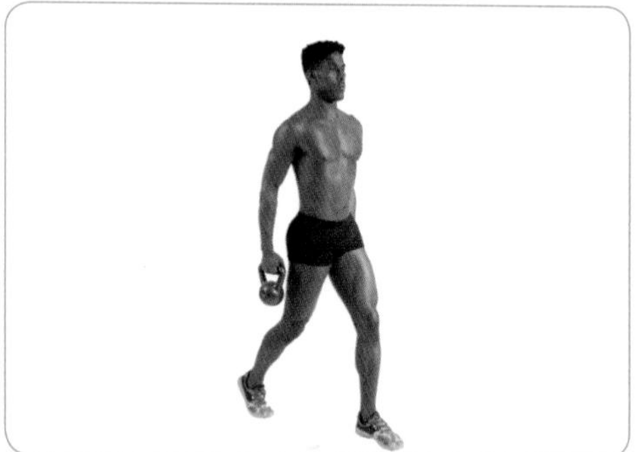
Farmer's Walk
pages 202–203

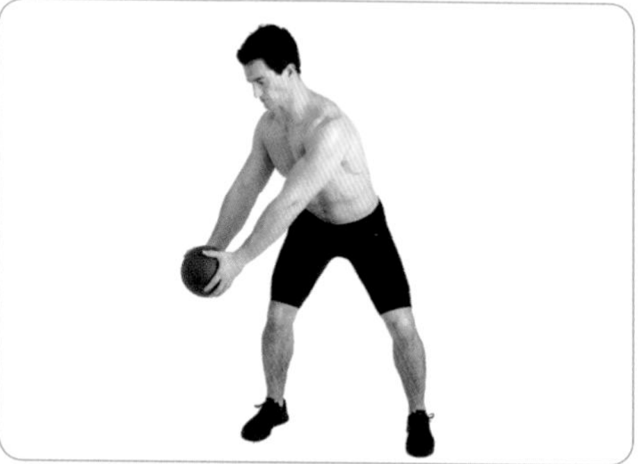
Figure 8
pages 286–287

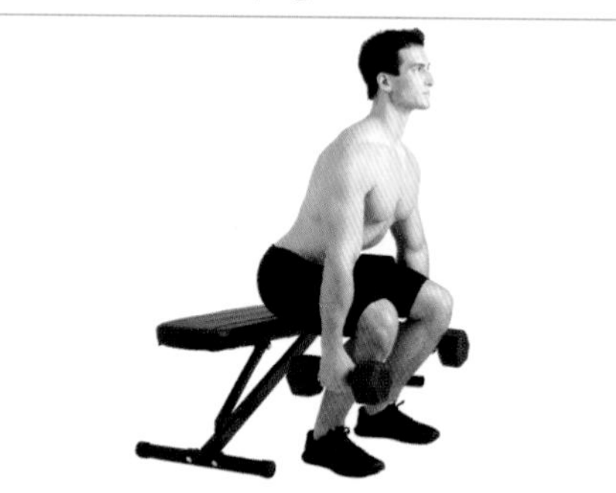
Flat Bench Dumbbell Squat
pages 206–207

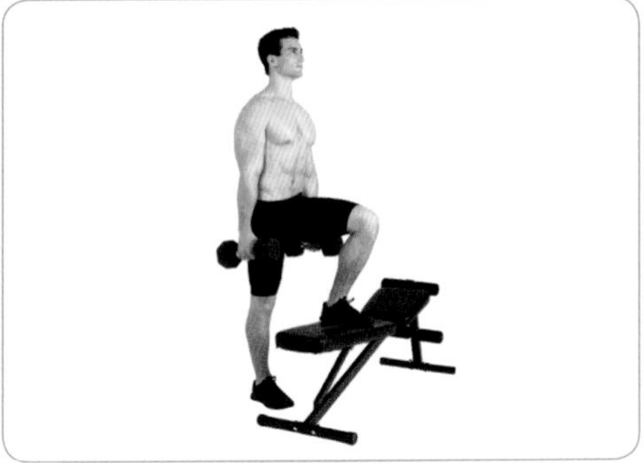
Flat Bench Step-Up
pages 208–209

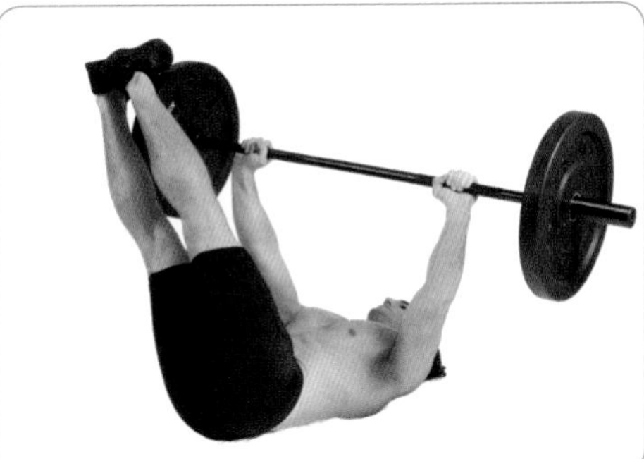
Floor Wiper
page 282

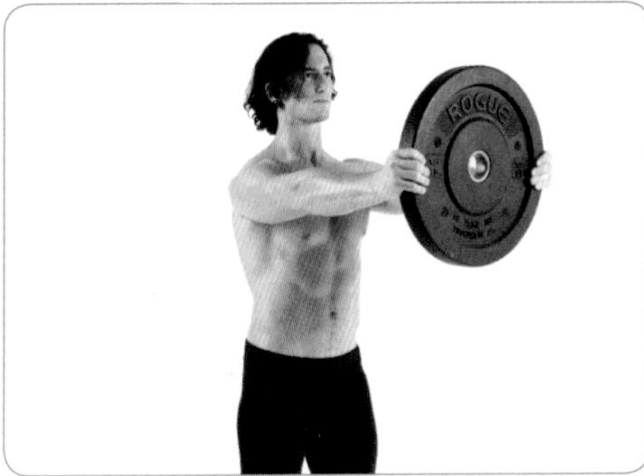

Front Plate Raise
pages 258–259

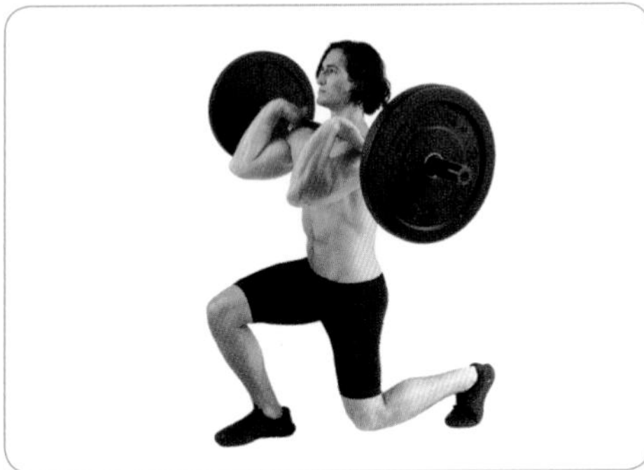
Front Rack Barbell Lunge
page 308

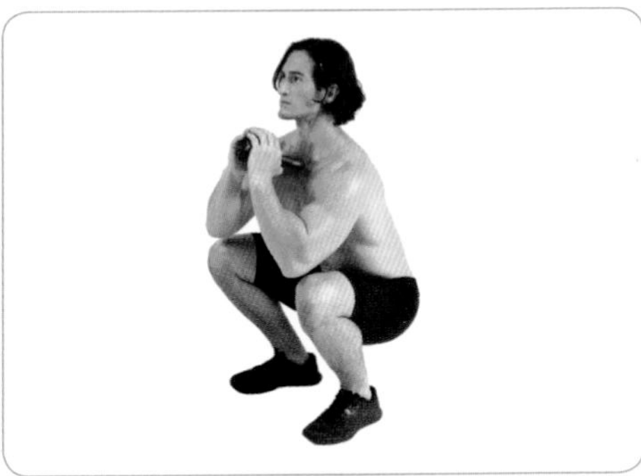
Goblet Squat
page 213

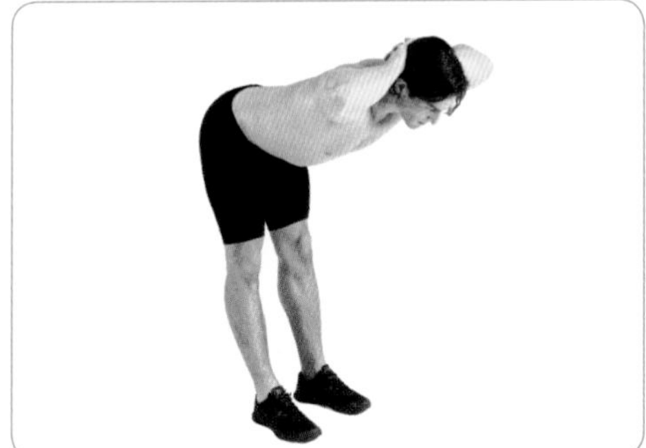
Good Morning
page 60

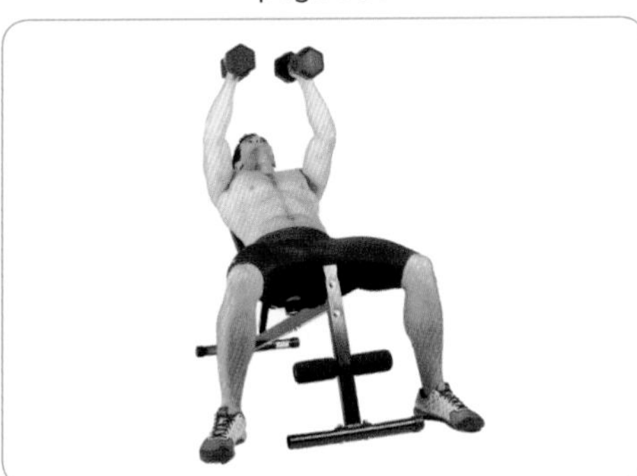
Hammer-Grip Press
pages 186–187

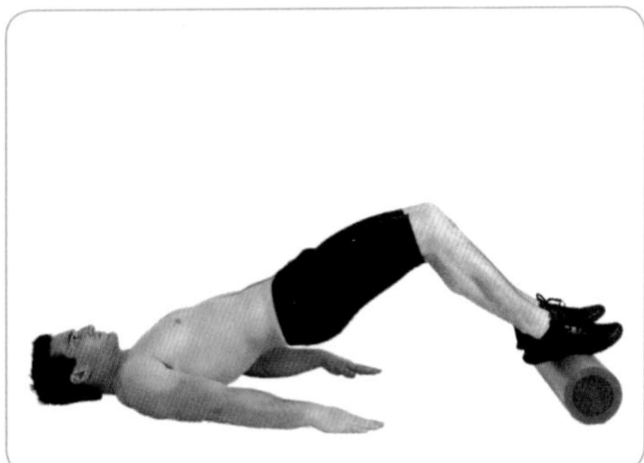
Hamstrings Pull-In
pages 304–305

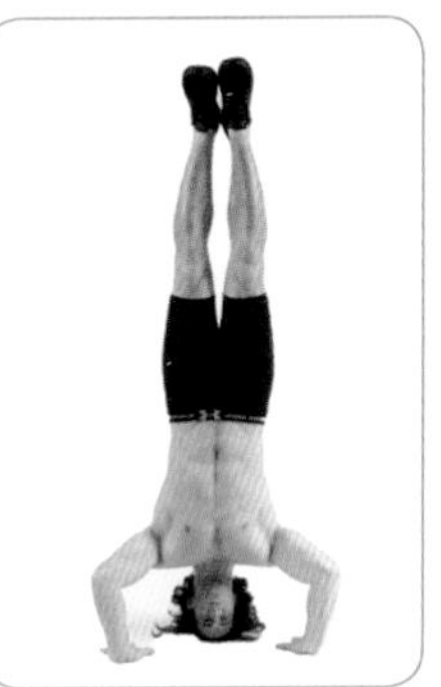
Handstand Push-Up
pages 74–75

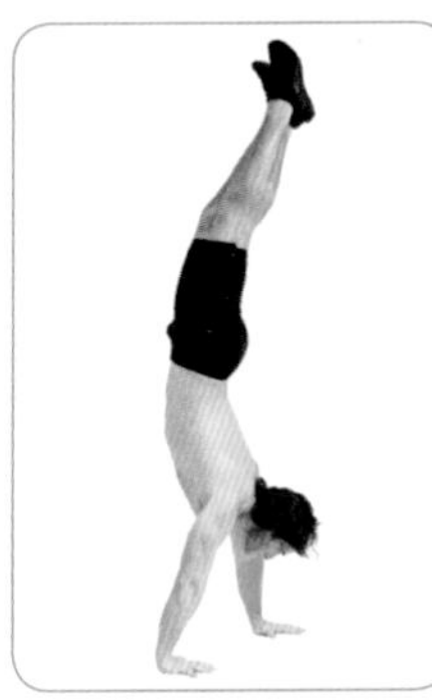
Handstand Walk
page 140

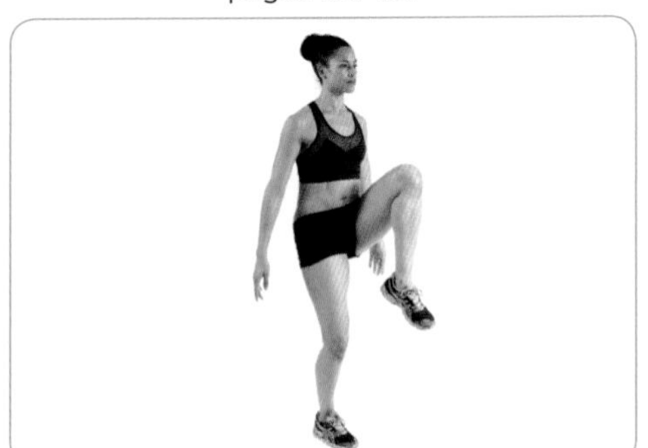
High Knees
pages 94–95

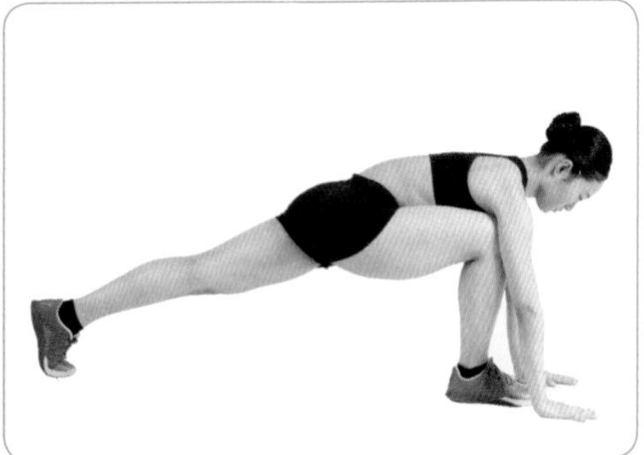
High Lunge
pages 38–39

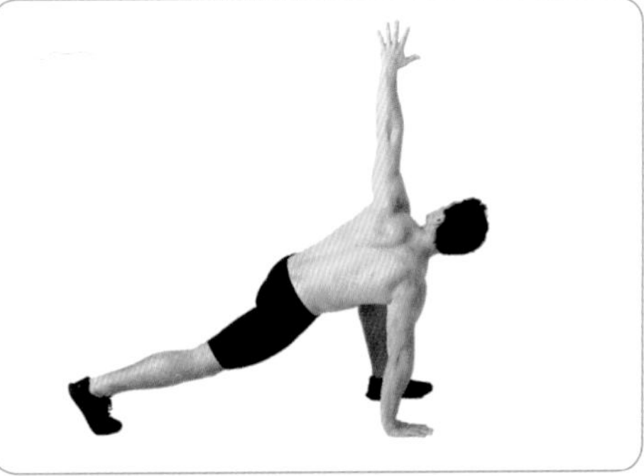
High Lunge with Twist
pages 114–115

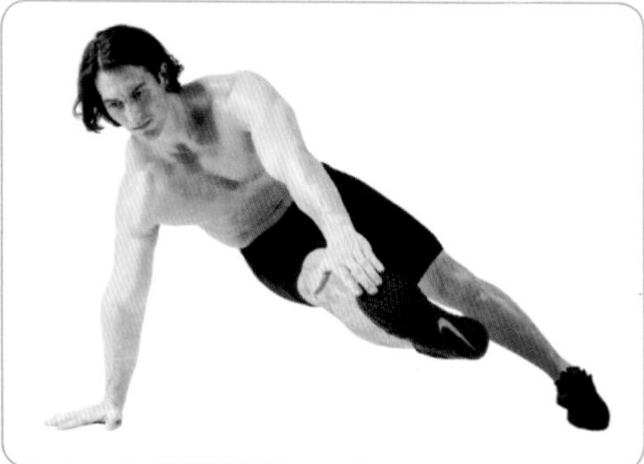
High Plank Kick-Through
page 143

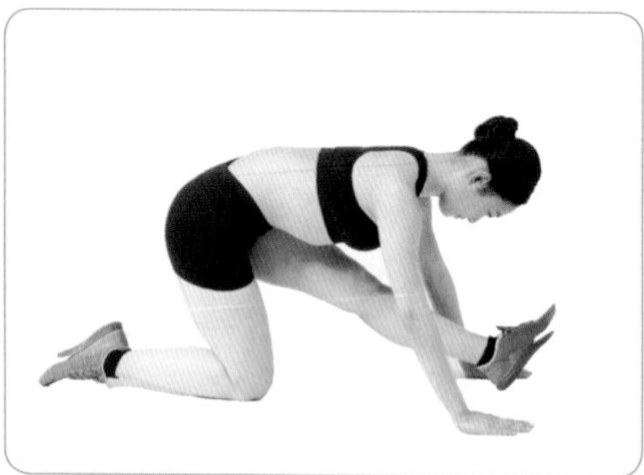
Hip Flexor Stretch
page 37

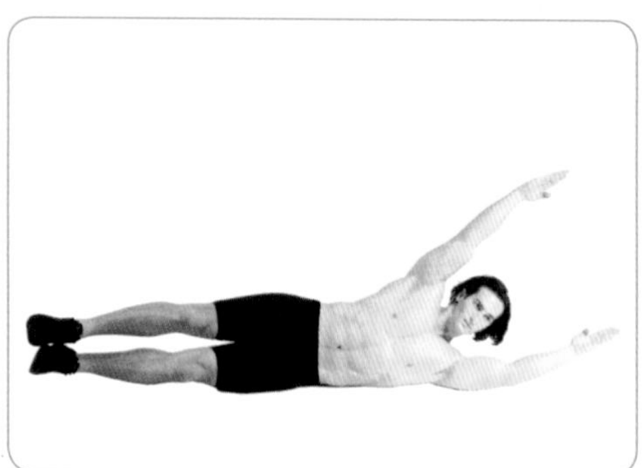
Hollow Hold to Superman
page 105

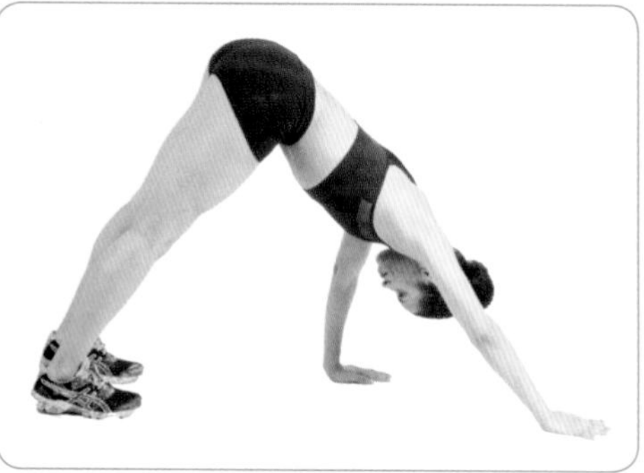
Inchworm
pages 66–67

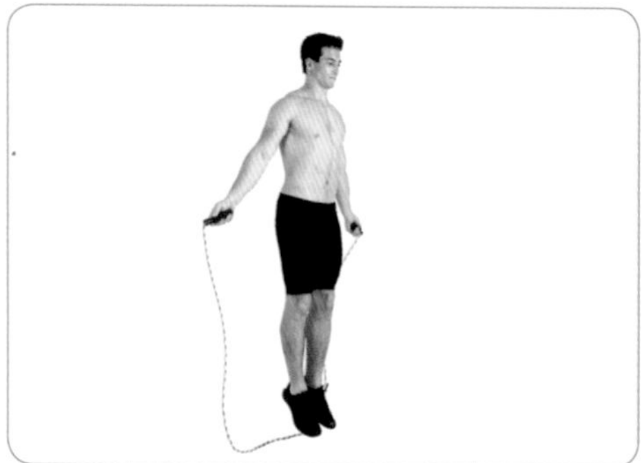
Jump Rope
pages 310–311

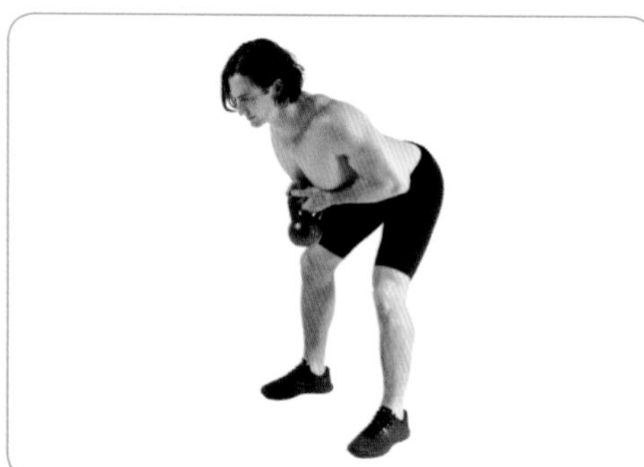
Kettlebell Bent-Over Row
page 149

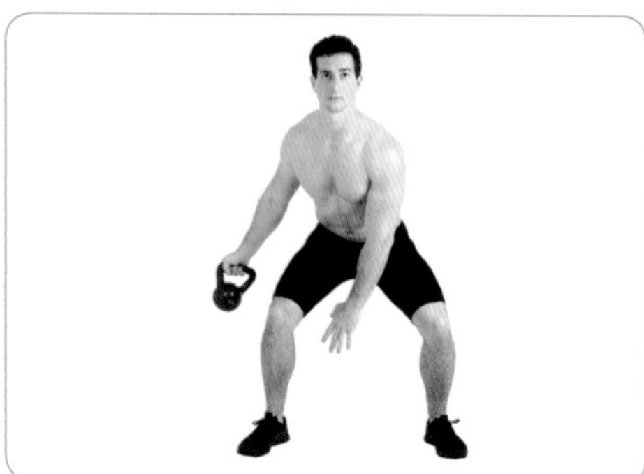
Kettlebell Figure 8
pages 218–219

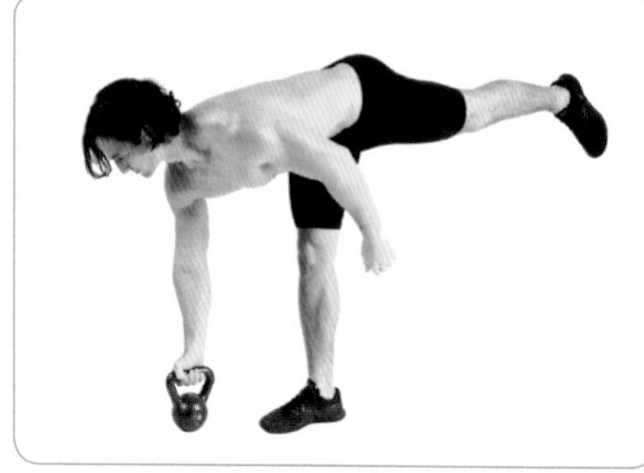
Kettlebell Single-Leg Russian Deadlift
page 212

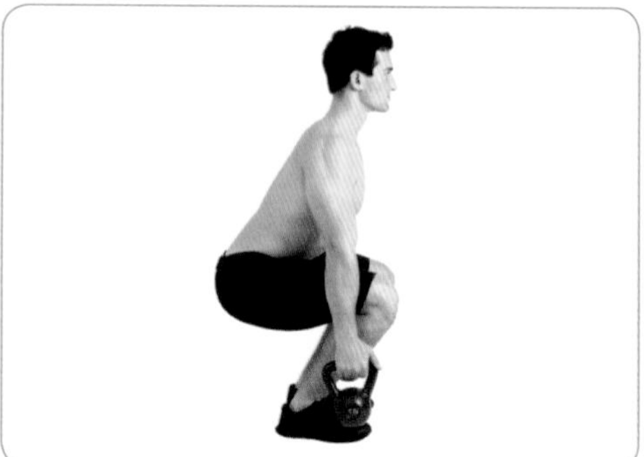
Kettlebell Squat
pages 220–221

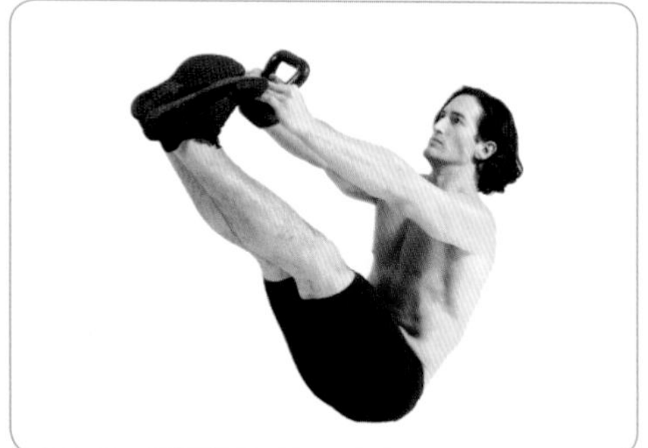
Kettlebell Toe Toucher
page 205

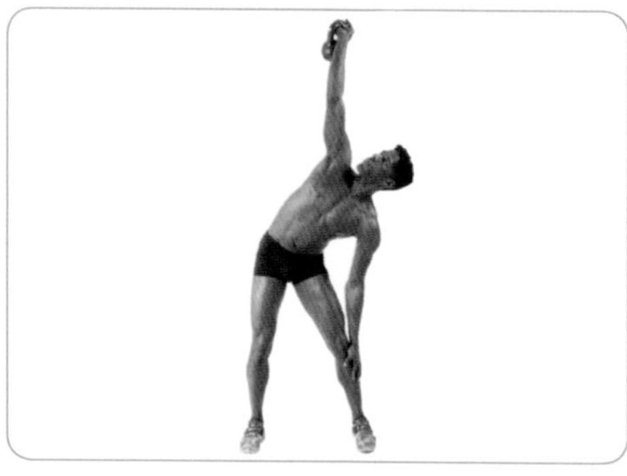
Kettlebell Windmill
pages 200–201

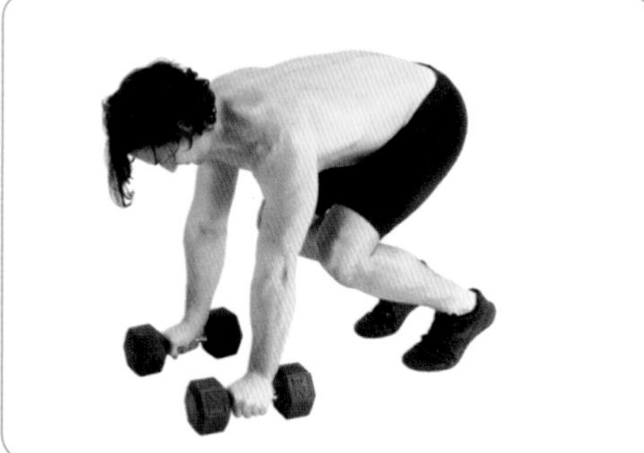
Kitchen Sink
pages 234–235

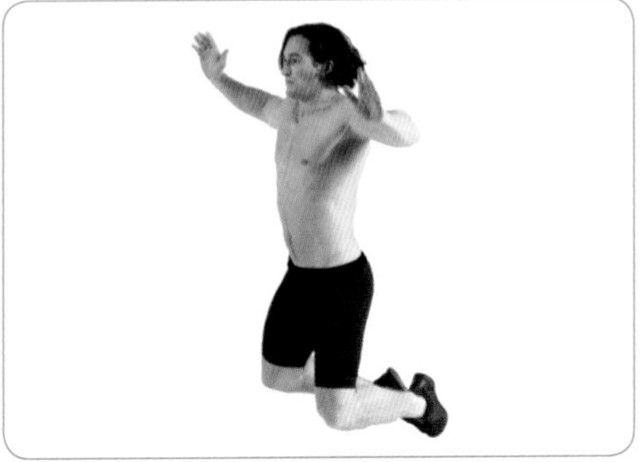
Kneeling Squat Jump
page 127

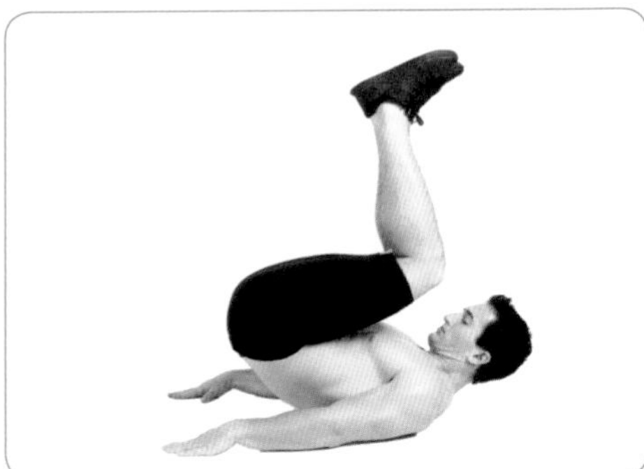
Knees to Chest
pages 98–99

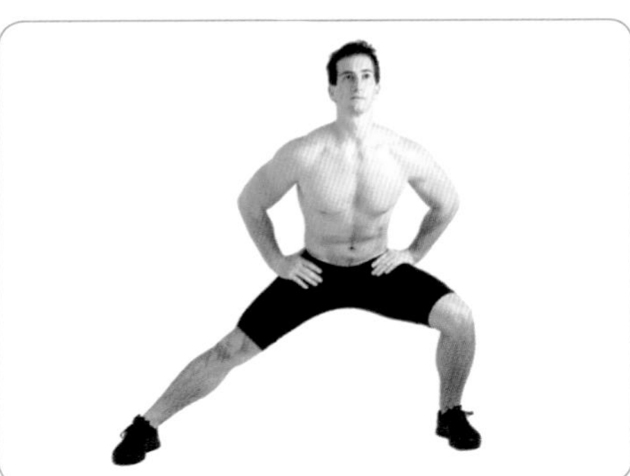
Lateral Lunge with Squat
pages 112–113

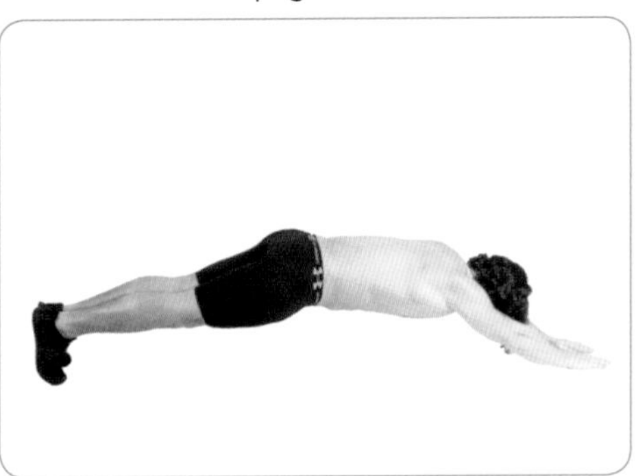
Layout Push-Up
page 61

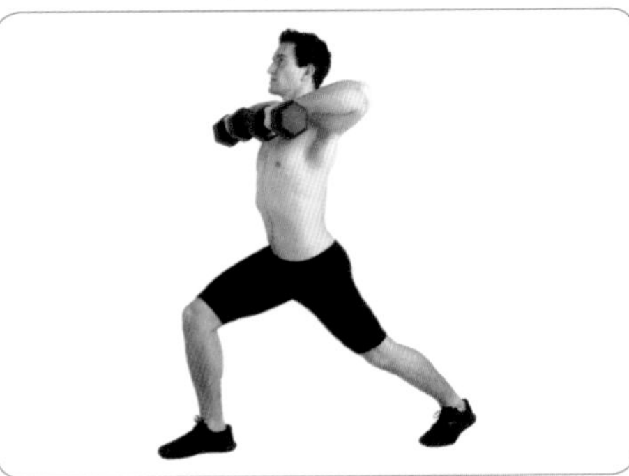
Lunge with Dumbbell Upright Row
pages 230–231

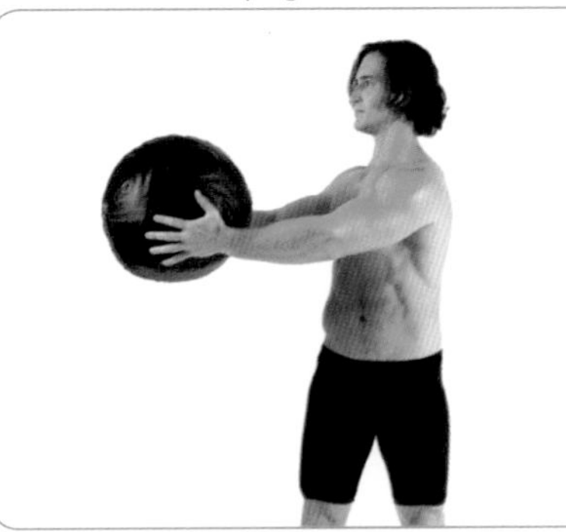
Medicine Ball Core Twist
page 283

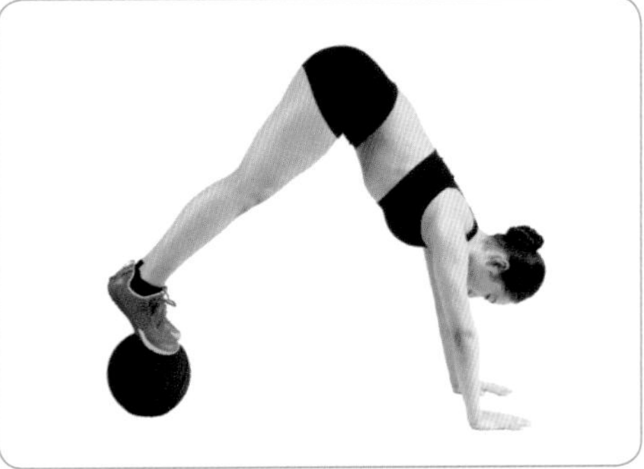
Medicine Ball Pike-Up
pages 294–295

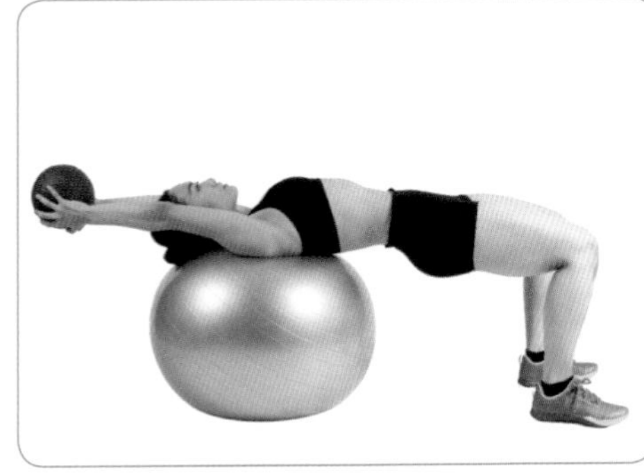
Medicine Ball Pullover on Swiss Ball
pages 252–253

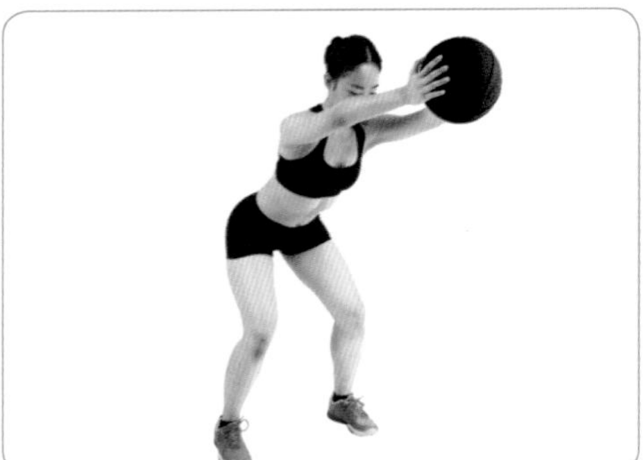
Medicine Ball Slam
pages 318–319

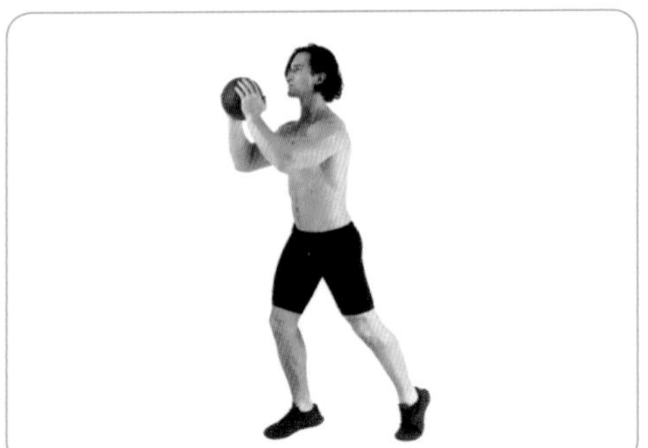
Medicine Ball Throw
pages 268–269

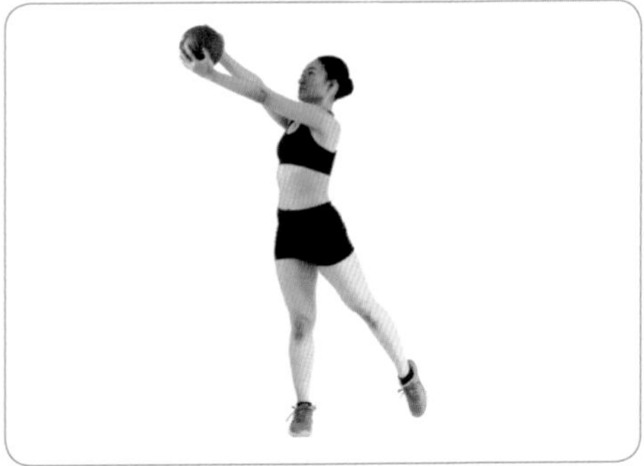
Medicine Ball Woodchop
pages 288–289

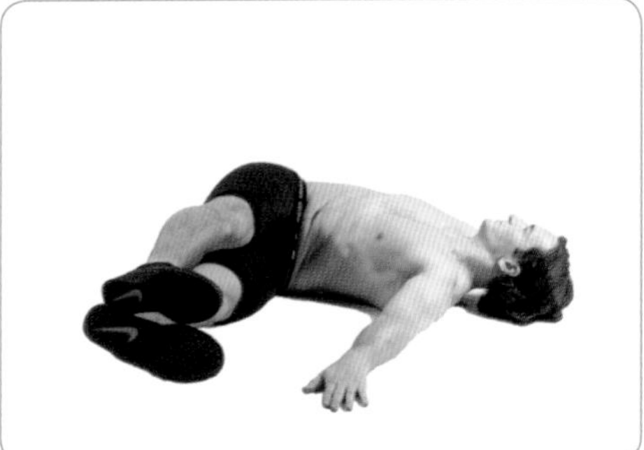
Metronome
page 104

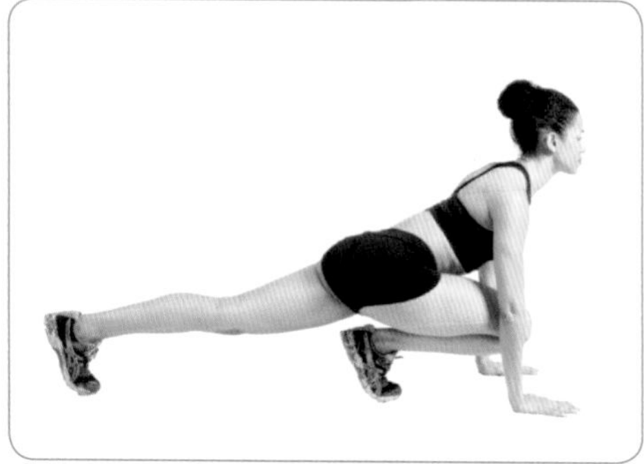
Mountain Climber
pages 138–139

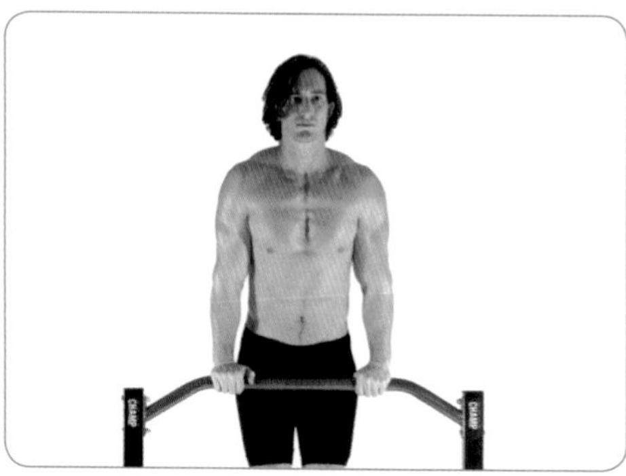
Muscle-Up
page 141

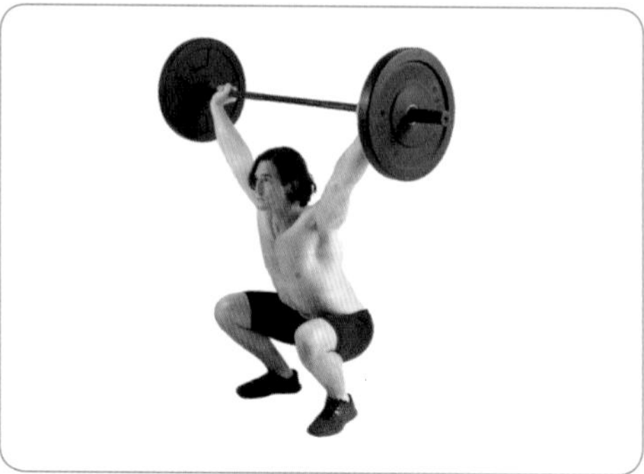
Overhead Squat
page 309

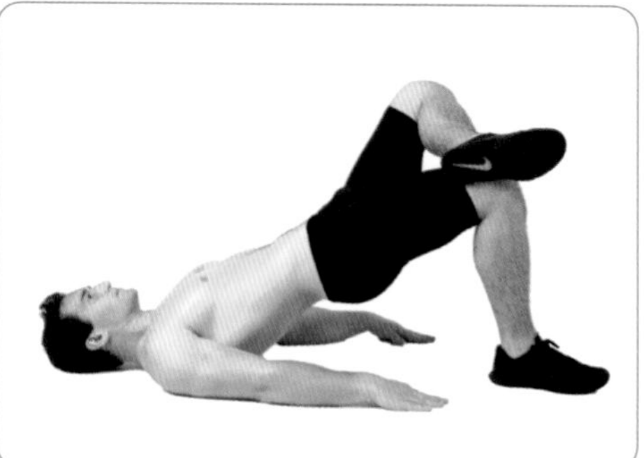
Piriformis Bridge
pages 30–31

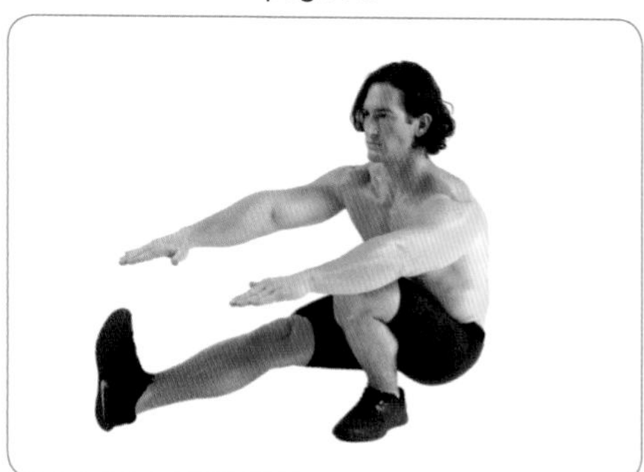
Pistol
page 123

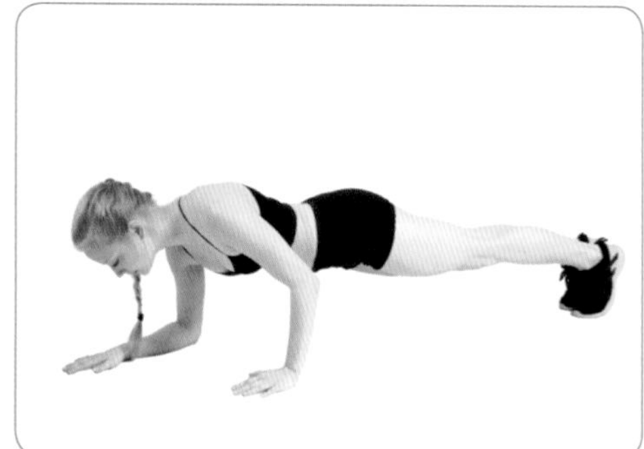
Plank-Up
pages 68–69

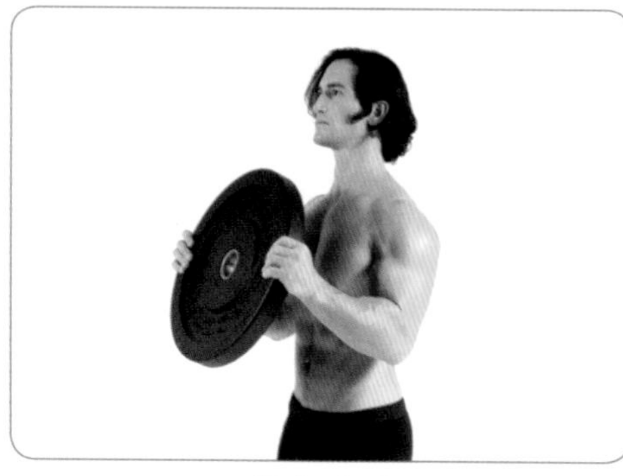
Plate Curl
pages 256–257

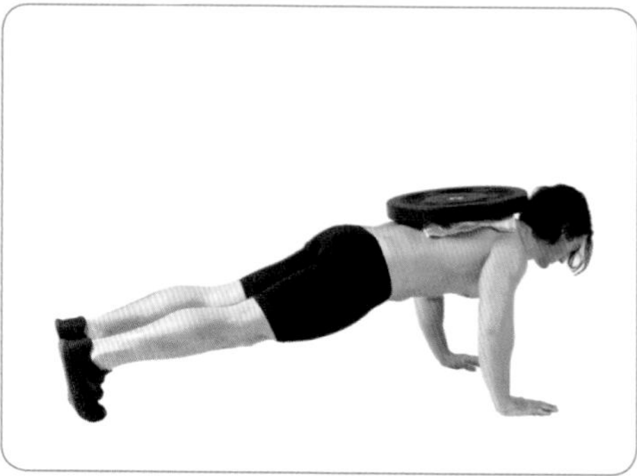
Plate Push-Up
pages 276–277

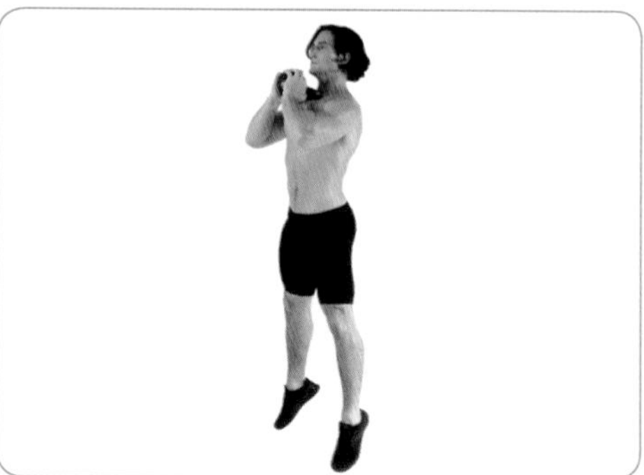
Plyo Goblet Squat
pages 214–215

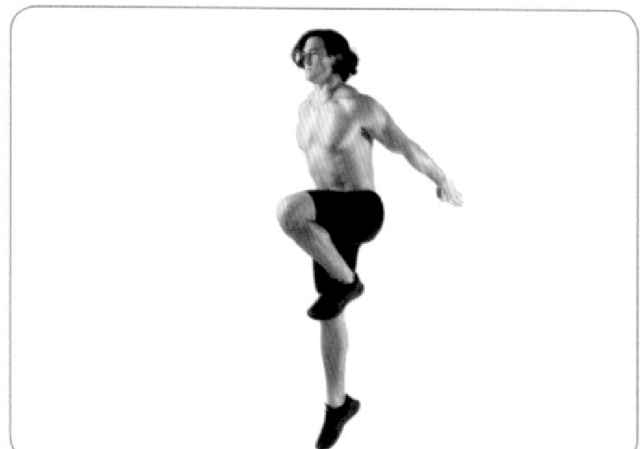
Plyo Knee Drive
page 122

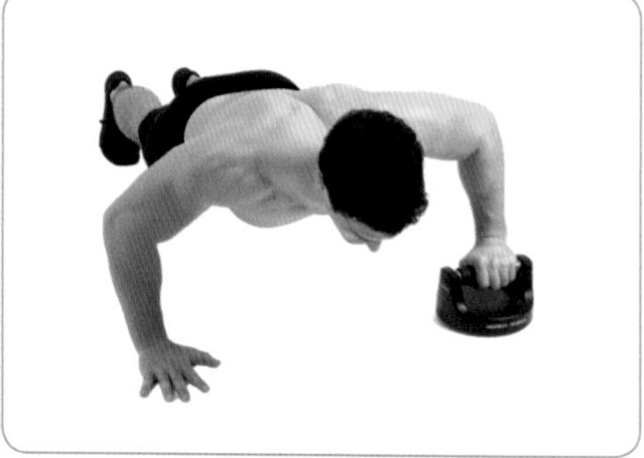
Plyo Power Stand Push-Up
pages 190–191

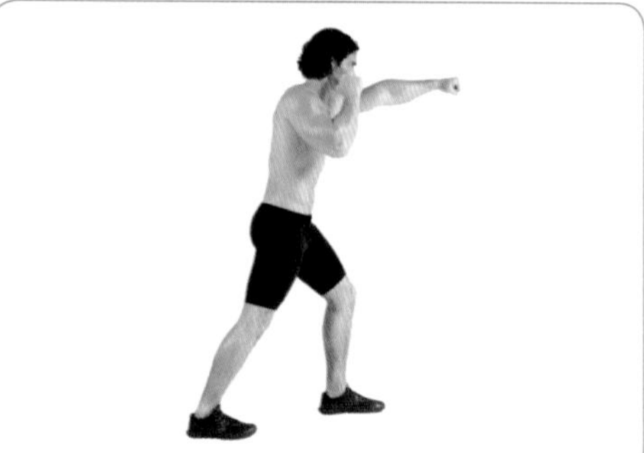
Power Punch
pages 70–71

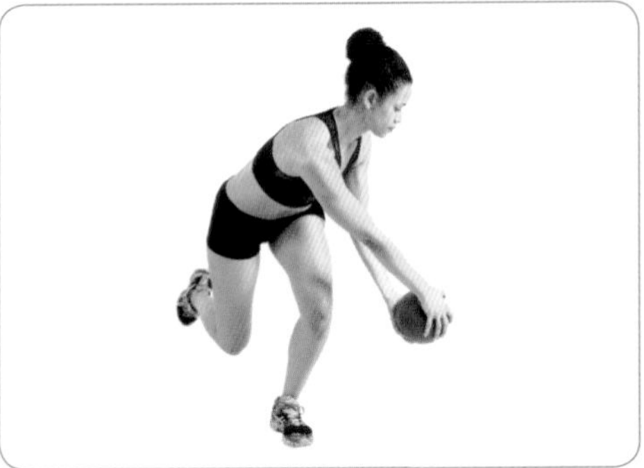
Power Squat
pages 300–301

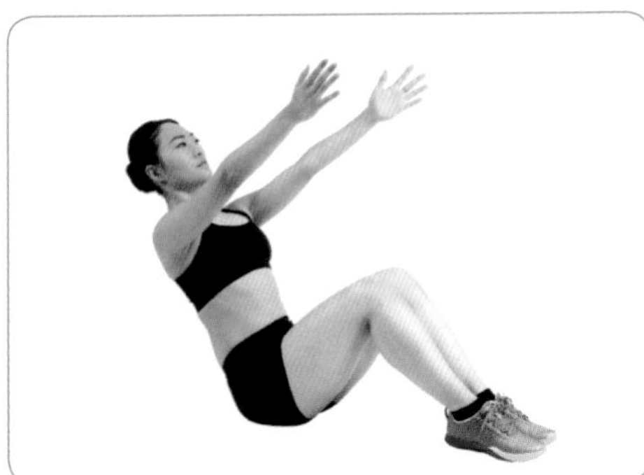
Pullover Pass
pages 290–291

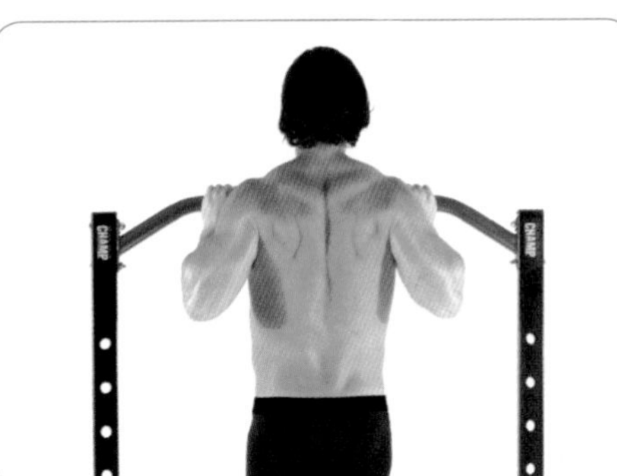

Pull-Up
pages 44–45

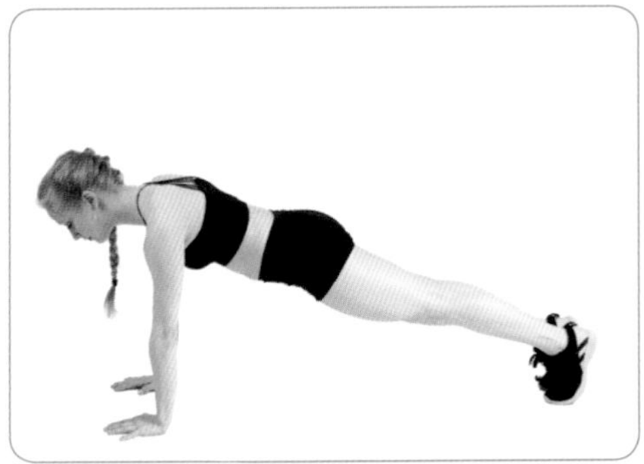
Push-Up
pages 76–77

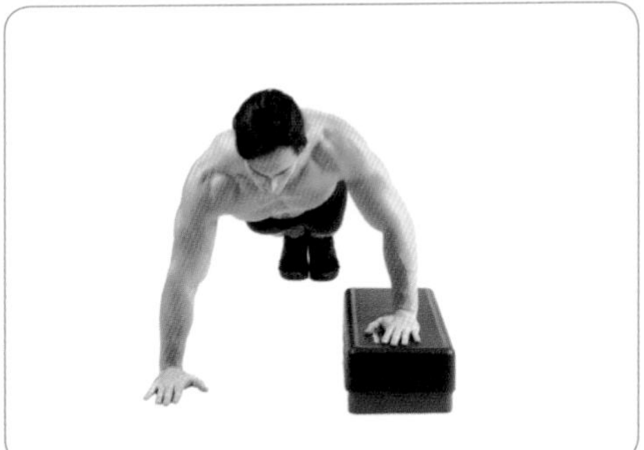
Push-Up Hand Walk-Over
pages 272–273

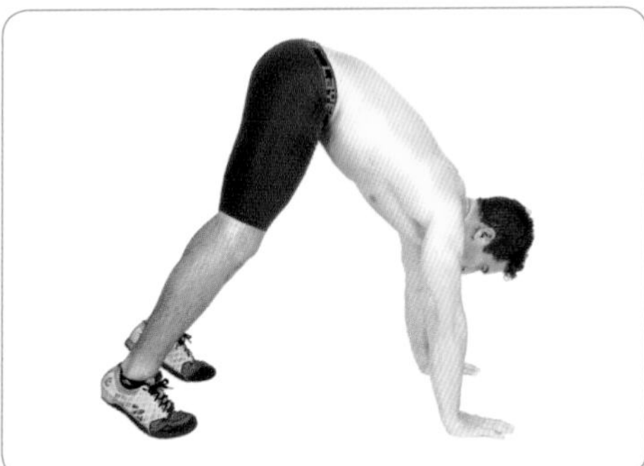
Push-Up Walkout
pages 26–27

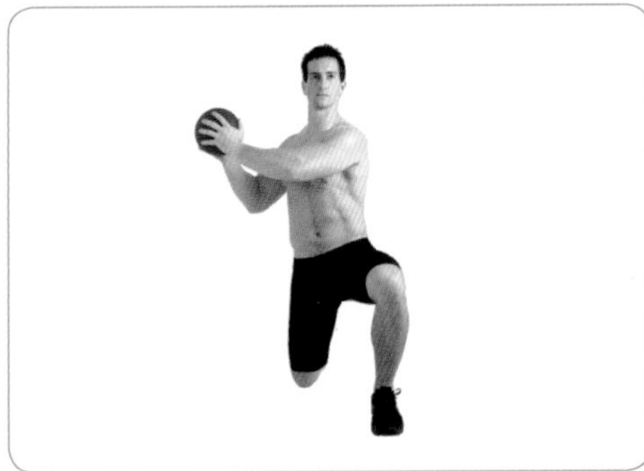
Reach-and-Twist Walking Lunge
pages 306–307

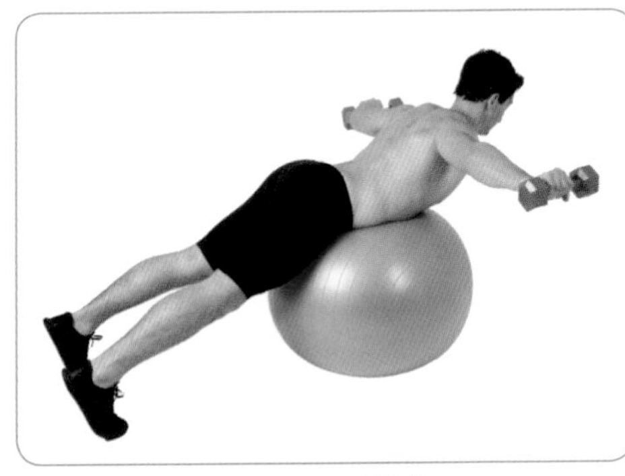
Rear Lateral Raise
pages 160–161

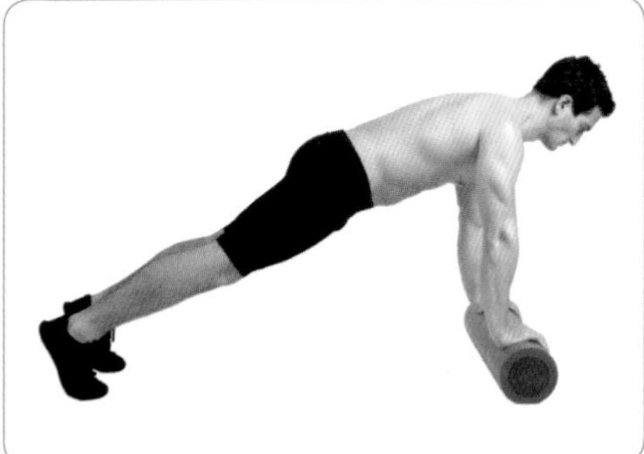
Roller Push-Up
pages 274–275

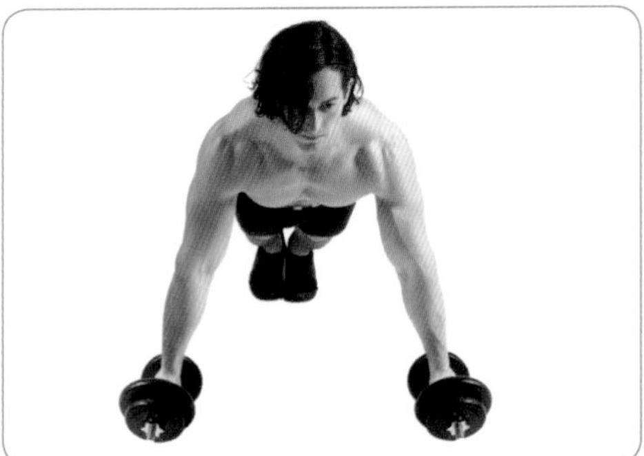
Rolling Dumbbell Fly
page 193

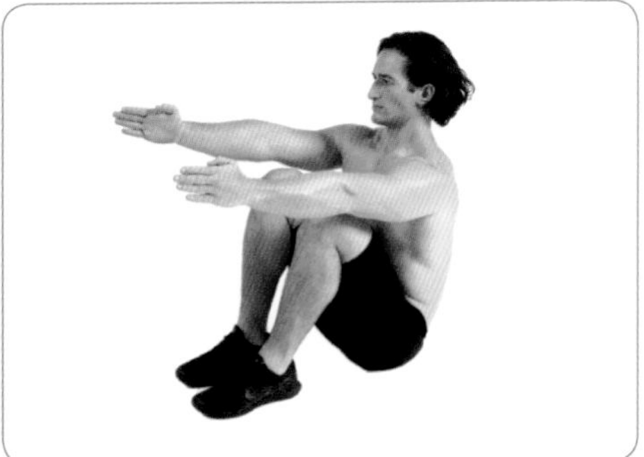
Roll-Up
page 142

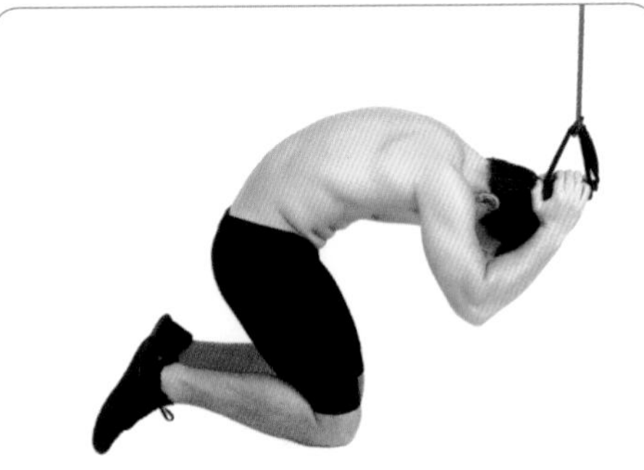
Rope Pull-Down
pages 284–285

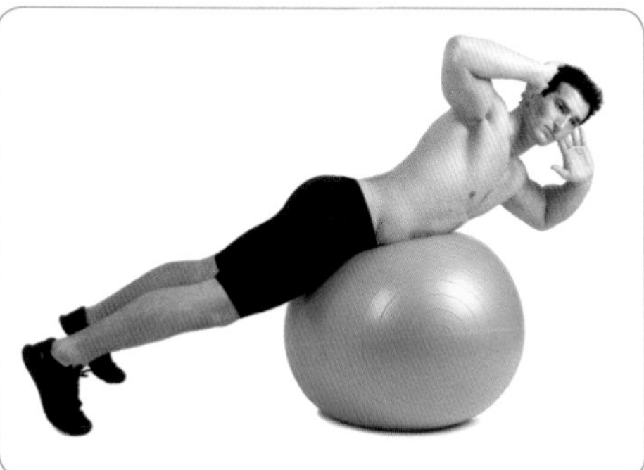
Rotated Back Extension
pages 58–59

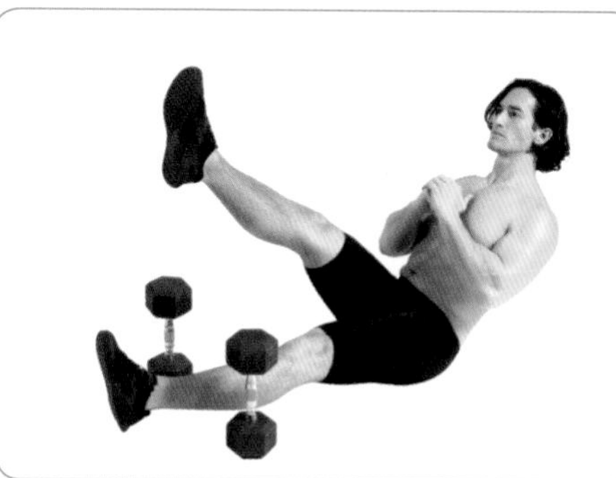
Scissors over Dumbbells
pages 194–195

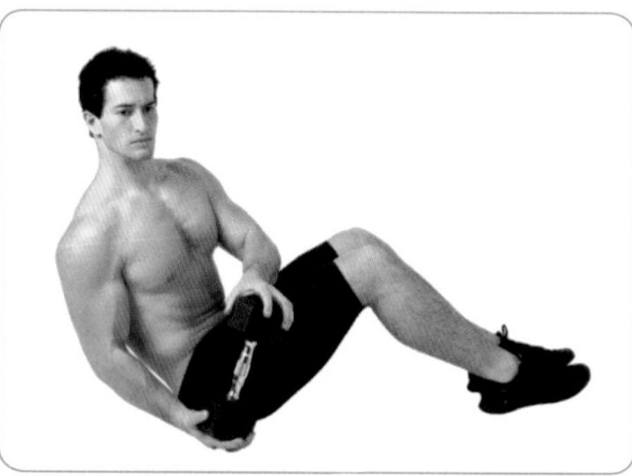
Seated Dumbbell Russian Twist
pages 198–199

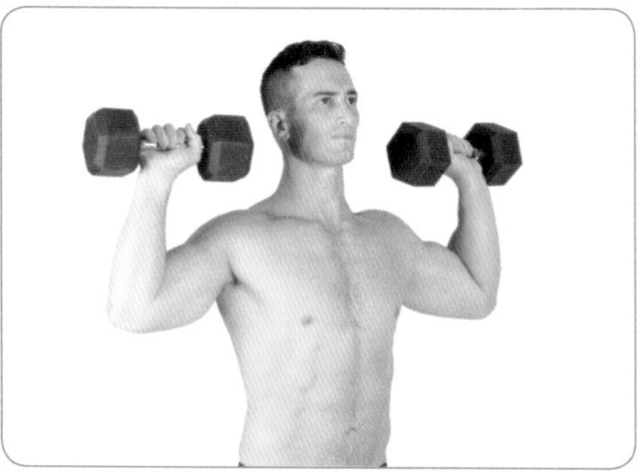
Shoulder Crusher
pages 176–177

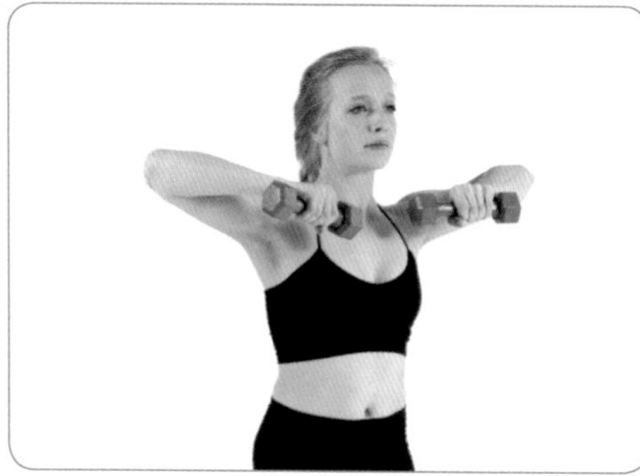
Shoulder Raise and Pull
pages 170–171

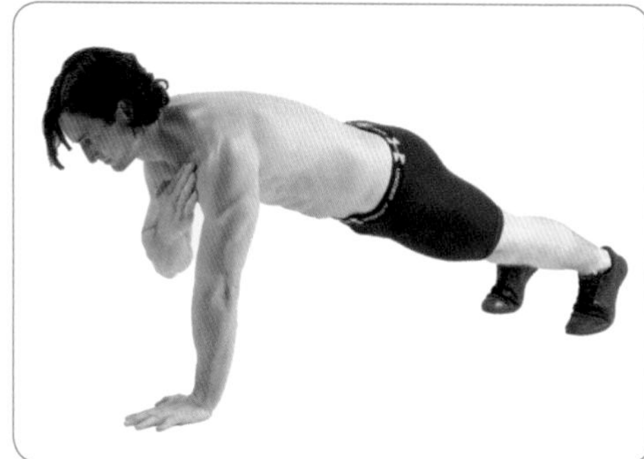
Shoulder-Tap Push-Up
pages 78–79

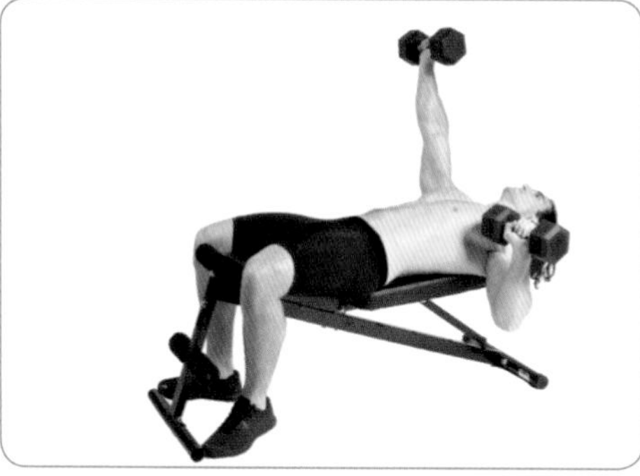
Single-Arm Dumbbell Press
page 182

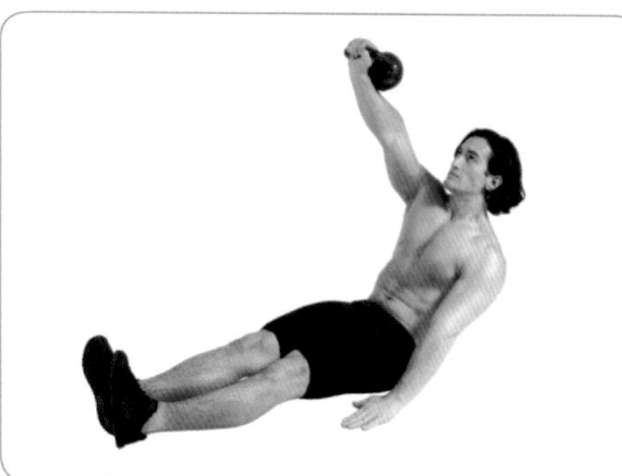
Single-Arm Kettlebell Press-Up
page 204

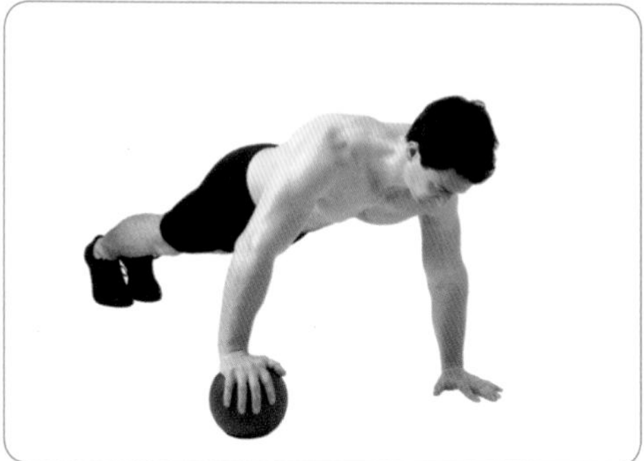
Single-Arm Medicine Ball Push-Up
page 280

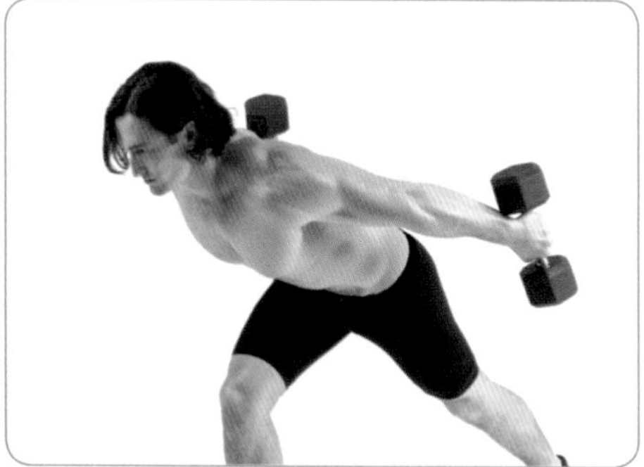
Double-Arm Triceps Kickback
page 180

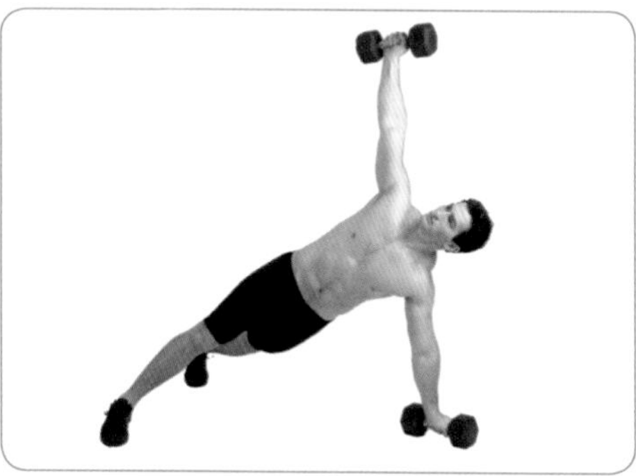
Single-Arm T-Row
page 152–153

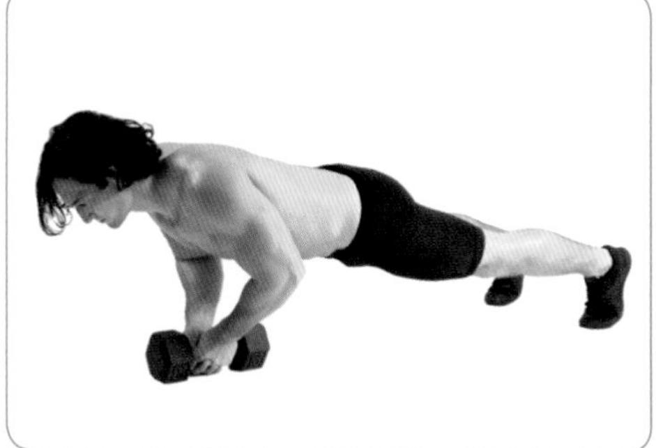
Single Dumbbell Push-Up
page 192

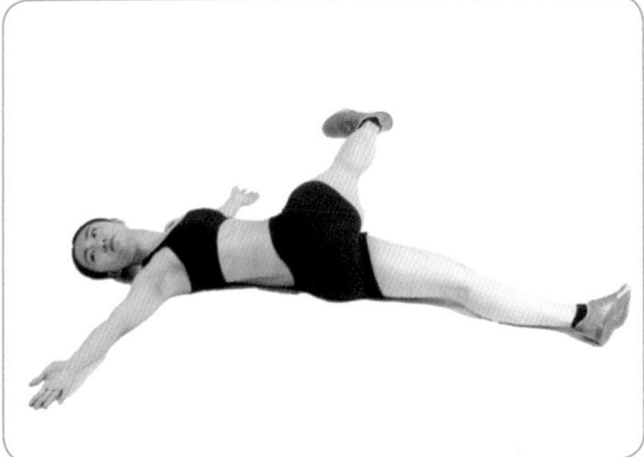
Single-Leg Crossover
pages 34–35

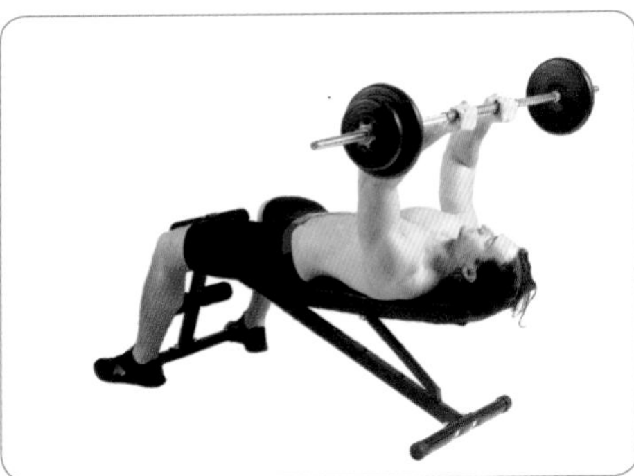
Skull Crusher
pages 260–261

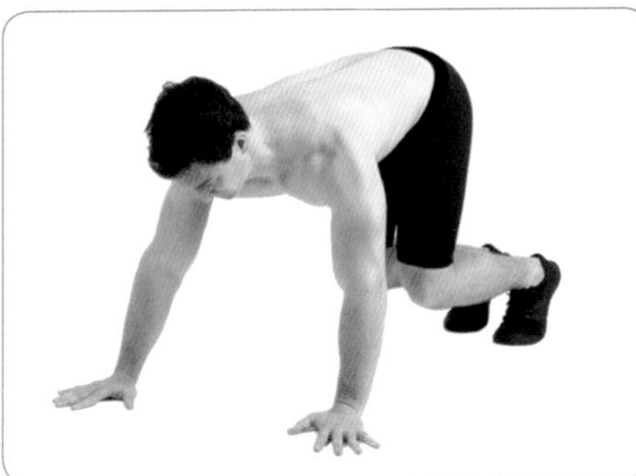
Slalom Skier
pages 136–137

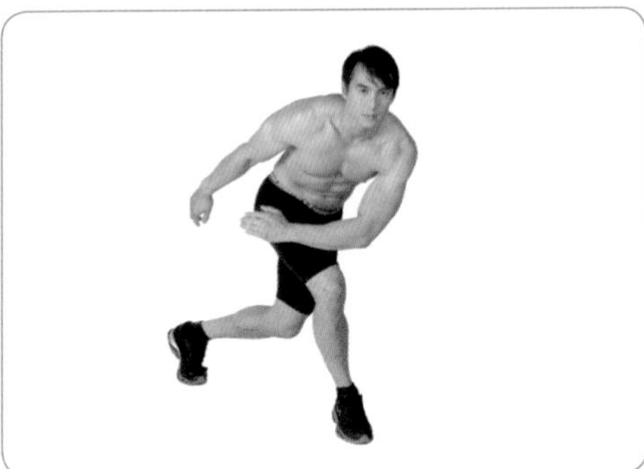
Speed Skater
pages 118–119

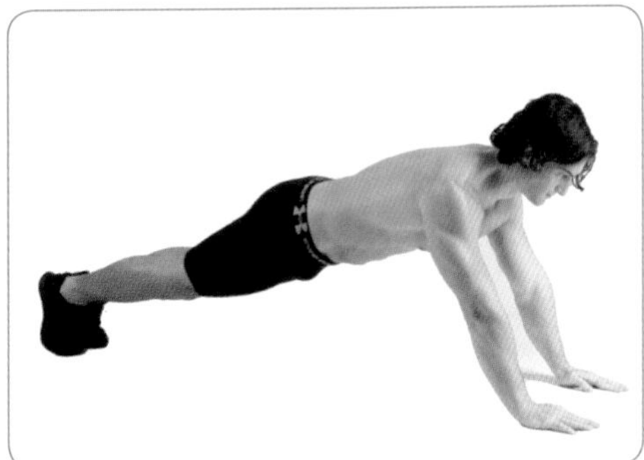
Sphinx Push-Up
page 88

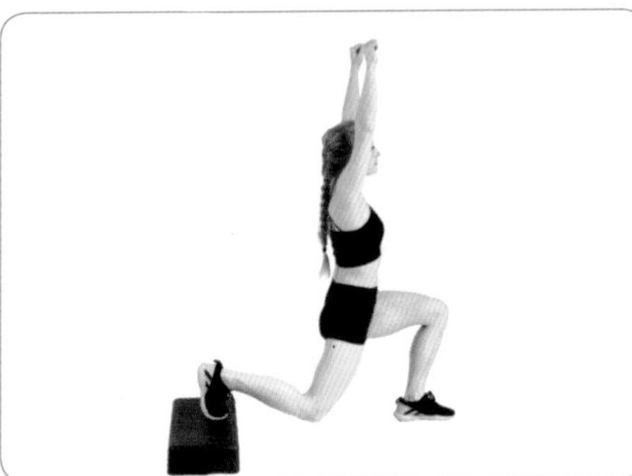
Split Squat with Overhead Press
pages 228–229

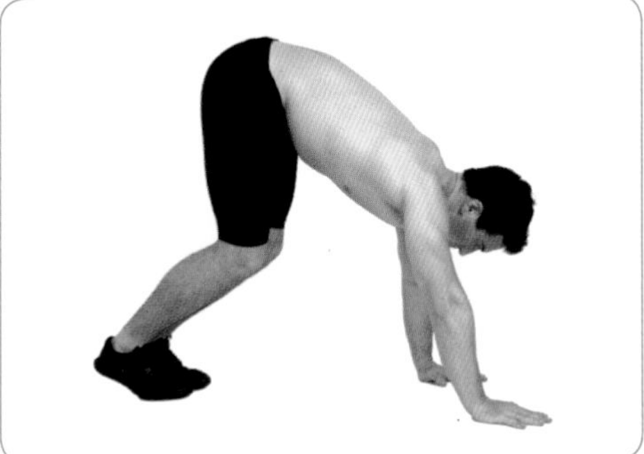
Sprawl Push-Up
pages 86–87

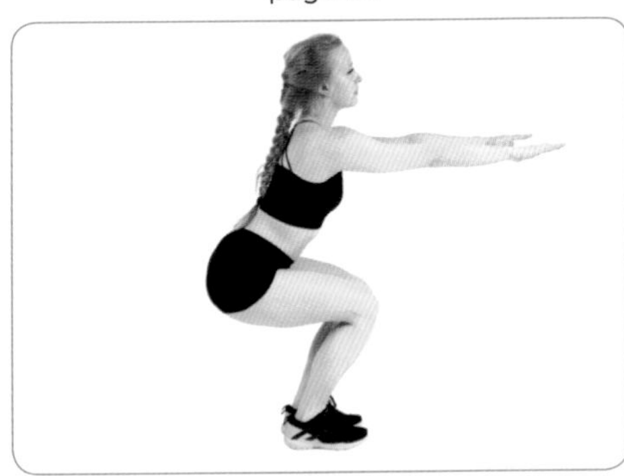
Squat
pages 106–107

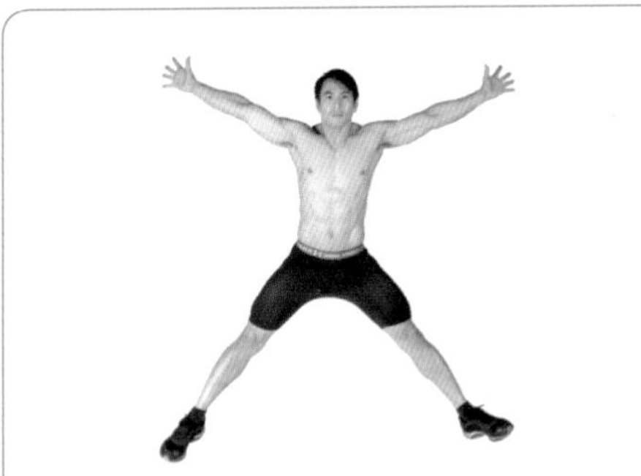
Star Jump
pages 130–131

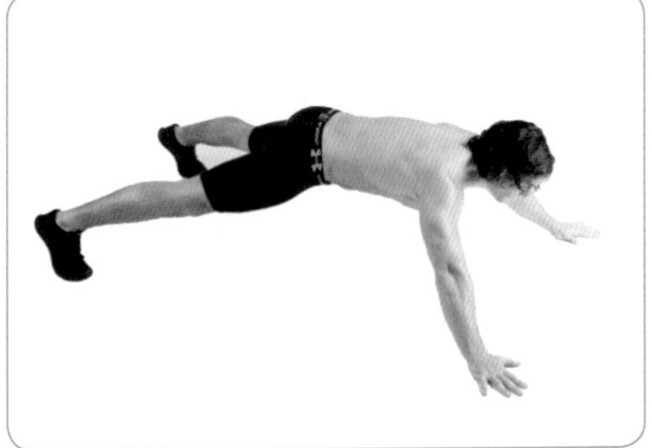
Star Push-Up
page 89

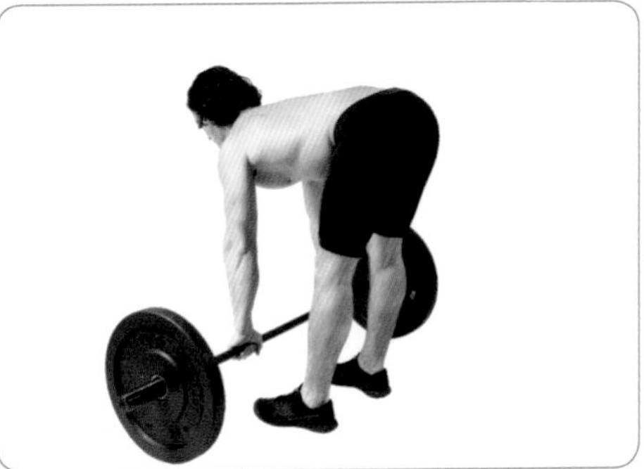
Stiff-Legged Barbell Deadlift
pages 242–243

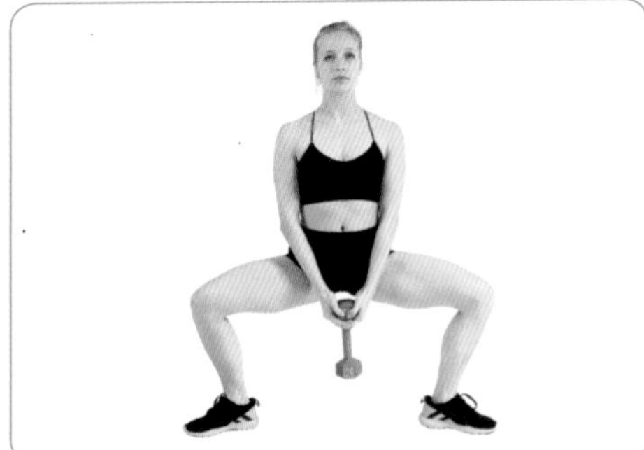
Sumo Squat with Dumbbell
pages 216–217

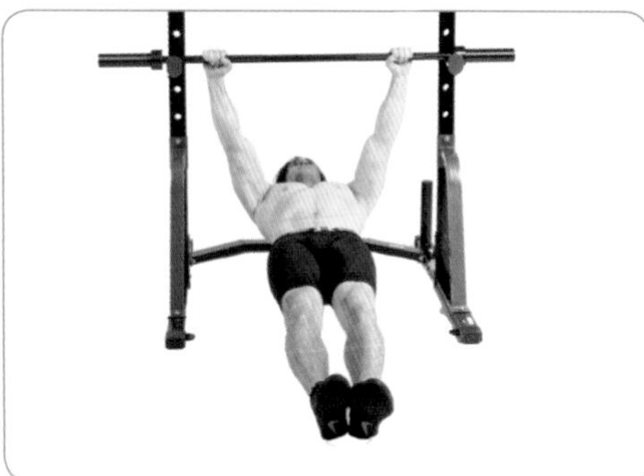

Supine Reverse-Grip Back Row
page 72

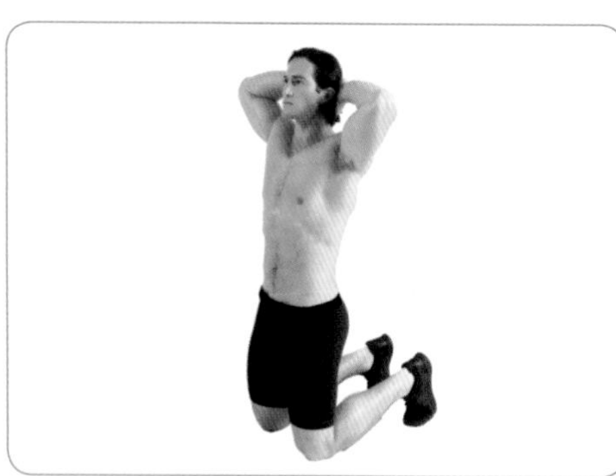

Surrender
page 126

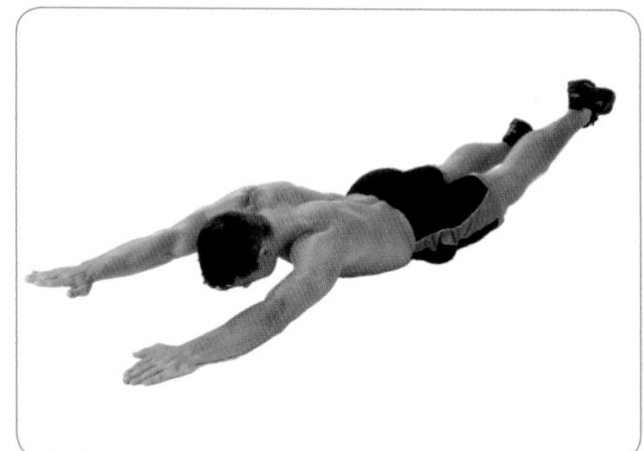

Swimmer
pages 50–51

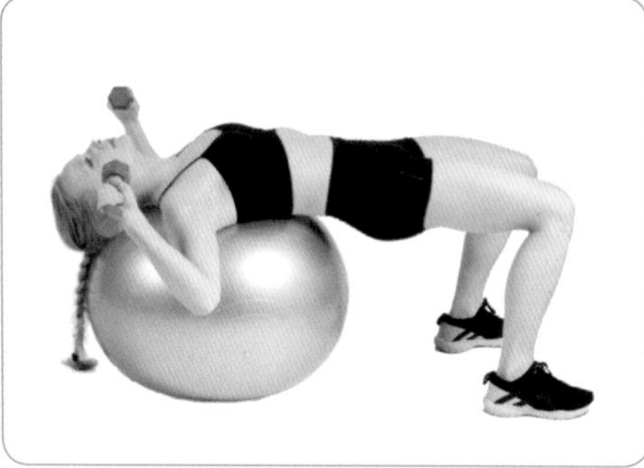

Swiss Ball Flat Dumbbell Press
pages 184–185

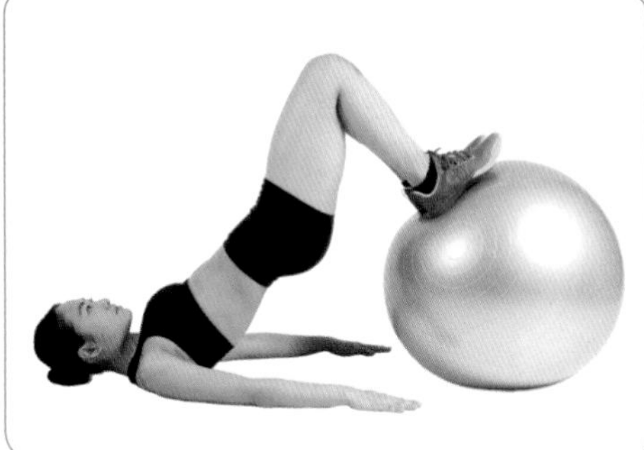

Swiss Ball Hamstrings Curl
pages 302–303

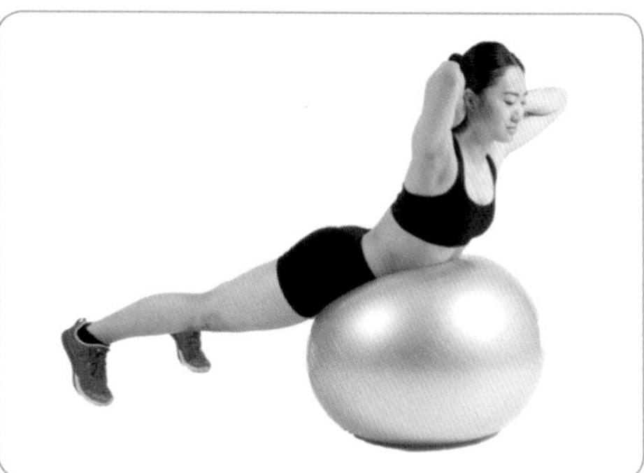

Swiss Ball Hyperextension
pages 56–57

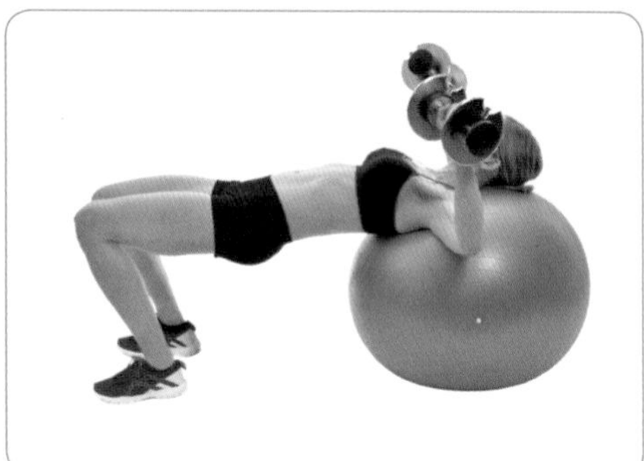

Swiss Ball Incline Dumbbell Press
page 183

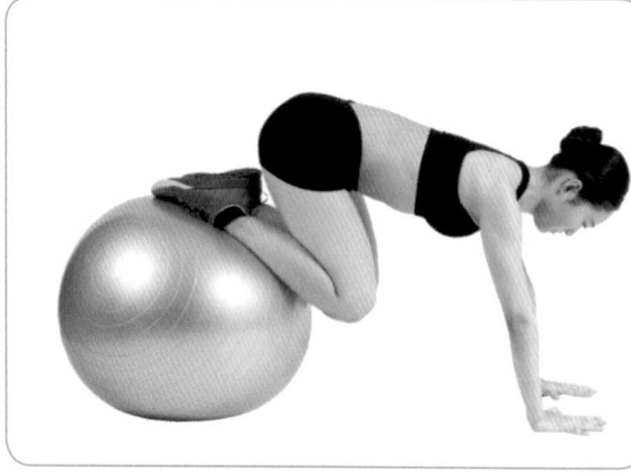

Swiss Ball Jackknife
pages 292–293

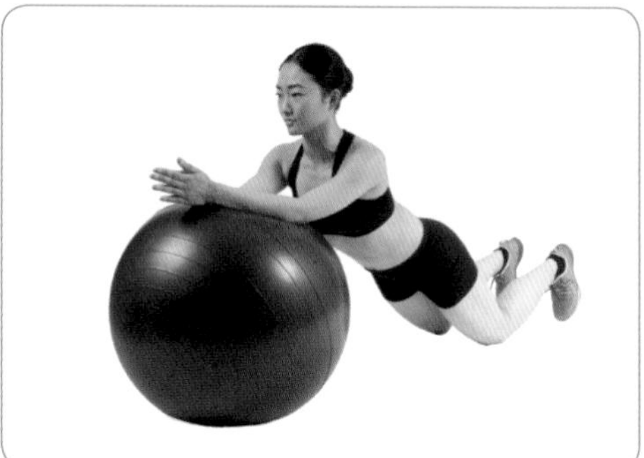

Swiss Ball Rollout
pages 296–297

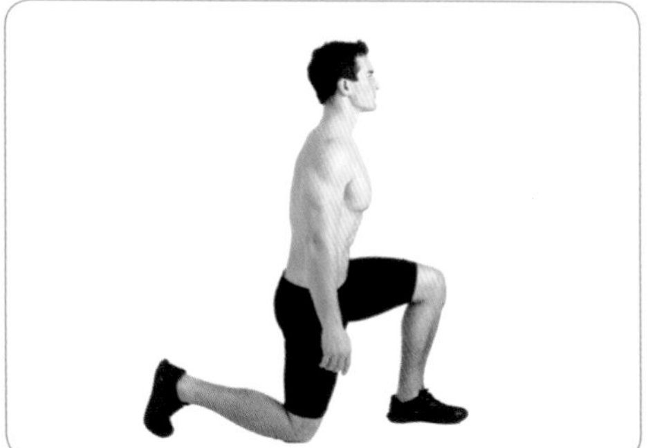

Switch Lunge
pages 110–111

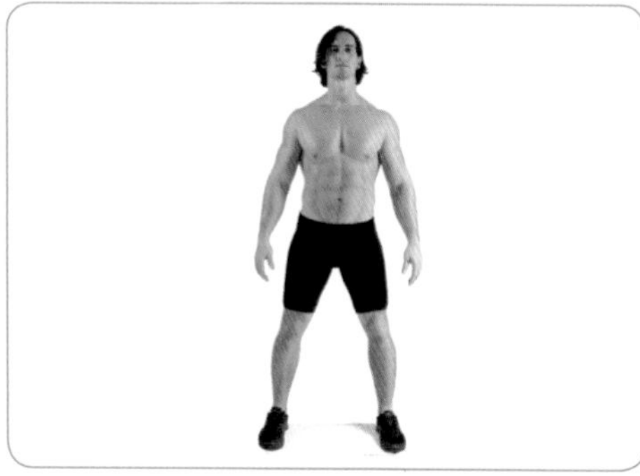

Towel Abduction and Adduction
page 125

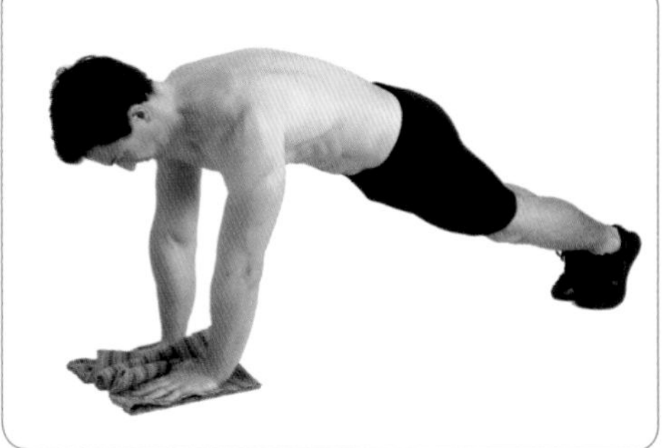

Towel Fly
pages 84–85

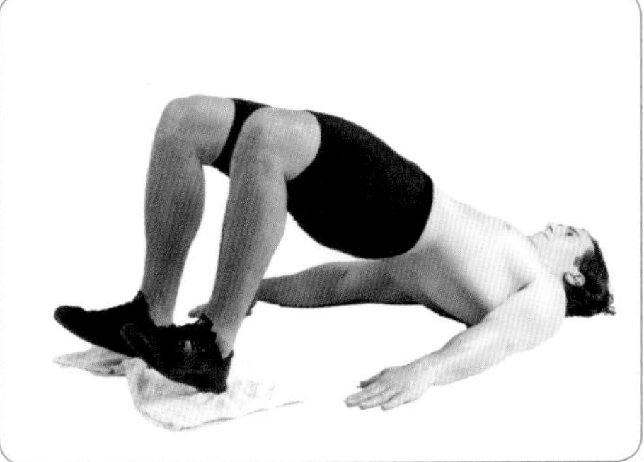
Towel Hamstrings Pull
page 124

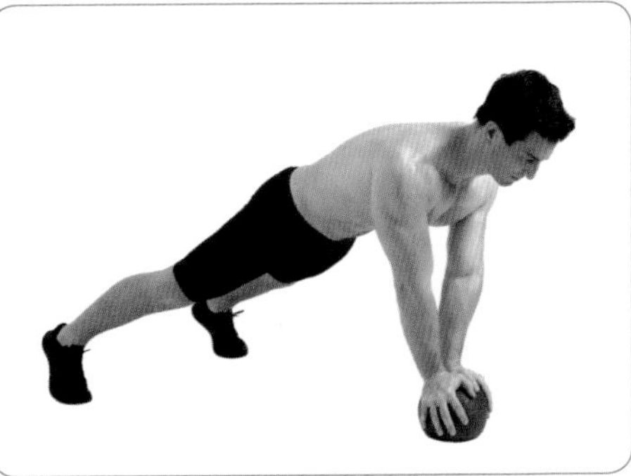
Triangle Push-Up with Medicine Ball
page 281

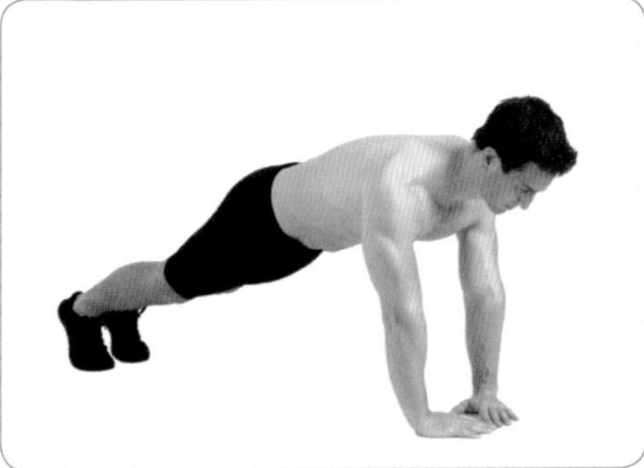
Triceps Push-Up
pages 64–65

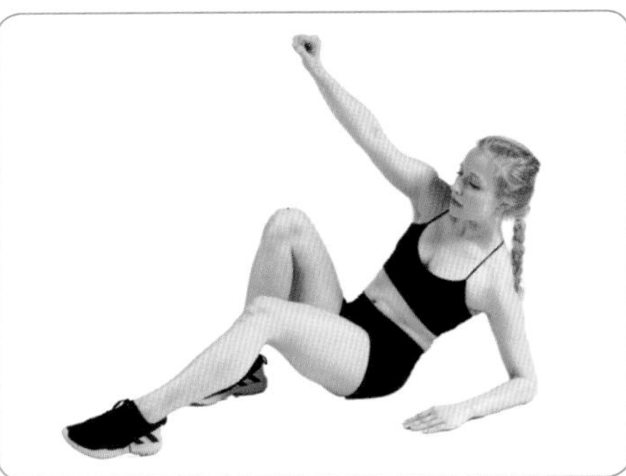
Turkish Get-Up
pages 144–145

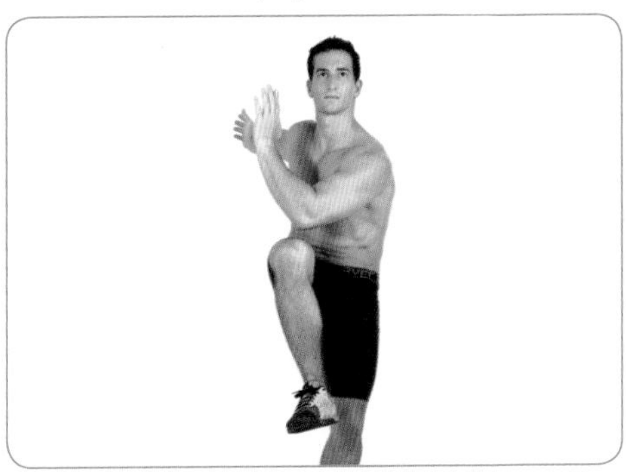
Twisting Knee Raise
pages 28–29

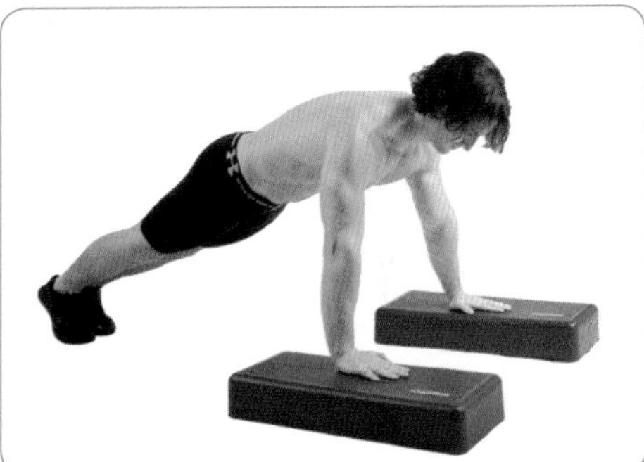
Two-Level Push-Up
pages 278–279

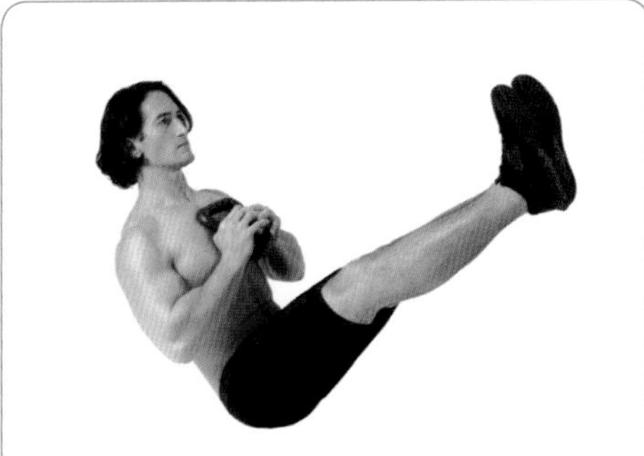
V-Sit Kettlebell Hold with Leg Lift
page 197

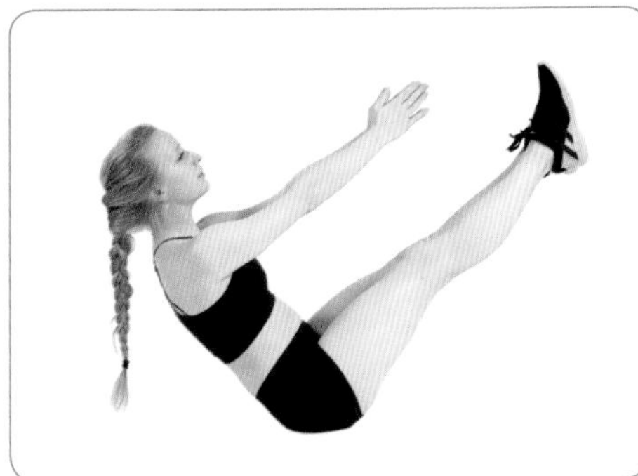
V-Up
pages 96–97

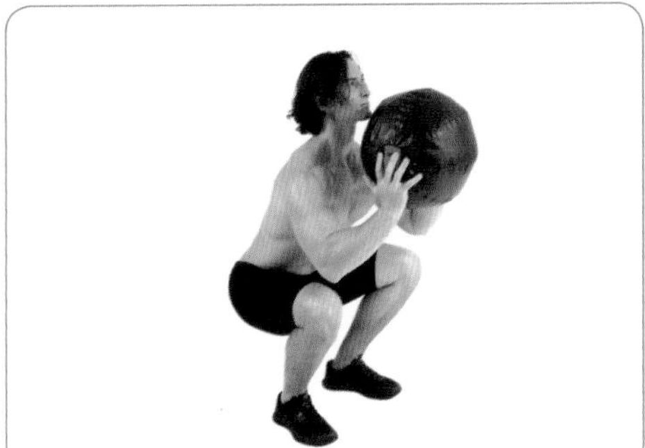
Wall Ball Shot
page 320

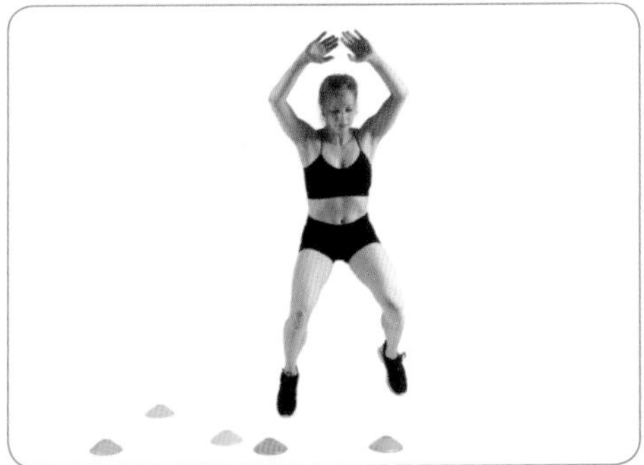
Warm-Up Obstacle Course
pages 32–33

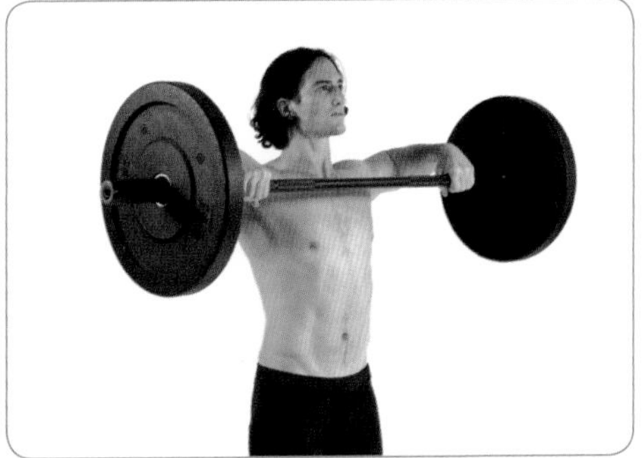
Wide-Grip High Pull
pages 250–251

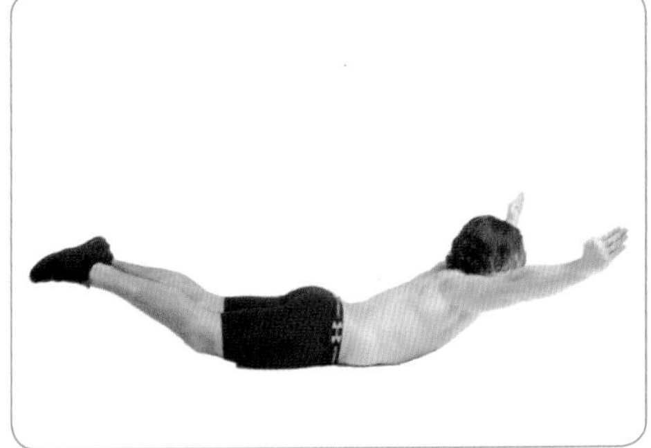
The Y
page 53

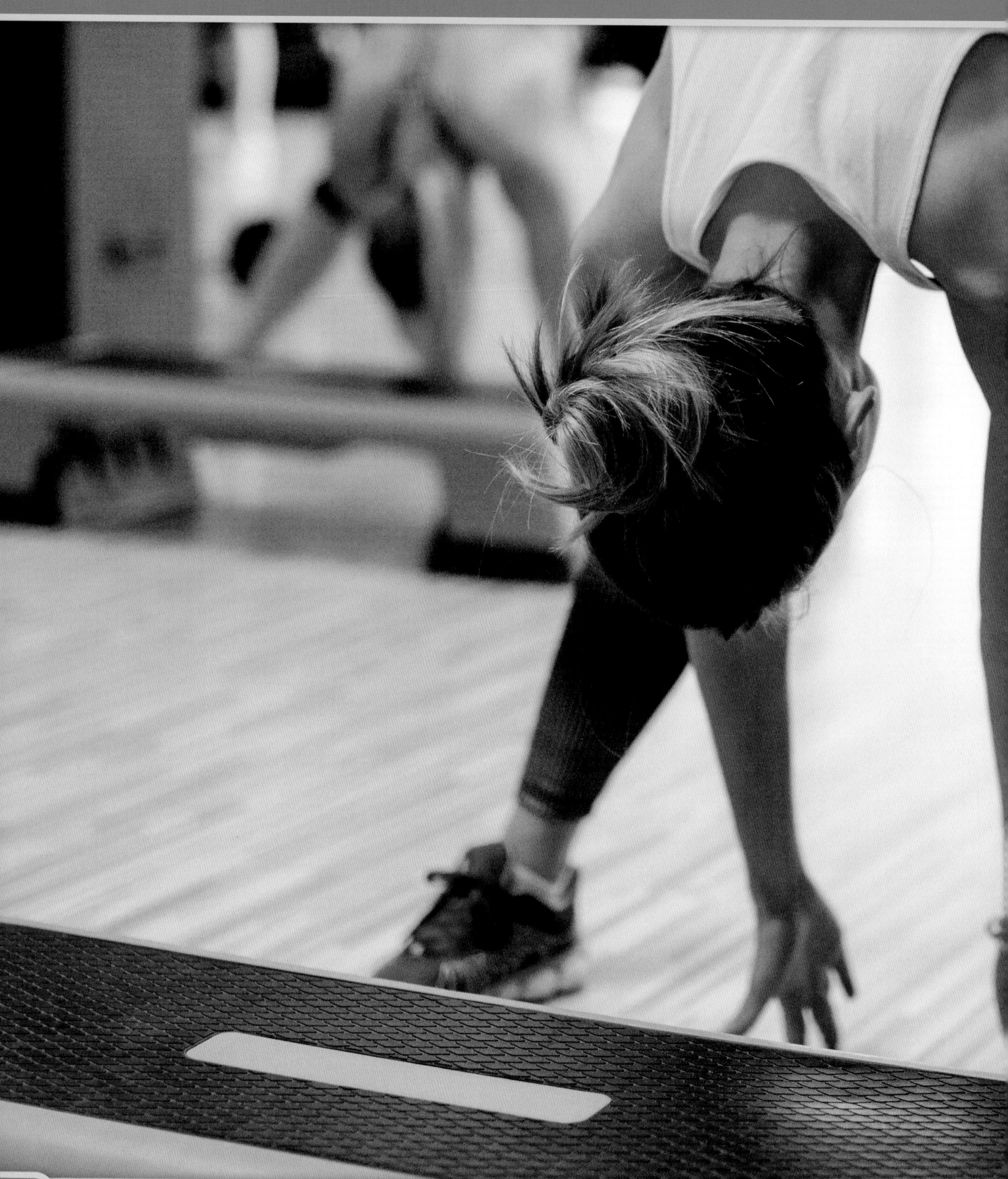

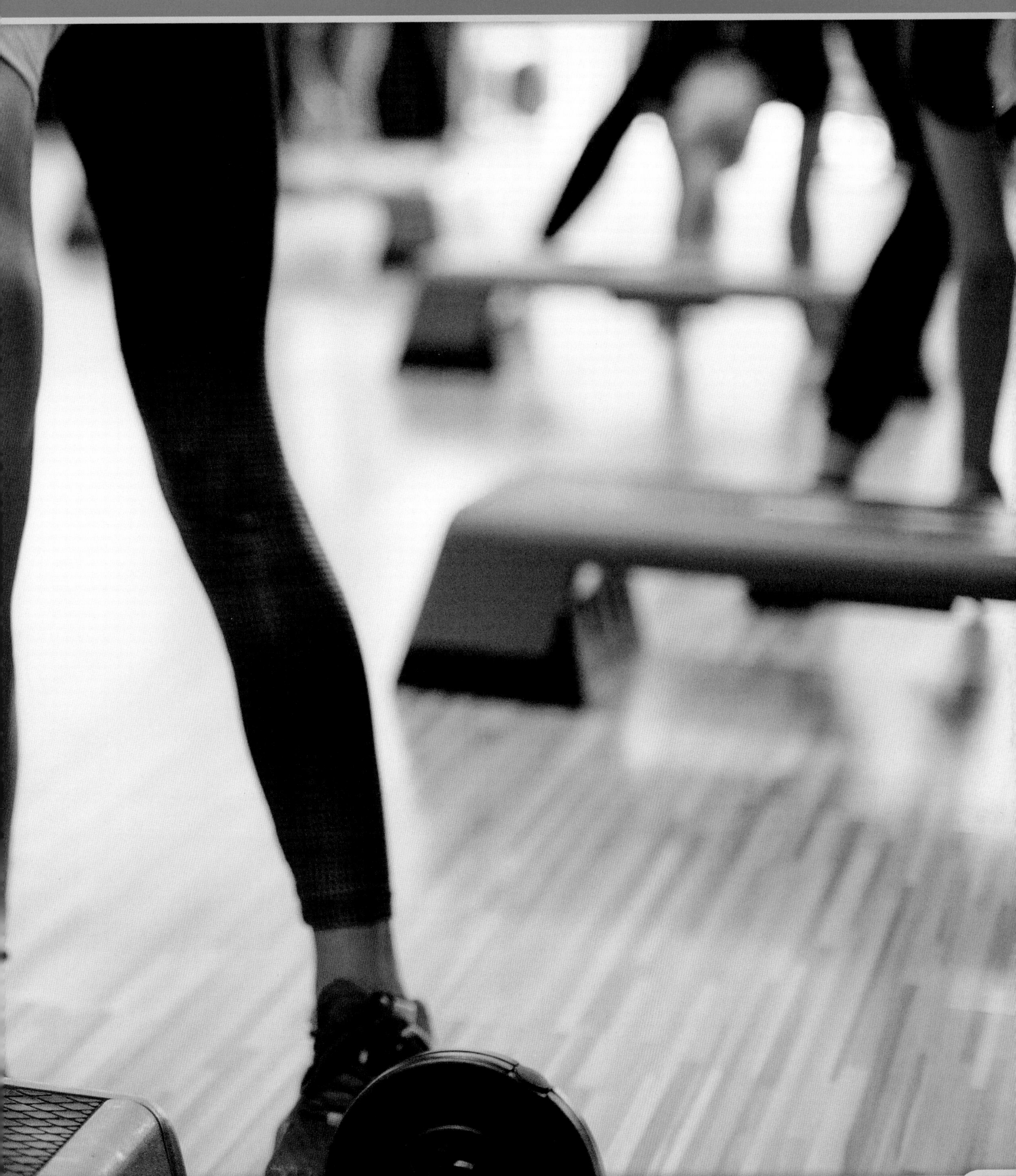

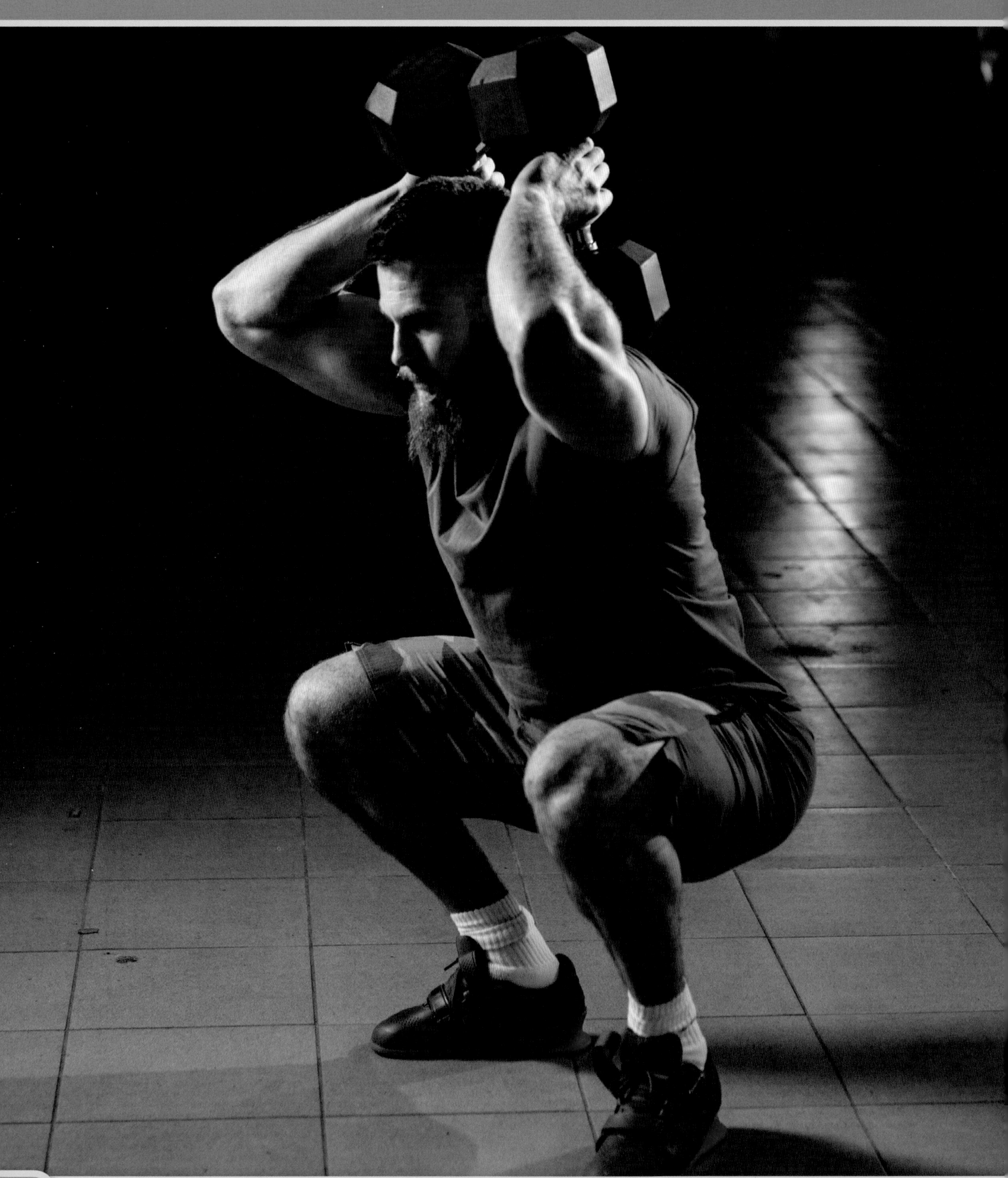

Index

A

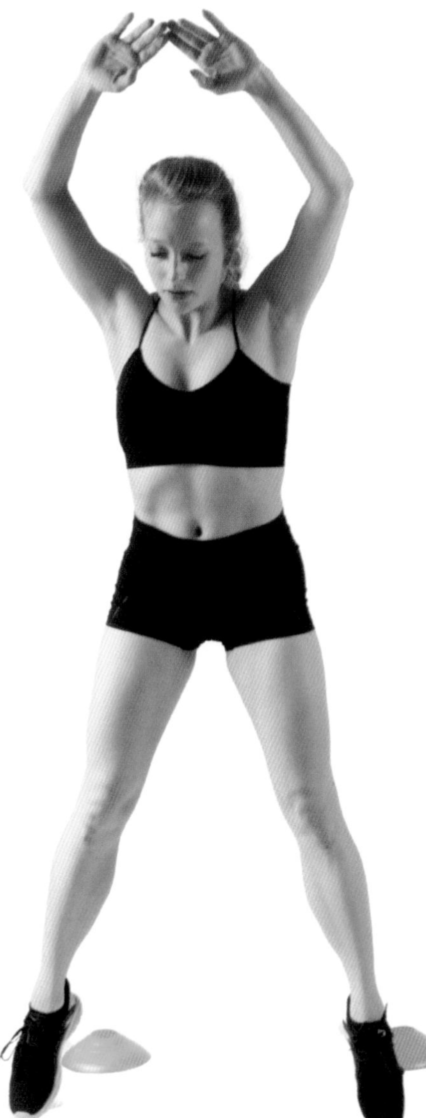

B

C

D

E

Q

R

S

T

V

W

Y

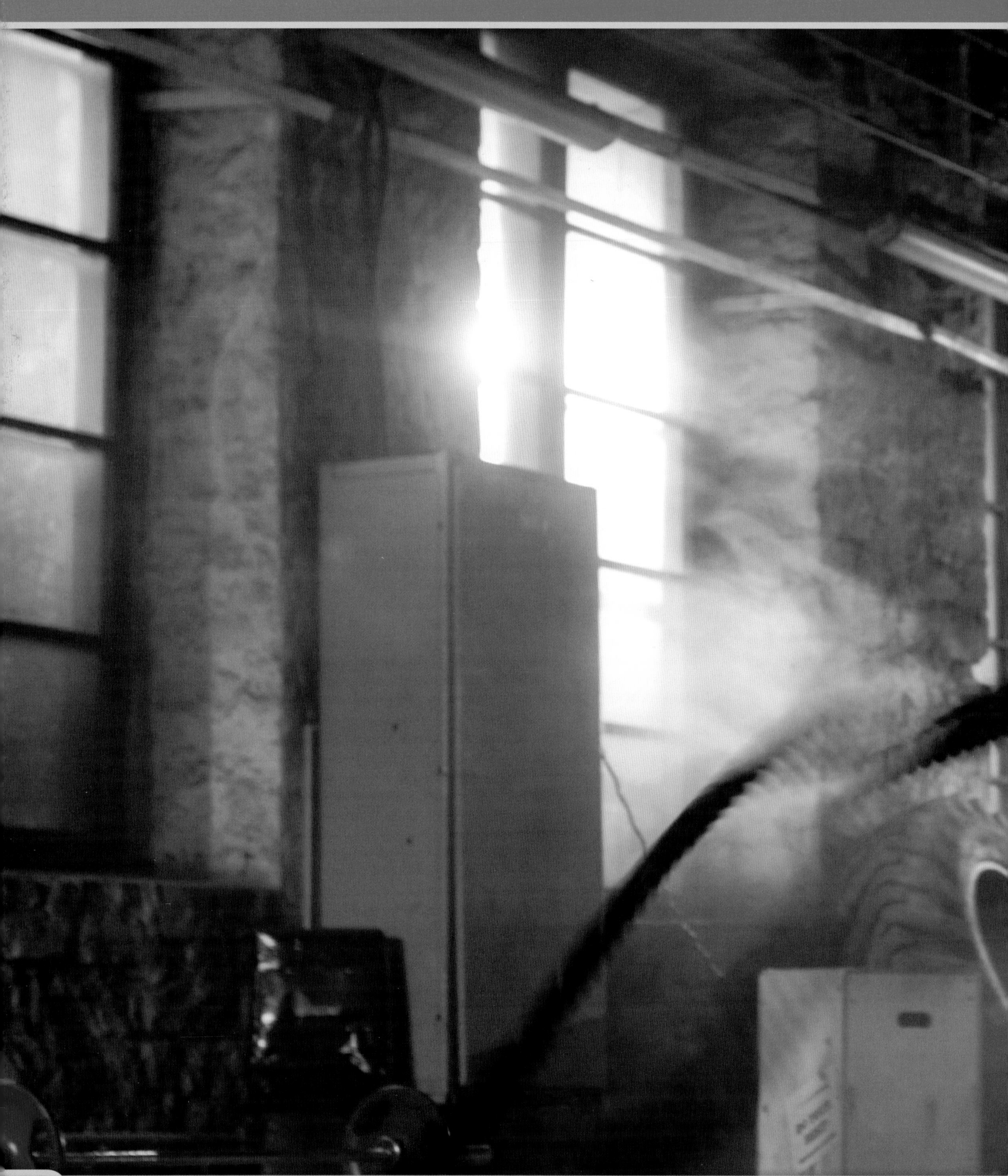

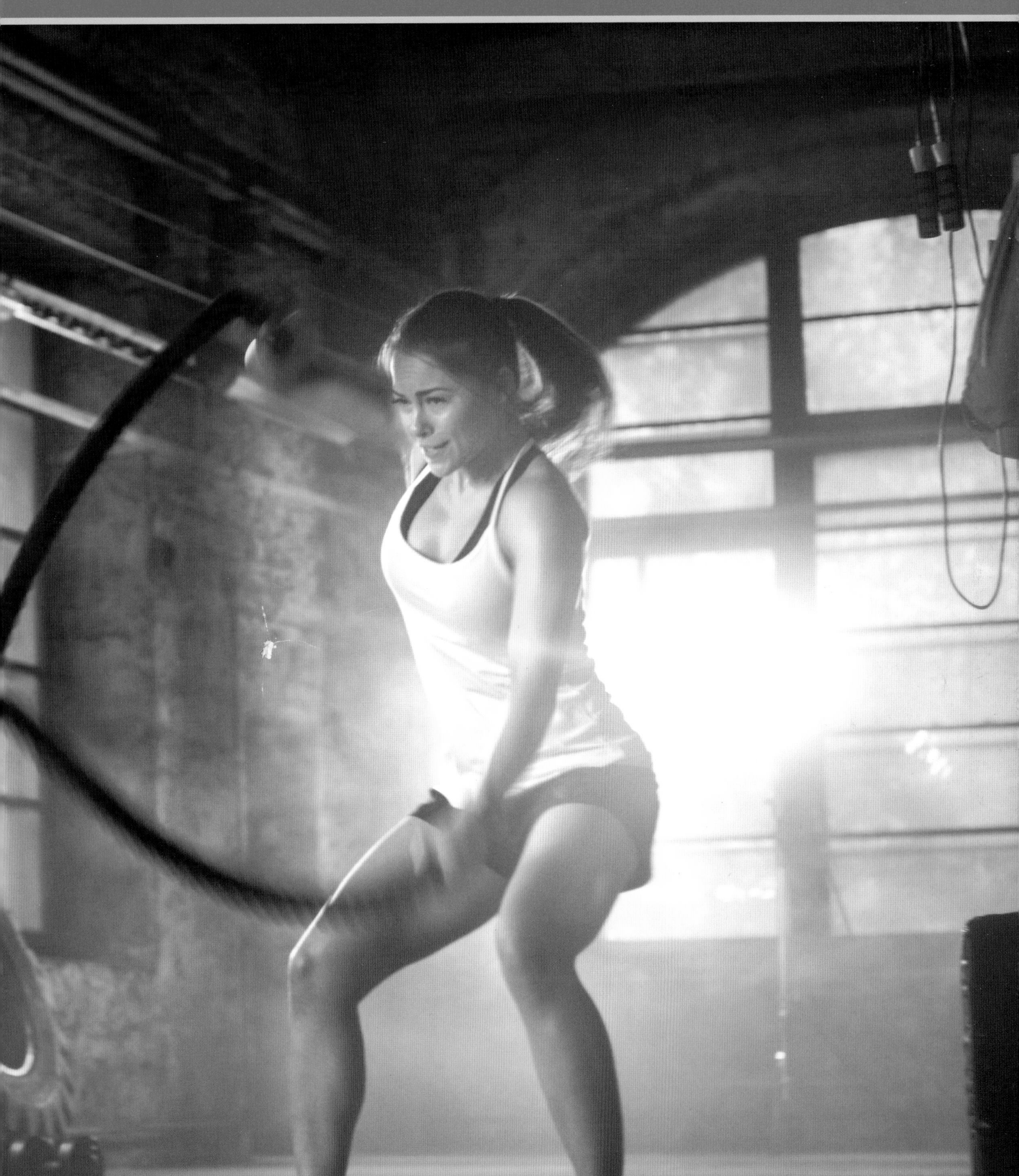

Credits & Acknowledgments

PHOTOGRAPHY

Naila Ruechel

MODELS

Philip Chan
Natasha Diamond-Walker
Jessica Gambellur
Alex Geissbuhler
Lloyd Knight
Larissa Terada

ADDITIONAL PHOTOGRAPHY

4 Volodymyr Tverdokhlib | Dreamstime.com
7 Andreadonetti | Dreamstime.com
8–9 Albertshakirov | Dreamstime.com
11 Albertshakirov | Dreamstime.com
13 Konstantin Yuganov | Dreamstime.com
16 top right, Zazamaza | Dreamstime.com
16 bottom right, Tina Zovteva | Dreamstime.com
17 Dojo666 | Dreamstime.com
18 top left, Paul Maguire | Dreamstime.com
18 bottom left, Scvoart | Dreamstime.com
19 Albertshakirov | Dreamstime.com
24–25 Vasyl Chipiha | Dreamstime.com
42–43 Khwaneigq | Dreamstime.com
146–147 Thamrongpat Theerathammakorn | Dreamstime.com
238–239 Maksym Protsenko | Dreamstime.com
324–325 107158287 | Dreamstime.com
372–373 MiniStocker | Shutterstock.com
392–393 shevtsovy | Shutterstock.com
394 Dusan Petkovic | Shutterstock.com
398–399 shevtsovy | Shutterstock.com

ILLUSTRATIONS

All anatomical illustrations by Adam Moore and Hector Diaz/
3DLabz Animation Limited. www.3dlabz.com
Full-body anatomy and insets by Linda Bucklin/Shutterstock.com

ABOUT THE AUTHOR

Alex Geissbuhler, CPT, CSCS, has spent the last decade helping people achieve their goals as a personal trainer accredited by the National Academy of Sports Medicine. Currently, Alex is attaining his doctorate in physical therapy with aspirations to continue to bring the best out of every body for decades to come.

ACKNOWLEDGEMENTS

I would like to dedicate this to all of the people whom I have worked with over the past 10 years—they have had just as much of an impact on me as I have on them. I am honored to have you in my life, and if any of the movements in this book look familiar, you know who you are!

Thank you to my wife, Josie, who has helped me over every hurdle and inspires me daily to bring out the best in myself. You have been my personal trainer all along, and I love you for it.

—Alex Geissbuhler